Practical and Professional Clinical Skills

Edited by

Vinod Patel BSc (Hons) MD FRCP MRCGP DRCOG

Associate Professor in Clinical Skills, Warwick Medical School, University of Warwick
Honorary Consultant in Endocrinology and Diabetes, General Internal Medicine, Medical
Obstetrics, George Eliot Hospital NHS Trust, Nuneaton, Warwickshire

John Morrissey MA MMEd MRCP

Honorary Associate Clinical Professor, Warwick Medical School, University of Warwick

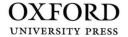
OXFORD
UNIVERSITY PRESS

OXFORD
UNIVERSITY PRESS

Great Clarendon Street, Oxford OX2 6DP

Oxford University Press is a department of the University of Oxford.
It furthers the University's objective of excellence in research, scholarship,
and education by publishing worldwide in

Oxford New York

Auckland Cape Town Dar es Salaam Hong Kong Karachi
Kuala Lumpur Madrid Melbourne Mexico City Nairobi
New Delhi Shanghai Taipei Toronto

With offices in

Argentina Austria Brazil Chile Czech Republic France Greece
Guatemala Hungary Italy Japan Poland Portugal Singapore
South Korea Switzerland Thailand Turkey Ukraine Vietnam

Oxford is a registered trade mark of Oxford University Press
in the UK and in certain other countries

Published in the United States
by Oxford University Press Inc., New York

British Library Cataloguing in Publication Data
Data available

Library of Congress Cataloging in Publication Data
Data available

Typeset by Sparks—www.sparkspublishing.com
Printed in Italy
on acid-free paper by
L.E.G.O. S.p.A—Lavis TN

ISBN 978-0-19-958561-8

1 3 5 7 9 10 8 6 4 2

Oxford University Press makes no representation, express or implied, that the drug
dosages in this book are correct. Readers must therefore always check the product
information and clinical procedures with the most up-to-date published product
information and data sheets provided by the manufacturers and the most recent codes of
conduct and safety regulations. The authors and the publishers do not accept responsibility
or legal liability for any errors in the text or for the misuse or misapplication of material in
this work. Except where otherwise stated, drug dosages and recommendations are for the
non-pregnant adult who is not breast-feeding.

Contents

vi

Contents

viii

Contents

Introduction

At the beginning of the twenty-first century we face the challenge of how to practise medicine in a way that is both evidence-based and patient-centred. Patients have many reasonable and justifiable expectations of their doctors. Not least they expect their doctors to be competent and professional, and to be safe in their care.

The main purpose of this book is to help senior medical students and newly qualified doctors become proficient in the wide range of skills they will need to practise medicine competently and safely. It will assist in preparation for OSCE assessments and clinical examinations, and we hope it will help build learners' confidence in their abilities in the early stages of their careers.

However, this book is not just of relevance to medical students and junior doctors. Unlike in years gone by, when the doctor was seen as the pre-eminent authority, patient care is now the responsibility of multidisciplinary teams. Many of the skills we describe and discuss will also be relevant to nurses and other health care professionals who are now performing roles previously the preserve of doctors.

We have organized these skills into four suites:

Suite 1, History and examination, comprises the most fundamental skills in the toolkit of any doctor. The chapters in this suite provide an overview of history taking and examination of the main body systems. We have also included brief guides to the application of these skills in more specialised situations: obstetrics, paediatrics, and psychiatry.

Suite 2, Procedures, consists of the bedside and near-patient practical procedures at which the newly qualified doctor will be expected to be proficient.

Suite 3, Emergency skills, covers not only resuscitation and cardiac arrest but also outlines the management of several acute medical conditions commonly requiring urgent admission to hospital.

Suite 4, Professional skills, is a more heterogeneous collection of mostly cognitive skills which are frequently not formally taught or assessed by medical schools but are skills that the newly qualified doctor will need after graduation. We have called these professional skills, since they are the preserve of health care professionals, but this is not to imply that the skills in the other three suites require any lesser standard of professionalism.

In 2009 the body which regulates medical education in the United Kingdom, the General Medical Council, published a revised edition of *Tomorrow's Doctors*, its guidance to teachers, students, and medical schools. In it the Council provides an exhaustive list of the learning outcomes required of UK medical graduates. The skills we describe and discuss in this book are closely mapped against this list.

It is not our intention to generalize the UK experience to the rest of the world. Patterns of ill health and disease, the culture of medical practice, and the organization of health care delivery vary greatly between countries. However, the vast majority of the skills we describe will be needed wherever medicine is practised.

The General Medical Council defines the 'overarching outcome' for medical graduates as follows: 'graduates will make the care of patients their first concern, applying their knowledge and skills in a competent and ethical manner'. This outcome comprises knowledge, skills, and attitudes. Our main concern in this book is with skills but these are underpinned by knowledge: skills cannot be exercised in a cognitive vacuum. The attitudes, and the behaviours to which they give rise, constitute professionalism.

Learning clinical skills

Skills can be learned opportunistically in the clinical setting, but this is not ideal. We advocate a structured programme of clinical skills teaching commencing soon after entry to medical school and continuing until graduation. The steps in skill acquisition are: (i) an appreciation of why that skill is necessary; (ii) an understanding of its anatomical, physiological, and pathological principles; (iii) instruction and demonstration by a tutor; followed by practice, assessment, and feedback, repeated as often as necessary; and (iv) certification as competent and safe.

The chapters of this book are structured to reflect this process. To assist learning through assessment and feedback each contains a clinical skills competency assessment checklist. This can be used at three levels of skill acquisition. First, by the individual student for revision and self-assessment. Second, by students working in pairs and small groups for peer assessment. Finally, for formal assessment by a clinical skills tutor and for certification. Since the precise details of how a skill or procedure is performed vary between institutions we have left blank lines in the checklists so additional items can be inserted if needed.

Each chapter also includes a small number of patient safety tips to help the student or junior trainee doctor avoid the more egregious errors and omissions.

The current emphasis on competencies and minimum acceptable standards is understandable and necessary, since instances of substandard care are regrettably common. When patient safety is compromised it is usually because something basic has not been done, or was done incorrectly. Checklists help to ensure that at least the basics are performed correctly. Harvard-based surgeon and writer Atul Gawande has persuasively argued for their key role in improving patient safety.

But the minimum should not become the maximum: as doctors we should not aspire to be just good enough and no more. Another aspect of professionalism is the drive to improve one's performance continually. Although our clinical skills competency assessment checklists represent the minimum acceptable standards, in the text we have at times included a little more detail than the student or recent graduate absolutely needs to know in the expectation of stimulating curiosity, interest, and self-directed learning.

The competencies required of health care professionals are constantly changing. Medicine changes as the evidence base grows and priorities for health care systems alter as new challenges arise. Likely priorities in the next few years will be patient safety, illness prevention and health promotion, and reducing health inequalities. All these will require health care professionals to acquire new and sometimes unfamiliar skills.

But professionalism itself is a constant, although it is elusive of definition. One element of it is competence. Others are honesty, integrity, and trustworthiness, but these are characteristics we expect in any individual whatever their walk in life. But one quality patients expect from those to whom they entrust their health, which perhaps they do not anticipate to the same degree from other professionals, is *kindness*. The nineteenth century novelist George Eliot – we both work at the hospital which bears her name – noted in *Middlemarch* that:

'Many of us ... would say that the kindest man we have ever known has been a medical man'

The 'man' is archaic since the majority of UK medical graduates are female, as was George Eliot, despite her male *nom de plume*. We hope tomorrow's doctors will be knowledgeable, exercise their skills competently, and above all treat their patients with kindness.

Vinod Patel

John Morrissey

How to use this book

Know your learning needs

From the start of your course be aware of the required learning outcomes: which skills you will need to acquire and by when.

- Familiarize yourself with the clinical skills teaching and assessment curriculum in your medical school or training programme.

- In the first instance be instructed by an accredited clinical skills tutor. You will observe practice in clinical areas but be aware that even the most experienced of professionals may be out of date or have acquired bad habits.

- The relevant chapter of this book can be read either before or after the teaching session, or both. The illustrations have been chosen to encourage reflection and discussion on the skills and the equipment used.

- Practise the skill, preferably in pairs or small groups. Early practice will likely involve simulation. Once proficiency at this level has been achieved, move on to practise on real patients, initially under expert supervision.

Formative Assessment

The main purpose of this type of assessment is to provide the learner with feedback. The clinical skills competency assessment checklists in this book can be used for:

- Revision, a guide to practice and self-assessment.
- Peer assessment by students working in pairs and small groups.
- Assessment by a clinical skills tutor.

The assessment checklists are all OSCE-style but fall into four main categories:

1 **The history or examination OSCE**, which requires interaction with a patient, real or simulated – for example, obstetric history taking or examination of the respiratory system. In the very early stages the 'patient' may well be another student, but move on to practise on real patients as soon as possible.

2 **The practical procedure OSCE**, which requires access to equipment in a clinical skills teaching facility – for example, bladder catheterization or emergency life support skills. Practice, self- and peer assessment should not be undertaken prior to instruction by a clinical skills tutor.

3 **Structured clinical questioning**, which takes the form of an interaction between a student and an assessor, and in which the student is required to produce short answers – for example, ECG rhythm recognition or prescribing. On the whole no information is required except this book. No equipment is needed except perhaps some stationery (for example, IVI charts or facsimile death certificates).

4 **Structured clinical discussion and reflection** is similar to (3) except there are no strictly correct or incorrect answers; topics may include health promotion or clinical leadership, for example. What is being tested here is the depth of understanding, insight, and judgment. Assessors will need to be familiar with the content and be able to guide the student to an appropriate answer if necessary.

The checklists can be used in the same way as in an OSCE. Beside each item is a box: check this if the item is performed correctly, leave it blank if it is omitted or performed incorrectly. There are four columns of boxes for successive assessments: self, peer (repeated if necessary) and tutor. These enable progress to be reviewed. We have not suggested a pass mark since this will depend on circumstances and the stage of the learner. However, a global assessment of competence can be recorded by circling U, B, S or E for unsatisfactory, borderline, satisfactory or excellent.

Summative assessment

This type of assessment seeks to make a formal determination of whether learning outcomes have been achieved.

- Formal summative assessment will vary between medical schools and training programmes. Most assessments do not test every learning outcome but depend on sampling. Passing the examination does not mean you have acquired all the necessary competencies: ensure you are also proficient at those skills on which you have not been formally assessed.

- Formal assessment, especially on procedures, is frequently on simulations. In that case arrange informal formative assessment by an expert on real patients to ensure proficiency before starting work.

- Miller's pyramid comprises four stages in skills acquisition: knowledge, understanding, demonstration and performance. You need to reach the apex of the pyramid!

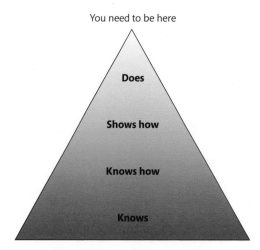

The checklists are available on the accompanying Online Resource Centre as downloadable PDFs. These resources are available at no cost but are password-protected. To access the resources simply visit the Online Resource Centre at www.oxfordtextbooks.co.uk/orc/patel_skills/ and enter the following username and password:

- Username: patel
- Password: ligature

All figures from the book are also available online, for access by adopting lecturers only.

Contributors and acknowledgements

Contributors

Clinical Skills Tutors:

Delia Carrasco, Louise Harmer, Lisa McDonnell, Rachael Greasley, Lorraine Thursby, Linda Tyrer

Linda Crinigan, Sandra Navas, Vanessa Threadgold, Alex McCurdie, Catherine Baldock

Julie Lyons, Clare Pahal, Dawn Hockley

Principal Clinical Photographer:

John Scullion

Senior Clinical Faculty:

Amitabh Palit, Consultant Radiologist
Sakera Shaikh, Senior Clinical Pharmacist
Michael Weinbren, Consultant Microbiologist
Linda Maxwell, Clinical Anatomist

John Berth-Jones, Consultant Dermatologist
Pachiappan Chellamuthu, Consultant in Acute Medicine
James Clayton, Consultant Microbiologist
Ian Fraser, Consultant Upper GI Surgeon
Alia Ghilani, Health Inequalities Pharmacist
Dilip Kumar, Consultant Ophthalmologist
George Mathew, Consultant Colorectal Surgeon
Maggie Morrissey, Blood Transfusion Practitioner
Rajiv Nair, Consultant in General Internal Medicine
Gavin Perkins, Professor in Critical Care Medicine
Mohan Ranganathan, Consultant Intensivist
Ponnusamy Saravanan, Consultant Endocrinologist
Rashmi Shukla, Regional Director of Public Health
Mike Stansbie, retired consultant ENT Surgeon
Asok Venkataraman, Consultant Cardiologist

Stephen Ayre, Clinical Librarian
Mandy Barnett, Consultant in Palliative Care
David Bennett-Jones, Consultant Renal Physician
Ivan Burchess, Consultant in Learning Disabilities
Geraldine Cassidy, Consultant in Learning Disabilities
Isobel Down, Organisation Consultant
James Egbuji, Consultant in Stroke Medicine
Julie Grant, Consultant in Palliative Care
Peter Handslip, Consultant Respiratory Physician
Jane Kidd, Director of MB ChB course, Warwick Medical School
Gary Lawrence, Consultant Obstetrician & Gynaecologist
Chris Marguerie, Consultant Rheumatologist
John Marriott, Professor of Clinical Pharmacology

Ram Nangalia, Consultant Breast Surgeon
Christine O'Brien, Consultant Respiratory Physician
Krishna Prasad, Consultant Urologist
Sankara Raman, Consultant Gastroenterologist
Adam Rennie, Consultant Radiologist
Carolyn Rodgers, Senior Clinical Teacher
Harbinder Sandhu, Assistant Professor in Health Psychology
Swaran Singh, Professor of Community Psychiatry
Rupan Somaiya, Consultant Anaesthetist
Andy Stein, Consultant Renal Physician
Heather Stirling, Consultant Paediatrician
Michael Walzman, Consultant in Genitourinary Medicine
Mahmud Wasfi, Consultant Cardiologist
David Watts, Clinical Audit Officer
Veronica Wilkes, General Practitioner
Gordon Wood, Consultant Gastroenterologist

Trainee Clinicians:

Sushil Agarwal, Isaac Chirwa, Subramanya Kumar, Rachel Nyambo, Abi Patel, Jamie Roebuck, Nithya Sukumar

Usman Ahmed, Mahboob Ali, Sayan Bhattacharya, Alistair Burn, Ram Chittal, Amy Evans, Anne-Marie Feely, Ruth Francis, Birgit Fruhstorfer, Emma Gordon, Raja Haq, Shazia Jaleel, Timothy Joseph, Sandhya Kulkarni, Priyanka Lakhani, James Lee, Konstantinos Lipas, Anil Kumar Miriyala, Ralph Mitchell, James Rainsbury, Tim Rattay, James Royle, Mahomed Saleh, Tom Sapsford, Rupa Sharma, Brian Shields, Mitesh Thanki, Carly Williams

Medical Students:

Aoife Abbey, Alfred Adiamah, Naomi Anderson, Sarah Green, Sarah Kinsman, Steven Laird, Tom Peachey

Siobhan Akhtar, Christopher Allen, Amy Attwater, Gudrun Asa Bjornsdottir, Claire Budd, Katherine Gallagher, Ayrton Goddard, Ashley Horsley, Francesca Hughes, Rebecca Jackson, Jennifer Johnson, Miriam Kay, Feyi Kunle-Hassan, Peter Mathias, Benjamin Miguras, Alexis Missick, Alex Murray, Gihan Nanayakkara, Siobhan Reilly, Sakib Rokadiya, Mandeep Sandhu, Fatima Shaik, Ursula Smith

Administrative Support:

Amitha Gopinath, Sarah North, Jo Moore, Karen Rouault, Kevin Lynch

Sam Cook, Ann Davies, Joanne Wilson, Theresa Ritchie, Maxine Knighton, Diane James, Judith Plester, Shelley Lapper, Lisa Cartwight, Eileen Taylor

The majority of the faculty above were drawn from Warwick Medical School, University of Warwick, and three local NHS Trusts (George Eliot Hospital NHS Trust, University Hospitals Coventry and Warwickshire NHS Trusts, South Warwickshire NHS Foundation Trust).

In the preparation of some chapters of this volume we referred extensively to two highly recommended books, both from Oxford University Press: *Clinical Skills* edited by Niall Cox and TA Roper (2005) and the *Oxford Handbook of Clinical Examination and Practical Skills* edited by James Thomas and Tanya Monaghan (2007).

Suite 1 History and examination skills

Unit 1   Introduction and history taking

1.1 History taking and examination skills: introduction

As doctors we have three ways of obtaining the information we need about our patients in order to help them: engaging in conversation with them, examining them, and carrying out investigations. Suite 1 of this book provides an overview of the first two of these. It is necessarily very abbreviated and is definitely not a substitute for a comprehensive textbook on these skills. For that we strongly recommend *Clinical Skills*, edited by Niall Cox and T A Roper (Oxford University Press, 2005).

The consultation

The consultation starts when the patient presents with what he or she believes to be a health problem or problems. It ends with agreement on a management plan that is acceptable to both patient and doctor. Consultations are almost infinite in their variety: part of the fascination of medicine is that no two are the same. Those in primary and secondary care are very dissimilar, not least because the former are usually much shorter, and the approach to an emergency situation is necessarily very different from one which is less acute.

But whatever the setting and the situation, the consultation must be *structured* (Figure 1.1). An aimless, unstructured consultation will not result in an accurate diagnosis, a successful management plan, or a satisfied patient. Many structures for the consultation have been proposed but our strong preference is for the Calgary-Cambridge model, which is used in most UK medical schools. It is fully described in *Skills for Communicating with Patients*, 2nd edition, by Jonathan Silverman, Suzanne Kurtz, and Juliet Draper (Radcliffe Publishing, 2005).

The Calgary-Cambridge model

This model organizes the consultation into five tasks that are performed in sequence: initiating the session, gathering information, physical examination, explanation and planning, and closing the session. To this we have added a further step, differential diagnosis, which in Calgary-Cambridge is subsumed into explanation and planning. In addition, there are two tasks that are continuous throughout the consultation: providing structure and building the doctor–patient relationship.

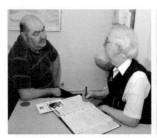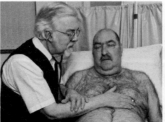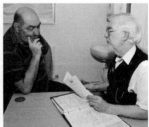

Figure 1.1 The consultation: the history, the physical examination, and explanation and care planning.

The Calgary-Cambridge model is applicable to almost any consultation, irrespective of the patient's problems or the setting. One of its great strengths is its integration of content – what the doctor does – and process – how he or she goes about it.

Content and process

Suite 1 of this book is chiefly concerned with two components of the Calgary-Cambridge model: gathering information and physical examination. With regard to the former we have reverted to traditional medical terminology: 'taking the history'. 'History' derives from the Latin *historia*, a story, and immersion in and interpretation of narrative is an essential part of the practice of medicine.

Our main focus is on the content of the consultation: in Figure 1.2 we map that content against the Calgary-Cambridge structure. But it must be stressed that mastery of process is as important as understanding of content. Process skills – also called communications skills – can only be acquired through experience, but it is also essential to refer to a good textbook. *Skills for Communicating with Patients* is excellent in this regard.

Providing structure   Building the relationship

Initiating the session

- Preparation
- Identifying the patient's problem(s)

Gathering information: taking the history

Biomedical perspective ('disease')	Patient's perspective ('illness')
• Sequence of events	• Ideas and beliefs
• Analysis of symptoms	• Concerns
• Review of relevant systems(s)	• Expectations
	• Effects of symptoms on life
	• Feelings

Context: background information

- Past medical history
- Treatment history and allergies
- Personal and social history
- Smoking, alcohol, and recreational drug use history
- Family history
- Review of other systems

Physical examination

- Explanation and consent
- Correct position and adequate exposure
- General inspection
- General examination
- System(s) examination(s)
- Additional examination

Differential diagnosis

- Biomedical
- Patient's perspective
- Social context

Explanation and planning

- Physician's plan of management
- Explanation and negotiation
- Shared decision-making and care planning
- Self-management by patient

Closing the consultation

- Forward planning
- Ensuring appropriate point of closure
- Documentation

Figure 1.2
The structure and content of the consultation.

History taking

The purpose of taking the history is twofold: first, to assemble the information required to make a diagnosis and, second, to understand the patient's perspective on the problem and assess the impact of the illness on his or her life. In the interest of both accuracy and immersion in the patient's experience it is necessary that he or she is encouraged to tell their story in their own fashion: the record of the consultation should also be in the patient's own words and not a translation into medical jargon.

History taking is undertaken in stages: the identification of the patient's immediate symptoms, then the detailed exploration of those symptoms, followed by their location in the wider circumstances of the patient's previous medical history and life in general. It is frequently stated that 80% of diagnostically useful information comes from the history and most of the rest from the investigations. Sometimes it is possible to make a diagnosis on the history alone. Alternatively, the history will suggest a range of diagnostic hypotheses – the differential diagnosis – which indicate what physical examination is necessary.

Physical examination

The purpose of examination is also twofold: first, to elicit signs which by their presence or absence help to confirm or refute diagnostic hypotheses erected on the basis of the history, and second, to assess the severity of the patient's condition. The examination is also performed in stages:

1 The general inspection, also called the 'general look' or 'end of the bed inspection'
2 The general examination, which is more or less the same in every patient
3 Examination of the body system in which the problem is thought to reside
4 Seeking additional relevant signs.

In the sections on systems examinations which follow, we have not sought primarily to describe each step in detail. Our main intention is to situate the main stages and elements of the examination in their clinical context: why they are necessary and how they contribute to the process of diagnosis. But each section includes a clinical skills competency assessment checklist, which lists the main steps in a basic systems examination.

This division of the body into systems, especially for purposes of the physical examination, is now near-universal practice. Organizing our understanding of the body and the information we gather from patients in this way makes the task more manageable. However, it is in many ways artificial. We do not interrogate or examine 'systems': we talk with and examine our patients. It is frequently necessary to examine more than one system and most patients admitted to hospital require comprehensive assessment by a full clinical history and physical examination.

Differential diagnosis

The process of using the information gathered from the history and the physical examination to arrive at a diagnosis or differential diagnosis is sometimes called 'clinical reasoning'. We have included differential diagnosis as a discrete step in the structure of the consultation. However, clinical reasoning is undertaken continually from its commencement as diagnostic hypotheses are erected, tested, confirmed or discarded. Even before greetings are exchanged, a patient's appearance or demeanour may suggest a possible diagnosis.

Diagnostic hypotheses may be anywhere on the spectrum from the totally confident to the extremely tentative. Constructing them requires consideration and analysis not only of the symptoms and signs of biomedical disease but also of the patient's perspective and the social context. The consultation then enters its final stage, the one which matters most to the patient: an explanation, however provisional, on what is troubling him or her and agreement on what is to be done about it.

1.2 Clinical history taking

Background

Gathering information about the patient's problems starts with listening to the history, the patient's own account of the events which led to their seeking medical attention. Taking an accurate and comprehensive history is the first step to diagnosis of the problems and therefore the most fundamental of clinical skills (Figure 1.3). However, in the emergency situation it is often necessary to institute management without the advantage of a detailed history: identification of the key facts may have to suffice.

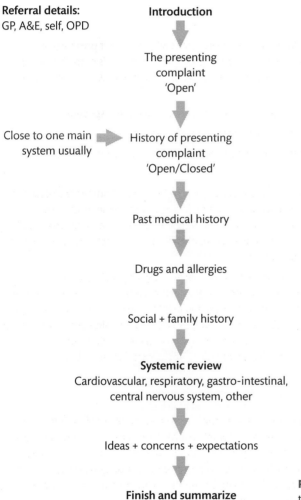

Referral details:
GP, A&E, self, OPD

Introduction

The presenting
complaint
'Open'

Close to one main
system usually

History of presenting
complaint
'Open/Closed'

Past medical history

Drugs and allergies

Social + family history

Systemic review
Cardiovascular, respiratory, gastro-intestinal,
central nervous system, other

Ideas + concerns + expectations

Finish and summarize

Figure 1.3 Outline of history taking: this should take around 10 minutes in most cases.

6 The sequence for history taking

History sequence	Clinical context
The presenting complaint	The first task is to identify the problem or problems. The symptom first mentioned by the patient is not necessarily the most important and there may be not one but several. Ask 'What else did you notice?' more than once if necessary
History of the presenting complaint	Gaining a full picture needs not just enquiry into the presenting symptom but also about all symptoms relevant to the system in which the problem might lie. It is often necessary to enquire into two or more systems
Past medical history	This is the start of contextualization, locating the current problem in the wider circumstances of the patient's life. Start with open questions – 'Anything else?' – and move to closed ones when the patient's recollection falters
Treatment history and allergies	An accurate list of current and recent medications is a precondition for safe prescribing: it also indicates diagnoses made previously and enables consideration of whether the current problem might be iatrogenic
Personal and social history	This contextualizes the problem further. It enables assessment of how the symptoms are affecting the patient's life and insight into the patient's view of the problem
Smoking, alcohol, and recreational drug use history	Smoking is a risk factor for cardiovascular and respiratory disease, alcohol mainly for liver disease and also for neurological, gastrointestinal, haematological, and cardiac problems
Family history	This is frequently non-contributory to the diagnosis but may be helpful, for example in relation to certain cancers, and may also encourage the patient to reveal concerns
Review of other systems	This series of closed questions may reveal evidence of co-morbidity, which is especially common in elderly people: it is also a safety net if you have forgotten anything
Ideas, concerns, and expectations	If you consider you still have not gained adequate insight into the patient's perspective then enquire specifically about 'ICE'.
To finish off the history	Ask 'Is there anything else you would like to tell me?' then summarize what you have heard and what are your thoughts

Common presentations

A few of the common presentations which result in urgent admission to hospital are:

- **Chest pain**: the priority is often to confirm or exclude a cardiac origin
- **Breathlessness**: due to heart failure, a respiratory cause, or anaemia
- **Abdominal pain**: the priority is usually to determine whether a surgical emergency is present
- **Unilateral weakness**: usually but not always due to stroke
- **Haematemesis and/or melaena**: these are characteristic symptoms of upper gastrointestinal bleeding
- **Feverishness**: commonly due to respiratory or urinary tract infection
- **Impairment or loss of consciousness**: the list of causes of coma is long but they can be categorized broadly as either neurological or metabolic
- **Non-specific symptoms**, especially in elderly people: impaired cognition ('confusion') and/ or mobility ('off legs').

Communication principles

The authors of the Calgary-Cambridge model list no fewer than 71 separate communication skills relevant to the consultation. Of course, it is not necessary to exercise all of them on every occasion! However, some important principles of communication are listed below.

- History taking must be structured and undertaken in stages, each clearly signposted to the patient.
- Taking the history is the best opportunity to start building a relationship based on mutual trust without which the likelihood of a positive therapeutic outcome is limited.
- Initially use open questions to allow the patient freely to relate their own version of events: move progressively to more closed questions when it becomes necessary to establish specific facts.
- As early as possible try to explore the problem from the patient's point of view ('illness') as well as from the biomedical perspective ('disease').

Patient safety tips

- ✔ A high proportion of medical errors are prescribing errors and many can be avoided by taking a full medication history and recording it accurately. It is impossible to prescribe safely without knowing which drugs the patient is presently taking and whether allergy or intolerance has occurred previously.
- ✔ Clear and legible notes are essential to safe practice.

Student name:	Medical school:	Year:				

History taking

Please take a clinical history from this patient.

		Self	Peer	Peer /tutor	Tutor
Initiating the consultation	● Greets patient, confirms patient's name	☐	☐	☐	☐
	● Introduces self, states role and purpose of interview, gains consent	☐	☐	☐	☐
	● Uses appropriate open question to elicit presenting complaint(s)	☐	☐	☐	☐
	●	☐	☐	☐	☐
The presenting complaint	● Fully explores presenting complaint: asks all questions appropriate to relevant system(s)	☐	☐	☐	☐
	● Uses open and closed questions appropriately, moving from open to closed	☐	☐	☐	☐
	● Listens attentively and minimizes interruptions	☐	☐	☐	☐
	● Seeks clarification when necessary	☐	☐	☐	☐
	● Uses clear, easily understood language and avoids jargon	☐	☐	☐	☐
	● Actively determines the patient's perspective: ideas and beliefs, concerns, expectations, effects of symptoms on life, feelings	☐	☐	☐	☐
	●	☐	☐	☐	☐
Background and context	● Explores the patient's past medical history	☐	☐	☐	☐
	● Explores treatment history and allergies	☐	☐	☐	☐
	● Explores personal and social history	☐	☐	☐	☐
	● Asks about smoking, alcohol, and recreational drug use	☐	☐	☐	☐
	● Explores family history	☐	☐	☐	☐
	● Undertakes full review of other systems	☐	☐	☐	☐
	●	☐	☐	☐	☐
Providing structure	● Structures history in a logical sequence	☐	☐	☐	☐
	● Progresses from one section to another using signposting	☐	☐	☐	☐
	● Summarizes at end of each section and confirms understanding	☐	☐	☐	☐
	● Attends to timing and keeps the interview on task	☐	☐	☐	☐
	●	☐	☐	☐	☐
Building the doctor–patient relationship	● Demonstrates appropriate non-verbal behaviour	☐	☐	☐	☐
	● Acknowledges patient's views and feelings	☐	☐	☐	☐
	● Makes empathic statements to communicate appreciation of the patients' feelings or predicament	☐	☐	☐	☐
	● Expresses concern and understanding	☐	☐	☐	☐
	● Attends to patient's physical comfort	☐	☐	☐	☐
	●	☐	☐	☐	☐
Finishing the history	● Asks the patient if there is anything they want to add	☐	☐	☐	☐
	● Summarizes the history, including the patient's perspective	☐	☐	☐	☐
	●	☐	☐	☐	☐

				Self	Peer	Peer/tutor	Tutor
Self-assessed as at least borderline:	Signature:	Date:		U B S E	U B S E	U B S E	U B S E
Peer-assessed as ready for tutor assessment:	Signature:	Date:		U B S E	U B S E	U B S E	U B S E
Tutor-assessed as satisfactory:	Signature:	Date:		U B S E	U B S E	U B S E	U B S E

Notes

Unit 2   Systems examination

2.1 General examination

Background

The 'general examination' is in two parts. The first part consists of measurement of the patient's vital signs: pulse rate, blood pressure, temperature, and respiratory rate. All are needed in the acutely ill patient, but the last two may be omitted in the patient who is basically well, provided the history indicates no specific need. The second part consists of examination of the hands, face, eyes, mouth, lymph nodes, and feet. The general examination follows assessment of the patient's appearance, condition, and surroundings by general inspection and precedes examination of the relevant body system or systems.

Common presentations

Numerous abnormalities can be detected on general examination. Which ones will be looked for in an individual patient will be guided by the diagnostic hypotheses erected on the basis of the history. However, six signs are traditionally sought in every patient:

- Jaundice
- Conjunctival pallor for anaemia
- Finger clubbing
- Peripheral and central cyanosis
- Oedema
- Lymphadenopathy.

Examination and diagnostic principles

The discovery of any of the above signs should prompt a search for other abnormalities that could be of diagnostic importance. For example, the finding of conjunctival pallor suggestive of anaemia should be followed by reassessment of the nails for koilonychia, examination of the mouth for angular stomatitis and glossitis, and a search for signs that might indicate the cause of the anaemia, which could well entail a full physical examination. Similarly, the discovery of mild jaundice not noticed or mentioned by the patient should prompt a look for other signs of liver disease, such as spider naevi and palmar erythema, an abdominal examination, and enquiry into elements of the history not previously considered relevant, such as the colour of the urine.

Patient safety tip

✔ In a patient with lymphadenopathy it is necessary to determine its distribution. If the lymph nodes are examined it is therefore essential to examine all of them: cervical, axillary, and inguinal. However, the last two are often wrongly omitted, perhaps because they are situated in intimate areas and the patient might find examination embarrassing. A logical point at which to palpate the axillary nodes is after examination of the hands and arms, as the focus of examination travels up towards the head. The best time to assess the inguinal nodes is after examination of the abdomen since the patient is now lying flat and the focus is moving down to the legs and feet.

The sequence for a general examination

Examination sequence	Clinical context
Explanation and consent	Wash your hands before contact with the patient
Correct position and adequate exposure	The examination is best performed with the patient reclining comfortably: ensure you can get behind the head of the bed to palpate the cervical lymph nodes
General inspection	The most important observations are those which can be made from the end of the bed. Do changes in skin colour immediately suggest jaundice, anaemia, or polycythaemia?
General examination	The temperature of the hands, cyanosis and capillary refill time are indications of the adequacy of the peripheral circulation

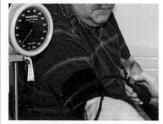

The causes of finger clubbing constitute the most famous list in medicine: it is most frequently seen in cryptogenic fibrosing alveolitis, bronchiectasis, and lung cancer

The pulse rate needs to be interpreted in the context of the clinical situation. In a sick hypotensive patient a tachycardia is probably an indication of hypovolaemia. In a less unwell patient an unexpectedly slow or rapid heart rate may be due to previously unsuspected thyroid disease

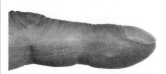

Always take the blood pressure even if there is no reason to suspect it to be abnormal: hypertension is usually asymptomatic and its treatment reduces the risk of kidney disease, heart failure and stroke

The clinical diagnosis of anaemia is difficult and confirmation with a blood count is necessary: the red cell indices will suggest the direction of further investigation

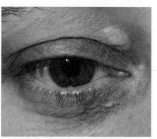

Jaundice is always abnormal and invariably requires investigation. However, mild jaundice in a well patient is most likely to be due to Gilbert's disease

Central cyanosis is usually an indication of severe hypoxia and may suggest the urgent need of oxygen therapy

Soft, tender, enlarged lymph nodes suggest infection; hard, irregular ones suggest cancer. Unexplained lymphadenopathy requires further investigation

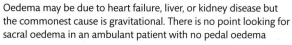

Oedema may be due to heart failure, liver, or kidney disease but the commonest cause is gravitational. There is no point looking for sacral oedema in an ambulant patient with no pedal oedema

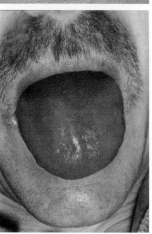

Additional examination	The history and the findings on general examination will suggest the need of examination of one or more body systems
Professionalism	Maintain patient dignity, communicate sensitively, thank the patient, wash hands, explain conclusions to the patient, document fully and accurately, communicate appropriately with colleagues

Student name:	Medical school:	Year:

General examination

Please perform a general examination on this patient.

		Self	Peer	Peer /tutor	Tutor
Explanation and consent	● Washes hands with alcohol gel or soap and water	☐	☐	☐	☐
	● Explains procedure to patient and obtains verbal consent	☐	☐	☐	☐
	●	☐	☐	☐	☐
Correct position and adequate exposure	● Patient reclining with trunk at 45°	☐	☐	☐	☐
	● Exposes arms, upper thorax, neck and head while maintaining patient dignity: exposes legs when appropriate	☐	☐	☐	☐
	●	☐	☐	☐	☐
General inspection	● Inspects patient from end of bed, commenting on any relevant findings	☐	☐	☐	☐
	● Inspects patient's surroundings for 'clues'	☐	☐	☐	☐
	●	☐	☐	☐	☐
General examination	● Examines hands for temperature, capillary refill time, peripheral cyanosis	☐	☐	☐	☐
	● Examines nails for clubbing, koilonychia, leuconychia, splinter haemorrhages	☐	☐	☐	☐
	● Palpates radial pulse for rate and rhythm	☐	☐	☐	☐
	● Takes the blood pressure	☐	☐	☐	☐
	● Comments on need to take temperature and assess respiratory rate	☐	☐	☐	☐
	● Palpates axillary lymph nodes	☐	☐	☐	☐
	● Inspects eyes for anaemia, jaundice, xanthelasmata, corneal arcus	☐	☐	☐	☐
	● Inspects face and mouth for malar flush, glossitis, hydration status, central cyanosis	☐	☐	☐	☐
	● Palpates cervical lymph nodes from behind	☐	☐	☐	☐
	● Sits patient forward and examines for sacral oedema	☐	☐	☐	☐
	● Lies patient flat and palpates inguinal lymph nodes	☐	☐	☐	☐
	● Inspects feet and palpates for pedal oedema	☐	☐	☐	☐
	●	☐	☐	☐	☐
Additional examination	● Comments on which system(s) examination is needed in light of the findings	☐	☐	☐	☐
	●	☐	☐	☐	☐
Professionalism	● Covers patient, thanks patient, washes hands	☐	☐	☐	☐
	●	☐	☐	☐	☐

Self-assessed as at least borderline:	Signature:	Date:	U B S E	U B S E	U B S E	U B S E
Peer-assessed as ready for tutor assessment:	Signature:	Date:	U B S E	U B S E	U B S E	U B S E
Tutor-assessed as satisfactory:	Signature:	Date:	U B S E	U B S E	U B S E	U B S E

Notes

2.2 Cardiovascular examination

Background

Patients with known or suspected cardiovascular disease make up a high proportion of the caseload in primary care, in the outpatients department and on the acute medical take. Even if the patient's symptoms are not due to cardiac disease, exclusion of it is frequently the first management priority. Assessment of the cardiovascular system is of particular importance in the acutely ill patient: the 'C' of the 'ABCDE' approach.

Common presentations

Patients with cardiovascular disease commonly present with:

- **Chest pain**: whether chest pain is of cardiac origin can usually be determined by a careful history but investigation is often needed for confirmation.
- **Breathlessness**: shortness of breath due to heart failure typically presents with characteristic symptoms and signs but investigation is usually required. Cardiac and respiratory causes of breathlessness frequently coexist in the same patient.
- **Palpitations**: these are usually benign but atrial fibrillation is common and modern management is aggressive.
- **Syncope**: there are many causes of this, ranging from the trivial to the life-threatening, and diagnosis depends mainly on a detailed history.

Anatomical and physiological principles

The apex beat, normally situated in the fifth intercostal space (ICS) within the mid-clavicular line, more or less corresponds to the apex of the left ventricle. The right ventricle lies mainly beneath the sternum and makes up the inferior border of the heart. The right heart border comprises the right atrium and the inferior and superior vena cava. The left heart border comprises the left atrium and the left ventricle. The mitral, tricuspid, aortic, and pulmonary auscultation areas do not correspond to the actual positions of those valves: they are some distance away in the direction of blood flow.

The sequence for a cardiovascular examination

Examination sequence	Clinical context
Explanation and consent	Wash your hands before contact with the patient
Correct position and adequate exposure	The patient should be positioned at 45°: this is of particular importance when assessing the jugular venous pressure (JVP)
General inspection	The most important observations are those which can be made on general inspection. Does the patient appear basically well, or is he or she clearly in pain, distressed, or breathless?
General examination	Splinter haemorrhages suggest a diagnosis of infective endocarditis. Capillary refill time is a useful measure of the peripheral circulation. Palpation of the radial pulse permits assessment only of the rate and rhythm. If an electronic reading of the blood pressure is unexpectedly abnormal consider checking it manually

Examination sequence	Clinical context
	Cyanosis is a subtle sign but when present indicates severe hypoxia. Anaemia may be the primary or an aggravating cause of shortness of breath
System examination	Palpation of the carotid artery permits assessment of the volume and character of the pulse, and timing of findings on cardiac auscultation in relation to the cardiac cycle. Attempt to elicit hepatojugular reflux in all patients, regardless of whether the JVP is visible or not
	Inspect the precordium carefully if you have not already done so. Scars from previous surgery are easily missed!
	The apex beat is impalpable in 50% of normal subjects but may yield useful information if it can be felt. Lateral displacement of the apex beat indicates left ventricular enlargement not hypertrophy: the latter produces an abnormal character ('heaving') of the apex beat which may be normally situated. Left parasternal heaves and thrills are rare
	The main purpose of auscultation is to detect valvular stenosis or incompetence
Additional examination	The chief signs of left ventricular failure are tachycardia and crackles at the lung bases. Biventricular failure produces these plus the signs of right ventricular failure: a raised JVP, hepatomegaly and peripheral oedema
Professionalism	Maintain patient dignity, communicate sensitively, thank the patient, wash hands, explain conclusions to the patient, document fully and accurately, communicate appropriately with colleagues

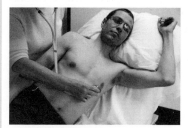

Mitral valve area: apex

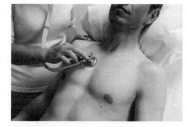

Aortic valve area: 2nd ICS right

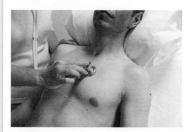

Pulmonary valve area: 2nd ICS left
Tricuspid valve area: 4th ICS left

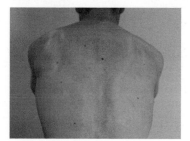

Auscultation of lung bases for cardiac failure

Patient safety tip

✔ Checking for asymmetry of the radial pulses is of importance only in patients with acute severe chest pain in whom aortic dissection is suspected. However, performing it routinely in all patients will ensure you do not forget it when it is really necessary.

Student name: Medical school: Year:

Examination of the cardiovascular system

Please examine this patient's cardiovascular system.

		Self	Peer	Peer /tutor	Tutor
Explanation and consent	● Washes hands with alcohol gel or soap and water	☐	☐	☐	☐
	● Explains procedure to patient and obtains verbal consent	☐	☐	☐	☐
	●	☐	☐	☐	☐
Correct position and adequate exposure	● Patient reclining with trunk at 45°	☐	☐	☐	☐
	● Adequately exposes chest	☐	☐	☐	☐
	● Offers to cover females until removal is appropriate	☐	☐	☐	☐
	●	☐	☐	☐	☐
General inspection	● Inspects patient from end of bed, commenting on any relevant findings	☐	☐	☐	☐
	● Inspects patient's surroundings for 'clues'	☐	☐	☐	☐
	●	☐	☐	☐	☐
General examination	● Examines hands for temperature, capillary refill time, peripheral cyanosis, Osler's nodes	☐	☐	☐	☐
	● Examines nails for clubbing, koilonychia, splinter haemorrhages	☐	☐	☐	☐
	● Palpates radial pulse for rate and rhythm	☐	☐	☐	☐
	● Examines for radioradial delay and for collapsing pulse	☐	☐	☐	☐
	● Takes the blood pressure	☐	☐	☐	☐
	● Inspects eyes for xanthelasmata, anaemia, corneal arcus	☐	☐	☐	☐
	● Inspects face and mouth for malar flush, glossitis, hydration status, central cyanosis	☐	☐	☐	☐
	●	☐	☐	☐	☐
System examination	● Inspects neck for jugular venous pulse and elicits hepatojugular reflux	☐	☐	☐	☐
	● Palpates carotid pulse for character and volume	☐	☐	☐	☐
	● Reinspects precordium more closely, commenting on any relevant findings	☐	☐	☐	☐
	● Palpates precordium for apex beat, left ventricular heave, thrills	☐	☐	☐	☐
	● Listens in all four areas, for mitral stenosis and aortic regurgitation, and over carotid arteries	☐	☐	☐	☐
	● If murmur is present, times with palpation of carotid artery	☐	☐	☐	☐
	●	☐	☐	☐	☐
Additional examination	● Auscultates lung bases for pulmonary oedema	☐	☐	☐	☐
	● Inspects lower back for sacral oedema	☐	☐	☐	☐
	● Examines abdomen for hepatomegaly, abdominal aortic aneurysm	☐	☐	☐	☐
	● Palpates feet for oedema, foot pulses	☐	☐	☐	☐
	●	☐	☐	☐	☐
Professionalism	● Covers patient, thanks patient, washes hands	☐	☐	☐	☐
	●	☐	☐	☐	☐

			Self	Peer	Peer /tutor	Tutor
Self-assessed as at least borderline:	Signature:	Date:	U B S E	U B S E	U B S E	U B S E
Peer-assessed as ready for tutor assessment:	Signature:	Date:	U B S E	U B S E	U B S E	U B S E
Tutor-assessed as satisfactory:	Signature:	Date:	U B S E	U B S E	U B S E	U B S E

Notes

2.3 Gastrointestinal examination

Background

Almost everybody has experienced gastrointestinal disturbance at some time. In many cases the causes are trivial, for example most instances of dyspepsia and altered bowel habit. However, serious intra-abdominal pathology is not uncommon and may present with apparently innocuous symptoms. Disorders outside the abdomen – hyperthyroidism for example – may present with symptoms which are initially attributed to gastrointestinal disease.

Common presentations

Common symptoms of gastrointestinal disorders are:

- Loss of appetite
- Weight loss
- Dysphagia
- Odynophagia
- Heartburn
- Dyspepsia
- Nausea and/or vomiting
- Haematemesis
- Jaundice
- Abdominal pain
- Altered bowel habit
- Flatulence and/or flatus
- Rectal bleeding
- Melaena.

In many instances a diagnosis can be made on the basis of a careful history and examination but investigation may be needed. There are well-established guidelines as to which patients can be treated symptomatically and those who need investigating. Conditions easily missed include coeliac disease, the presentation of which can be very non-specific, and Crohn's disease, which may be misdiagnosed as irritable bowel syndrome.

Anatomical and physiological principles

The abdomen is separated from the thorax superiorly by the lower costal margin, and its inferior borders are the inguinal ligaments and the superior edge of the superior pubic rami.

The abdomen can be divided into four quadrants by a horizontal and a vertical line through the umbilicus. Clinically the abdomen is divided into nine areas. Figure 2.1 shows the structures beneath your fingers when you palpate these nine areas.

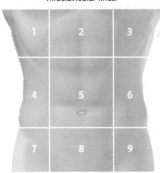

The vertical lines are the midclavicular lines.

The upper horizontal line is at the level of the gastric pylorus (L1 vertebra), and is known as the transpyloric plane.

The lower horizontal line is at the level of the iliac tubercles (L5 vertebra), and is known as the transtubercular plane.

1 **Right hypochondrium:** The lower border of the liver and gallbladder
2 **Epigastrium:** The distal stomach
3 **Left hypochondrium:** The spleen
4 **Right lumbar/loin:** The right kidney
5 **Umbilical:** The small bowel and aorta
6 **Left lumbar/loin:** The left kidney
7 **Right inguinal:** The appendix, terminal ileum and caecum
8 **Suprapublic:** The bladder, and in females the uterus
9 **Left inguinal:** The sigmoid colon.

Figure 2.1 Areas of palpation in the abdomen and anatomical correlates.

The sequence for a gastrointestinal examination

Examination sequence	Clinical context
Explanation and consent	Wash your hands before contact with the patient
Correct position and adequate exposure	Lay the patient flat with one pillow behind the head. Expose the entire abdomen but expose the chest only when needed and keep the lower half of the patient's body covered
General inspection	The most important observations are those which can be made on general inspection. Does the patient appear basically well, or is there evidence of dehydration, jaundice, wasting, or abdominal distension?
General examination	The main purpose of inspecting the hands is for signs of chronic liver disease – clubbing, Dupuytren's contracture, palmar erythema, leuconychia, liver flap
	Jaundice is invariably an abnormal finding and always needs investigation. Anaemia is commonly the result of gastrointestinal blood loss
	An enlarged lymph node in the left supraclavicular fossa (Virchow's node) may be a sign of metastatic gastric cancer
System examination	Reinspect the abdomen to make sure you missed nothing from the end of the bed! Look closely for scars from previous surgery which the patient forgot to mention
	Palpation is done in three stages: light for areas of tenderness, deep for masses, then specifically for enlarged organs
	If the abdomen is distended look for signs of ascites: shifting dullness and a fluid thrill.
	The acute abdomen is one of the few situations in which the examination may yield more information than the history. Findings of rigidity, rebound tenderness, and absent bowel sounds are diagnostically more significant than the patient's symptoms
Additional examination	Consider whether it is necessary to examine the hernial orifices and external genitalia, and perform a rectal examination. Testicular torsion and strangulated hernia can both present with abdominal pain

Examination sequence	Clinical context
Professionalism	Maintain patient dignity, communicate sensitively, thank the patient, wash hands, explain conclusions to the patient, document fully and accurately, communicate appropriately with colleagues

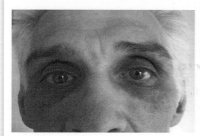

Dupuytren's contracture

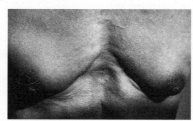

Bilateral gynaecomastia

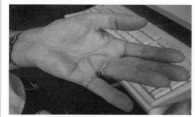

Jaundice: best discerned from upper sclera

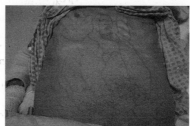

Ascites and distended veins in portal hypertension

Patient safety tip

✔ When taking the history the most important 'red flag' symptom is weight loss. Failure to ask about this is a very serious omission. Significant unintentional weight loss must always be taken very seriously, even if the symptoms are otherwise non-specific and apparently minor.

Student name:	Medical school:	Year:

Examination of the gastrointestinal system

Please examine this patient's gastrointestinal system.

		Self	Peer	Peer/tutor	Tutor
Explanation and consent	• Washes hands with alcohol gel or soap and water	☐	☐	☐	☐
	• Explains procedure to patient and obtains verbal consent	☐	☐	☐	☐
	•	☐	☐	☐	☐
Correct position and adequate exposure	• Positions patient flat with one pillow	☐	☐	☐	☐
	• Adequately exposes the abdomen while maintaining patient dignity	☐	☐	☐	☐
	•	☐	☐	☐	☐
General inspection	• Inspects patient from end of bed, commenting on any relevant findings	☐	☐	☐	☐
	• Inspects patient's surroundings for 'clues'	☐	☐	☐	☐
	•	☐	☐	☐	☐
General examination	• Examines hands for palmar erythema, Dupuytren's contracture, and liver flap	☐	☐	☐	☐
	• Examines nails for clubbing, leuconychia, and koilonychia	☐	☐	☐	☐
	• Takes the pulse and blood pressure	☐	☐	☐	☐
	• Assesses axillary lymph nodes	☐	☐	☐	☐
	• Inspects eyes for jaundice and anaemia	☐	☐	☐	☐
	• Examines mouth for dentition, angular stomatitis, aphthous ulcers, hydration status, pigmentation, telangiectasia, and candidiasis	☐	☐	☐	☐
	• Assesses cervical lymph nodes, paying particular attention to the left supraclavicular fossa	☐	☐	☐	☐
	• Inspects chest for spider naevi and in male subjects for gynaecomastia	☐	☐	☐	☐
	•	☐	☐	☐	☐
System examination	• Reinspects abdomen more closely, commenting on any relevant findings	☐	☐	☐	☐
	• Asks permission to palpate the abdomen, enquires about areas of tenderness, and starts as far away from these as possible	☐	☐	☐	☐
	• Palpates lightly then deeply in all nine areas	☐	☐	☐	☐
	• Palpates for liver, spleen, kidneys, bladder, and for abdominal aortic aneurysm	☐	☐	☐	☐
	• Percusses for liver, spleen, bladder, and shifting dullness	☐	☐	☐	☐
	• Auscultates for bowel sounds	☐	☐	☐	☐
	•	☐	☐	☐	☐
Additional examination	• Assesses the inguinal lymph nodes	☐	☐	☐	☐
	• Comments on need to examine hernial orifices and external genitalia, and perform rectal examination	☐	☐	☐	☐
	• Examines for peripheral oedema	☐	☐	☐	☐
	•	☐	☐	☐	☐
Professionalism	• Covers patient, thanks patient, washes hands	☐	☐	☐	☐

				Self	Peer	Peer/tutor	Tutor
Self-assessed as at least borderline:	Signature:	Date:		U B S E	U B S E	U B S E	U B S E
Peer-assessed as ready for tutor assessment:	Signature:	Date:		U B S E	U B S E	U B S E	U B S E
Tutor-assessed as satisfactory:	Signature:	Date:		U B S E	U B S E	U B S E	U B S E

Notes

2.4 Respiratory examination

Background

Respiratory disease is the second biggest cause of death in the UK and the largest single cause of emergency hospital admissions. All patients admitted to hospital will need at least a basic respiratory examination. Since much respiratory disease is related to smoking, this area of medicine offers many opportunities for primary and secondary prevention and anticipatory care.

Common presentations

Patients with respiratory disease commonly present with:

- **Cough**: it must be determined first whether the cough is acute (less than 2 months duration or chronic (more than 2 months).
- **Sputum**: green sputum does not necessarily indicate chest infection – it may also occur in allergic conditions, notably asthma.
- **Haemoptysis**: blood in the sputum may be the result of bronchitis but its occurrence for the first time almost always needs investigation to exclude lung cancer.
- **Wheeze**: you need to ensure that your patient's understanding of 'wheeze' is the same as yours. True wheeze indicates small airways obstruction, such as in asthma or chronic obstructive pulmonary disease.
- **Breathlessness**: differentiating between a respiratory and a cardiac cause may need investigation and both may coexist in the same patient.
- **Chest pain**: determination of the origin of chest pain requires a careful history.

Anatomical and physiological principles

When you examine the back of the chest you are mainly over the lower lobes of the lungs: disease here may also produce signs in the axillae. Disease in the upper lobes produces signs in the upper chest anteriorly, high up on the back of the chest and sometimes also in the axillae. Disease in the right middle lobe produces signs in the right lower chest anteriorly but not over the back.

The sequence for a respiratory examination

Examination sequence	Clinical context
Explanation and consent	Wash your hands before contact with the patient
Correct position and adequate exposure	The patient should be positioned at 45° if breathlessness permits
General inspection	The most important observations are those which can be made on general inspection. Does the patient appear basically well, or is he or she clearly cyanosed, breathless, or using the accessory muscles of respiration? If a sputum pot has been used, inspect the contents (see Figure 2.2)
General examination	The unexpected discovery of clubbing in a smoker with chest symptoms of recent onset suggests lung cancer
	When taking the radial pulse consider whether it is bounding in character. CO_2 retention may be confirmed by the finding of a flapping tremor but this is an unreliable sign
	Recording the respiratory rate is a crucial part of the assessment of the acutely ill patient. However, it must be done surreptitiously since patients alter their breathing pattern if they know it is being observed

System examination	Ask the patient to take a deep breath and observe the chest movements. If there is asymmetry, the abnormal side is the one which moves less
	The combination of dullness to percussion and reduced or absent breath sounds usually indicates a pleural effusion. However, it may also be caused by consolidation with an occluded airway
	There is usually no need to examine for both tactile vocal fremitus and vocal resonance, and the latter is easier to elicit
	One of the most <u>ominous signs in medicine</u> is a silent chest in a patient with asthma: this patient is very ill and may need assisted ventilation
Additional examination	The finding of pedal oedema in a patient with chronic respiratory disease prompts consideration of right heart failure but does not confirm it: most oedema is gravitational in origin
Professionalism	Maintain patient dignity, communicate sensitively, thank the patient, wash hands, explain conclusions to the patient, document fully and accurately, communicate appropriately with colleagues

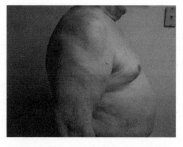

Increased anteroposterior diameter of chest in chronic obstructive pulmonary disease

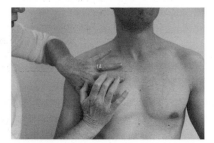

Chest percussion

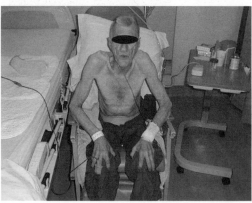

- Observe for discomfort /dyspnoea/tachypnoea
- Cachexia
- Pursed lips breathing
- Supplementary oxygen
- ?Are there any inhalers/nebulizers nearby?
- Accessory muscle of respiration: extra support gained by holding onto knees
- Sputum jar (?blood, colour. etc.)
- Continuous pulse oximetry monitoring
- Increased AP diameter of chest
- Nutritional supplements
- Bedside micturition aid
- Wasting of hands
- ? tar–stained fingers
- Dilated veins left shoulder ? axillary vein thrombosis
- ? upper clothing removed due to fever
- Check for Horner's syndrome

Figure 2.2 Inspection in respiratory patient – a large array of signs can be gleaned from detailed observation alone.

Patient safety tip

✔ Tracheal deviation is a subtle sign that is difficult to elicit. However, its detection in a patient who is *in extremis* with a tension pneumothorax may be life-saving.

Student name: Medical school: Year:

Examination of the respiratory system

Please examine this patient's respiratory system.

	Self	Peer	Peer/tutor	Tutor
Explanation and consent				
Washes hands with alcohol gel or soap and water	☐	☐	☐	☐
Explains procedure to patient and obtains verbal consent	☐	☐	☐	☐
	☐	☐	☐	☐
Correct position and adequate exposure				
Positions patient with trunk at 45°	☐	☐	☐	☐
Adequately exposes chest and arms	☐	☐	☐	☐
Offers to cover females until removal is appropriate	☐	☐	☐	☐
	☐	☐	☐	☐
General inspection				
Inspects patient from end of bed, commenting on any relevant findings	☐	☐	☐	☐
Inspects patient's surroundings for 'clues'	☐	☐	☐	☐
	☐	☐	☐	☐
General examination				
Examines hands for peripheral cyanosis, tremor, muscle wasting, tar staining, and CO_2 retention flap	☐	☐	☐	☐
Examines nails for clubbing	☐	☐	☐	☐
Palpates radial pulse for rate and rhythm	☐	☐	☐	☐
Assesses respiratory rate and pattern	☐	☐	☐	☐
Takes the blood pressure	☐	☐	☐	☐
Assesses axillary lymph nodes	☐	☐	☐	☐
Inspects eyes for anaemia and Horner's syndrome	☐	☐	☐	☐
Inspects face and mouth for swelling, hydration status, central cyanosis	☐	☐	☐	☐
Inspects neck for jugular venous pulse and elicits hepatojugular reflux	☐	☐	☐	☐
Assesses cervical lymph nodes	☐	☐	☐	☐
	☐	☐	☐	☐
System examination				
Reinspects anterior chest wall more closely, commenting on any relevant findings	☐	☐	☐	☐
Asks patient to take a deep breath and assesses chest movement	☐	☐	☐	☐
Palpates the trachea and for apex beat position	☐	☐	☐	☐
Palpates for chest expansion anteriorly, comparing both sides: considers palpation for tactile vocal fremitus	☐	☐	☐	☐
Percusses the chest anteriorly, including the clavicles and axillae, comparing both sides	☐	☐	☐	☐
Auscultates the chest anteriorly, including the supraclavicular fossae and axillae, comparing both sides	☐	☐	☐	☐
Assesses vocal resonance anteriorly, comparing both sides	☐	☐	☐	☐
Repeats inspection, palpation, percussion, auscultation posteriorly	☐	☐	☐	☐
	☐	☐	☐	☐
Additional examination				
Palpates for sacral and pedal oedema	☐	☐	☐	☐
Assesses the inguinal lymph nodes	☐	☐	☐	☐
Offers to measure peak expiratory flow rate if necessary	☐	☐	☐	☐
	☐	☐	☐	☐
Professionalism				
Covers patient, thanks patient, washes hands	☐	☐	☐	☐
	☐	☐	☐	☐

	Signature:	Date:	Self	Peer	Peer/tutor	Tutor
Self-assessed as at least borderline:			U B S E	U B S E	U B S E	U B S E
Peer-assessed as ready for tutor assessment:			U B S E	U B S E	U B S E	U B S E
Tutor-assessed as satisfactory:			U B S E	U B S E	U B S E	U B S E

Notes

2.5 Neurology I: general and cranial nerves examination

Background

Most non-specialists find neurological assessment daunting. However, neurological symptoms are common and it essential to master the history and a basic examination. Headaches are a near-universal phenomenon: most are benign but it is important to identify accurately the small proportion of patients who need further investigation, sometimes urgently. Cranial nerve disorders are not unusual: Bell's palsy is frequently seen in primary care and others may be encountered, especially in patients with diabetes.

Common presentations

A general principle in neurology is that whereas the examination locates the lesion in the nervous system it is the history – especially the timing of symptoms, for example whether of sudden onset or slowly progressive – which gives the best clue to the nature of the pathology. Vascular pathologies usually have a sudden onset of symptoms, space-occupying or inflammatory pathologies a more insidious onset. Common symptoms in the head with which patients present are:

- Visual loss
- Hearing loss
- Disturbance of smell or taste
- Headache
- Blackouts and syncope
- Dizziness and vertigo

All of these symptoms may also arise from non-neurological causes.

Anatomical and physiological principles

The cranial nerves are 12 pairs of nerves that originate from the brain and innervate the head and neck. Some provide the same motor and sensory functions as the spinal nerves do to the trunk and limbs but others are responsible for the special senses: smell, vision, taste, and hearing. The olfactory and optic nerves are not actually nerves at all but forward protrusions of the central nervous system. The 12 pairs of cranial nerves are numbered according to the location of their nuclei in the brain stem. For instance, oculomotor nerve (CN III) leaves the brainstem at a higher position than the hypoglossal nerve (CN XII), whose origin is situated more caudally.

The sequence for a general neurology and cranial nerves examination

Examination sequence	Clinical context
Explanation and consent	Wash your hands before contact with the patient
Correct position and adequate exposure	The examination is best performed with the patient and the examiner sitting face to face at arm's length: expose the face, neck, and shoulders
General inspection	The most important observations are those which can be made on general inspection. Does the patient wear glasses or a hearing aid? Is there evidence of facial asymmetry, ptosis, or any abnormality of speech?
General examination	A general examination is always necessary. Finger clubbing and lymphadenopathy in a smoker with headache suggest cerebral metastases from lung cancer

System examination	**CNI**	Bilateral anosmia is usually due to a nasal not a neurological cause. Unilateral anosmia may result from head injury or subfrontal meningioma
	CNII	The visual field abnormalities most commonly detected are the homonymous hemianopia, frequently seen in stroke, and the bitemporal hemianopia, typically caused by a pituitary tumour
	CNIII, CNIV, CNVI	Severe unilateral ptosis suggests a IIIrd nerve palsy, although a partial ptosis may be seen in Horner's syndrome. The only common cause of bilateral ptosis is myasthenia gravis.
		The most frequent cause of a IIIrd nerve palsy is a diabetic mononeuritis: usually the pupil is spared
	CNV	Wasting of the muscles of mastication occurs in motor neurone disease
	CNVII	A VIIth nerve palsy is the most commonly encountered cranial nerve lesion. It is imperative to distinguish between a lower (for example, Bell's palsy) and an upper motor neurone lesion (for example, stroke). In the latter the forehead is spared
	CNVIII	Conductive deafness is usually due to disease of the outer or middle ear. The commonest causes of sensorineural deafness are presbycusis and noise-induced deafness: both are irreversible.
	CNIX CNX CNXI CNXII	Lesions of the lower cranial nerves usually occur in combination. Bulbar palsy comprises bilateral lower motor neurone lesions of CNIX, X, and XII: the usual cause is motor neurone disease. Pseudobulbar palsy is due to bilateral upper motor neurone lesions consequent upon multiple sclerosis or bilateral strokes
Additional examination		Fundoscopy is most conveniently performed at the end of the examination. The most important abnormality to recognize is papilloedema but its absence does not exclude raised intracranial pressure
		All patents will need neurological assessment of the limbs as well
Professionalism		Maintain patient dignity, communicate sensitively, thank the patient, wash hands, explain conclusions to the patient, document fully and accurately, communicate appropriately with colleagues

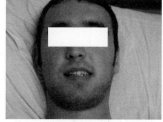

Facial asymmetry due to left Bell's palsy

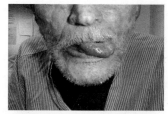

Hypoglossal nerve lesion on left

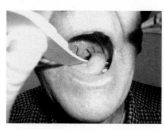

Deviated uvula

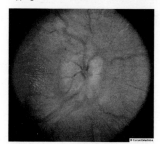

Papilloedema: blurred optic disc margin

Patient safety tip

✔ A cause of headache which is sometimes overlooked is giant-cell arteritis (GCA). This must be considered in any patient over the age of 55 years with headache, especially if there is scalp or temporal artery tenderness. The erythrocyte sedimentation rate (ESR) is typically markedly elevated. Left untreated there is a risk of sudden blindness, consequently high-dose steroid therapy must be commenced immediately if GCA is suspected. Temporal artery biopsy may confirm the diagnosis but a negative result does not exclude it.

Student name:	Medical school:	Year:

Examination of the cranial nerves

Please examine this patient's cranial nerves.

		Self	Peer	Peer /tutor	Tutor
Explanation and consent	● Washes hands with alcohol gel or soap and water	☐	☐	☐	☐
	● Explains procedure to patient and obtains verbal consent	☐	☐	☐	☐
	●	☐	☐	☐	☐
Correct position and adequate exposure	● Sits opposite patient at arm's length	☐	☐	☐	☐
	● Exposes patient's face, neck, and shoulders	☐	☐	☐	☐
	●	☐	☐	☐	☐
General inspection	● Makes general inspection of patient, commenting on any relevant findings	☐	☐	☐	☐
	● Inspects patient's surroundings for 'clues'	☐	☐	☐	☐
	●	☐	☐	☐	☐
General examination	● Comments on need for a general examination	☐	☐	☐	☐
	●	☐	☐	☐	☐
System examination	● **Olfactory (I)**: Asks about changes in senses of smell or taste: comments on need for formal testing if necessary	☐	☐	☐	☐
	● **Optic (II)**: Inspects eyes closely	☐	☐	☐	☐
	● **Optic (II)**: Assesses visual acuity with Snellen's chart: comments on need to assess colour vision (Ishihara's chart)	☐	☐	☐	☐
	● **Optic (II)**: Assesses visual fields by confrontation	☐	☐	☐	☐
	● **Optic (II) and oculomotor (III)**: Checks direct and consensual pupillary light reflexes and near reflex	☐	☐	☐	☐
	● **Optic (II)**: Mentions that fundoscopy will be performed at the end of the examination	☐	☐	☐	☐
	● **Oculomotor (III), trochlear (IV), abducens (VI)**: Assesses ocular movements, asks about diplopia and checks for nystagmus	☐	☐	☐	☐
	● **Trigeminal (V)**: Assesses facial sensation (ophthalmic, maxillary, mandibular), and power of muscles of mastication (masseters and temporalis)	☐	☐	☐	☐
	● **Trigeminal (V)**: Comments on need to test jaw jerk (positive in bilateral upper motor neurone lesions above the pons) and corneal reflex (motor component is facial)	☐	☐	☐	☐
	● **Facial (VII)**: Assesses power of muscles of facial expression (frontalis, orbicularis oculi, buccinator, orbicularis oris, naso-labial)	☐	☐	☐	☐
	● **Vestibulocochlear (VIII)**: Assesses hearing, comments on need to perform Weber's and Rinne's tests	☐	☐	☐	☐
	● **Glossopharyngeal (IX) and vagus (X)**: Assesses patient's voice, movement of soft palate and mentions gag reflex	☐	☐	☐	☐
	● **Accessory nerve (XI)**: Assesses power of trapezius and sternomastoid	☐	☐	☐	☐
	● **Hypoglossal nerve (XII)**: Inspects tongue, assesses position and power, ? fasciculation	☐	☐	☐	☐
	●	☐	☐	☐	☐
Additional examination	● Performs fundoscopy	☐	☐	☐	☐
	● Comments on need of neurological assessment of limbs	☐	☐	☐	☐
	●	☐	☐	☐	☐
Professionalism	● Covers patient, thanks patient, washes hands	☐	☐	☐	☐
	●	☐	☐	☐	☐

				Self	Peer	Peer/tutor	Tutor
Self-assessed as at least borderline:	Signature:		Date:	U B S E	U B S E	U B S E	U B S E
Peer-assessed as ready for tutor assessment:	Signature:		Date:	U B S E	U B S E	U B S E	U B S E
Tutor-assessed as satisfactory:	Signature:		Date:	U B S E	U B S E	U B S E	U B S E

Notes

2.6 Neurology II: examination of the limbs

Background

Stroke is by far the commonest major neurological disease and the one most frequently requiring urgent hospital admission. However, the non-specialist will not infrequently be required to manage patients with Parkinson's disease, multiple sclerosis or motor neurone disease when they develop concurrent problems, often a chest or urinary infection. The cause of stroke in about 80% of cases is thromboembolic. Haemorrhagic stroke is less common because of more effective treatment of its main risk factor, hypertension.

Common presentations

The patient with a neurological problem affecting one or more limbs will usually present with:

- Pain
- Paraesthesia
- Numbness
- Muscle weakness.

Anatomical and physiological principles

When testing power in the upper limbs many muscle groups can be assessed but a minimum set, since each root level is tested at least once, is: shoulder abduction (C5), shoulder adduction (C5, 6, 7), elbow flexion (C5, 6), elbow extension (C7), wrist dorsiflexion (C7), wrist palmar flexion (C7,8), grip (C8), and finger abduction (T1). The minimum to be tested in the lower limbs is: hip flexion (L1, 2), hip extension (L5, S1), knee flexion (S1), knee extension (L3, 4), ankle dorsiflexion (L4), and ankle plantar flexion (S1, 2).

A quick screening assessment of sensation in the upper limbs is to test for light touch on the upper arm medially and laterally, on the lower arm medially and laterally, on each digit, followed by vibration and position sense on a finger. In the lower limbs test light touch on the thigh medially and laterally, on the calf medially and laterally, on the dorsum of the foot, the tip of the big toe, the lateral border of the foot, then vibration sense at the medial malleolus and position sense on the big toe.

Patient safety tip

✔ Embolism from the heart is a common cause of stroke, up to 30% of cases in some studies. Cardiological assessment is therefore as important as neurological and most patients will need an echocardiogram. Atrial fibrillation increases the risk of stroke fivefold, consequently much effort is directed to returning the patient to sinus rhythm, although the fibrillation frequently recurs. In the meantime the risk of stroke can be reduced by anticoagulation with warfarin. However, the decision to anticoagulate a frail elderly patient can be a difficult one since the dangers may be perceived to outweigh the benefit. In such cases aspirin is safer but less effective.

The sequence for a neurological examination of the limbs

Examination sequence	Clinical context
Explanation and consent	Wash your hands before contact with the patient
Correct position and adequate exposure	The arms may be examined with the patient sitting or, if unable to sit, propped up in bed. For examination of the legs the patient must be supine. The limbs should be fully exposed

General inspection	The most important observations are those that can be made on general inspection. Involuntary movements may be an important clue to the diagnosis. Walking aids or a wheelchair are obvious indications of a problem with use of the legs	
General examination	A general examination is always necessary. Patients with stroke are frequently hypertensive and exhibit other evidence of vascular disease	
System examination	Muscle bulk	Generalized muscle weakness may simply result from malnutrition or cachexia. Localized weakness and wasting suggest a lower motor neurone lesion and may be associated with fasciculation
	Tone	Clasp-knife spasticity is characteristic of an upper motor neurone lesion, lead-pipe rigidity of extrapyramidal disease. The cogwheel rigidity of Parkinson's disease is due to a combination of rigidity and tremor
	Power	Weakness may result from a problem with the upper motor neurone, the lower motor neurone, the neuromuscular junction or the muscle. Marked variation in weakness with dramatic worsening after activity suggests myasthenia gravis
	Reflexes	The tendon reflexes are increased with an upper motor neurone lesion, reduced with a lower motor neurone lesion. Reflexes cannot be deemed to be absent unless they are absent with reinforcement
	Sensation	The patterns of sensory loss commonly encountered are (i) in the distribution of a nerve root or peripheral nerve, (ii) hemianaesthesia due to a lesion in the contralateral cerebral hemisphere, (iii) over the lower part of the body with a sensory level due to a spinal cord lesion, and (iv) the glove and stocking distribution of peripheral neuropathy
	Coordination	Intention tremor, past-pointing and dysdiadokokinesis are features of a cerebellar lesion. Romberg's is a test for sensory ataxia
	Function	Function in the hands may be assessed by asking the patient to write, undo and redo a button or pick up coins. Assessment of the gait is an essential element of examination of the lower limbs
Additional examination	If an upper motor neurone lesion is suspected, clonus and an extensor plantar response are confirmatory signs	
	All patents will need assessment of the cranial nerves as well	
Professionalism	Maintain patient dignity, communicate sensitively, thank the patient, wash hands, explain conclusions to the patient, document fully and accurately, communicate appropriately with colleagues	

Median nerve is compressed at the wrist, resulting in numbness or pain

Carpal tunnel syndrome: weakness of abductor pollicis brevis and opponens pollicis, loss of sensation in lateral three and half digits

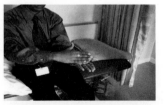

Coordination: checking for dysdiadochokinesia

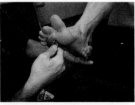

Babinski reflex: plantar extension indicates upper motor neurone lesion

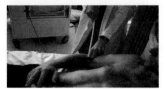

Reflexes: note tendon hammer is held at the very end, correct swinging action essential to deliver short sharp knock

Student name:	Medical school:	Year:

Examination of the upper and lower limbs

Please perform a neurological examination of this patient's upper and lower limbs.

		Self	Peer	Peer /tutor	Tutor
Explanation and consent	● Washes hands with alcohol gel or soap and water	☐	☐	☐	☐
	● Explains procedure to patient and obtains verbal consent	☐	☐	☐	☐
	●				
Correct position and adequate exposure	● Positions patient appropriately: sitting or propped up in bed for upper limbs, supine for lower limbs	☐	☐	☐	☐
	● Achieves adequate exposure while maintaining patient dignity	☐	☐	☐	☐
	●				
General inspection	● Makes general inspection of patient, commenting on any relevant findings	☐	☐	☐	☐
	● Inspects patient's surroundings for 'clues'	☐	☐	☐	☐
	●				
General examination	● Comments on need for a general examination	☐	☐	☐	☐
	●				
System examination	● Alternates between sides throughout examination	☐	☐	☐	☐
	● Inspects upper limbs and assesses muscle bulk by palpation	☐	☐	☐	☐
	● Assesses tone at shoulder, elbow, and wrist	☐	☐	☐	☐
	● Assesses muscle power in upper limbs, proximally to distally	☐	☐	☐	☐
	● Tests biceps, triceps, and supinator reflexes	☐	☐	☐	☐
	● Tests light touch, pain, vibration and position sense in upper limbs	☐	☐	☐	☐
	● Performs finger-nose test and assesses alternating hand movements	☐	☐	☐	☐
	● Assesses function in hands	☐	☐	☐	☐
	● Inspects lower limbs and assesses muscle bulk by palpation	☐	☐	☐	☐
	● Assesses tone at hip, knee and ankle	☐	☐	☐	☐
	● Assesses muscle power in lower limbs, proximally to distally	☐	☐	☐	☐
	● Tests knee and ankle reflexes	☐	☐	☐	☐
	● Tests light touch, pain, vibration and position sense in lower limbs	☐	☐	☐	☐
	● Performs heel-shin and Romberg's tests	☐	☐	☐	☐
	● Assesses gait	☐	☐	☐	☐
	●				
Additional examination	● Comments on need to test plantar reflex and for clonus	☐	☐	☐	☐
	● Comments on need to examine cranial nerves	☐	☐	☐	☐
	●				
Professionalism	● Covers patient, thanks patient, washes hands	☐	☐	☐	☐
	●				

				Self	Peer	Peer/tutor	Tutor
Self-assessed as at least borderline:	Signature:		Date:	U B S E	U B S E	U B S E	U B S E
Peer-assessed as ready for tutor assessment:	Signature:		Date:	U B S E	U B S E	U B S E	U B S E
Tutor-assessed as satisfactory:	Signature:		Date:	U B S E	U B S E	U B S E	U B S E

Notes

Unit 3   Musculoskeletal examination

3.1   GALS assessment

Background

Rheumatological conditions are extremely common and account for about 10% of consultations in primary care. After mental health problems they are the second commonest cause of time lost from work in the UK. Since prevalence rises with age it can be predicted that the burden of arthritis and other rheumatological conditions will increase with a progressively ageing population.

Common presentations

The main symptoms referable to the joints with which patients present are:

- Pain
- Stiffness
- Swelling
- Deformity
- Loss of function.

However, since many rheumatological conditions are multisystem disorders patients may also present with extra-articular problems, such as rashes or Raynaud's syndrome.

Examination of the joints mostly follows the sequence look → feel → move but it is sometimes necessary to deviate slightly from this. GALS – **G**ait **A**rms **L**egs **S**pine – is a quick screening assessment for musculoskeletal disorders.

Anatomical and physiological principles

Most of the joints of the limbs exhibit a wide range of movement and are synovial joints. Such joints are surrounded by a fibrous capsule lined on the inside by a synovial membrane. The latter secretes synovial fluid which occupies the joint cavity. The ends of the bones are covered in cartilage which facilitates their movement relative to each other. The joints of the vertebral column are cartilaginous joints: they have no cavity and move only slightly. Fibrous joints, such as those between the bones of the skull, do not move at all.

The sequence for a GALS assessment

Examination sequence	Clinical context		
Explanation and consent	Wash your hands before contact with the patient		
Adequate exposure	The patient should be clad in light underclothes		
General inspection	Observe the patient's general appearance and posture, and note the presence of any aids		
General examination	Perform a general examination if there are unusual features in the history or on general inspection, for example, weight loss, feverishness, or if the patient appears generally unwell.		
Joint examination	The four components of the GALS assessment can be performed in any order, depending on the circumstances		
	Gait	There are numerous causes of an abnormal gait. Trendelenburg's gait is usually due to chronic hip disease	
	Arms	Inspection of the hands may reveal characteristic changes of osteoarthritis or rheumatoid arthritis	
		Rheumatoid arthritis typically affects the metacarpophalangeal joints first: local warmth indicates active inflammation	
		Pain in the joints of the hands, deformity or neurological disorder may all cause impairment of function and loss of dexterity	
	Legs	Limitation of internal rotation is often the earliest sign of hip disease	
		Knee swelling may be due to fluid, synovial inflammation or bony growth	
		Callosities on the feet may be the consequence of long-standing abnormal weight-bearing on walking	
	Spine	Exaggerated thoracic kyphosis with loss of lumbar lordosis is typical of ankylosing spondylitis	
		Tenderness over the mid-supraspinatus is common in fibromyalgia	
		Lateral flexion of the cervical spine is usually the first movement to be affected by degenerative changes	
Additional examination	Proceed to detailed assessment of individual joint(s) if any problem is detected		
Professionalism	Maintain patient dignity, communicate sensitively, thank the patient, wash hands, explain conclusions to the patient, document fully and accurately, communicate appropriately with colleagues		

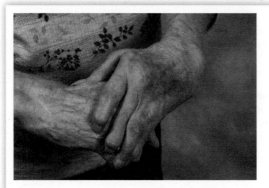

Rheumatoid hands: often have distinct changes such as swan-neck and boutonnière's deformity and rheumatoid nodules. © Stan Rohrer/iStockphoto

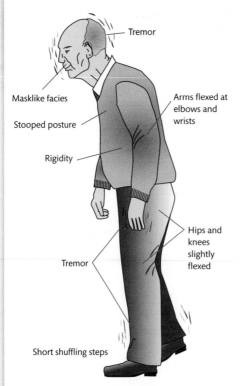

Typical gait and demeanour of a patient with Parkinson's disease

Patient safety tip

✔ The GALS assessment is not a comprehensive rheumatological examination: its purpose is screening. If the patient experiences no symptoms from a joint, it looks normal and its range of movement is satisfactory it is reasonable to conclude that it is a normal joint. However, if any of these conditions do not apply, the joint must be formally examined in detail.

Student name:	Medical school:	Year:

GALS assessment

Please perform a GALS assessment on this patient.

		Self	Peer	Peer/tutor	Tutor
Explanation and consent	● Washes hands with alcohol gel or soap and water	☐	☐	☐	☐
	● Explains procedure to patient and obtains verbal consent	☐	☐	☐	☐
	● Asks about any particularly painful or tender areas	☐	☐	☐	☐
	●	☐	☐	☐	☐
Adequate exposure	● The patient should be clad in light underwear	☐	☐	☐	☐
	●	☐	☐	☐	☐
General inspection	● Assesses patient's appearance and posture, commenting on any relevant findings	☐	☐	☐	☐
	● Inspects patient's surroundings for 'clues'	☐	☐	☐	☐
	●	☐	☐	☐	☐
General examination	● Comments on whether a general examination is required	☐	☐	☐	☐
	●	☐	☐	☐	☐
Joints examination	● Observes patient's gait	☐	☐	☐	☐
	● With patient sitting, *'arms straight'*: tests active elbow extension, supination and pronation	☐	☐	☐	☐
	● *'Put hands behind head'*: tests active shoulder external rotation	☐	☐	☐	☐
	● Inspects hands	☐	☐	☐	☐
	● Palpates metacarpophalangeal joints	☐	☐	☐	☐
	● *'Put index finger on thumb'*: tests pincer grip	☐	☐	☐	☐
	● Assesses function in hands	☐	☐	☐	☐
	● With patient supine, inspects legs	☐	☐	☐	☐
	● If any knee swelling tests for effusion	☐	☐	☐	☐
	● Tests passive knee flexion and extension	☐	☐	☐	☐
	● Tests passive hip flexion and internal rotation	☐	☐	☐	☐
	● Inspects feet	☐	☐	☐	☐
	● Palpates metatarsophalangeal joints	☐	☐	☐	☐
	● With patient standing, inspects spine from behind and from the sides	☐	☐	☐	☐
	● Palpates over mid-supraspinatus	☐	☐	☐	☐
	● *'Tilt head towards shoulder'*: tests cervical spine lateral flexion	☐	☐	☐	☐
	● *'Touch your toes'*: tests hip and lumbar spine flexion	☐	☐	☐	☐
	●	☐	☐	☐	☐
Additional examination	● Comments on whether detailed examination of any joint(s) is necessary in view of findings	☐	☐	☐	☐
	●	☐	☐	☐	☐
Professionalism	● Assists patient to dress, thanks patient, washes hands	☐	☐	☐	☐
	●	☐	☐	☐	☐

Self-assessed as at least borderline:	Signature:	Date:	U B / S E	U B / S E	U B / S E	U B / S E
Peer-assessed as ready for tutor assessment:	Signature:	Date:	U B / S E	U B / S E	U B / S E	U B / S E
Tutor-assessed as satisfactory:	Signature:	Date:	U B / S E	U B / S E	U B / S E	U B / S E

Notes

3.2 Knee examination

Background

A painful swollen knee is a problem commonly encountered, especially in the accident and emergency department. Acute pain and swelling in a fit young person is usually due to trauma. However, the knee can be affected by all the common arthritides including osteo-arthritis, rheumatoid arthritis, septic arthritis, and gout.

Common presentations

The patient with a knee problem will typically present with:

- Pain: trauma to the knee or a mechanical problem cause localized pain, whereas in arthritis it is usually more diffuse.
- Swelling: depending on its aetiology this may be acute or chronic.
- Functional impairment: walking, climbing stairs, and getting in and out of chairs may be difficult.

Other symptoms which patients may report are:

- Locking and unlocking: these are due to a loose body in the joint, often a torn meniscus.
- 'Giving way': this may be due to ruptured ligaments or patellar instability.

Anatomical and physiological principles

The knee is a hinge joint with a rather complex structure consequent on the need to maintain its stability. The anterior cruciate ligament prevents the tibia slipping forwards on the femur and the posterior cruciate prevents it slipping backwards. The medial and lateral collateral ligaments prevent sideways movement. The medial and lateral menisci are unfortunately susceptible to degeneration and tearing.

The sequence for a knee examination

Examination sequence	Clinical context
Explanation and consent	Wash your hands before contact with the patient
Adequate exposure	The lower limbs should be fully exposed
General inspection	Observe the patient's general appearance and gait. Instability of the knee may be evident on walking. Note the presence of walking aids
General examination	Perform a general examination if there are unusual features in the history or on general inspection, for example, weight loss, feverishness, or if the patient appears generally unwell

Examination sequence		Clinical context
Joint examination	Look	Genu valgum (knock knees) is sometimes seen in rheumatoid arthritis and genu varum (bow legs) in osteoarthritis
		Swelling of the knee may be due to trauma, an effusion, fluid in a bursa, synovial inflammation or bony growth
		Wasting of the quadriceps muscle may result from any long-standing painful knee condition
	Feel	If the knee is swollen test for an effusion using the bulge test or the patellar tap
		Especially if the knee is painful and/or unstable, test the integrity of the collateral and cruciate ligaments
	Move	The prone-lying test will reveal a fixed flexion deformity as in tight hamstrings or a locked knee consequent upon a torn meniscus
		Quadriceps lag is due to weakness of the muscle
		Pain on movement and/or restricted range of movement may occur in any acute or chronic knee condition
Additional examination		If a meniscal tear is suspected the specific tests are Apley's and McMurray's. If in doubt ask an orthopaedic surgeon
Professionalism		Maintain patient dignity, communicate sensitively, thank the patient, wash hands, explain conclusions to the patient, document fully and accurately, communicate appropriately with colleagues

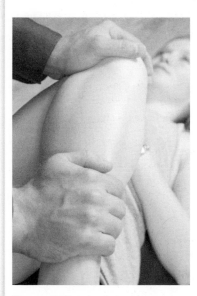

Knee examination: draw test

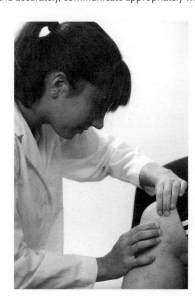

Examination for effusion

Patient safety tip

✔ An acutely painful swollen knee is not necessarily due to trauma: the differential diagnosis includes septic arthritis and gout. The former must be considered especially if the patient is feverish or systemically unwell. The most important investigation is joint aspiration. If doubt remains then the patient should be treated for septic arthritis. Untreated sepsis can result in irrevocable damage to the joint within days.

Student name:	Medical school:	Year:

Examination of the knees

Please examine this patient's knees.

		Self	Peer	Peer /tutor	Tutor
Explanation and consent	● Washes hands with alcohol gel or soap and water	☐	☐	☐	☐
	● Explains procedure to patient and obtains verbal consent	☐	☐	☐	☐
	● Asks about tenderness in either knee	☐	☐	☐	☐
	●	☐	☐	☐	☐
Adequate exposure	● Exposes lower legs fully while maintaining patient dignity	☐	☐	☐	☐
	●	☐	☐	☐	☐
General inspection	● Assesses patient's appearance, posture and gait, commenting on any relevant findings	☐	☐	☐	☐
	● Inspects patient's surroundings for 'clues'	☐	☐	☐	☐
	●	☐	☐	☐	☐
General examination	● Comments on whether a general examination is required	☐	☐	☐	☐
	●	☐	☐	☐	☐
Joint examination	● With patient standing inspects knees from the front, sides, and back	☐	☐	☐	☐
	● With patient supine commences palpation on the unaffected side	☐	☐	☐	☐
	● Palpates both knees	☐	☐	☐	☐
	● If swelling is present tests for effusion	☐	☐	☐	☐
	● Tests medial and lateral collateral ligaments	☐	☐	☐	☐
	● Tests anterior and posterior cruciate ligaments	☐	☐	☐	☐
	● Performs prone-lying test	☐	☐	☐	☐
	● With patient supine tests for active hyperextension	☐	☐	☐	☐
	● Tests for quadriceps lag	☐	☐	☐	☐
	● Assesses active flexion, passive extension, and passive flexion	☐	☐	☐	☐
	●	☐	☐	☐	☐
Additional examination	● Comments on need to test for meniscal tears	☐	☐	☐	☐
	●	☐	☐	☐	☐
Professionalism	● Covers patient, thanks patient, washes hands	☐	☐	☐	☐
	●	☐	☐	☐	☐

Self-assessed as at least borderline:	Signature:	Date:	U B S E	U B S E	U B S E	U B S E
Peer-assessed as ready for tutor assessment:	Signature:	Date:	U B S E	U B S E	U B S E	U B S E
Tutor-assessed as satisfactory:	Signature:	Date:	U B S E	U B S E	U B S E	U B S E

Notes

3.3 Hip examination

Background

The hip is frequently affected by osteoarthritis, the commonest disease of the joints. Symptomatic osteoarthritis is three times commoner in women than in men and the mean age of onset is 50 years. However, other disorders may also cause pain in the hip and/or limping. Hip replacement is one of the most frequently performed orthopaedic procedures.

Common presentations

The patent with a hip problem will typically present with:

- Pain: this is usually felt in the groin but may radiate to the knee.
- A limp: in association with pain a limp is a compensatory mechanism to take weight off the joint. A painless limp may be due to instability of the hip or to differing leg lengths.
- Functional impairment: sitting down, standing up, walking, and climbing stairs may all be uncomfortable and difficult because of stiffness and pain.

Anatomical and physiological principles

The hips are ball and socket joints and carry the weight of the upper body. The joint lies deep beneath layers of muscle, consequently disease of the hip produces less in the way of visible external signs than disorders of most other joints. Similarly it is not really possible to palpate the hip joint, but disease may result in tenderness around the mid-point of the inguinal ligament. With ageing, the neck of the femur becomes osteoporotic and is the commonest site of a hip fracture.

The sequence for a hip examination

Examination sequence	Clinical context
Explanation and consent	Wash your hands before contact with the patient
Adequate exposure	The lower limbs should be fully exposed
General inspection	Observe the patient's general appearance and gait. The nature of a limp may give a clue to the diagnosis
General examination	Perform a general examination if there are unusual features in the history or on general inspection, for example, weight loss, feverishness, or if the patient appears generally unwell

Joint examination	Look	Inspect the pelvis from in front and behind for deformity, muscle wasting and pelvic tilt
		Trendelenburg's sign -- the pelvis on the unaffected side drops when the patient stands on the affected leg -- indicates chronic hip disease
		Unequal apparent leg lengths despite equal true leg lengths indicate a problem with the hip joint, pelvis or spine
	Feel	Many patients complaining of 'hip pain' have trochanteric bursitis which may be detected by finding tenderness over the greater trochanter
	Move	Limitation of external and internal rotation is often the earliest sign of hip disease
		Thomas's test will detect any spinal movement compensating for a fixed flexion deformity of either hip
Additional examination		If you suspect a muscle strain or tendon problem, test resisted movements to see if they cause discomfort: for example, resisted hip flexion may be painful in a patient with a 'groin strain'
Professionalism		Maintain patient dignity, communicate sensitively, thank the patient, wash hands, explain conclusions to the patient, document fully and accurately, communicate appropriately with colleagues

(A)   (B)

Trendelenburg's test: (A) is abnormal as pelvis has dropped on one leg standing. The pelvis rise in (B) is normal

Patient safety tip

✔ Do not assume that pain in the hip is always due to osteoarthritis. Serious or even life-threatening disease may be responsible, for example septic arthritis or a secondary deposit in the pelvis or femur. It is important not to focus on examination of the joint immediately but to make a general assessment of the patient first. If necessary perform a full physical examination and investigate appropriately.

Student name:	Medical school:	Year:

Examination of the hips

Please examine this patient's hips.

		Self	Peer	Peer /tutor	Tutor
Explanation and consent	• Washes hands with alcohol gel or soap and water	☐	☐	☐	☐
	• Explains procedure to patient and obtains verbal consent	☐	☐	☐	☐
	• Asks about any particularly painful or tender areas	☐	☐	☐	☐
	•	☐	☐	☐	☐
Adequate exposure	• Exposes patient's legs fully while maintaining patient dignity	☐	☐	☐	☐
	•	☐	☐	☐	☐
General inspection	• Assesses patient's appearance and gait, commenting on any relevant findings	☐	☐	☐	☐
	• Inspects patient's surroundings for 'clues'	☐	☐	☐	☐
	•	☐	☐	☐	☐
General examination	• Comments on whether a general examination is required	☐	☐	☐	☐
	•	☐	☐	☐	☐
Joint examination	• With patient standing straight with arms at sides inspects pelvis from front and behind	☐	☐	☐	☐
	• Performs Trendelenburg's test	☐	☐	☐	☐
	• With patient supine measures true and apparent leg lengths	☐	☐	☐	☐
	• Commences palpation on the unaffected side	☐	☐	☐	☐
	• Palpates around midpoint of inguinal ligament and over both greater trochanters	☐	☐	☐	☐
	• Assesses hip flexion and performs Thomas's test	☐	☐	☐	☐
	• Assesses internal and external rotation	☐	☐	☐	☐
	• Assesses abduction and adduction	☐	☐	☐	☐
	• With patient prone assesses hip extension	☐	☐	☐	☐
	•	☐	☐	☐	☐
Additional examination	• Tests resisted movements for possible discomfort	☐	☐	☐	☐
	•	☐	☐	☐	☐
Professionalism	• Covers patient, thanks patient, washes hands	☐	☐	☐	☐
	•	☐	☐	☐	☐

				Self	Peer	Peer /tutor	Tutor
Self-assessed as at least borderline:	Signature:		Date:	U B S E	U B S E	U B S E	U B S E
Peer-assessed as ready for tutor assessment:	Signature:		Date:	U B S E	U B S E	U B S E	U B S E
Tutor-assessed as satisfactory:	Signature:		Date:	U B S E	U B S E	U B S E	U B S E

Notes

3.4 Spine examination

Background

Back pain is extremely common. It is usually due to trauma, such as twisting injury or injudicious heavy lifting, or to degenerative or mechanical causes. However, on occasions it may be the first manifestation of serious or even life-threatening disease. The vast majority of cases are managed in primary care but patients with a new severe episode sometimes refer themselves to the accident and emergency department.

Common presentations

Patients will usually present with:

● Back pain: radiation to a limb may occur and may be significant.

Inquiry must also be made about:

● Neurological symptoms: in particular weakness or sensory disturbance in the limbs.

Anatomical and physiological principles

The vertebral column is divided into the cervical, thoracic, and lumbar spine: the neck the upper back, and the lower back, respectively. The vertebral column is a complex structure that protects the spinal cord and provides scaffolding for the limbs, and the intervertebral discs are shock absorbers which dampen vibration on walking. The cervical spine can move in all directions. The main movement of the thoracic spine is rotation and that of the lumbar spine is flexion and extension. In the adult the spinal cord extends to the upper part of the second lumbar vertebra – lower in children – and is drawn upwards when the spine is flexed. The functional anatomy of the spine is shown in Figure 3.1.

The sequence for a spine examination

Examination sequence	Clinical context
Explanation and consent	Wash your hands before contact with the patient
Adequate exposure	If the whole spine is to be examined the patient should disrobe to his or her underwear
General inspection	Observe the patient's general appearance, posture and gait, and note the presence of a wheelchair or a walking aid
General examination	Perform a general examination if there are suspicious features in the history or on general inspection: the back pain could be due to inflammation, infection or secondary deposits.

Examination sequence		Clinical context
Joints examination	Look	Note especially any abnormality of the spinal curvature. Exaggerated thoracic kyphosis with loss of lumbar lordosis – the 'question mark spine' – is typical of ankylosing spondylitis. An angular kyphosis suggests vertebral fracture or infection. Scoliosis may result from trauma, developmental abnormalities, disease of the vertebral bodies, or muscle abnormality
	Feel	Tenderness over a vertebra is significant and may indicate collapse, infection or tumour. Use gentle percussion
	Move	Lateral flexion of the cervical spine is usually the first movement to be affected by degenerative changes
		Lhermitte's or reverse Lhermitte's sign (paraesthesiae in the arms on neck flexion or extension, respectively) indicates neurological disease: the former occurs in multiple sclerosis, the latter in cervical myelopathy.
		Rotation of the thoracic spine is best viewed from above with the patient seated.
		Schober's test measures flexion of the lumbar spine: increase of less than 5 cm indicates limitation. This is often seen in ankylosing spondylitis
	Special tests	Restriction of straight leg raising to <60° or a positive sciatic stretch test suggests lumbar disc prolapse, usually at the L4/5 or L5/S1 level
		The sacroiliac joints can be assessed by determining whether pressure simultaneously applied to both anterior superior iliac spines produces sacroiliac discomfort. Sacroiliitis may be a manifestation of enteropathic arthritis
Additional examination		Complete examination of the cervical and lumbar spine requires neurological assessment of the upper and lower limbs, respectively
Professionalism		Maintain patient dignity, communicate sensitively, thank the patient, wash hands, explain conclusions to the patient, document fully and accurately, communicate appropriately with colleagues

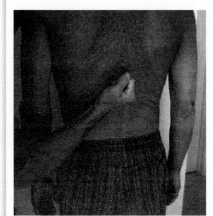

Percussion of lumbar spine to detect local tenderness

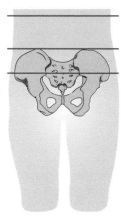

10 cm above iliac crest

Iliac crest line

5 cm below iliac crest

Schober's test: posterior view

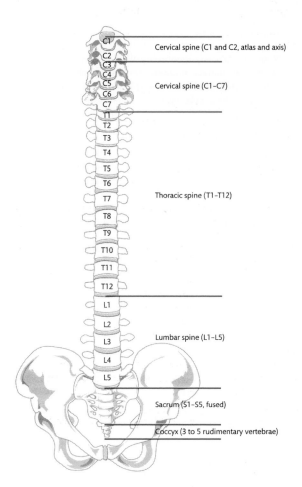

Figure 3.1 Functional anatomy of the spine

Patient safety tip

✔ It is easy to jump to the conclusion that back pain is due to a traumatic, mechanical or degenerative cause: serious pathology can therefore be missed. Warning symptoms and signs in a patient with back pain include fever, unexplained weight loss, abnormal gait, progressive neurological deficit, bladder or bowel dysfunction, and saddle anaesthesia. Such patients require full physical and neurological examination and usually urgent investigation.

Student name:	Medical school:	Year:				

Examination of the spine

Please examine this patient's spine.

		Self	Peer	Peer /tutor	Tutor
Explanation and consent	Washes hands with alcohol gel or soap and water	☐	☐	☐	☐
	Explains procedure to patient and obtains verbal consent	☐	☐	☐	☐
	Asks about any particularly painful or tender areas	☐	☐	☐	☐
		☐	☐	☐	☐
Adequate exposure	Exposes spine fully while maintaining patient dignity	☐	☐	☐	☐
		☐	☐	☐	☐
General inspection	Assesses patient's appearance, posture and gait, commenting on any relevant findings	☐	☐	☐	☐
	Inspects patient's surroundings for 'clues'	☐	☐	☐	☐
		☐	☐	☐	☐
General examination	Comments on whether a general examination is required	☐	☐	☐	☐
		☐	☐	☐	☐
Joints examination	With patient standing inspects spine from behind and from the sides	☐	☐	☐	☐
	Assesses cervical spine flexion, extension, lateral flexion and rotation	☐	☐	☐	☐
	Stabilizes pelvis and assesses thoracic spine rotation	☐	☐	☐	☐
	Assesses lumbar spine flexion, extension and lateral flexion	☐	☐	☐	☐
	Performs Schober's test	☐	☐	☐	☐
	With patient sitting palpates cervical vertebral spines and muscles alongside	☐	☐	☐	☐
	With patient prone palpates thoracic and lumbar vertebral spines and muscles alongside, over sacroiliac joints and upper buttock muscles	☐	☐	☐	☐
	Performs femoral stretch test	☐	☐	☐	☐
	With patient supine estimates straight leg raising and performs sciatic stretch test	☐	☐	☐	☐
	Assesses sacroiliac joints	☐	☐	☐	☐
		☐	☐	☐	☐
Additional examination	Comments on need of a neurological examination	☐	☐	☐	☐
		☐	☐	☐	☐
Professionalism	Covers patient, thanks patient, washes hands	☐	☐	☐	☐
		☐	☐	☐	☐

			U B S E	U B S E	U B S E	U B S E
Self-assessed as at least borderline:	Signature:	Date:				
Peer-assessed as ready for tutor assessment:	Signature:	Date:	U B S E	U B S E	U B S E	U B S E
Tutor-assessed as satisfactory:	Signature:	Date:	U B S E	U B S E	U B S E	U B S E

Notes

3.5 Hands examination

Background

The small joints of the hands are commonly affected at an early stage in both the common polyarthritides: osteoarthritis and rheumatoid arthritis. However, the pattern of joint involvement is different in the two conditions. The appearance of advanced rheumatoid changes in the hands is characteristic and can often be recognized immediately. The hands may also be affected by rarer rheumatological conditions, including psoriatic arthropathy, scleroderma, and systemic lupus erythematosus (SLE).

Common presentations

Patients with arthritis in the hands typically present with pain, swelling, and stiffness in the joints, and deformity may follow.

- Osteoarthritis typically presents with pain in the joints aggravated by movement and worse as the day proceeds: the joints most commonly affected are the distal interphalangeal (DIP) and the first metacarpophalangeal (MCP).
- Rheumatoid arthritis most commonly presents with pain, stiffness, and swelling of the hands and feet, especially in the morning. The MCP joints are typically involved first and the other joints follow.

Anatomical and physiological principles

The DIP, proximal interphalangeal (PIP), and MCP joints can all readily be assessed individually. However, it is easy to forget the thumb. Carpometacarpal joint tenderness here can be detected by palpation in the anatomical snuffbox. It is also necessary to examine the wrists and look at the elbows. Muscle groups which require attention are the interossei and those of the thenar and hypothenar eminences. The nerve supply to the hand is via the radial, ulnar, and median nerves.

Patient safety tip

✔ Generalized wasting of the muscles of the hands may occur in any chronic arthritis consequent upon disuse. However, specific wasting due to a mononeuropathy may also occur. A median nerve palsy in particular may complicate rheumatoid arthritis: the outward sign of this may be wasting of the thenar eminence. A lesion of the ulnar nerve causes wasting of the interossei and the hypothenar eminence with sparing of the thenar. The diagnoses can be confirmed by the findings of muscle weakness and characteristic areas of sensory loss. Examination of the joints of the hands should therefore always include a neurological assessment.

The sequence for a hands examination

Examination sequence	Clinical context
Explanation and consent	Wash your hands before contact with the patient
Correct position and adequate exposure	The arms should be exposed to above the elbows
General inspection	Observation may reveal psoriatic plaques or a cushingoid appearance due to chronic steroid therapy, or suggest a diagnosis of systemic sclerosis or SLE. Note the presence of any aids which indicate a problem with use of the hands

General examination		Many arthritides, including rheumatoid arthritis, are multisystem disorders and the patient will need assessment with a full physical examination
Joints examination	Look	Inspect the fingernails: pitting occurs in psoriatic arthropathy, ridging in rheumatoid arthritis
		The distribution of swelling of the joints is of diagnostic significance: DIP joints in osteoarthritis and MCP joints in rheumatoid arthritis
		The deformity of the hands in advanced rheumatoid arthritis is mainly consequent upon subluxation of the joints: at the MCP joints this produces the typical ulnar deviation of the fingers
	Feel	Hard osteophytes around the joint margins develop in osteoarthritis, e.g. Heberden's nodes around the DIP joints. Soft tissue swelling suggests synovitis: local warmth may be detectable with the back of the hand
		Tenderness in the anatomical snuffbox may indicate a problem with the thumb carpometacarpal joint: this is commonly affected by osteoarthritis
		Inspect and palpate the elbows and forearms for rheumatoid nodules and gouty tophi
	Move	Restricted range of movement will result in the patient being unable to bury their nails in their palms when they make a fist
		Swelling of the MCP joints due to synovitis, as in rheumatoid arthritis, results in loss of the gutters between the metacarpal heads when the fist is clenched
		Restricted wrist dorsiflexion or palmar flexion may be due to pain or swelling
	Function	This can be tested by, for example, asking the patient to undo and redo a button, or pick up coins. Loss of dexterity may be due to pain, deformity or neurological disorder
Additional examination		Screen for nerve problems by assessing thumb abduction (median nerve), little finger abduction (ulnar nerve) and sensation. If carpal tunnel syndrome is suspected perform Tinel's test and Phalen's test
Professionalism		Maintain patient dignity, communicate sensitively, thank the patient, wash hands, explain conclusions to the patient, document fully and accurately, communicate appropriately with colleagues

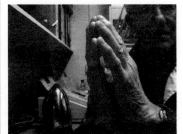

Prayer sign positive in diabetic cheiroarthropathy: associated with carpal tunnel syndrome

Osteoarthritis of the hands with Heberden's and Bouchard's nodes

Student name:	Medical school:	Year:

Examination of the hands

Please examine this patient's hands.

		Self	Peer	Peer /tutor	Tutor
Explanation and consent	● Washes hands with alcohol gel or soap and water	☐	☐	☐	☐
	● Explains procedure to patient and obtains verbal consent	☐	☐	☐	☐
	● Asks about areas of tenderness in the hands	☐	☐	☐	☐
	●	☐	☐	☐	☐
Adequate exposure	● Exposes arms to above elbows	☐	☐	☐	☐
	●	☐	☐	☐	☐
General inspection	● Assesses patient's appearance commenting on any relevant findings	☐	☐	☐	☐
	● Inspects patient's surroundings for 'clues'	☐	☐	☐	☐
	●	☐	☐	☐	☐
General examination	● Comments on whether a general examination is required	☐	☐	☐	☐
	●	☐	☐	☐	☐
Joints examination	● With patient's hands on a pillow inspects back of both hands, then palms	☐	☐	☐	☐
	● Using back of hands palpates for heat in the joints	☐	☐	☐	☐
	● Asks patient to make fists of both hands and comments on any lack of full movement	☐	☐	☐	☐
	● Inspects backs of clenched fists	☐	☐	☐	☐
	● Palpates DIP, PIP, and MCP joints, and in anatomical snuff box in both hands	☐	☐	☐	☐
	● Tests for trigger fingers by asking the patient to open their closed fists quickly	☐	☐	☐	☐
	● Checks pincer grip and thumb opposition	☐	☐	☐	☐
	● Assesses wrist dorsiflexion and palmar flexion	☐	☐	☐	☐
	● Palpates both wrists	☐	☐	☐	☐
	● Inspects and palpates both elbows and forearms	☐	☐	☐	☐
	● Assesses function in hands	☐	☐	☐	☐
	●	☐	☐	☐	☐
Additional examination	● Assesses thumb abduction, little finger abduction, and light touch and pinprick sensation	☐	☐	☐	☐
	● Comments on need to perform Tinel's test and Phalen's test	☐	☐	☐	☐
	●	☐	☐	☐	☐
Professionalism	● Thanks patient, washes hands	☐	☐	☐	☐
	●	☐	☐	☐	☐

			Self	Peer	Peer/tutor	Tutor
Self-assessed as at least borderline:	Signature:	Date:	U B S E	U B S E	U B S E	U B S E
Peer-assessed as ready for tutor assessment:	Signature:	Date:	U B S E	U B S E	U B S E	U B S E
Tutor-assessed as satisfactory:	Signature:	Date:	U B S E	U B S E	U B S E	U B S E

Notes

Unit 4   Specialized examination

4.1 Breast examination

Background

Breast cancer is the second most common cancer in women after lung. Detection of a lump understandably causes fear and apprehension. Meticulous examination of the breast can both increase the likelihood of correct diagnosis and help to allay some of the patient's fears.

Common presentations

The usual indications for breast examination are:

- A new breast lump
- Change in the appearance of the nipple or nipple discharge
- Changes in the breast contour or skin dimpling
- Pain in the breast.

Anatomical and physiological principles

The base of the female breast extends from the 2nd to the 6th rib vertically and from the sternum to the midaxillary line horizontally. Most of the breast rests on the pectoralis muscles. Breast tissue may extend into the axilla to form the axillary tail: it is important to remember this during examination. The majority of the lymphatic drainage of the breast is to the axillary nodes: involvement of these is an important prognostic feature in breast cancer.

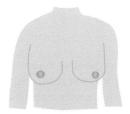

1: Inspection from front and side: Ensure adequate exposure, maintain comfort and dignity.

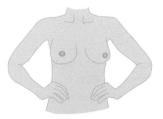

3: Ask the patient to push her hands into hips to contract pectoral muscles.

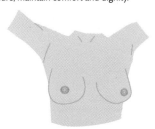

2: Ask the patient to lift her hands above her head and hold head from behind.

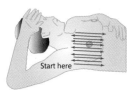

Start here

4: Palpation: With the patient lying down at 45 °, and arm resting on her forehead or hand behind the head. Palpate all four quadrants in a stepwise fashion using the pulps of three fingers, not the tips.

Figure 4.1 Inspection and palpation of the breasts.

The sequence for a breast examination

Examination sequence	Clinical context
Explanation and consent	Informed consent is especially important for intimate examinations and documentation in the notes is advisable. Obtain a chaperone if necessary. Wash hands before contact with the patient
Correct position and adequate exposure	The patient should be sitting on the edge of the examination couch and exposed to the waist
Inspection (see Figure 4.1)	Do not be in too much of a hurry to palpate the breast: much useful information can be gained from inspection
	Asymmetry, abnormal contour and skin dimpling may suggest the presence of cancer
Palpation (see Figure 4.1)	Reposition the patient at 45° with her hands behind her head
	The two methods of palpation commonly used are 'concentric circles' and the 'lawnmower'
	On each side palpate the breast, axillary tail, axilla and supraclavicular fossa. The axillary nodes are usually examined with the clinician supporting the arm to relax the muscles
	If a lump is detected note its position, size, shape, surface, consistency, mobility, tenderness, temperature, any skin changes, and its relations to overlying skin and underlying muscle
	Cancers are typically hard with an irregular shape and surface, and may be tethered or fixed to skin or muscle
Professionalism	Maintain patient dignity, communicate sensitively, thank the patient, wash hands, explain conclusions to the patient, document fully and accurately, communicate appropriately with colleagues

Upper outer quadrant | Upper inner quadrant
Central
lower outer quadrant | Lower inner quadrant

Patient safety tip

✔ Clinical examination of the breast will often yield a clear indication whether the problem is cancer or not. However, it is not totally reliable and overconfidence must be avoided. Many breast lumps will require further investigation with imaging and fine needle aspiration. When in doubt, refer. Most National Health Service (NHS) trusts have fast-track clinics for the urgent assessment of breast lumps.

✔ In larger breasted women, inspection should be carried out with the woman leaning forward. A pillow behind the shoulder blade will aid palpation by allowing the breast to spread over the chest wall.

Student name: Medical school: Year:

Breast examination

Please perform a breast examination on this manikin and talk to it as if it was a real patient.

		Self	Peer	Peer /tutor	Tutor
Explanation and consent	Explains procedure to patient, obtains verbal consent, considers need of chaperone	☐	☐	☐	☐
	Washes hands	☐	☐	☐	☐
		☐	☐	☐	☐
Correct position and adequate exposure	Positions patient appropriately	☐	☐	☐	☐
	Exposes neck, breasts, chest wall, and arms	☐	☐	☐	☐
		☐	☐	☐	☐
Inspection	Inspection from front and sides	☐	☐	☐	☐
	Assesses symmetry and comments on any skin or nipple changes	☐	☐	☐	☐
	Asks patient to slowly elevate hands above head and repeats inspection	☐	☐	☐	☐
	Asks patient to press hands against hips and repeats inspection	☐	☐	☐	☐
		☐	☐	☐	☐
Palpation	Lies patient back at 45° with hands behind head	☐	☐	☐	☐
	Starts palpation on asymptomatic side	☐	☐	☐	☐
	Systematically palpates whole breast including areola and nipple	☐	☐	☐	☐
	Palpates axillary tail	☐	☐	☐	☐
	Palpates axilla for lymphadenopathy	☐	☐	☐	☐
	Repeats palpation for symptomatic side	☐	☐	☐	☐
	Palpates supraclavicular fossae for lymphadenopathy	☐	☐	☐	☐
	Checks for nipple discharge	☐	☐	☐	☐
		☐	☐	☐	☐
Professionalism	Covers patient, thanks patient	☐	☐	☐	☐
	Washes hands	☐	☐	☐	☐
		☐	☐	☐	☐

				U B S E	U B S E	U B S E	U B S E
Self-assessed as at least borderline:	Signature:		Date:				
Peer-assessed as ready for tutor assessment:	Signature:		Date:	U B S E	U B S E	U B S E	U B S E
Tutor-assessed as satisfactory:	Signature:		Date:	U B S E	U B S E	U B S E	U B S E

Notes

4.2 **Thyroid examination**

Background

Thyroid disease is extremely common and many forms of it can be managed successfully in primary care. The diagnosis of hyper- or hypothyroidism is always confirmed on thyroid function tests before treatment is commenced. However, a high level of clinical suspicion is always necessary otherwise the diagnosis is easily missed. The purpose of the thyroid examination is twofold: first, to determine whether the patient is hyper-, hypo-, or euthyroid; and second, to establish whether the gland is enlarged and if so what the characteristics of that enlargement are.

Common presentations

Thyroid disease is notorious for its extremely wide range of presentations. The patient may complain of a lump in the neck or of a variety of symptoms which may erroneously be ascribed to disease of other systems. For example, the agitation of hyperthyroidism or the depression of hypothyroidism may be attributed to psychiatric illness, palpitations to cardiac disease, or altered bowel habit to gastrointestinal disorder.

Anatomical and physiological principles

The thyroid gland is located anteriorly in the neck at the level of the C5–T1 vertebrae: it consists of two lateral lobes joined across the thyroid cartilage and trachea by the isthmus. The gland lies within the pretracheal fascia, which blends superiorly into the larynx: this causes it to move upwards on swallowing. Thyroid hormone abnormalities are usually due to disease of the gland itself. However, hypothyroidism may occur as part of hypopituitarism, although hyperthyroidism due to pituitary disease is extremely rare.

The sequence for a thyroid examination

Examination sequence	Clinical context
Explanation and consent	Wash your hands before contact with the patient
Correct position and adequate exposure	The patient should be seated with the neck and upper thorax exposed
General inspection	The typical facial appearances of Graves' disease and hypothyroidism can suggest the diagnosis even before you touch the patient

General examination	In hyperthyroidism the hands are usually warm and sweaty, in hypothyroidism the skin is scaly and dry
	The pulse rate and rhythm are important signs: resting tachycardia suggests hyperthyroidism, bradycardia indicates hypothyroidism. Atrial fibrillation may be the first presentation of hyperthyroidism
	Lid retraction and lid lag are eye signs of hyperthyroidism. Exophthalmos occurs specifically in Graves' disease – in about 50% of patients – but the patient may be hyper-, hypo-, or euthyroid
Thyroid examination	If the thyroid is enlarged, palpation should establish whether it is smooth, multinodular, or a single nodule is present. A smooth toxic goitre suggests Graves' disease. Multinodular goitre is usually euthyroid but may be toxic. Around 10% of solitary thyroid nodules are malignant
	A bruit over the thyroid is characteristic of the hyperthyroid goitre of Graves' disease
	Suspected retrosternal extension of a goitre may be confirmed by Pemberton's sign: raising the arms above the head produces signs of venous compression
Additional examination	Slow-relaxing ankle reflexes are pathognomonic of hypothyroidism
Professionalism	Maintain patient dignity, communicate sensitively, thank the patient, wash hands, explain conclusions to the patient, document fully and accurately, communicate appropriately with colleagues

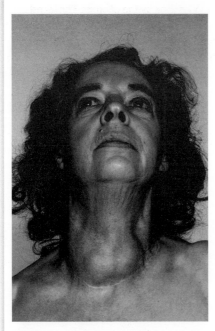

Goitre can be difficult to spot, note left lobe larger than right ? soft (lips), firm (tip of nose) or hard (frontal bone)

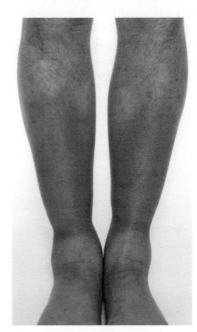

Pre-tibial myxoedema – rarely seen in hyperthyroidism

Patient safety tip

✔ Thyroid cancer is uncommon but can be very aggressive. The typical presentation is as a solitary thyroid nodule. Cancer is especially likely if a nodule is greater than 4 cm in diameter; 90% of solitary thyroid nodules are benign but all require investigation with ultrasound and fine needle aspiration with cytology.

Student name:	Medical school:	Year:

Examination and assessment of the thyroid gland

Please examine this patient's thyroid gland and clinically assess the thyroid status.

		Self	Peer	Peer /tutor	Tutor
Explanation and consent	● Washes hands with alcohol gel or soap and water	☐	☐	☐	☐
	● Explains procedure to patient and obtains verbal consent	☐	☐	☐	☐
	●	☐	☐	☐	☐
Correct position and adequate exposure	● Patient in appropriate seated position	☐	☐	☐	☐
	● Adequate exposure of neck and upper thorax and any jewellery removed	☐	☐	☐	☐
	●	☐	☐	☐	☐
General inspection	● Inspects patient for signs of hypo- or hyperthyroidism, commenting on any relevant findings	☐	☐	☐	☐
	●	☐	☐	☐	☐
General examination	● Examines hands for sweating, clubbing and onycholysis	☐	☐	☐	☐
	● Examines hands specifically for tremor	☐	☐	☐	☐
	● Feels pulse for rate and rhythm	☐	☐	☐	☐
	● Inspects eyes and tests specifically for lid lag	☐	☐	☐	☐
	●	☐	☐	☐	☐
Thyroid examination	● Inspects neck for swellings and scars	☐	☐	☐	☐
	● Palpates thyroid gland from behind	☐	☐	☐	☐
	● Tests for movement of mass on swallowing	☐	☐	☐	☐
	● Palpates cervical lymph nodes	☐	☐	☐	☐
	● Percusses over upper sternum for retrosternal goitre	☐	☐	☐	☐
	● Auscultates over thyroid for bruit	☐	☐	☐	☐
	●	☐	☐	☐	☐
Additional examination	● Inspects lower legs for pretibial myxoedema	☐	☐	☐	☐
	● Tests ankle reflexes	☐	☐	☐	☐
	●	☐	☐	☐	☐
Professionalism	● Covers patient, thanks patient, washes hands	☐	☐	☐	☐
	●	☐	☐	☐	☐

				U B S E	U B S E	U B S E	U B S E
Self-assessed as at least borderline:	Signature:	Date:					
Peer-assessed as ready for tutor assessment:	Signature:	Date:					
Tutor-assessed as satisfactory:	Signature:	Date:					

Notes

4.3 Digital rectal examination

Background

It is sometimes tempting to omit digital rectal examination to avoid embarrassment. However, prostate cancer is the commonest malignancy in men and colorectal cancer is the second commonest cause of cancer death in the UK. Failure to perform rectal examination when it is indicated risks missing vital diagnostic information with a disastrous effect on the outcome for the patient.

Common presentations

Digital rectal examination (DRE) is indicated in:

- Gastrointestinal examination, especially when there is altered bowel habit, anaemia, bleeding per rectum, tenesmus or pruritis ani.
- Investigation of urological symptoms for assessment of the prostate.
- Assessment of the colour and consistency of the faeces in altered bowel habit or gastro-intestinal bleeding.
- Assessment of anal sphincter tone in neurological disorders

Anatomical and physiological principles

The perianal region is first inspected and any abnormalities palpated: the positions around the anus are described by clock positions, 12 o'clock being towards the perineum and 6 o'clock towards the natal cleft. The rectum is approximately 12 cm long and connects the sigmoid colon (at the level of the third sacral vertebra, S3) to the anus. Despite the meaning of rectum (from the Latin meaning, 'straight'), the human rectum is actually a curved structure both anteroposteriorly and laterally. Within the rectum are three transverse mucosal folds, the lowest sometimes palpable on DRE (referred to as the 'valves of Houston'). Of note is the fact that the rectum is an important site of portosystemic anastomosis, between the superior rectal vein (portal) and the middle/inferior rectal veins (systemic), thus predisposing to haemorrhoids. The rectum has both sympathetic (contracts smooth muscle sphincters, relaxes bowel wall and transmits pain) and parasympathetic (relaxes smooth muscle sphincters, contracts bowel wall, transmits fullness/distension) innervation.

On rectal examination the rectal mucosa and in a male patient the prostate are assessed. Normal rectal mucosa is uniformly smooth and pliable to palpation. The posterior surface of the prostate can be assessed due to its close opposition to the anterior rectal wall. Palpable are the two lateral lobes separated by the median sulcus. The normal prostate is 3 cm across, protrudes 1 cm into the rectum and has a smooth, rubbery consistency.

The sequence for a DRE

Examination sequence	Clinical context
Explanation and consent	Informed consent is especially important for intimate examinations and documentation in the notes is advisable. Obtain a chaperone if necessary. Wash hands and apply gloves before contact with the patient
Correct position and adequate exposure	The patient should be in the left lateral position with knees drawn up to the chest and buttocks as close as possible to the edge of the bed, covered above the waist and below the upper thighs
Perianal examination	Inspection may reveal skin tags, warts, pilonidal sinuses, fissures, fistulae, external haemorrhoids, or prolapsed rectal mucosa. Perianal lesions in a patient with abdominal pain and persistent diarrhoea suggest Crohn's disease
DRE	Anal sphincter tone can be assessed as the finger is inserted. If necessary ask the patient to clench on your finger
	Benign or malignant tumours may manifest as polyps, nodules, masses, or areas of unusual hardness. Extreme tenderness suggests the presence of an abscess
	In benign prostatic hypertrophy the gland is usually symmetrically enlarged, smooth, and rubbery in consistency with a preserved median sulcus. In prostate cancer it may be asymmetrical, nodular or hard with loss of the sulcus
Professionalism	Maintain patient dignity, communicate sensitively, thank the patient, wash hands, explain conclusions to the patient, document fully and accurately, communicate appropriately with colleagues

Patient safety tip

✔ Ideally a chaperone should always be present when an intimate examination is performed: this helps to avoid misunderstandings and reassures the patient. In everyday practice this is considered absolutely necessary only when the doctor is male and the patient female. However, the need of a chaperone should be considered seriously in other circumstances as well.

Student name: Medical school: Year:

Digital rectal examination

Please perform a DRE on this manikin and talk to it as if it were a real patient.

		Self	Peer	Peer /tutor	Tutor
Explanation and consent	● Explains procedure to patient, obtains verbal consent, considers need of chaperone	☐	☐	☐	☐
	● Washes hands and applies gloves	☐	☐	☐	☐
	●	☐	☐	☐	☐
Correct position and adequate exposure	● Positions patient appropriately	☐	☐	☐	☐
	● Exposes perineum adequately while maintaining patient dignity	☐	☐	☐	☐
	●	☐	☐	☐	☐
Perianal examination	● Enquires about tenderness then gently separates buttocks	☐	☐	☐	☐
	● Inspects perianal region and palpates any abnormal areas	☐	☐	☐	☐
	●	☐	☐	☐	☐
Digital rectal examination	● Applies lubrication and warns patient of insertion of finger	☐	☐	☐	☐
	● Presses pulp of fingertip against anal verge at 6 o'clock position and gently introduces finger	☐	☐	☐	☐
	● Comments on anal tone	☐	☐	☐	☐
	● Examines posterior, left and right lateral and anterior walls of rectum covering full 360°	☐	☐	☐	☐
	● Assesses prostate	☐	☐	☐	☐
	● Withdraws finger and checks glove tip for stool and blood	☐	☐	☐	☐
	● Wipes excess lubricant or stool from anus with swab or paper towel	☐	☐	☐	☐
	●	☐	☐	☐	☐
Professionalism	● Covers patient, thanks patient, invites patient to get dressed	☐	☐	☐	☐
	● Disposes waste appropriately and washes hands	☐	☐	☐	☐
	●	☐	☐	☐	☐

			Self	Peer	Peer/tutor	Tutor
Self-assessed as at least borderline:	Signature:	Date:	U B S E	U B S E	U B S E	U B S E
Peer-assessed as ready for tutor assessment:	Signature:	Date:	U B S E	U B S E	U B S E	U B S E
Tutor-assessed as satisfactory:	Signature:	Date:	U B S E	U B S E	U B S E	U B S E

Notes

4.4 Scrotum and hernia examination

Background

Problems in the scrotum range from those of little significance, such as the epididymal cyst, to the life-threatening, such as testicular cancer. The latter is the commonest malignancy in males aged 15–44 years and when disease is detected early cure rates are high. Groin hernias are common and it is important to be able to distinguish clinically between the three main types, not least because of their different risks of strangulation.

Common presentations

The most common problem to present in this region is a **lump**, which may or may not be **painful**. A lump which is present intermittently, in particular on standing or coughing, is likely to be a hernia.

Anatomical and physiological principles

The inguinal canal, which permits passage of the spermatic cord, runs obliquely from the internal ring, situated above the midpoint of the inguinal ligament, to the external ring, above and medial to the pubic tubercle. An inguinal hernia is defined as a protrusion of visceral tissue through a weakness in the abdominal wall into the inguinal canal. An indirect inguinal hernia travels through the internal ring into the canal and may pass through the external ring into the scrotum. A direct inguinal hernia simply bulges forward at the site of the external ring.

The femoral canal lies beneath the inguinal ligament medial to the femoral vein, artery, and nerve. The femoral hernia travels through this into the upper thigh. Unlike inguinal hernias, femoral hernias do not reduce, feel like fatty lumps and usually have no cough impulse. Since femoral and indirect hernias pass through narrow openings – the femoral canal and the internal ring, respectively – they are likely to strangulate. However, direct inguinal hernias rarely do so.

Patient safety tip

✔ Physical examination is not an exact science and presentations are not always typical. Do not dismiss the possibility of serious or life-threatening disease unless you can exclude it with complete confidence. Assume that any acute painful swelling of the testis is torsion until proved otherwise, and any lump not clearly separate from the testis is cancer until proved otherwise.

The sequence for a scrotum and hernia examination

Examination sequence	Clinical context
Explanation and consent	Informed consent is especially important for intimate examinations and documentation in the notes is advisable. Obtain a chaperone if necessary. Wash hands before contact with the patient
Correct position and adequate exposure	The patient should be exposed from the waist down, but the lower legs can be covered if lying flat. For examination of a hernia it is often necessary for the patient to stand
Inspection	The most likely visible abnormality is a lump but others may be evident, for example the female pubic hair distribution and testicular atrophy of chronic liver disease
Palpation	Inguinal lymph nodes greater than 1 cm in diameter are probably pathological and need explanation
	If a lump is present in the scrotum, the three key features are whether one can get above it, whether it includes or is separate from the testis, and if it is cystic or solid. Transillumination may help confirm whether a lump is cystic
	If one cannot get above the lump, it is a hernia. If testicular and cystic it is probably a hydrocoele: if separate and cystic probably an epididymal cyst. If testicular and solid it may well be a tumour
	Identify the pubic tubercle on both sides. Check that there is no hernia on the other side. Then feel above the symptomatic side for a palpable impulse on coughing to confirm the diagnosis.
	If the testis is painful, swollen, and very tender to palpation, the differential diagnosis is orchitis or torsion. These can be difficult to distinguish clinically and the latter is a surgical emergency
Hernia examination	If the neck of the hernia is above and medial to the pubic tubercle it is an inguinal hernia, if below and lateral, a femoral hernia
	If reduction of the hernia can be maintained by pressure over the internal ring, it is an indirect inguinal hernia. A direct inguinal hernia will pop out again
	If it is difficult to decide about a hernia when the patient is examined supine, repeat the examination standing up
Additional examination	Examination of the abdomen and perineum, and a DRE may also be needed
Professionalism	Maintain patient dignity, communicate sensitively, thank the patient, wash hands, explain conclusions to the patient, document fully and accurately, communicate appropriately with colleagues

Student name:	Medical school:	Year:

Groin and scrotum examination

Please examine this patient's groins and scrotum, and demonstrate how you would proceed if you suspected the presence of a hernia.

		Self	Peer	Peer /tutor	Tutor
Explanation and consent	● Explains procedure to patient, obtains verbal consent, considers need of chaperone	☐	☐	☐	☐
	● Washes hands	☐	☐	☐	☐
	● Enquires about any tender or painful areas	☐	☐	☐	☐
	●	☐	☐	☐	☐
Correct position and adequate exposure	● Patient supine with one pillow	☐	☐	☐	☐
	● Patient exposed from waist to knees	☐	☐	☐	☐
	●	☐	☐	☐	☐
Inspection and palpation	● Inspects groin and scrotum	☐	☐	☐	☐
	● Palpates inguinal lymph nodes	☐	☐	☐	☐
	● Palpates each hemiscrotum, commencing on the normal side	☐	☐	☐	☐
	● Transilluminates hemiscrotum if necessary	☐	☐	☐	☐
	●	☐	☐	☐	☐
Hernia examination	● Inspects groins and asks patient to cough	☐	☐	☐	☐
	● Palpates for cough impulse, commencing on the normal side	☐	☐	☐	☐
	● Identifies the pubic tubercle and the relationship of the hernia neck to the tubercle	☐	☐	☐	☐
	● Reduces hernia and determines whether control is achieved by pressure over internal ring	☐	☐	☐	☐
	● If no hernia demonstrated, repeats examination with patient standing	☐	☐	☐	☐
	●	☐	☐	☐	☐
Additional examination	● Comments on need for examination of abdomen, perineum, and digital rectal examination	☐	☐	☐	☐
	●	☐	☐	☐	☐
Professionalism	● Covers patient, thanks patient	☐	☐	☐	☐
	● Washes hands	☐	☐	☐	☐
	●	☐	☐	☐	☐

		Self	Peer	Peer /tutor	Tutor
Self-assessed as at least borderline:	Signature:	Date:	U B S E	U B S E	U B S E	U B S E
Peer-assessed as ready for tutor assessment:	Signature:	Date:	U B S E	U B S E	U B S E	U B S E
Tutor-assessed as satisfactory:	Signature:	Date:	U B S E	U B S E	U B S E	U B S E

Notes

4.5 Pelvic examination

Background

Pelvic examination is an essential part of the gynaecological examination and is commonly performed in general practice, sexual health clinics (family planning/genitourinary medicine) and in obstetrics and gynaecology. It may also be relevant to general surgery and general medicine.

Pelvic examination is used to assess a woman's lower genitourinary (reproductive) tract. It involves an external and internal examination. Speculum examination allows the inspection of the vaginal walls and cervix, and enables the examiner to obtain vaginal, endocervical, and cervical swabs. Cusco's (bivalve) speculum is used for inspecting the cervix, and a Sim's speculum (two right angle bends) is used to hold back the posterior vaginal wall. Bimanual examination provides information on size, position, mobility and texture of a woman's reproductive organs including the vagina, cervix, uterus, fallopian tubes, and ovaries.

Many women find pelvic examination a painful, undignified, and embarrassing process. By having a good basic knowledge, following the suggested steps and showing professionalism, patient anxiety can be greatly reduced and important diagnostic information elicited.

Common indications

Assessment and diagnosis

- Vaginal discharge, pruritus, pelvic pain and dyspareunia, abnormal bleeding
- External genitalia, vagina, cervix, uterus and adnexae
- Colposcopy, hysteroscopy and cervical biopsy, endometrial biopsy
- Pregnancy and labour
- Uterine and vaginal prolapse
- Incontinence

Screening tests

- Sexually transmitted infections, vaginal swabs
- Cervical cytology

Treatment

- Removal of a foreign body, removal of polyps,
- Fitting of ring pessaries
- Fitting of contraception devices (IUCD)
- Endometrial ablation
- Evacuation of retained products of conception
- Manual removal of placenta.

General aspects of examination

Warming a metal speculum under a warm tap makes examination more comfortable.

It is not easy to select the appropriate size of speculum prior to the bimanual vaginal examination. This difficulty can be overcome by considering the patient's obstetric/gynaecological history, previous examination(s), use of tampons or coitus, and assessment of introitus (presence of hymen).

A general and abdominal examination should be considered part of the complete pelvic examination and undertaken as part of the assessment.

Always keep the discussion relevant and do not make unnecessary personal comments.

Reassure the patient at each stage of the examination if all is normal

GMC guidance on chaperones (*Maintaining Boundaries*)

- Wherever possible, you should offer the patient the security of having an impartial observer (a 'chaperone') present during an intimate examination. This applies whether or not you are the same gender as the patient.
- A chaperone does not have to be medically qualified but will ideally:
  - ○ Be sensitive, and respectful of the patient's dignity and confidentiality
  - ○ Be prepared to reassure the patient if they show signs of distress or discomfort
  - ○ Be familiar with the procedures involved in a routine intimate examination
  - ○ Be prepared to raise concerns about a doctor if misconduct occurs.

In some circumstances, a member of practice staff, or a relative or friend of the patient may be an acceptable chaperone. If either you or the patient does not wish the examination to proceed without a chaperone present, or if either of you is uncomfortable with the choice of chaperone, you may offer to delay the examination to a later date when a chaperone (or an alternative chaperone) will be available, if this is compatible with the patient's best interests.

You should record any discussion about chaperones and its outcome. If a chaperone is present, you should record that fact and make a note of their identity. If the patient does not want a chaperone, you should record that the offer was made and declined.

Anatomical principles

- **Vagina**: a fibromuscular tube 8–12 cm long, starting at the vaginal orifice and extending up and back, ending in fornices **anterior and posterior** to the cervix. It is lined with stratified squamous epithelium.
- **Cervix**: connects uterine cavity to vagina, and consists of three areas: external os, cervical canal, and internal os. Changes from squamous to columnar epithelium at the transition zone.
- **Uterus**: a thick-walled muscular organ in the midline between the bladder and rectum. Consists of the body and cervix. Superiorly fallopian tubes project laterally and open into peritoneal cavity immediately adjacent to ovaries.

Blood supply of the pelvis and perineum

- Internal iliac artery, originating from the common iliac artery.
- Divides into anterior (superior gluteal, lateral sacral, iliolumbar arteries) and posterior trunks (uterine artery, inferior gluteal artery, internal pudendal, vesical artery, rectal artery).
- Ovarian artery originates from the abdominal aorta.

Figure 4.2(a) shows the external female genitalia and Figure 4.2(b) shows the internal pelvic organs and blood supply.

The venous drainage in the pelvis follows the course of all branches of the internal iliac artery except for the umbilical artery and the ilio-lumbar artery. The venous drainage bilaterally is into the common iliac veins via the internal iliac veins. The ovarian veins drain to the inferior vena cava.

Lymphatic drainage from the pelvis

- Lymphatics from most pelvic viscera drain mainly into lymph nodes distributed along the internal iliac and external iliac arteries. From here drainage is via nodes associated with the common iliac arteries to the lateral aortic nodes to the origin of the thoracic duct.
- Lymphatics from the ovaries and fallopian tubes drain via vessels that accompany the ovarian arteries directly into lateral aortic nodes and pre-aortic nodes.

Anatomical relations

It is vital to consider the anatomical relations of the internal genitals as it is relevant to bimanual examination (palpating cervix, uterus, and adnexae), and other structures such as bladder,

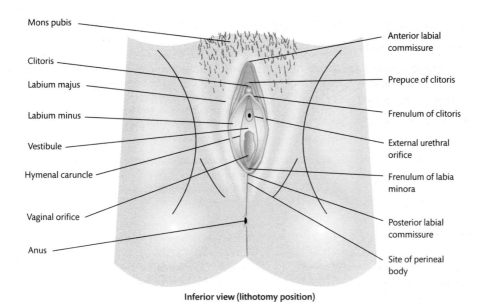

Inferior view (lithotomy position)

Posterior view

Figure 4.2 (a) The external female genitalia, and (b) the internal pelvic organs and blood supply.

rectum, and peritoneal reflections in terms of pain, fistula formation, and referred symptoms (see Table 4.1). The ovaries lie on the posterior aspect of the broad ligament and, together with the distal ends of the fallopian tubes, are normally located in the recto-uterine pouch.

Table 4.1 Anatomical relations of the internal genitals

	Anterior	**Posterior**	**Lateral**
Vagina	Base of bladder and urethra	Anal canal, rectum, recto-uterine pouch	Levator ani, pelvic fascia, ureters
Uterus and cervix	Vesico-uterine pouch, superior surface bladder	Recto-uterine pouch (pouch of Douglas)	Broad and cardinal ligaments, uterine vessels, ureters

The sequence for a pelvic examination

Examination sequence	Clinical context
Explanation and consent	Explain why an examination is necessary and give the patient an opportunity to ask questions. Informed consent is especially important for intimate examinations and documentation in the notes is advisable.
	Always explain to the patient what you are about to do before moving on to the next stage of the examination and be prepared to discontinue the examination if the patient asks you to
	Show the patient the speculum if she has not seen one before. Explain how you will use it
Correct position and adequate exposure	Before examining the patient it is essential to have a good light source and a suitable couch. The patient's bladder should be empty. They should remove their clothing from the waist down, they will feel less exposed if their knees and thighs are partially covered with a sheet. There are several positions which may be used to carry out a pelvic examination: (1) left lateral (2) full lithotomy, and used most commonly is (3) the dorsal position. In this position the patient's knees are bent and legs allowed to fall apart, with feet together. Wash hands, non-sterile gloves are sufficient
External vaginal examination	Announce what you are going to do.
	Inguinal region: palpate for any inguinal lymphadenopathy. Inspect the outer genitalia by examining each part of the genital tract in a logical sequence
	Pubic hair: assess distribution and any sign of infestations
	Vulva: inspect for swelling, inflammation, ulceration. Note the size/site/shape/consistency of any swelling
	Urethral orifice: inspect for inflammation and discharges (urethritis), caruncle
	Vaginal orifice (introitus) for discharge (and note origin/consistency/colour/if mal-odorous) and swellings such as Bartholin's cyst or an abscess. (See 'Swab taking during speculum examination') Ask the patient to cough or strain and any prolapse or stress incontinence is noted
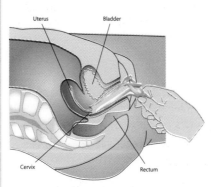 Speculum and digital examination	Separate the labia minora between thumb and index finger. Using a sterile, lubricated, closed, bivalve speculum, insert blades of speculum into vaginal orifice. Handle may be either up or down. Advance along posterior vaginal wall, at an approximate 45° angle, towards sacrum. Open the speculum a few centimetres and look for the cervix, it should drop down into view between the open blades. Secure the speculum open when the cervix and cervical os are exposed and visible. When examination complete close the speculum gradually, under direct vision, as you withdraw it, to avoid trapping the cervix

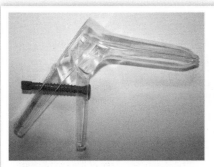

This is the common type of disposable speculum used in everyday practice, not the one shown in the figure above.

If sampling is appropriate then correct order is as follows:

Vaginal swabs (herpes [HVS], *Candida*, *Trichomonas vaginalis*)

pH and amine (bacterial vaginosis)

cervical cytology if required

cervical swabs – other (gonorrhoea/chlamydia)

Digital examination: can almost always be satisfactorily performed by using the index finger alone. This causes less discomfort and muscles spasms. If the vagina is long or voluminous a second finger may be indicated.

Introduce the gloved lubricated index finger of your dominant hand into the vagina and place your other hand on the patient's lower abdomen. Note: the condition of the vaginal walls

Palpate the cervix with your index finger noting size, shape, and consistency. Gently move the cervix side to side noting its mobility and any tenderness

Palpate the uterus by pushing the cervix backwards, this rotates the body of the uterus downwards and forwards. Note whether the uterus is anteverted or retroverted

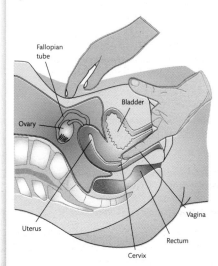

Bimanual palpation

Palpate the pelvic organs: done predominantly by the abdominal hand, which is placed at the umbilical level. Gradually move this hand down towards the suprapubic region and gently press downward and palpate the uterus (if possible) Note the size, consistency, shape, mobility, presence of masses, or tenderness on pressure

Fornices: the finger in the vagina is now moved into the right lateral fornix, the hand on the abdomen follows to explore for any enlargement or tenderness of the tubes or ovaries. Repeat this sequence in the left adnexa. Normal fallopian tubes are never palpable without significant pathology

Recto-vaginal examination may be necessary in some cases, e.g. prolapse, fistula, pelvic pain, or retroverted uterus

Professionalism

Throughout the examination communicate sensitively. Keep discussion relevant and do not make unnecessary personal comments. When finished wipe away any lubricant or discharge with cotton wool or gauze. Thank the patient and ensure tissues available for patient to wipe herself before getting dressed. Wash hands, explain conclusions to the patient, document fully and accurately

Patient safety tip

✔ Always tell the patient what you are about to do before you do it.

✔ Particularly in sexual health settings explain about confidentiality.

✔ It is usual and preferable, especially for male doctors, to have a chaperone present during examination. This helps to avoid misunderstandings and reassures the patient.

✔ Insert the speculum obliquely to avoid the clitoris and urethra.

✔ The speculum is not usually lubricated if cytology testing is undertaken to avoid contamination of the sample. It may be sufficient to use water alone.

✔ Ensure that swabs/smears are placed in the correct pathology department containers and despatched quickly.

Student name:	Medical school:	Year:

Pelvic examination

Please perform pelvic examination on this manikin and talk to it as if it were a real patient.

		Self	Peer	Peer /tutor	Tutor
Explanation and consent	● Explains procedure to patient and why it is considered necessary, obtains verbal consent, considers need of chaperone	☐	☐	☐	☐
	● Washes hands and applies gloves	☐	☐	☐	☐
	● Shows speculum to patient	☐	☐	☐	☐
	●	☐	☐	☐	☐
Correct position and adequate exposure	● Positions patient appropriately	☐	☐	☐	☐
	● Exposes external genitalia adequately while maintaining patient dignity	☐	☐	☐	☐
	●	☐	☐	☐	☐
External examination	● Palpates for inguinal lymphadenopathy	☐	☐	☐	☐
	● Thoroughly inspects the labia, urethral, and vaginal orifices	☐	☐	☐	☐
	● Asks the patient to cough to identify any prolapse	☐	☐	☐	☐
	●	☐	☐	☐	☐
Speculum examination	● Selects appropriate size and type of speculum, lubricates speculum	☐	☐	☐	☐
	● Inserts speculum at correct orientation and angle with minimal discomfort to patient	☐	☐	☐	☐
	● Identifies cervix and locks speculum	☐	☐	☐	☐
	● Assesses appearance of the vaginal walls and cervix. Obtains swabs if appropriate	☐	☐	☐	☐
	● Closes the speculum gradually, under direct vision ensuring that the cervix is not being trapped in it	☐	☐	☐	☐
	●	☐	☐	☐	☐
Bi-manual examination	● Uses lubricated gloved finger to assess condition of vaginal wall and cervix	☐	☐	☐	☐
	● Applies pressure to cervix and palpates for uterus with hand on patient's abdomen	☐	☐	☐	☐
	● Notes any cervical excitation. Determines size, consistency, shape, mobility, and presence of masses or any tenderness of uterus	☐	☐	☐	☐
	● Moves internal finger and abdominal hand in correspondence to check left and right adnexa	☐	☐	☐	☐
	● Comments whether uterus is anteverted or retroverted	☐	☐	☐	☐
	●	☐	☐	☐	☐
Professionalism	● Talks patient through the procedure explaining each step	☐	☐	☐	☐
	● Explains any important findings of examination to patient	☐	☐	☐	☐
	● Uses gauze to wipe away discharge or lubricant from external genitalia	☐	☐	☐	☐
	● Gives patient sufficient time to get dressed and sit comfortably before clinical discussion and end to consultation	☐	☐	☐	☐
	●	☐	☐	☐	☐

				U B S E	U B S E	U B S E	U B S E
Self-assessed as at least borderline:	Signature:		Date:				
Peer-assessed as ready for tutor assessment:	Signature:		Date:				
Tutor-assessed as satisfactory:	Signature:		Date:				

Notes

4.6 Eye examination

Background

Eye problems are common in the general population. Approximately 1.5% of all consultations in general practice will be about ophthalmological problems – this equates to about 50 consultations per 1000 population per year. About two million people in the UK have a sight problem. Many common and significant systemic diseases (e.g. hypertension, diabetes) affect the eye. Ophthalmological examination is necessary in a number of other medical and surgical specialties, including general medicine, paediatrics, accident and emergency, ENT, neurology, and neurosurgery.

Common indications

A general ophthalmological examination consisting of an assessment of the pupillary size and reflexes, presence of xanthelasma, corneal arcus and cataract should be undertaken in the majority of patients having a full medical examination. Specifically in relation to various systems and specialty examinations, a more detailed external eye examination and direct ophthalmoscopy is often indicated as in the examples below:

- **Diabetes**: cataract, diabetic retinopathy (see the grading chart in Table 4.2), corneal arcus (dyslipidaemia)

- **Endocrinology**: Graves' ophthalmopathy with exophthalmos/diplopia, cataract (Cushing's or long-term steroid use)

- **Cardiology**: hypertensive retinopathy (grade 1, arteriolar narrowing [copper or silver wiring]; grade 2, arteriovenous nipping; grade 3, haemorrhages or exudates; grade 4 papilloedema); endocarditis with Roth spots (retinal haemorrhagic infarcts), familial dyslipidaemias (corneal arcus, xanthelasma, lipaemia retinalis)

Table 4.2 Diabetic retinopathy (DR) grading chart

Level 0: No DR	
Level 1: Background DR	Microaneurysm(s) or retinal haemorrhage(s) ± any exudate not within the definition of maculopathy
Level 2: Pre-proliferative DR	Venous beading, venous loop, or reduplication intraretinal microvascular abnormality (IRMA) multiple deep, round or blot haemorrhages, cotton wool spots
Level 3: Proliferative DR (and advanced DR)	New vessels on disc
	New vessels elsewhere
	Pre-retinal or vitreous haemorrhage
	Pre-retinal fibrosis ± tractional retinal detachment
Maculopathy (M)	Exudate within 1 disc diameter (DD) of the centre of the fovea, circinate or group of exudates within the macula, retinal thickening within 1 DD of the centre of the fovea (if stereo imaging available), any microaneurysm or haemorrhage within 1 DD of the centre of the fovea only if associated with a best visual acuity of ≤6/12 (if no stereo)
Photocoagulation (P)	Evidence of focal/grid laser to macula or evidence of peripheral scatter laser
Unclassifiable (U)	Unobtainable/ungradable

Adapted from the National Screening Programme for Diabetic Retinopathy website.

- **Infection**: bacterial or viral conjunctivitis, human immunodeficiency virus (HIV) retinopathy, syphilis (vasculitis, uveitis, unequal pupils that accommodate but do not react normally to light – Argyll Robertson pupils)
- **Neurology**: transient loss of vision with retinal artery atheroma embolus (Hollenhorst plaque) in the amaurosis fugax type of transient ischaemic attack, homonymous hemianopia in some strokes, transient loss of vision in migraine, papilloedema due to raised intracranial pressure in any cause of space-occupying lesion, inflammation or reduced cerebrospinal fluid (CSF) drainage, optic atrophy due to multiple sclerosis or longstanding localized raised intracranial pressure, ptosis in myasthenia gravis, Horner's syndrome due to multiple causes including Pancoast's tumour in lung cancer. A preretinal haemorrhage is sometimes seen in subarachnoid haemorrhage
- **Rheumatology**: scleritis, iritis, uveitis, and dry eyes in many conditions such as rheumatoid arthritis, Sjögren's syndrome and other arthropathies.

For images of patients with eye conditions, see the eyes section of the clinical picture suite in the colour plate section.

Anatomical and physiological principles

- **Bony orbit and eyelids**: these enclose the eye. Apart from the eyeball itself, the orbit contains blood vessels, nerves (including CNII, III, IV, VI), extraocular muscles, and the lacrimal gland. There is also soft tissue, especially fat that cushions the eyeball.
- **Globe (eyeball)**: bounded in the most part by the sclera, apart from anteriorly, where the cornea takes its place. The conjunctiva covers the visible part of the sclera, and is continuous with the conjunctiva of the eyelids. The globe can be rotated in any direction by the six extraocular muscles.
- **Three globe compartments**: internally, the globe is divided into anterior and posterior chambers, and vitreous compartment. The anterior and posterior chambers are partially separated by the iris and lens. Aqueous humour is produced in the posterior chamber and circulates into the anterior chamber communicating through the pupil, where it drains at the angle of the iris and cornea (canal of Schlemm). The vitreous is a clear jelly-like substance that helps to maintain the shape of the eye – around 80% of the eyeball is separated from the anterior segment by the lens and zonule.
- **Lens**: this is a clear, flexible structure that is suspended from a ring of smooth muscle, the ciliary body. This contracts and relaxes to change the shape of the lens, focusing the light on the retina. The amount of light allowed into the eye is controlled by the iris, which dilates and contracts. The central opening of the iris is the pupil. The clarity and flexibility of the lens decreases with age.
- **Retina**: this lines the inside of the vitreous compartment. It is composed of light sensitive nerve-endings that carry information to the optic nerve. The most sensitive part of the retina is the macula – this provides our most central, acute vision. There are two main types of nerve cells: rods, which are sensitive to light (but cannot distinguish colour); and cones, which can differentiate colour (but require more light to function).
- **Optic disc**: this is the part of the optic nerve that is visible at the back of the eye on direct ophthalmoscopy. Radiating from the optic disc is a network of blood vessels. These lie on the surface of the retina covered by the internal limiting membrane, there is additional vasculature in the choroid layer, between the retina and sclera.
- **Retinal circulation**: this is clearly visible on direct ophthalmoscopy. At the optic disc the veins are dark red with no visible wall and the arteries are more orange and narrower. Arterioles and venules imperceptibly merge into each in the peripheral retina.
- **Extraocular muscles**: there are six in each eye (lateral and medial rectus, superior and inferior rectus, superior and inferior oblique) which allow conjugate movement in two planes only, up-down and medial-lateral.

Examination sequence	Clinical context
Explanation and consent	Informed consent is especially important for an examination that necessitates being in very close facial proximity to the patient in a darkened room. Arrange a chaperone if necessary. Wash hands before contact with the patient
Correct position and adequate exposure	The patient should be sitting comfortably, ideally with the patient's eye level should be 10–30 cm below yours in the examining position
General inspection	What clinical observations can be made on general inspection alone?
	Pay attention to spectacles – magnifying lens with long-sight (hypermetropia) and demagnifying lens with short-sight (myopia), thyrotoxic/hypothyroid features, hemiparesis, facial asymmetry, pupil size, xanthelasma, corneal arcus, foot ulcers (diabetes)
Assessment of vision	Assess each eye individually using a patch or card to cover the non-test eye. Spectacles or contact lenses should be used if worn. Use pinhole to attempt to correct for any refraction problem
	Visual acuity (**VA**): Use Snellen's chart to record the patient's best vision, express as 6/6, 6/12, 6/36, etc. depending on the smallest print line that can be read at least 50%. For example: right 6/9; left 6/9 means that the patient has a VA at 6 m that a person without a VA problem would have at 9 m. VA can be assessed grossly by asking the patient to read some 12 font print at normal reading distance
	Visual fields by confrontational field testing
External examination	**Lids** (symmetry, inflammation, skin changes, swellings), **conjunctiva** (injection, chemosis, discharge, pallor)
	Cornea (abrasion, ulceration – use 1% fluorescein if available), **anterior chamber** (cloudy, hypopyon, hyphaema)
Assessment of ocular function	**Ocular position**: from in front, above, and the sides. Look for proptosis, exophthalmos, and enophthalmos.
	Ocular movement: lid lag, ocular palsy, nystagmus. Ask about diplopia, test for diplopia (check both eyes have adequate vision!)
	Ocular alignment: assess symmetry of corneal reflection. Use the cover test to look for manifest and latent squints
	Pupils: Look for inequality of size and shape. Assess direct and consensual reflexes, and accommodation-convergence reflex. Look for relative afferent pupillary defect.

Examination sequence	Clinical context
Direct ophthalmoscopy	Use short-acting mydriatic if detailed examination necessary (e.g. 0.5% or 1% tropicamide drops)
	Dim the lights. Ask patient to remove spectacles (contact lenses can be left in situ) and look straight ahead. Examine the right eye with your right eye and vice versa
	Hold ophthalmoscope onto your medial orbital ridge – 'integrate' ophthalmoscope into your visual axis and focus to read fine print. Start about 1 m away and about 30° lateral to the vertical plane. Look for **red reflex** (note any opacities particularly cataracts)
	Move in very close to the patient (only 1–3 cm apart) until the retina comes into focus. Ophthalmoscope lens may need adjustment for myopia (– lenses will correct), or hypermetropia (+ lenses will correct)
	Examine the optic disc for colour, margins, cup/disc ratio (papilloedema, disc cupping)
	Systematically examine the four quadrants of the **retina** (examine initially with the patient in the neutral position and then consider asking patient to look up, down, lateral, medial) and **macula** (after initial look, turn down light a little if possible and ask patient to 'look at the light'). Look for haemorrhages, exudates, cotton wool spots, pigmentation changes, scarring, drusen, etc. Examine **vessels** (emboli, proliferative retinopathy, IRMA, silver/copper wiring, arteriovenous nipping)
	Finally examine the peripheral retina clockwise starting at the 12 o'clock position looking for peripheral lesions, especially retinitis pigmentosa or previous laser treatment
Additional examination	Consider intraocular pressure testing especially in atypical headache or any red eye
	Consider formal assessment of visual acuity (Snellen's chart), visual fields (perimetry) and colour vision (Ishihara charts)
Professionalism	Maintain dignity of patient, communicate sensitively with patient, thank the patient, wash hands, write appropriate record of findings, communicate appropriately with colleagues

Patient safety tips

✔ Think acute glaucoma with any atypical headache or red eye – late diagnosis can result in permanent visual loss. Similarly be aware of not missing temporal arteritis in patients with headache or scalp tenderness.

✔ The green light setting on the ophthalmoscope is particularly useful for retinal examination, blood will look black so papilloedema and any haemorrhages are easier to spot.

Student name:	Medical school:	Year:

Eye examination

Please examine this patient's eyes. Please include direct ophthalmoscopy. Consider using manikin if available.

Category	Item	Self	Peer	Peer/tutor	Tutor
Explanation and consent	Washes hands with alcohol gel or soap and water	☐	☐	☐	☐
	Explains procedure to patient and obtains verbal consent	☐	☐	☐	☐
		☐	☐	☐	☐
Correct position	Comfortably seated, patient's eye level appropriate	☐	☐	☐	☐
		☐	☐	☐	☐
General inspection	Inspects patient commenting on any relevant findings: checks for thyroid disorders, facial asymmetry, pupil size, xanthelasma, corneal arcus	☐	☐	☐	☐
	? Spectacles – magnifying lens with long sight or demagnifying lens with short sight	☐	☐	☐	☐
		☐	☐	☐	☐
Assessment of vision	Uses Snellen's chart and records patient's best vision	☐	☐	☐	☐
	Expresses vision as: right 6/x, left 6/y; explains meaning	☐	☐	☐	☐
	States how to do gross testing of VA	☐	☐	☐	☐
	Assesses each eye individually using a patch or card to cover the non-test eye	☐	☐	☐	☐
	Uses pinhole to attempt to correct for any refraction problem	☐	☐	☐	☐
	Visual fields by confrontational field testing	☐	☐	☐	☐
		☐	☐	☐	☐
External examination	Inspects lids, conjunctiva, cornea, and anterior chamber, and names one clinical condition for each site	☐	☐	☐	☐
		☐	☐	☐	☐
Assessment of ocular function	Checks ocular position: looks for proptosis, exophthalmos, and enophthalmos	☐	☐	☐	☐
	Checks ocular movement: lid lag, ocular palsy, nystagmus, diplopia	☐	☐	☐	☐
	Checks ocular alignment: assesses symmetry of corneal reflection. Uses the cover test for squints	☐	☐	☐	☐
	Examines pupils: ? inequality in size and shape. Assesses direct and consensual reflexes, and accommodation-convergence reflex. Looks for relative afferent pupillary defect	☐	☐	☐	☐
		☐	☐	☐	☐
Direct ophthalmoscopy	Considers using short-acting mydriatic if detailed examination necessary (e.g. tropicamide drops)	☐	☐	☐	☐
	Asks patient to remove spectacles (contact lenses can be left *in situ*) and look straight ahead. Examine the right eye with your right eye and vice versa	☐	☐	☐	☐
	Looks for red reflex and states why (? cataracts)	☐	☐	☐	☐
	Adjusts ophthalmoscope lens if necessary and corrects position relative to patient	☐	☐	☐	☐
	Examines the optic disc for colour, margins, cup/disc ratio (papilloedema, disc cupping)	☐	☐	☐	☐
	Systematically examines four quadrants of retina, periphery, and specifically the macula	☐	☐	☐	☐
	States looking for: haemorrhages, exudates, cotton wool spots, pigmentation changes, scarring, drusen	☐	☐	☐	☐
	Examines vessels for: emboli, proliferative retinopathy, IRMA, silver/copper wiring, arteriovenous nipping	☐	☐	☐	☐
		☐	☐	☐	☐
Additional examination	Considers intraocular pressure testing ? headache or red eye	☐	☐	☐	☐
	Considers formal assessment of visual acuity (Snellen's chart), visual fields (perimetry) and colour vision (Ishihara's charts)	☐	☐	☐	☐
		☐	☐	☐	☐
Professionalism	Thanks the patient, writes appropriate record of findings. Communicates appropriately with colleagues	☐	☐	☐	☐
		☐	☐	☐	☐
Clinical images	Recognizes and discusses each of the clinical pictures briefly	☐	☐	☐	☐
		☐	☐	☐	☐

	Signature:	Date:	U B S E	U B S E	U B S E	U B S E
Self-assessed as at least borderline:						
Peer-assessed as ready for tutor assessment:	Signature:	Date:	U B S E	U B S E	U B S E	U B S E
Tutor-assessed as satisfactory:	Signature:	Date:	U B S E	U B S E	U B S E	U B S E

Notes

4.7 Ear examination

Background

ENT pathologies account for 10–20% of consultations in general practice, and this figure rises to about 50% in GP consultations involving children. ENT referrals currently constitute the third largest group of patients referred to hospital specialist clinics. ENT examination also plays a part in general paediatrics, plastic surgery, neurology and neurosurgery, dermatology, and general medicine. Hence, a good working knowledge of ENT and a basic competence in examination of the head and neck is essential for many doctors.

Anatomy and physiology

- **Three divisions**: external ear (pinna and ear canal), middle ear (malleus, incus, stapes) and inner ear (cochlea, vestibule, and semicircular canals).
- **External auditory meatus** (ear canal) is an elongated S-shaped tubular structure lined by skin and ending blindly at the tympanic membrane (ear drum). The outer third has a cartilaginous skeleton continuous with that of the pinna, a thick dermis, and contains hair follicles, ceruminous glands (modified apocrine sweat glands), and sebaceous glands, which together produce cerumen (wax). The skin of the inner two-thirds is thin, lines the bony external meatus of the temporal bone, and bears no hair follicles or accessory glands.
- **The squamous epithelium of the ear canal** exhibits the phenomenon of migration of its maturing cells towards the outer end of the canal. This means that the inner two-thirds of the canal is normally free of contained keratin and other material. Wax is produced only in the outer canal and is therefore not to be found in the inner two-thirds of the canal unless it has been displaced there by the patient's attempts to clean the canal.
- **The thin skin of the inner two-thirds of the meatus** is exquisitely sensitive to touch, while the thicker skin of the outer canal is very much less so. This is important with regard to the manipulation of instruments in the canal.
- **The sensory innervation** of the ear involves C2, the mandibular division of the trigeminal nerve, and glossopharyngeal and vagus nerves. Pain may therefore be referred to the ear from any other area innervated with sensory fibres by these nerves, and these areas must be assessed fully in any patient complaining of otalgia in whom otological examination is normal.
- **Facial nerve** passes through the temporal bone on its way from the posterior cranial fossa to the stylomastoid foramen, beyond which it enters the parotid gland. In the internal acoustic meatus it accompanies the vestibulocochlear nerve and supplies the stapedius, to prevent hyperacusis to loud noise. Three branches of the facial nerve are given off within the temporal bone and may be affected by disease of the ear or temporal bone.
- **Sound** is conducted through the external auditory meatus, tympanic membrane, and ossicular chain into the oval window and thence into the cochlea, where sound energy is transformed into nerve impulses which are transmitted to the brain along the vestibulo-cochlear nerve. Conduction of sound through the tympanic membrane and ossicular chain is optimal only if the middle ear contains air at atmospheric pressure.
- **Conductive and sensorineural deafness**: hearing loss involving a defect of transmission of sound from the exterior to the oval window is defined as conductive while one involving pathology of the cochlea or its central connections is defined as sensorineural hearing loss.
- **Balance**: the organ of balance is the vestibular apparatus (semicircular ducts, saccule and utricle). It senses rotational and linear acceleration and also transmits information to the brain via the vestibulocochlear nerve.

- Features of the tympanic membrane seen on otoscopy include the pars tensa, pars flaccida, umbo, light reflex, malleus (handle and lateral process), and sometimes the chorda tympani, long process of the incus, and stapedius tendon.

For images of infected ears, see the ears section of the clinical picture suite in the colour plate section.

The sequence for an ear examination

Examination of the ears	Sequence
Introduction, explanation, consent, position	Wash hands, introduce yourself, explain what you would like to do and gain verbal consent, seat patient comfortably on a chair (small children on parent's lap), ask which is the better hearing ear and start with this side. Ask if there is any tenderness
General inspection and examination	Look for hearing aids, dysmorphic features, and non-otological evidence of lesions of cranial nerves, e.g. facial palsy, nystagmus, dysarthria, dysphonia
Examination of pinna and mastoid	Inspect using a torch or preferably a headlight, which frees both hands for other instrumentation Compare the pinnae for symmetry of position and shape Examine the pinna and surrounding area for scars, skin lesions, accessory auricles, sinuses, discharge, inflammation, and swellings
Auroscopy	**Basic tips**: use largest speculum that fits comfortably in the outer meatus. Hold otoscope in the same hand as the ear being examined, with its handle pointing upwards and forwards away from the ear. Hold handle between the thumb and index with little finger braced against the patient's face to minimize uncontrolled movement of the speculum within the external meatus **Straighten meatus for best view**: use free hand to pull the pinna superiorly, laterally and posteriorly in adults or inferiorly and posteriorly in young children **Speculum**: insert into meatus under direct vision to avoid missing any lesions in wall of outer meatus. End of speculum should not be positioned beyond the hair bearing meatus as contact with the very sensitive wall of the deep meatus may produce a reflex response from the patient which could damage meatal skin or the tympanic membrane **Ear canal**: full length of canal and ear drum should be examined systematically. Failure to achieve this may result from atresia or narrowing of part or the whole of the meatus or from occlusion of the lumen by wax, foreign body, discharge, space-occupying lesion of the meatal wall, or an inflammatory polyp or other lesion arising in the middle ear. The shape of the bony wall of the deep meatus may make it impossible to view the anterior part of ear drum and the anterior recess of the deep meatus **Meatal occlusion**: nature of the occlusion should be recorded and, in the case of any discharge, its nature, amount, colour, and consistency noted. If wax, foreign body, or discharge prevents a full examination of the meatus and drum, consider clearing it using a wax hook or loop, mopping with small wisps of cotton wool attached to a wool carrier, microsuction, or syringing. Consider the ability of the patient to be cooperative and your experience and expertise. In any case of doubt an ENT specialist should be consulted.

Examination of the ears	Sequence
	Colour and vascularity of meatal wall: normal variation is considerable, meatal instrumentation, syringing and the crying of a child may result in a marked hyperaemia which may be misinterpreted as inflammation
	Ear drum: orientation is by identification of the handle and lateral process of the malleus. Note: abnormalities of colour and translucency, thinning, bulging, discharge, granulations, crusting, and perforations. During Valsalva's manoeuvre, the identification of a meatal hissing sound may help confirm the presence of a small drum perforation or indicate a perforation not previously identified
	Light reflex: this is dependent on the reflectivity of the ear drum, the contour and angulation of the surface of the ear drum relative to the long axis of the meatus and incident angle of the light source. Although the reflex is usually conical and directed anteroinferior to the umbo it may appear in other areas of a normal ear drum, or even be absent. Its clinical usefulness is therefore minimal

Hearing tests

The gold standard test of hearing is provided by pure tone audiometry. It can, however, be backed up by other clinical techniques using tuning forks and voice tests of hearing which, although inherently less accurate, are still to a degree quantitative and can usefully be included in the standard clinical assessment of patients with otological problems.

A pure tone audiogram is a graphical representation of the thresholds of hearing in decibels of hearing level below a standard of 0 dB at frequencies between 125 Hz and 8000 Hz. In Figure 4.3 the responses in the right ear are represented by the O–O graph and those in the left ear by △–△ graph. The colour coding and the annotation on the right of the chart indicate the degrees of deafness represented by hearing thresholds at various levels below the 0 dB line.

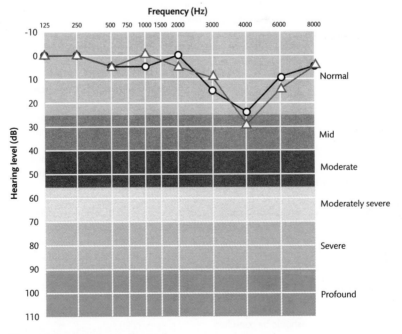

Figure 4.3 A pure tone audiogram.

Tuning fork tests

These are performed using a tuning fork of 512 cycles/second and are really reliable only if the meati are clean and a single pathology is present, i.e. a conductive or sensorineural deficit in one ear.

- **Weber test**: The tuning fork is struck and placed firmly over the bony midline vertex or forehead. The patient is asked to say whether the sound is heard centrally in the head or better in one ear. (See Figure 4.4.)

- **Rinne test**: The tuning fork is struck and placed close to one ear with the axis of vibration of the prongs in line with the axis of the meatus (air conduction). If the patient hears the sound he or she is asked to indicate when it is no longer audible and the fork is then placed firmly on the mastoid process (bone conduction). The patient is asked whether or not the sound is again audible. (See Figure 4.5.)

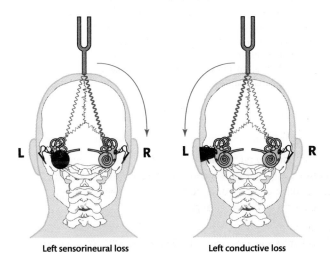

Left sensorineural loss   Left conductive loss   **Figure 4.4** Weber test.

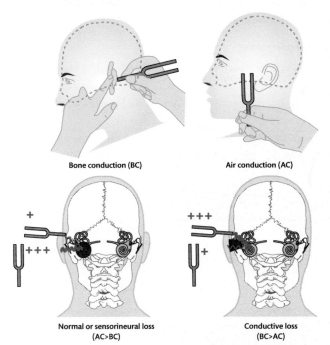

Bone conduction (BC)   Air conduction (AC)

Normal or sensorineural loss   Conductive loss
(AC>BC)   (BC>AC)   **Figure 4.5** Rinne test.

Logic table for interpreting findings of Weber's and Rinne's tests

Clinical findings		
Weber: normal central response	Both ears normal or →	Symmetrical sensorineural loss: R and L
Sound referred to R	Sensorineural loss L or →	Conductive loss R
Sound referred to L	Sensorineural loss R or →	Conductive loss L
Rinne: air conduction better (positive Rinne) (L or R ear individually)	Normal L ear or →	Sensorineural loss L
	Normal R ear or →	Sensorineural loss R
Bone conduction better (negative Rinne) (L or R ear individually)	Conductive loss L or →	Conductive loss R

Interpretation

Normal   **R Sensorineural**   **L Sensorineural**   **R Conductive**   **L Conductive**

Conduct both tests and tick all that are possible

Only one possibility will emerge with the proviso that the tests only apply if a single pathology is present. NB In severe sensorineural loss, there may be a false negative Rinne test. This is because there is a conductive or sensorineural loss or deafness in one ear only

An abbreviated form of the Rinne test involves placing the tuning fork first near the meatus and then on the mastoid process and asking the patient in which position the sound is heard the louder. The interpretation is as above.

Voice test of hearing

This test is reliable only if the meati are clean. If well performed it gives a useful semiquantitative assessment of the range of hearing loss present in each ear.

Free field voice test for assessment of hearing

- Instruct the patient on the procedure, testing each ear in turn. Follow steps 1 to 4 (see Table 4.3) if needed.
- Use tragal masking (rubbing the tragus firmly against the outer meatus) to eliminate the non-test ear from the assessment.
- **Whisper** multi-syllable numbers in the test ear at arm's length distance (approximately 60 cm). Ensure patient is unable to lip read the examiner (stand behind the patient).

Table 4.3 Free field voice test – simple adaptation for non-specialist examination

Technique and clinical findings	Interpretation
1 **Whisper**: at arm's length. Patient repeats the numbers correctly. If not OK →	Normal hearing (better than 30 dB). The second ear is then tested
2 **Whisper**: Mouth positioned close to the test ear. If not OK →	Hearing is between 30 and 50 dB and the second ear is tested
3 **Normal spoken voice**: Mouth positioned close to the test ear. If not OK →	Hearing loss is between 50 and 90 dB and the second ear is tested
4 **If still cannot hear, use 90 dB, loud voice, mouth positioned close to ear**:	Hearing loss is greater than 90 dB. The second ear is then tested

Patient safety tip

✔ Good hearing is profoundly important to quality of life (and general patient safety in the home) and therefore tests of hearing should be undertaken far more often than is the current norm in clinical practice. Even removal of wax will markedly improve hearing.

✔ Pure tone audiometry will be needed to complete a full assessment, and hearing aids if indicated

✔ Conduct a full ENT examination if the complaint is of otalgia and otological examination is normal. Conduct nasal and oral examination if a middle ear effusion is suspected.

✔ Change in voice should be investigated if persisting for longer than a few weeks: common causes include laryngeal malignancy, damage to recurrent laryngeal nerve or hypothyroidism.

✔ Conduct a full cranial nerve examination if a sensorineural deafness of uncertain cause is identified.

Student name:	Medical school:	Year:

Ear examination

Please examine this patient's ears.

		Self	Peer	Peer /tutor	Tutor
Washes hands	• Washes hands with alcohol gel or soap and water	☐	☐	☐	☐
	•	☐	☐	☐	☐
Introduction and explanation	• Introduces herself/himself	☐	☐	☐	☐
	• Explains what they would like to do	☐	☐	☐	☐
	•	☐	☐	☐	☐
Asks permission	• Obtains verbal consent from the patient	☐	☐	☐	☐
	•	☐	☐	☐	☐
Appropriate position	• Seats patient comfortably on a chair	☐	☐	☐	☐
	• Asks which is the better hearing ear and starts with this side	☐	☐	☐	☐
	• Asks if there is any tenderness before touching patient	☐	☐	☐	☐
	•	☐	☐	☐	☐
General inspection and examination	• Looks for hearing aids, facial palsy, dysmorphic features	☐	☐	☐	☐
	•	☐	☐	☐	☐
Examination of pinna and mastoid	• Uses pen torch or head light	☐	☐	☐	☐
	• Looks in front and behind pinna	☐	☐	☐	☐
	• Inspects mastoid process	☐	☐	☐	☐
	• Palpates for tenderness over mastoid, pinna, and tragus	☐	☐	☐	☐
	•	☐	☐	☐	☐
Otoscopy	• Holds otoscope in same hand as the ear, which is examined	☐	☐	☐	☐
	• Holds the handle of otoscope between thumb and index finger with little finger braced against side of patient's face	☐	☐	☐	☐
	• Pulls the pinna superiorly, laterally, and posteriorly (adults) with the other hand	☐	☐	☐	☐
	• Pulls the pinna inferiorly and posteriorly (children) with the other hand	☐	☐	☐	☐
	• Inspects ear canal and comments on appearance and need for cleaning. Indicates limitations of further assessment if meatus is not cleared	☐	☐	☐	☐
	• Systematically examines tympanic membrane (pars tensa and flaccida) and comments on findings	☐	☐	☐	☐
	•	☐	☐	☐	☐
Clinical hearing Tests	• Performs free field voice test	☐	☐	☐	☐
	• Performs Rinne's test and interprets correctly	☐	☐	☐	☐
	• Performs Weber's test and interprets correctly	☐	☐	☐	☐
	•	☐	☐	☐	☐
Essential extras	• Conducts cranial nerve examination (particulary CNVII)	☐	☐	☐	☐
	• Considers formal audiological testing	☐	☐	☐	☐
	•	☐	☐	☐	☐
Ending the examination	• Thanks patient	☐	☐	☐	☐
	• Washes hands	☐	☐	☐	☐
	• Presents findings appropriately	☐	☐	☐	☐
	•	☐	☐	☐	☐
Professionalism	• Maintains dignity of patient	☐	☐	☐	☐
	• Communicates sensitively with patient	☐	☐	☐	☐
	•	☐	☐	☐	☐
Clinical images	• Recognizes and discusses each of the ear examination clinical pictures briefly	☐	☐	☐	☐
	•	☐	☐	☐	☐

				Self	Peer	Peer /tutor	Tutor
Self-assessed as at least borderline:	Signature:	Date:		U B S E	U B S E	U B S E	U B S E
Peer-assessed as ready for tutor assessment:	Signature:	Date:		U B S E	U B S E	U B S E	U B S E
Tutor-assessed as satisfactory:	Signature:	Date:		U B S E	U B S E	U B S E	U B S E

Notes

Unit 5   Specialities history and examination

5.1 Paediatrics

Background

Paediatrics is a dynamic speciality. Children and young people are constantly changing and developing as they grow from birth through infancy into childhood and adolescence. The approach and the examination required will vary according to the age of the child. In this section we have tried to cover the type of examination you might be expected to know about in a clinical assessment and we have also included elements of acute paediatrics which may be more useful in a clinical setting.

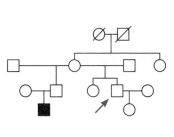

Many clinical conditions in paediatrics will require a detailed family history: Patient indicated with an arrow: □ is male, O is female, shaded is affected by the condition, a line through at 45° indicates death.

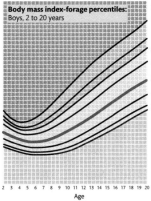

Growth charts will be different for boys and girls. There are also some ethnicity specific charts.

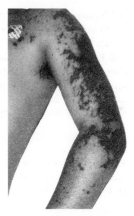

Always look out for red flag examination signs such as this purpuric rash. Others include silent chest, inactive child, confusion, pale, mottled skin.

Figure 5.1 Paediatric history and examination

Box 5.1 Basic observations

Age	Heart rate (beats per min)	Respiratory rate (breaths per min)	Systolic blood pressure (mmHg)
<1 year	120–160	30–60	60–95
1–3	90–140	24–40	95–105
3–5	75–110	18–30	95–110
8–12	75–100	18–30	90–110
12–16	60–90	12–16	112–130

History taking

Presenting Complaint

- Allow the parents or child to explain their concerns in their own words
- Establish accurate timing of symptoms. (Many illnesses such as bronchiolitis follow a pattern)
- Identify exacerbating and relieving factors
- Discuss impairment of function, what can't they do that they used to be able to do?
- Is the child thriving or has there been any weight loss?
- Identify any alterations in diet, fluid intake, sleep pattern, micturition and bowel habits.
- Has there been exposure to anyone else who is unwell or any foreign travel?

Past Medical History

- Personal Child Health Record (Red Book)
- Issued to every child at birth, records immunizations, health visits and growth
- Birth - gestation, mode, admission to neonatal unit (relevant in babies and children but may not be relevant in adolescents)
- Immunizations
- Frequency of exacerbations (e.g. Asthma)
- Previous treatments
- Hospital or PICU admissions

Development

- There are 4 main areas - gross motor, fine motor, language and social development
- Document key milestones
- When did he first...
  - Smile, fix and follow (6 weeks)
  - Sit unaided, grasp objects, babble (6 months)
  - 1st steps, 1st words (12 months)
  - Runs, kicks, 2 word sentences (2 yrs)

Growth and nutrition

- Always ask to see the Red Book
- Are they gaining/losing weight?
- If concerns regarding stature calculate mid parent height. (mother's height + father's height/2, + 7cm for boys, - 7cm for girls)
- Diet. (In babies - type of milk, quantity and frequency)

Drug History

- Current medications
- Do they know how to use them? Ask for parents or child to demonstrate use of medicines such as inhalers.
- Allergies (include food allergies)
- Degree of allergic response e.g. Rash, swelling, anaphylaxis

Family History

- Many hereditary conditions present in childhood
- Take a detailed family history particularly of childhood illnesses
- Draw a family tree
- Are parents consanguineous?

Social History

- Who is the main carer?
- Does the child go to nursery or school
- Who lives in the child's home? (including relatives, friends, partners)
- Are parents separated or together?
- Has the family ever had any involvement with family (social) services?

Child Protection Red Flags

- Delay in presentation
- Injury inconsistent with history
- Varying history
- Fractures in non-ambulant infants
- Frequent attendances to A + E particularly if at different hospitals

Physical examination

General inspection

- Observe child at play prior to formal examination.
- Measure weight and height.
- Plot on appropriate centile chart.
- Note any dysmorphic features.
- Observe the child's appearance, including any signs of neglect or injury
- Rashes - blanching, non-blanching, distribution, macular/papular, etc.

Respiratory examination

Inspection:

- Effort of breathing:
  - ○ Respiratory rate
  - ○ Use of accessory muscles
  - ○ Grunting
  - ○ Stridor
  - ○ Recession.
- Efficacy of breathing:
  - ○ Chest expansion
  - ○ Breath sounds
  - ○ Oxygen saturations.
- Effect of breathing
  - ○ Heart rate
  - ○ Cyanosis
  - ○ Conscious level.
- Chest shape.

Palpation:

- Palpate for lymphadenopathy
  - ○ Posterior and anterior cervical areas, axilla, and groin.

Percussion:

- Dull – collapse/consolidation
- Stony dull – pleural effusion
- Hyperresonant – pneumothorax.

Auscultation:

- Compare both sides.
- Vesicular breath sounds – 'rustling' sound heard in normal airways, that increases during inspiration and decreases in expiration.
- Bronchial breath sounds – harsh sounding, expiratory and inspiratory phase are of equal length with a pause in the middle. Indicates areas of consolidation or fibrosis.
- Wheeze (rhonchi) – high or low pitch musical sounds that indicate a narrowing of the bronchi.
- Crackles (crepitations) – due to secretions or the reopening of small airways with each breath. Crackles due to secretions may alter following coughing. Widespread fine crackles are common in bronchiolitis. Localized coarse crackles are indicative of local changes such as pneumonia.
- Absent breath sounds may occur in severe asthma.

Ears and throat

Inspect the back of the throat, tonsils, and tympanic membranes. This is best left to the end of an examination as it is not well tolerated.

Box 5.2 Acute asthma in children aged over 2 years (*British Guideline on the Management of Asthma, British Thoracic Society, 2009*)

....

Acute severe:
● Peak expiratory flow 33–50%
● Oxygen saturations <92%
● Can't complete sentences in one breath or too breathless to talk or feed
● Pulse >125 (>5 years), >140 (2–5 years)
● Respiration >30 breaths/min (>5 years), >40 per min (2–5 years).

Life-threatening asthma:
● Oxygen saturations <92%
● Peak expiratory flow <33% best or predicted
● Hypotension
● Exhaustion
● Confusion
● Coma
● Silent chest
● Cyanosis
● Poor respiratory effort.

Cardiovascular examination

Inspection:

● Cyanosis:
  ○ Indicates impaired pulmonary flow and right to left shunting, e.g. pulmonary stenosis with ventricular septal defect
● Respiratory distress:
  ○ May be present in heart failure
● Surgical scars.

Palpation:

● Pulse:
  ○ Rate, character, and volume
  ○ Radial and brachial are most commonly used
  ○ Femoral pulses may be absent in aortic coarctation
● Apex beat:
  ○ A forceful apex beat displaced laterally indicates left ventricular hypertrophy and is called a 'heave'.
  ○ A 'thrill' is a palpable murmur and should be palpable over where a murmur is heard loudest
● Liver edge:
  ○ Displaced in heart failure.

Auscultation:

● Heart murmurs are common in paediatrics; they indicate turbulent blood flow.
● Assess murmurs in terms of grade, timing (systolic/diastolic), location, radiation, palpable thrills.
● Systolic versus diastolic:
  ○ Difficult to assess, particularly when heart rates are fast
  ○ Most paediatric murmurs are systolic
  ○ Timing the murmur with the pulse can help determine whether it is diastolic or not.

Innocent murmurs:

- Very faint
- Grade 1 or 2
- Have no associated features (radiation, tachypnoea)
- Disappear when the child moves position.

Chest signs:

- Listen at both lung bases for bilateral basal crackles.

Gastrointestinal examination

Inspection:

- Jaundice, anaemia, mouth ulcers, failure to thrive
- Any scars and hernias should be noted.

Palpation:

- Make sure the child is comfortable and your hands warm
- Palpate lightly in all areas before performing deep palpation
- Identify normal organs, the liver may be palpable in a healthy infant, 1 cm below the right costal margin.
- Masses

  Organomegaly – kidneys, liver, or spleen

  Tumours, e.g. nephroblastoma, neuroblastoma

  Faecal masses are indentable.
- Tenderness

  Children can be stoical and may deny painful symptoms particularly if they are not keen on staying in hospital

  Key features include children who are quiet, pale, unwilling to move or be examined and rebound tenderness
- Rectal exam is rarely called for in children, however, inspection of the external anus may be useful.
- Pubertal staging (Tanner staging) is an important part of paediatrics but beyond the remit of this text.

Box 5.3 Dehydration (*Diarrhoea and Vomiting in Children Under 5*. National Institute for Health and Clinical Excellence, clinical guideline 84, April 2009)

Moderate dehydration:
- Altered responsiveness (e.g. irritable or lethargic)
- Sunken eyes or sunken fontanelle
- Dry mucous membranes
- Reduced skin turgor
- Tachycardia and tachypnoea .

Severe dehydration/shock
- A decreased level of consciousness
- Prolonged capillary refill time
- Cool peripheries
- Pale or mottled skin
- Tachycardia and tachypnoea
- Weak peripheral pulses
- Hypotension.

Neurological examination

Inspection:

Observation of children at play will yield most of the information required for developmental assessment and will give clues to any neurological impairment.

Conscious level:

- AVPU:
  - ○ **A**lert
  - ○ responsive to **V**oice
  - ○ responsive to **P**ain
  - ○ **U**nresponsive .
- Responsive to pain corresponds approximately to 8/15 on the Glasgow Coma Scale (GCS) and should raise concerns that the child cannot protect their airway effectively.

Gait:

- Ask child to walk back and forth
- Observe any abnormal position or flexion of joints, foot drop, or ataxia.

Tone, power, reflexes:

- Assess upper and lower limbs
- Compare both sides
- Reflexes include triceps, brachial, supinator, knee jerk, ankle jerk, and plantar response
- Examine primitive reflexes in babies, e.g. Moro reflex, should disappear at 4–5 months.

Cerebellar signs:

- Coordination, i.e. finger pointing, dysdiadokinesis
- Nystagmus.

Patient safety tips

- ✔ Familiarize yourself with national guidelines such as NICE or British Thoracic Society guidelines. These are a useful resource and aim to provide an evidence base to support current practice. They also provide guidance on the standard of care that can be expected of clinicians.
- ✔ Take time over your communication: whether with parents, children, or colleagues; written or verbal.
- ✔ Check all dosages and routes of administration carefully: incorrect doses of medication can be unsafe because of over-treatment with significant complications, or due to under-dosing and ineffective treatment.
- ✔ Senior clinician involvement: have a low threshold for senior involvement. If you are unsure or are new to paediatrics you should always discuss your cases with a senior colleague.
- ✔ Create safety nets: when discharging patients ensure they have a safety net, i.e. a clear plan of what to do and who to contact if symptoms reoccur or child becomes more unwell.
- ✔ Child protection red flags: be vigilant for possible child protection issues. Child protection red flags include: history from parent or guardian not consistent with clinical picture, late presentations, bruising in distribution unlikely to be due to purely accidental injury, and injuries which could be due to cigarette burns.

Student name:	Medical school:	Year:

Paediatric history and examination

Please take a history and examine this child.

		Self	Peer	Peer /tutor	Tutor
Initiating the consultation	Greets patient and parents, confirms patient's name and age	☐	☐	☐	☐
	Introduces self, states role and purpose of interview, gains consent	☐	☐	☐	☐
	Uses body language and manner appropriate for the age of the child	☐	☐	☐	☐
	Uses appropriate open question to initiate interview	☐	☐	☐	☐
		☐	☐	☐	☐
History	Allow the parents or child to explain their concerns in their own words	☐	☐	☐	☐
	Asks appropriate follow-up questions	☐	☐	☐	☐
	Takes a birth history	☐	☐	☐	☐
	Takes a developmental history	☐	☐	☐	☐
	Lists immunizations	☐	☐	☐	☐
	Explores treatment history and allergies	☐	☐	☐	☐
	Explores social history, main carer, home occupants, school, etc.	☐	☐	☐	☐
	Asks about smoking within the home and alcohol, and recreational drug use, if appropriate	☐	☐	☐	☐
	Takes family history	☐	☐	☐	☐
	Draws family tree	☐	☐	☐	☐
	Listens attentively and minimises interruptions	☐	☐	☐	☐
	Seeks clarification when necessary	☐	☐	☐	☐
	Asks to see red book	☐	☐	☐	☐
		☐	☐	☐	☐
Explanation and consent	Washes hands with alcohol gel or soap and water	☐	☐	☐	☐
	Explains examination procedure to patient and obtains verbal consent	☐	☐	☐	☐
		☐	☐	☐	☐
General inspection	Observes child at rest or at play prior to examination	☐	☐	☐	☐
	Inspects patient's surroundings for 'clues'	☐	☐	☐	☐
		☐	☐	☐	☐
General examination	Plots weight and height with centile chart	☐	☐	☐	☐
	Observes general appearance including rashes and any signs of neglect or non-accidental injury	☐	☐	☐	☐
	Appropriate exposure	☐	☐	☐	☐
		☐	☐	☐	☐
Respiratory	Comments on respiratory rate and work of breathing	☐	☐	☐	☐
	Percusses in a symmetrical fashion	☐	☐	☐	☐
	Auscultates in a symmetrical fashion including axillae	☐	☐	☐	☐
	Asks to examine ears and throat	☐	☐	☐	☐
		☐	☐	☐	☐
Cardiovascular	Comments on systemic signs and any scars	☐	☐	☐	☐
	Examines pulse and requests blood pressure	☐	☐	☐	☐
	Auscultates heart sounds	☐	☐	☐	☐
	Auscultates chest and palpates for liver edge	☐	☐	☐	☐
		☐	☐	☐	☐
Gastrointestinal	Comments on systemic signs	☐	☐	☐	☐
	Looks in mouth	☐	☐	☐	☐
	Examines abdomen systematically	☐	☐	☐	☐
	Asks to examine genitalia and anus	☐	☐	☐	☐
		☐	☐	☐	☐
Neurological	Comments on development while the child is at play	☐	☐	☐	☐
	Observes gait	☐	☐	☐	☐
	Assesses tone, power, and reflexes	☐	☐	☐	☐
	Assesses coordination	☐	☐	☐	☐
		☐	☐	☐	☐
Professionalism	Thanks child carer, records clinical findings	☐	☐	☐	☐
		☐	☐	☐	☐

				U B S E	U B S E	U B S E	U B S E
Self-assessed as at least borderline:	Signature:		Date:				
Peer-assessed as ready for tutor assessment:	Signature:		Date:				
Tutor-assessed as satisfactory:	Signature:		Date:				

Notes

5.2 Obstetrics

Background

The aim of obstetric management is to maintain or improve the health of the mother and to produce as normal a pregnancy and as safe a delivery as possible. History taking and examination therefore focus on:

- Highlighting any previous medical, surgical or obstetric complications
- Identification of actual and potential risks to the pregnancy and delivery
- Formulation of the management pathway for the current pregnancy.

Management objectives by trimester

First trimester (1–13 weeks)

- Record details and dates of the pregnancy.
- Identify any existing medical problems.
- Assess risks to pregnancy and explore lifestyle.
- Assess need for additional services.

Second trimester (14–26 weeks)

- Monitor maternal health.
- Monitor growth of baby.
- Assess for any new problems.

Third trimester (27 weeks to term)

- Monitor overall health and progress.
- Monitor growth of baby.
- Plan childbirth.

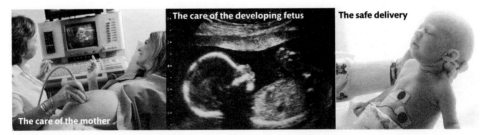

The care of the developing fetus

The safe delivery

The care of the mother

Figure 5.2 Images in obstetrics: history, examination, and care planning. Left © Banana Stock; middle © Isabelle Limbach/iStockphoto; right © Corbis/Digital Stock

History taking

Personal History

- Personal details: Age, Marital status: single, partnership or married.
- Gravid: the number of all pregnancies including the current one.
- Parity: the number of births beyond 24 weeks.
- Last menstrual period (LMP) first day and expected date of delivery (EDD). Naegele's Rule: add one year and seven days to the LMP and subtract three months. Dating scans are more accurate.
- Previous menstrual cycle history: regular or irregular.
- Relevant Reproductive System History: Recent use of oral contraception, History of subfertility, Sexually transmitted diseases, Previous cervical smears, Female circumcision, Urinary and/or faecal incontinence.
- Identify any need for an interpreter.

Current obstetric health

- Hospital admissions during current pregnancy.
- Foetal movements after 20 weeks.
- Date and detail of first scan.
- Results of other scans.
- Results of other laboratory tests.
- Subsequent antenatal check ups.

Past obstetric history:

- Outcome of previous pregnancies:
- Antepartum, intrapartum or postpartum complications.
- Gestational age at delivery.
- Labour: spontaneous, induced or planned caesarean section.
- Mode of delivery : normal, assisted, breech or caesarean section
- Birth weight and health of baby since delivery..
- Previous miscarriages, ectopic pregnancies or terminations.
- Causes of early and late pregnancy losses, if known.

Current and past medical history

- General: Anaemia, urinary tract infections, tuberculosis exposure, back problem, asthma, thromboembolism, epilepsy.
- CVD: Heart disease, Hypertension.
- Diabetes and Endocrine: Type 1 or type 2 diabetes mellitus, thyroid disorders.
- Any other medical condition.

Mental health history

- Present or past mental health problems.
- Depression, especially postnatal.
- Personality disorder.
- Suicidal tendency.
- Details of treatment, if any.

Surgical history

- Previous Obstetrics or Gynaecology surgery: Caesarean section, myomectomy, cervical cone biopsy, large Loop Excision of Transformation Zone (LLETZ), cervical cerclage.
- Bowel surgery or any laparotomy.
- Anaesthetic complications.

Drug History

- Intake of any teratogenic drugs, e.g. warfarin, ACE-inhibitors, statins, ARBs.
- Any other drugs, e.g. beta blockers which may impair foetal growth.
- Alcohol or smoking or recreational drugs.
- Previous referral to a substance misuse or smoking cessation advisor.

Allergies

- Drug.
- Food.
- Latex.
- Any others.

Social History

- Housing and/or employment issues.
- Support from partner, friends and family.
- Religion.
- Social issues, including language difficulties.
- Domestic violence.

Family history

- Diabetes mellitus.
- Thromboembolism.
- Hypertension.
- Pre-eclampsia / HELLP.
- Congenital hip disorders.
- Neural tube defects.
- Down's syndrome.
- Cystic fibrosis.
- Thalassemia.
- Congenital abnormalities.
- Metabolic disorders.
- Mental health problems.
- Any other familial disorders.
- Twins.
- Consanguinity.
- Passive smoking.

Physical examination

The physical examination will differ depending on what stage of pregnancy the mother is at. Table 5.1 details the examinations needed at each trimester.

Table 5.1 Physical examination by trimester

Examination	1st trimester	2nd trimester	3rd trimester	Labour
BMI	✓		✓ if BMI >40	
General examination including blood pressure and urinalysis	✓	✓	✓	✓
Abdominal	Tenderness or mass	Tenderness Symphysio-fundal height Fetal heart sounds	Tenderness Symphysio-fundal height Presentation Fetal heart sounds	Tenderness Symphysio-fundal height Presentation Fetal heart sounds Monitor for contractions
Cardiovascular system	✓	✓	✓	✓
Respiratory system	✓	✓	✓	✓
Breast	✓			
Thyroid	✓			
Vaginal	Indicated only if bleeding, vaginal discharge, ruptured membranes, suspected labour/active labour			
Reflexes			If pre-eclampsia	
Fundoscopy	If pre-eclampsia, headache, or diabetes			

General examination

- General appearance
- Weight, height and body mass index (BMI), temperature
- Cardiovascular examination: pulse, blood pressure in the semi-recumbent position or at 45°, heart, and lungs
- Breast and thyroid, especially for nodules
- Reflexes if pre-eclampsia
- Fundoscopy if history of headaches, pre-eclampsia, or diabetes

Abdominal examination

Inspection

- Scars
- Overdistension: multiple pregnancy, polyhydramnios, fibroids, or ovarian cysts
- Asymmetrical distension: fibroids
- Visible fetal movements
- Rash
- Scratch marks
- Striae.

Palpation

- Tenderness or mass: localized or generalized tenderness in the 2nd or 3rd trimester may indicate placental abruption.
- Uterine size: the uterus should be palpable at the symphysis at 13 weeks and at the umbilicus at 20–22 weeks. Up to 22 weeks uterine size is assessed as 13 plus 1 week per fingerbreadth above the symphysis pubis. From 24 weeks symphyso-fundal height (SFH) is measured in centimetres from the pubic symphysis to the highest point on the fundus: it should be recorded every 2–3 weeks.
  - ○ Increased SFH: multiple pregnancy, fibroid, ovarian cyst, macrosomia, polyhydramnios
  - ○ Reduced SFH: fetal growth restriction, small for gestational age, oligohydramnios.
- Fetal lie: is defined as the relationship of the long axis of the fetus to the long axis of the uterus. It can be: longitudinal, transverse, or oblique.
- Fetal presentation: is defined as the fetal part which lies over the pelvic brim. It can be: cephalic, breech, hand, footling, cord, compound, e.g. hand presenting with head.
- The four grips of Leopold's manoeuvre are palpation of:
  - ○ The uterine fundus
  - ○ The uterine sides
  - ○ The fetal presenting part between two hands
  - ○ The presenting part between index finger and thumb to assess for fetal descent and engagement (two-fifth or less palpable).

Percussion

This is not generally used in obstetric examination but a fluid thrill may be demonstrated in polyhydramnios.

Auscultation

Use a hand-held Doppler over the anterior fetal shoulder to auscultate the heart for 1 minute: normal is 110–160 beats per minute.

Vaginal examination: speculum and digital

This is not a part of routine obstetric examination and is indicated only when there is:

- Suspected bleeding
- Ruptured membranes
- Offensive vaginal discharge
- Suspected labour or active labour.

Plan of care

- Identify risks to the pregnancy with a detailed history and examination.
- Diagnose and treat any medical disorders.
- Offer a multidisciplinary team approach.
- Individualize the management plan in accordance with need and the severity of any disorder.
- Monitor health of the mother and baby.
- Monitor growth of the baby.
- Plan safe delivery.
- Give adequate information to the woman to enable her to make informed choices.

Patient safety tips

✔ Always take the history in a logical sequence and take care to avoid inadvertent omissions of detail.

✔ Refer to the medical team and offer a multidisciplinary approach in case of possible medical, surgical, or anaesthetic problems.

✔ Establish good communication with the woman and consider all her needs.

✔ List all her problems and make a care plan for each one before she leaves.

✔ Vary the history taking template according to the clinical problem.

✔ Always obtain consent before carrying out examination and use a chaperone.

✔ Each examination should be tailored to the woman's circumstances.

✔ Never carry out a vaginal examination in undiagnosed vaginal bleeding or if placenta praevia is suspected or known.

✔ Carry out a speculum examination if suspected ruptured membranes, bleeding, or threatened preterm labour.

✔ Avoid digital vaginal examination with ruptured membranes unless the woman is in labour.

✔ Always seek advice and senior support when necessary.

Student name:	Medical school:	Year:

Pregnancy assessment

Please make an assessment of this woman's pregnancy.

		Self	Peer	Peer /tutor	Tutor
Initiating the consultation	• Greets patient, confirms patient's name and age	☐	☐	☐	☐
	• Introduces self, states role and purpose of interview, gains consent	☐	☐	☐	☐
	• Uses appropriate open question to initiate interview	☐	☐	☐	☐
	•	☐	☐	☐	☐
History	• Establishes gravidity, parity, last menstrual period, and estimated delivery date	☐	☐	☐	☐
	• Explores history of current pregnancy	☐	☐	☐	☐
	• Uses open and closed questions appropriately, moving from open to closed	☐	☐	☐	☐
	• Explores past obstetric history	☐	☐	☐	☐
	• Explores current and past medical history	☐	☐	☐	☐
	• Explores treatment history and allergies	☐	☐	☐	☐
	• Explores personal and social history	☐	☐	☐	☐
	• Asks about smoking, alcohol, and recreational drug use	☐	☐	☐	☐
	• Explores family history	☐	☐	☐	☐
	• Listens attentively and minimizes interruptions	☐	☐	☐	☐
	• Seeks clarification when necessary	☐	☐	☐	☐
	• Actively determines the patient's perspective: ideas and beliefs, concerns, expectations, effects of pregnancy on life, feelings	☐	☐	☐	☐
	•	☐	☐	☐	☐
Explanation and consent	• Washes hands with alcohol gel or soap and water	☐	☐	☐	☐
	• Explains examination procedure to patient and obtains verbal consent	☐	☐	☐	☐
	•	☐	☐	☐	☐
Adequate exposure	• Achieves adequate exposure while maintaining patient dignity	☐	☐	☐	☐
	•	☐	☐	☐	☐
General inspection	• Assesses patient's appearance, commenting on any relevant findings	☐	☐	☐	☐
	• Inspects patient's surroundings for 'clues'	☐	☐	☐	☐
	•	☐	☐	☐	☐
General examination	• Comments on need to check weight and height	☐	☐	☐	☐
	• Performs appropriate general examination	☐	☐	☐	☐
	• Checks blood pressure	☐	☐	☐	☐
	•	☐	☐	☐	☐
Obstetric examination	• Inspects abdomen	☐	☐	☐	☐
	• Palpates abdomen for tenderness	☐	☐	☐	☐
	• Establishes uterine size	☐	☐	☐	☐
	• Determines fetal lie and presentation	☐	☐	☐	☐
	• Auscultates fetal heart sounds	☐	☐	☐	☐
	•	☐	☐	☐	☐
Additional examination	• Comments on need to perform vaginal examination	☐	☐	☐	☐
	•	☐	☐	☐	☐
Professionalism	• Covers patient, thanks patient, washes hands	☐	☐	☐	☐
	•	☐	☐	☐	☐

			Self	Peer	Peer/tutor	Tutor
Self-assessed as at least borderline:	Signature:	Date:	U B S E	U B S E	U B S E	U B S E
Peer-assessed as ready for tutor assessment:	Signature:	Date:	U B S E	U B S E	U B S E	U B S E
Tutor-assessed as satisfactory:	Signature:	Date:	U B S E	U B S E	U B S E	U B S E

Notes

5.3 Psychiatry

Background

All practising clinicians should be able to take a basic psychiatric history and perform a basic mental state examination. Psychiatric disorders, especially depression and anxiety, are common. Psychiatric and organic disorders frequently coexist in the same patient and each may aggravate the other. Some organic diseases, especially endocrine, for example thyroid disease, may present with psychiatric symptoms. On the other hand, mental health disorders not infrequently manifest with symptoms apparently of organic origin.

Common presentations

For each major and common condition there are a few key symptoms about which you must enquire:

Depression

- Low mood
- Loss of interest and enjoyment
- Sleep and appetite disturbance
- Loss of energy, increased fatigability and reduced activity
- Negative, pessimistic or guilty thoughts
- Hopelessness

Schizophrenia

- Hearing voices: sometimes as a running commentary
- Belief that thoughts are being inserted or withdrawn or that they are being broadcasted
- Belief that their speech, volition, bodies are being controlled
- Belief that they are being persecuted or followed
- Delusional perception
- Negative symptoms: apathy, paucity of speech, blunting or incongruity of emotional responses, usually resulting in social withdrawal

Mania

- Elevation of mood
- Increased energy and activity
- Decreased need for sleep
- Grandiose ideas
- Disinhibition and impaired judgement

Anxiety disorders

- Physical symptoms (autonomic arousal): muscle weakness, dry mouth, tremors, pilo-erection, dysaesthesia, tension, increased frequency of micturition or defaecation, increased sweating, hyperventilation
- Emotional symptoms: nervousness, anxiety, panic, tension, feeling low
- Thoughts: that something terrible is about to happen, disproportional worries

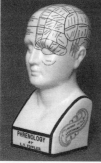
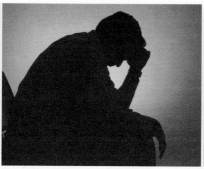
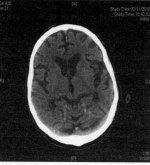

The human mind:
the most complex organ

Depression will affect 10–15% of all of us

Dementia:
an ever increasing idiopathic problem
and cardiovascular disease complication

Figure 5.3 Images in psychiatry.

Mental state examination

The mental state examination is your assessment in the present moment, not what you have learned from the history.

Appearance and Behaviour	**Speech**
• General appearance • Behaviour and body language • Abnormal motor behaviour • Attitude to examiner	• Amount • Rate • Volume • Tone
Mood and affect	**Thought**
• Subjective : how the patient says they are feeling • Objective : how your observations suggest the patient is actually feeling • Emotional reactivity to environment	• Thought form : the process of the patient's thinking • Thought content : worries, preoccupations, obsessions, over-valued ideas, delusions, suicidal thoughts
Perception	**Cognition**
• Hallucinations • Illusions	• Level of consciousness • Orientation • Memory • Concentration
Insight	
• Does the patient believe he or she has a problem?	

The mental state examination should be followed by a full physical examination.

History taking

Before starting
- Introduce yourself to the patient and make every effort to ensure they are at ease

The presenting complaint and history of the presenting complaint
- What has brought you to hospital today?
- Onset and duration of symptoms
- Progression
- Precipitating or aggravating factors
- How the symptoms are affecting the patient's life
- Mood, abnormal thoughts or abnormal experiences

Past Psychiatric History
- Any episodes of psychiatric illness
- Psychiatric in-patient episodes
- History of self-neglect, self harm or suicide attempts
- History of violence

Past medical history
- Any previous physical illness

Treatment History
- Regular medications
- Allergies
- Intolerances

Family History
- Psychiatric illness
- Physical illness
- Suicide
- Any recent significant events in the family

Personal History

Birth and early development
- Gestation and delivery
- Developmental milestones

Family background and early childhood
- Emotional and / or behavioural problems
- Friends
- Prolonged separation from parents

Education
- Educational achievements
- Enjoyment of school
- Relationship with teachers and peers

Occupation
- Chronological list of employment history
- Reasons for leaving
- Relationship with bosses and colleagues

Psychosexual and relationships
- Past and present partners, including same sex partners
- Difficulties in relationships
- Sexual problems
- Any physical or sexual abuse

Substance misuse
- Alcohol
- Smoking
- Recreational drugs

Forensic history
- Have you ever been in trouble with the police?

Social history
- Social support
- Housing
- Finances
- Self – care

Premorbid personality
- Personality before onset of symptoms
- How would your friends and family describe you?

Collateral history
- It is important to speak to others to gain further insight into the patient's presentation.

Box 5.4 Mental state tests

• Mini-Mental State Examination (MMSE)

The MMSE is a screening assessment of cognitive function. It is scored out of 30: a score of 21–26 indicates mild to moderate and of <20 more severe cognitive impairment.

MMSE (adapted from the original Folstein Test 1979)	Maximum score
Orientation	
What is the: date, day, month, year, season?	5 points
Where are we?: country, county, town, hospital, ward	5 points
Registration	
Name three objects only once, e.g. pen, chair, money, and ask the patient to repeat them. Then repeat until the patient learns all three in order to test recall later on	3 points
Attention and calculation	
Serial 7s: ask the patient to subtract 7 from 100 (= 93), then 93 – 7 (=86) and then three more times, or serial 9s or Ask the patient to spell WORLD backwards (D-L-R-O-W)	5 points
Recall	
Ask the patient to repeat the names of the three objects learnt in the registration test	3 points
Language	
Ask the patient to name two common objects shown, e.g. pen, watch, pillow	2 points
Ask the patient to repeat a complex phrase	1 point
Ask the patient to follow a three-stage command e.g. 'Take this pen in your left hand and put it in this cup'	3 points
Write 'Touch your nose' on a piece of paper and ask the patient to read it and do what it says	1 point
Repeat with 'Write down your address'	1 point
Ask the patient to copy the intersecting pentagons or hexagons	1 point

Score
≥25   Normal
21–24   Mild cognitive impairment
10–20   Moderate cognitive impairment
≤9   Severe cognitive impairment

Total score   / 30

The mental state examination should be followed by a full physical examination.

- Abbreviated Mental Test (adapted from Hodkinson 1972)

This is a quick screening test of cognition: it is scored out of 10. A score of 6 or under would suggest delirium or dementia.

Question	Score 1 for every correct answer
Age	
Time to the nearest hour	
(Address recall: repeat '42 West Street' until the patient understands)	
Year	
Name of this place	
Identification of two persons (doctor, nurse)	
Date of birth	
Year of the first world war or another important historical date	
Name of the present monarch	
Count backwards from 20 to 1	
Ask the patient to recall the address '42 West Street'	
	Score = / 10

A score of 6 or less suggests delirium or dementia

Dementia

The general medical take will inevitably include some patients with dementia. This is defined as an acquired chronic progressive cognitive impairment: it is not a normal part of ageing. In a patient with symptoms of dementia it is important first to rule out any organic cause. Basic investigations are:

Bloods

- Blood count for evidence of anaemia or infection
- U&Es for evidence of dehydration, renal failure or hyponatraemia
- Glucose for diabetes or hypoglycaemia
- Thyroid function tests for hypothyroidism
- LFTs for alcohol abuse
- B_{12} and folate : deficiency can cause reversible cognitive impairment
- Calcium for hyperparathyroidism

Sepsis screen

- MSU
- Chest X-ray
- Blood cultures

Consider

- CT or MRI of head especially if there are unusual features
- Further endocrine investigation for Addison's disease or Cushing's syndrome

- Capacity

Capacity is the ability of a patient to make decisions about their care. Simply making a decision with which you do not agree does not mean a patient lacks capacity. The assessment of capacity is a judgement only for the present and relates only to a specific decision. To have capacity, the patient must:

- Understand the information relevant to the decision
- Retain that information
- Use that information to formulate a decision
- Communicate their decision to you by any means

If any of these are lacking then the patient does not have capacity: management may then be undertaken according to considerations of what is in the patient's best interests.

Compulsory admission under the UK Mental Health Act 2007

Table 5.2 Sections from the Mental Health Act (MHA) 2007, and Police and Criminal Evidence Act.

	Table 5.2 Compulsory admissions: brief summary		
Section	**Purpose**	**Maximum duration**	**Recommendation**
MHA 2	Admission for assessment	28 days	2 doctors (at least one section 12(3) approved)
MHA 3	Admission for treatment	6 months	2 doctors (at least one section 12(3) approved)
MHA 5 (2)	Holding order for a patient already on the ward	72 hours	1 doctor (responsible medical officer or deputy)
PACE 136	Police order to remove a person appearing to suffer from a 'mental disorder' from a public place to a place of safety. AMHP (Approved Mental Health Professional) and nearest relative must consent	72 hours	Police officer (to allow assessment by medical practitioner)

* An approved Mental Health Practitioner will often take the lead in assessment and application together with the doctors.

Patient safety tips

✔ An essential part of the psychiatric history and examination is the risk assessment: whether the patient may be at risk of harming themselves or others. Suicide risk should be accessed directly but sensitively. Has the patient experienced thoughts of self-harm or suicide? If so, has he or she made a specific plan? Is there a previous history of self-harm? In the UK, patients who are deemed to be a risk to themselves or others can be admitted to hospital compulsorily under the Mental Health Act 2007.

	Student name:	Medical school:	Year:

Mental state examination

Please take a psychiatric history and perform a mental state examination on this patient.

	Self	Peer	Peer /tutor	Tutor
Initiating the consultation				
● Greets patient, confirms patient's name	☐	☐	☐	☐
● Introduces self, states role, and purpose of interview, gains consent	☐	☐	☐	☐
● Uses appropriate opening question to elicit presenting complaint(s)	☐	☐	☐	☐
●	☐	☐	☐	☐
The presenting complaint				
● Fully explores presenting complaint: asks about other relevant symptoms	☐	☐	☐	☐
● Uses open and closed questions appropriately, moving from open to closed	☐	☐	☐	☐
● Listens attentively and minimizes interruptions	☐	☐	☐	☐
● Seeks clarification when necessary	☐	☐	☐	☐
● Uses clear easily understood language and avoids jargon	☐	☐	☐	☐
● Actively determines the patient's perspective: ideas and beliefs, concerns, expectations, effects of symptoms on life, feelings	☐	☐	☐	☐
●	☐	☐	☐	☐
Background and context				
● Explores the patient's past psychiatric history	☐	☐	☐	☐
● Explores the patient's past medical history	☐	☐	☐	☐
● Explores treatment history and allergies	☐	☐	☐	☐
● Explores personal and social history	☐	☐	☐	☐
● Asks about smoking, alcohol and recreational drug use	☐	☐	☐	☐
● Explores forensic history	☐	☐	☐	☐
● Explores family history	☐	☐	☐	☐
● Enquires about premorbid personality	☐	☐	☐	☐
●	☐	☐	☐	☐
Providing structure				
● Structures history in a logical sequence	☐	☐	☐	☐
● Progresses from one section to another using signposting	☐	☐	☐	☐
● Summarizes at end of each section and confirms understanding	☐	☐	☐	☐
● Attends to timing and keeps the interview on task	☐	☐	☐	☐
●	☐	☐	☐	☐
Building the doctor–patient relationship				
● Demonstrates appropriate non-verbal behaviour	☐	☐	☐	☐
● Acknowledges patient's views and feelings	☐	☐	☐	☐
● Makes empathic statements to communicate appreciation of the patients' feelings or predicament	☐	☐	☐	☐
● Expresses concern and understanding	☐	☐	☐	☐
● Attends to patient's physical comfort	☐	☐	☐	☐
●	☐	☐	☐	☐
Finishing the history				
● Asks the patient if there is anything they want to add	☐	☐	☐	☐
● Summarizes the history including the patient's perspective	☐	☐	☐	☐
●	☐	☐	☐	☐
Mental state examination				
● Assesses appearance and behaviour	☐	☐	☐	☐
● Assesses speech	☐	☐	☐	☐
● Assesses mood	☐	☐	☐	☐
● Assesses thought	☐	☐	☐	☐
● Assesses perception	☐	☐	☐	☐
● Assesses cognition	☐	☐	☐	☐
● Assesses insight	☐	☐	☐	☐
●	☐	☐	☐	☐
Additional history and examination				
● Comments on need of collateral history	☐	☐	☐	☐
● Comments on need of physical examination	☐	☐	☐	☐
●	☐	☐	☐	☐

			Self	Peer	Peer /tutor	Tutor
Self-assessed as at least borderline:	Signature:	Date:	U B S E	U B S E	U B S E	U B S E
Peer-assessed as ready for tutor assessment:	Signature:	Date:	U B S E	U B S E	U B S E	U B S E
Tutor-assessed as satisfactory:	Signature:	Date:	U B S E	U B S E	U B S E	U B S E

Notes

5.4 Diabetes

Background

Three million people in the UK are known to have diabetes and there are undoubtedly many more undiagnosed. Around 10% have type 1 diabetes and 90% type 2: there are many other causes of diabetes but they are rare. The prevalence of type 2 diabetes is increasing rapidly due to rising rates of obesity. With recent changes in chronic disease management most routine diabetes care in the UK is now undertaken in primary care.

Common presentations

The classical symptoms of hyperglycaemia are:

- Thirst
- Polydipsia
- Polyuria
- Weight loss.

Patients with new type 1 diabetes may present acutely in ketoacidosis. By contrast, individuals with type 2 diabetes may be asymptomatic and not present until a complication develops, for example retinopathy, neuropathy, or a vascular event. The propensity of type 2 diabetes to cause damage for many years prior to diagnosis has led to calls for routine screening of high-risk groups.

Anatomical and physiological principles

Type 1 and type 2 diabetes are usually regarded as two different diseases. The former is a state of absolute insulin deficiency consequent upon pancreatic β-cell failure probably due to autoimmunity. The latter results from a complex interaction between genetic and environmental factors: it is primarily characterized by markedly increased cardiovascular risk accompanied by a wide range of metabolic abnormalities including insulin resistance and hyperglycaemia.

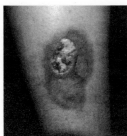 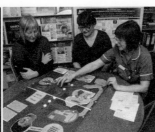 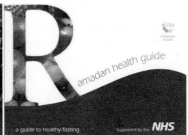

Necrobiosis lipoidica diabetocorum Associated with poor glycaemic control

Patient education and self-management is the most important aspect of care

Diabetes Care and Ramadan: fasting from sunrise to sunset entails change in many diabetes treatments and doses, such as tds treatment to bd, insulin dose changes, lower doses of antihypertensives

Figure 5.4 Images in diabetes care. Right image © Crown Copyright.

History and examination sequence	Clinical context
History	
Current problems	Start with an open question: 'What concerns do you have about your diabetes?' The answer may be unexpected, e.g. erectile dysfunction or weight gain
Assessment of glycaemic control	Many patients will self-monitor their blood glucose but the results cannot always be trusted!
	Episodes of hypoglycaemia are common in those on insulin or oral agents and may not be volunteered by the patient. Specific enquiry is needed and treatment change will be necessary
Symptoms of established and potential complications	The main risk factors for microvascular complications are long duration of diabetes, poor glycaemic control and hypertension
Medication	Most patients with diabetes are on polypharmacy and adherence is often poor
Lifestyle	Many patients with type 2 diabetes are obese and will need assistance with weight management and advice about exercise. Those who smoke must be helped to quit
Examination	
Correct position and adequate exposure	The examination is best performed with the patient reclining comfortably on the couch. The legs should be fully exposed but can be kept covered initially
General inspection	Many patients with type 2 diabetes exhibit truncal obesity: consider measuring BMI and waist circumference
	General inspection may offer a clue to a possible secondary cause of diabetes, for example Cushing's syndrome, hyperthyroidism or acromegaly
General examination	A large majority of patients with type 2 diabetes have raised blood pressure
	A resting tachycardia and/or postural hypotension (a >20 mmHg drop in systolic blood pressure on standing) suggest autonomic neuropathy
	Rashes on the shins are not uncommon in diabetes: consider pretibial diabetic dermopathy and necrobiosis lipoidica
Diabetes examination	In insulin-treated patients, examine the injection sites for lipohypertrophy and lipoatrophy
	Meticulous examination of the feet, neurovascular assessment, and patient education are essential to prevent ulceration and amputation. Asymptomatic neuropathy is common, especially in those with long-standing diabetes
	Direct fundoscopy has now largely been supplanted by digital retinal photography
	Background retinopathy is not a minor problem: it indicates that the patient has already sustained significant microvascular damage

Additional examination	Cardiovascular examination may reveal evidence of left ventricular hypertrophy secondary to hypertension or cardiac failure consequent upon coronary heart disease
Professionalism	Maintain patient dignity, communicate sensitively, thank the patient, wash hands, explain conclusions to the patient, document fully and accurately, communicate appropriately with colleagues

Patient safety tips

✔ Do not assume that a patient presenting with new diabetes who is not young must have type 2. Type 1 diabetes may occur at any age. The decision to treat with insulin is based on clinical assessment and on the severity of hyperglycaemia not on a guess, educated or not, whether this is type 1 or type 2.

✔ As an *aide-memoire*, all the main aspects of diabetes care can be recalled by use of the 'alphabet strategy for diabetes care':

   ○ **Advice**: smoking, weight, physical activity, diet, influenza vaccination

   ○ **Blood pressure**: usual target <130/80 mmHg

   ○ **Cholesterol and creatinine care**: usual cholesterol target is low-density lipoprotein (LDL) <2.0 mmol/L. Check renal function and test for microalbuminuria annually

   ○ **Diabetes control**: optimize HbA_{1c}% individualized to patient usually <7.5%

   ○ **Eye examination**: retinal examination yearly and appropriate referral if indicated

   ○ **Feet examination**: yearly examination of peripheral pulses and neuropathy

   ○ **Guardian drugs**: appropriate use of drugs for cardiovascular disease and renal protection such as angiotensin-converting enzyme (ACE) I, statins, aspirin, and angiotensin receptor blockers (ARBs).

Student name:	Medical school:	Year:				

Diabetes assessment

Please clinically assess this patient with diabetes.

		Self	Peer	Peer /tutor	Tutor
Initiating the consultation	● Greets patient, confirms patient's name	☐	☐	☐	☐
	● Introduces self, states role and purpose of interview, gains consent	☐	☐	☐	☐
	● Uses appropriate opening question to elicit current symptoms and patient's concerns	☐	☐	☐	☐
	●	☐	☐	☐	☐
History	● Fully explores current symptoms and patient's concerns	☐	☐	☐	☐
	● Assesses glycaemic control and asks about hypoglycaemia	☐	☐	☐	☐
	● Enquires about symptoms of complications	☐	☐	☐	☐
	● Enquires about medication and adherence	☐	☐	☐	☐
	● Asks about diet, smoking and exercise	☐	☐	☐	☐
	●	☐	☐	☐	☐
Explanation and consent	● Washes hands with alcohol gel or soap and water	☐	☐	☐	☐
	● Explains examination procedure to patient and obtains verbal consent	☐	☐	☐	☐
	●	☐	☐	☐	☐
Correct position and adequate exposure	● Patient in appropriate reclining position	☐	☐	☐	☐
	● Achieves adequate exposure while maintaining patient dignity	☐	☐	☐	☐
	●	☐	☐	☐	☐
General inspection	● Inspects patient from end of bed, commenting on any relevant findings	☐	☐	☐	☐
	● Inspects patient's surroundings for 'clues'	☐	☐	☐	☐
	● Comments on need to measure weight, BMI, and waist circumference	☐	☐	☐	☐
	●	☐	☐	☐	☐
General examination	● Takes pulse and blood pressure	☐	☐	☐	☐
	● Checks for postural hypotension	☐	☐	☐	☐
	● Inspects skin for rashes	☐	☐	☐	☐
	●	☐	☐	☐	☐
Diabetes examinations	● Examines injection sites	☐	☐	☐	☐
	● Inspects legs and feet	☐	☐	☐	☐
	● Palpates foot pulses and checks capillary refill time	☐	☐	☐	☐
	● Assesses light touch and vibration sensation, and checks ankle reflexes	☐	☐	☐	☐
	● Performs fundoscopy	☐	☐	☐	☐
	●	☐	☐	☐	☐
Additional examination	● Considers urine test for albuminuria and fingerprick blood glucose	☐	☐	☐	☐
	● Considers cardiovascular examination	☐	☐	☐	☐
	●	☐	☐	☐	☐
Professionalism	● Covers patient, thanks patient, washes hands	☐	☐	☐	☐
	●	☐	☐	☐	☐

			Self	Peer	Peer /tutor	Tutor
Self-assessed as at least borderline:	Signature:	Date:	U B S E	U B S E	U B S E	U B S E
Peer-assessed as ready for tutor assessment:	Signature:	Date:	U B S E	U B S E	U B S E	U B S E
Tutor-assessed as satisfactory:	Signature:	Date:	U B S E	U B S E	U B S E	U B S E

Notes

5.5 Endocrine disorders

Background

Endocrine disorders present with multifarious symptoms and signs, and there is no 'endocrine examination'. This section provides an overview of the main endocrine conditions other than diabetes and thyroid disease, which are covered elsewhere in this suite. Hyperlipidaemia and chronic fatigue syndrome are included since these are frequently seen in endocrine clinics.

Common presentations

Important areas of enquiry in the history include:

- When were you last your normal self?
- Growth, height, weight, pubertal development, development of sexual characteristics
- Menstruation, hair, skin, mood, change in body size
- Tiredness, weakness, changes in appetite, libido, lack of drive
- What main changes have you or others noticed in yourself?

Close attention to a detailed general examination is needed: major but subtle clues may be found, for example, in the patient's general demeanour or the appearance of the face. With regard to the latter, old photographs of the patient are often helpful.

The history and examination sequence for a patient with an endocrine disorder

History	Examination
Adrenal cortex	
Adrenal insufficiency (Addison's disease):	
Weakness, fatigue, sleepiness	Pigmentation of skin especially palmar creases, scars, lips, buccal mucosa: vitiligo possible
Dizziness on standing	Postural hypotension
Pallor	Hypoglycaemia
Weight loss or gain	
Abdominal pain	
Glucocorticoid excess (Cushing's syndrome):	
See pituitary gland	
Aldosterone excess (Conn's syndrome):	
Often no specific symptoms	Hypertension
Headache	Tachycardia
Androgen excess: females: (adrenal and ovary)	Hirsutism: lips, face, peri-areolar area, abdomen, acanthosis nigricans, skin tags
	Facial acne with greasy skin
	Increased shoulder girdle muscle bulk, obesity
	Clitoromegaly

History	Examination
Adrenal medulla	
Catecholamine excess (phaeochromocytoma):	
Headaches	Hypertension
Sweating	Tachycardia
Palpitations	Restlessness
Anxiety	Neuromas
Anterior pituitary	
Prolactin excess (hyperprolactinaemia):	
Female:	
Menstrual irregularity	Galactorrhoea
Infertility	Visual field defect (bitemporal hemianopia), diplopia, corneal reflex reduced (all rarer than in male)
Galactorrhoea	
Headaches	
Low mood, tiredness	
Male:	
Galactorrhoea, gynaecomastia	Galactorrhoea, gynaecomastia
Erectile dysfunction	Visual field defect (bitemporal hemianopia), diplopia, corneal reflex reduced
Headaches	
Low mood, tiredness	
Glucocorticoid excess (Cushing's syndrome):	
(pituitary and adrenal)	
Weight gain	Central obesity with proximal muscle wasting
Depression	'Moon face' with plethora
Weakness	Abdominal striae
Infection	Acne, hirsutism
Easy bruising	Bruising
Gonadotrophin deficiency:	
Female:	
Amenorrhoea, oligomenorrhoea	Breast atrophy
Infertility, lack of libido	Reduced or absent secondary sexual characteristics
Dyspareunia	
Breast atrophy	
Loss of secondary sexual hair	
Male:	
Low libido/erectile dysfunction	Testicular atrophy
Infertility	Reduced or absent secondary sexual characteristics
Testicular atrophy/softness	
Loss of secondary sexual hair	

History	Examination
Growth hormone excess (acromegaly):	
Enlargement of tissues: larger hands, rings not fitting, clothes size change	Coarse facies with soft tissue enlargement: nose, lips, tongue (macroglossia), goitre
Sweating	Supra-orbital ridge enlargement
Headaches	Prognathism with teeth separation
Arthritis	Hypertension
	Visual field defect (bitemporal hemianopia), diplopia, corneal reflex reduced
	Kyphosis, osteoarthritis
	Tall if pre-pubertal condition
Growth hormone deficiency:	
Low mood, tiredness	Truncal obesity with increased waist hip ratio
Social isolation	Reduction in muscle strength
Weight gain	Low mood on full mental state examination
Reduced stamina and strength	
Thyroid-stimulating hormone deficiency:	
As for hypothyroidism	
Adrenocorticotropic hormone deficiency:	
As for adrenocortical insufficiency	

Posterior pituitary

Anti-diuretic hormone (ADH) deficiency (diabetes insipidus)

Polyuria, polydipsia	Carries water bottle
Nocturia	
Copious light coloured urine	

Hyperlipidaemia

Family history of atherosclerotic disease	Corneal arcus, xanthelasmata
Atherosclerotic disease symptoms: angina, transient ischaemic attack, stroke, peripheral vascular disease	Tendon xanthomata (Achilles, extensor tendons of hands)
	Eruptive xanthomata (especially buttocks and palms)
	Atherosclerotic disease
	Lipaemia retinalis

Chronic fatigue syndrome (myalgic encephalomyelitis)

Fatigue, especially post-exertion	Look tired/exhausted
Sleep disturbance	Dark glasses (photophobia)
Pain: myalgia, fibromyalgia	Tender lymph nodes
Headaches, neuropathic pain	Postural hypotension
General poorer cognition	Low temperature
Photophobia, phonophobia	Reduced reflexes, atonic pupils, reduced reflexes
Dizziness, abnormal thermoregulation, sweating	
Recurrent infections	

For images of patients with endocrine disorders, see the endocrine section of the clinical picture suite in the colour plate section.

Patient safety tips

Some memorable missed diagnoses include:

✔ Hypothyroidism: misdiagnosed as cardiac failure, depression or stroke

✔ Addison's disease or diabetic ketoacidosis: acute abdomen

✔ Ovarian malignancy: hirsutism and weight gain

✔ Hypopituitarism: depression

✔ Diabetes mellitus: recurrent infections, incontinence, and poor vision

✔ Phaeochromocytoma: anxiety with mild hypertension

✔ Chronic fatigue syndrome/myalgic encephalomyelitis (ME): myasthenia gravis, Addison's disease, systemic lupus erythematosus, multiple sclerosis, vitamin D deficiency.

Student name:	Medical school:	Year:

Endocrinology examination

This assessment will be based around a discussion of clinical histories and examination findings in patients with endocrinological and related disorders such as hyperlipidaemia and chronic fatigue syndrome.

	Self	Peer	Peer /tutor	Tutor

How would you start to take an endocrinology history?

	Self	Peer	Peer /tutor	Tutor
● Greets patient, confirms patient's name and age	☐	☐	☐	☐
● Introduces self, states role and purpose of interview, gains consent	☐	☐	☐	☐
● Uses appropriate open question to initiate interview, such as:				
● When were you last your normal self?				
● Growth, height, weight, pubertal development, development of sexual characteristics				
● Menstruation, hair, skin, mood, change in body size	☐	☐	☐	☐
● Tiredness, weakness, changes in appetite, libido, lack of drive				
● What main changes have you or others noticed in yourself?				
●	☐	☐	☐	☐

Asks less open questions specifically in relation to the following endocrinological conditions.
After aspects of history, states and discuss potential examination findings:

	Self	Peer	Peer /tutor	Tutor
● Adrenal: Addison's disease	☐	☐	☐	☐
● Adrenal: Phaechromocytoma	☐	☐	☐	☐
● Adrenal: Conn's (including retinal changes)	☐	☐	☐	☐
● Ovary: Polycystic ovary syndrome	☐	☐	☐	☐
● Testes: Hypogonadism	☐	☐	☐	☐
● Pituitary: Prolactinoma	☐	☐	☐	☐
● Pituitary: Excess growth hormone	☐	☐	☐	☐
● Pituitary: Cushing's disease	☐	☐	☐	☐
● Pituitary: Prolactinoma	☐	☐	☐	☐
● Pituitary: Diabetes insipidus	☐	☐	☐	☐
● Pituitary: Pan-hypopituitarism	☐	☐	☐	☐
● Thyroid: Hypothyroidism	☐	☐	☐	☐
● Thyroid: Hyperthyroidism	☐	☐	☐	☐
● Cushing's syndrome (non-pituitary)	☐	☐	☐	☐
● Chronic fatigue syndrome	☐	☐	☐	☐
● Hyperlipidaemia	☐	☐	☐	☐
●	☐	☐	☐	☐

	Signature:	Date:	U B S E	U B S E	U B S E	U B S E
Self-assessed as at least borderline:	Signature:	Date:	U B / S E	U B / S E	U B / S E	U B / S E
Peer-assessed as ready for tutor assessment:	Signature:	Date:	U B / S E	U B / S E	U B / S E	U B / S E
Tutor-assessed as satisfactory:	Signature:	Date:	U B / S E	U B / S E	U B / S E	U B / S E

Notes

5.6 Dermatology

Background

The skin is the most visible and accessible of all organs. An estimated 20% of consultations in primary care relate to the skin. Skin disease encompasses a very broad spectrum of pathology including allergy, autoimmune disease, degenerative changes, infections, neoplasia, and tumours. In addition to thousands of different 'skin diseases', the skin is often involved in systemic disorders such as endocrine, metabolic, and neoplastic disease.

Anatomy

- The skin comprises the epidermis and dermis, supported by subcutaneous connective tissue and fat.
- The most functionally important layer of the epidermis is the stratum corneum, the complex 'barrier', on the very surface of the skin, derived from the end-products of keratinocyte differentiation. This barrier serves many purposes, not least keeping out microorganisms. The main purpose of the rest of the epidermis is to constantly regenerate the stratum corneum.
- The dermis serves to support and nourish the epidermis.
- Additional vital functions of the dermis include sensation and thermoregulation. These are mediated via the dermal vasculature and nerve endings.
- Adnexal structures which span the epidermis and dermis include sweat glands, sebaceous glands, and hair follicles. These contribute further to the sensory and thermoregulatory functions of the skin.
- Hair and nails are also products of keratinocyte differentiation.
- The appearance of the skin, hair, and nails is of paramount importance but is usually taken for granted until disturbed by disease.

Terminology

- **Bulla**   A fluid filled elevated lesion on the surface of the skin >5 mm diameter
- **Comedo**   A keratin plug in a hair follicle, the hallmark of acne vulgaris
- **Crust**   Dried exudate
- **Cyst**   A cavity lined by epithelium
- **Erosion**   Partial thickness epidermal loss
- **Erythema**   Red or blue discoloration due to dilated capillaries
- **Exudate**   Fluid on the skin surface 'exuding' from the tissue
- **Hirsutes**   Excess hair in a secondary sexual distribution
- **Hypertrichosis** Excess hair
- **Keloid**   Scar tissue growing in a tumour-like manner beyond the site of the original causative injury
- **Macule**   A flat area of colour or textural change <2 cm diameter
- **Nodule**   A solid elevated lesion >5 mm diameter
- **Papule**   A solid elevated lesion up to 5 mm diameter
- **Patch**   A large macule >2 cm in diameter
- **Petechia**   A purpuric lesion up to 2 mm in diameter

- **Plaque**   A palpable, elevated, flat-topped, patch or large macule
- **Poikiloderma** A skin appearance comprising hyperpigmentation, atrophy, and telangiectasia
- **Purpura**   Red or purple discoloration due to extravasation of erythrocytes
- **Pustule**   A dense liquid accumulation of extravasated neutrophils
- **Scale**   A detachable fragment of thickened keratin
- **Ulcer**   A discontinuity of epidermis
- **Vesicle**   A fluid filled lesion on the skin surface up to 5 mm diameter
- **Wheal**   A transient, elevated area of dermal oedema, the hallmark of urticaria

History and examination

Introduction

- Shake hands and introduce yourself.
- Consider the need for a chaperone.

History

- Enquire about presenting complaint and duration.
- Ascertain the patient's main concern about the condition (e.g. appearance, fear of cancer, pain, itching, etc.). Itching is usually the most prominent feature of atopic eczema, scabies, and dermatitis herpetiformis. Always remember that itching may also be caused by non-cutaneous disease (Hodgkin's disease, iron deficiency, thyroid dysfunction, etc.)
- If an eruption is extensive, ask how and where it began.
- Also enquire about:
  - Previous skin disease (broadly rashes and tumours)
  - Other previous medical disorders
  - Family history of skin disease
  - Drug history and allergies
  - Occupation and hobbies (e.g. gardening) may be relevant
  - Pets.

General inspection and examination

- Seat patient comfortably in a good light, preferably daylight.
- Clean your hands discreetly before and after the examination.
- Wear examination gloves if there is any suspicion of infection or infestation and when examining genitalia.

For images of patients with dermatological conditions, see the dermatology section of the clinical picture suite in the colour plate section.

Describing rashes

- Examine as much of the skin surface as practical, examine the hair and nails.

Record

- Distribution and pattern of the rash. Well-marginated? Diffuse? Discrete lesions?
- Colour and pigmentation. Erythema blanches, purpura does not blanch. Brown pigment may be haemosiderin or melanin. Drugs may also stain the skin.
- Erythema may be faint, livid, pink, red, blue, purple, violaceous, etc.

- Scaling. Large or small scales? Adherent? Continuous or at the periphery of lesions?
- Dryness, exudation, vesiculation (lesions <5 mm), bullae (lesions >5 mm)
- Is there erosion (partial loss of epidermis) or ulceration (full thickness loss)?
- Is the eruption flat and impalpable (macular) or palpable due to induration (hardening) or elevation (papules or plaques)?

Describing lumps

Record

- Location/distribution, size, shape, colour(s) and symmetry of lesion(s).
- Papules are <5 mm diameter, nodules are >5 mm diameter.
- Depth. Epidermal? Dermal? Within fat? Subcutaneous?
- Is the lesion tender?

Nail changes

- Onycholysis is separation of the nail plate from the nail bed. This is a characteristic feature of psoriasis.
- Pitting of the nails is seen in numerous dermatoses such as psoriasis, eczema, alopecia areata, lichen planus.
- Subungual haemorrhage may mimic melanoma (or vice versa). Splinter haemorrhages may occur in psoriasis, or result from sepsis (e.g. infective endocarditis). Both are usually due to trauma (which is more likely if splinters are acral).

Potassium hydroxide (KOH) preparation

- Obtain a generous sample of scale from the edge of the rash. Place this on a microscope side. Cover with a cover slip. Place a drop or two of 10% KOH at the edge of the cover slip and allow to run under the cover slip by capillary action. The KOH will dissolve the keratin in a few minutes, leaving fungal hyphae intact. Examine under the microscope (×20 or ×40 magnification) for fungal hyphae.
- This 'prep' is frequently invaluable for rapid diagnosis of dermatophyte infection.
- Placing a drop of KOH on top of a burrow, gently scraping the roof off the borrow and examining the contents in the same way can provide rapid and incontrovertible confirmation of scabies.

Examination using Woods (ultraviolet) lamp

Wood's light is an ultraviolet lamp used to:

- Highlight contrast in subtle pigmentary changes
- Elicit green fluorescence in tinea capitis infection with microsporum canis
- Elicit coral pink fluorescence in erythrasma.

Elicitation of dermographism

Although the triple response (erythema, wheal, and flare) is normal, it is exaggerated in dermographism. This is the commonest variety of physical urticaria (i.e. an urticarial eruption with a physical trigger) and often accompanies chronic idiopathic urticaria.

Stroke the skin on the back firmly (but not so hard as to cause any bleeding) with an orange stick or similar blunt pointed instrument. A positive test manifests as a palpable wheal developing at the site, usually within 5 minutes.

Student name:	Medical school:	Year:				

Dermatology

Please take a history and perform an examination on this patient with a skin disorder

		Self	Peer	Peer /tutor	Tutor
Initiating the consultation	● Greets patient, confirms patient's name	☐	☐	☐	☐
	● Introduces self, states role and purpose of interview, gains consent	☐	☐	☐	☐
	● Uses appropriate opening question to elicit presenting complaint(s)	☐	☐	☐	☐
	●	☐	☐	☐	☐
The presenting complaint	● Fully explores presenting complaint	☐	☐	☐	☐
	● Ascertains the patient's main concern about the condition	☐	☐	☐	☐
	●	☐	☐	☐	☐
Background and context	● Inquires about previous skin disease	☐	☐	☐	☐
	● Explores the patient's past medical history	☐	☐	☐	☐
	● Inquires about family history of skin disease	☐	☐	☐	☐
	● Explores drug history and allergies	☐	☐	☐	☐
	● Inquires about occupation and hobbies	☐	☐	☐	☐
	●	☐	☐	☐	☐
General inspection	● Washes hands with alcohol gel or soap and water	☐	☐	☐	☐
	● Expains procedure to patient and obtains verbal consent	☐	☐	☐	☐
	● Seats patient comfortably in a good light	☐	☐	☐	☐
	● Considers need of a chaperone	☐	☐	☐	☐
	● Wears examination gloves if appropriate	☐	☐	☐	☐
	●	☐	☐	☐	☐
Dermatological examination	● Examines as much of the skin surface as is practical	☐	☐	☐	☐
	● Accurately and fully describes any rash	☐	☐	☐	☐
	● Accurately and fully describes any lumps	☐	☐	☐	☐
	● Accurately and fully describes any nail changes	☐	☐	☐	☐
	●	☐	☐	☐	☐
Additional examination	● Can explain use of potassium hydroxide preparation	☐	☐	☐	☐
	● Can explain use of Wood's light	☐	☐	☐	☐
	● Can explain elicitation of dermographism	☐	☐	☐	☐
	●	☐	☐	☐	☐
Professionalism	● Covers patient, thanks patient, washes hands	☐	☐	☐	☐
	●	☐	☐	☐	☐
Self-assessed as at least borderline:	Signature:	Date:	U B S E	U B S E	U B S E	U B S E
Peer-assessed as ready for tutor assessment:	Signature:	Date:	U B S E	U B S E	U B S E	U B S E
Tutor-assessed as satisfactory:	Signature:	Date:	U B S E	U B S E	U B S E	U B S E

Notes

Unit 6   The full consultation

Background

It will often be necessary to take a full clinical history and perform a complete physical examination. The sequence has many variants, especially the examination, and our suggested one is presented in the clinical assessment at the end of this chapter. In practice you will rarely have more than 20–30 minutes to complete the whole process!

Throughout the consultation

- Provide structure and undertake in stages, each clearly signposted to the patient
- Establish rapport and build the relationship.

Initiating the session

- Hand washing (Figure 6.1), professional attire and readiness.
- Greet the patient and confirm their name.
- Introduce yourself, state your role and, if necessary, the purpose of the session.
- Obtaining consent may be appropriate if, for example, you rather than the patient have initiated the consultation.
- Identification of the patient's presenting complaint(s).

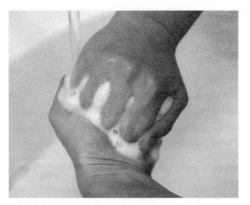

Figure 6.1 Every consultation should begin by washing your hands.

Taking the history

- The history of the presenting complaint
- Past medical history
- Treatment history and allergies
- Personal and social history
- Smoking, alcohol and recreational drugs
- Family history
- Review of other systems
- Ideas, concerns and expectations.

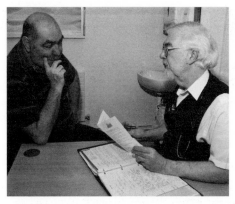

Figure 6.2 History taking.

Physical examination

With the patient reclining at 45°

- General inspection
- Examination of the hands and nails
- Pulse and blood pressure
- Palpation of the axillae for lymph nodes
- Examination of the eyes, face, mouth, and tongue
- Examination of the neck for lymph nodes, thyroid, trachea, jugular venous pressure, and carotid pulse
- Inspection, palpation, and auscultation of the precordium
- Inspection, palpation, percussion, and auscultation of the chest anteriorly.

Then sit the patient forward

- Inspection, palpation, percussion, and auscultation of the chest posteriorly
- Examination of the lumbosacral region.

Then lie the patient flat

- Inspection, palpation, percussion, and auscultation of the abdomen
- Examination of the groins, inguinal lymph nodes, hernial orifices and, if appropriate, the external genitalia
- Examination of the legs and feet.

Neurological, musculoskeletal, and breast examinations

- Neurological and musculoskeletal examinations are frequently omitted if the patient has no joint or neurological symptoms and general inspection reveals nothing to suggest disease.
- If necessary the GALS assessment (see Unit 3) can be used as a quick screen for musculo-skeletal problems.
- Routine examination of the female breasts is no longer advocated and is performed only if the patient reports a specific problem.
- If any of these examinations are required they are best performed after the general inspection and general examination and before examination of other systems.

Finally

- Consider rectal or vaginal examination
- Perform urine dipstick test: blood, glucose, protein, leucocytes, ketones

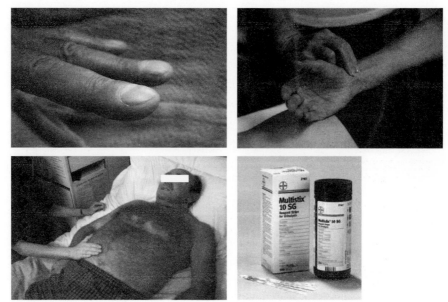

Figure 6.3 Physical examination.

Differential diagnosis

- **Biomedical**: working diagnoses based on clinical states and pathophysiology.
- **Patient's perspective**: an exploration of the patient's ideas, concerns, and expectations.
- **Social context**: factors that will or could impact on management (see Figure 6.4).

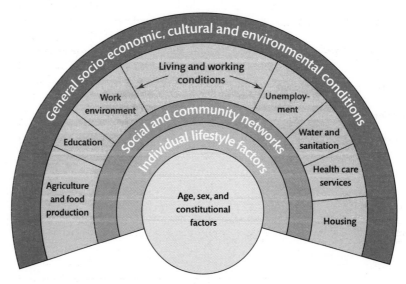

Figure 6.4 Dahlgren and Whitehead's model of the determinants of social health. From Dahlgren G and Whitehead M (1991): Policies and Strategies to Promote Social Equity in Health. Stockholm: Institute for Future Studies

Explanation and planning

- Give comprehensive information appropriate to the patient's needs
- Achieve a shared understanding that incorporates the patient's perspective.
- Involve the patient in decision making to the level they wish
- Negotiate a mutually acceptable management plan (Figure 6.5) and discuss medication.

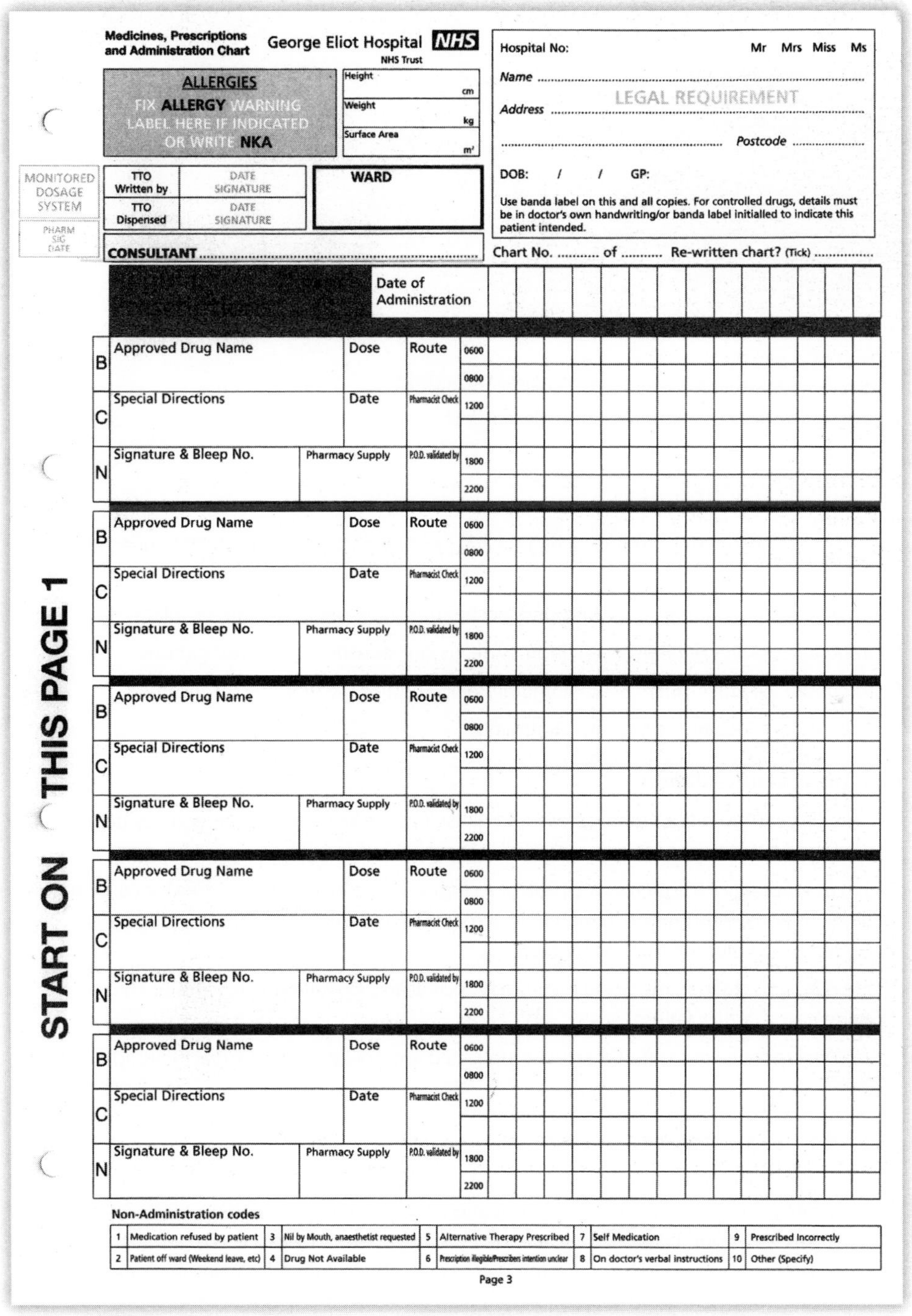

Figure 6.5 Drug chart.

Closing the consultation

- Agree the next steps for clinician and patient.
- Establish necessary safety nets.
- Summarize conclusions and check that the patient is satisfied.
- Complete all necessary documentation (Figure 6.6): legible and consistent with local and national standards.

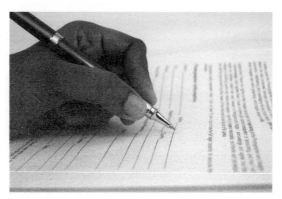

Figure 6.6 Clinician completing required documentation.

Presentation of findings

The Warwick four-point presentation is a succinct and organized way in which to present your findings. It consists of:

- *An introductory statement*: background, occupation, how referred, main problem
- *Important positive findings*: main findings on history, examination, investigations
- *Important 'negative' findings*: what findings help confirm the working diagnoses
- *The clinical conclusion*: a succinct summary.

Example of a presentation

- 'This 73-year-old retired miner presented himself to the accident and emergency department with a 2-hour history of severe central chest pain.'
- 'His description of the pain was typical of a cardiac origin. He has risk factors for coronary heart disease: hypertension, hypercholesterolaemia and a 45-pack year smoking history. His ECG shows ST elevation in leads V3–V6.'
- 'He is in sinus rhythm, his blood pressure is normal and examination reveals no clinical evidence of cardiac failure.'
- 'In conclusion, he has suffered an uncomplicated anterolateral myocardial infarction.'

Patient safety tips

✔ Safety nets are crucial. Do not assume that if you request a scan it will be carried out: request forms can go astray. A system in which a patient's survival may depend on a histology report finding its way from the pathology laboratory to the doctor's in-tray is not safe. Advise patients to contact you if they have not received an appointment for investigations within a specified period of time. Arrange a follow-up appointment to tie up loose ends unless you are totally confident that no further intervention is needed. *'I'll look at your test results and send you an appointment if I need to see you again'* is not safe management.

Student name: Medical school: Year:

The full consultation

This assessment will be based on taking a complete history and examination of a patient of your or the tutor's choice.

	Self	Peer	Peer /tutor	Tutor

Initiating the session

	Self	Peer	Peer/tutor	Tutor
● Hand washing, professional attire, and readiness	☐	☐	☐	☐
● Greet the patient and confirm their name	☐	☐	☐	☐
● Introduction, role and purpose	☐	☐	☐	☐
● Consent	☐	☐	☐	☐
● Identification of the patient's presenting complaint(s)	☐	☐	☐	☐
●				

Taking the history

	Self	Peer	Peer/tutor	Tutor
● The history of the presenting complaint	☐	☐	☐	☐
● Past medical history	☐	☐	☐	☐
● Treatment history and allergies	☐	☐	☐	☐
● Personal and social history	☐	☐	☐	☐
● Smoking, alcohol, and recreational drugs	☐	☐	☐	☐
● Family history	☐	☐	☐	☐
● Review of other systems	☐	☐	☐	☐
● Ideas, concerns and expectations	☐	☐	☐	☐
●				

Physical examination

With the patient reclining at 45°:

	Self	Peer	Peer/tutor	Tutor
● General inspection, hands, nails	☐	☐	☐	☐
● Pulse and blood pressure	☐	☐	☐	☐
● Palpation of the axillae for lymph nodes	☐	☐	☐	☐
● Examination of the eyes, face, mouth, and tongue	☐	☐	☐	☐
● Examination of the neck for lymph nodes, thyroid, trachea, jugular venous pressure, and carotid pulse	☐	☐	☐	☐
● Inspection, palpation and auscultation of the precordium	☐	☐	☐	☐
● Inspection, palpation, percussion and auscultation of the chest anteriorly	☐	☐	☐	☐
●				

Then sit the patient forward:

	Self	Peer	Peer/tutor	Tutor
● Inspection, palpation, percussion and auscultation of the chest posteriorly	☐	☐	☐	☐
● Examination of the lumbosacral region	☐	☐	☐	☐
●				

Then lie the patient flat:

	Self	Peer	Peer/tutor	Tutor
● Inspection, palpation, percussion and auscultation of the abdomen	☐	☐	☐	☐
● Groins, inguinal lymph nodes, hernial orifices and, if appropriate, the external genitalia	☐	☐	☐	☐
● Examination of the legs and feet	☐	☐	☐	☐
●				

Neurological, musculoskeletal, and breast examinations:

	Self	Peer	Peer/tutor	Tutor
● Can be omitted if patient has no joint or neurological symptoms and general inspection reveals nothing to suggest disease	☐	☐	☐	☐
● Consider GALS assessment	☐	☐	☐	☐
● Examine a female patient's breasts only if she reports a specific problem	☐	☐	☐	☐
●				

Finally:

	Self	Peer	Peer/tutor	Tutor
● Consider rectal or vaginal examination	☐	☐	☐	☐
● Perform urine dipstick test: blood, glucose, protein, leucocytes, ketones	☐	☐	☐	☐
●				

Differential diagnosis

	Self	Peer	Peer/tutor	Tutor
● Biomedical:	☐	☐	☐	☐
● Patient's perspective:	☐	☐	☐	☐
● Social context:	☐	☐	☐	☐
●				

Explanation and planning

- Give comprehensive information appropriate to the patient's needs   ☐ ☐ ☐ ☐
- Achieve a shared understanding which incorporates the patient's perspective   ☐ ☐ ☐ ☐
- Involve the patient in decision making to the level they wish   ☐ ☐ ☐ ☐
- Negotiate a mutually acceptable management plan   ☐ ☐ ☐ ☐
-

Closing the consultation

- Agree the next steps for clinician and patient   ☐ ☐ ☐ ☐
- Establish necessary safety nets   ☐ ☐ ☐ ☐
- Summarize conclusions and check patient satisfaction   ☐ ☐ ☐ ☐
- Complete all necessary documentation: legible and consistent with local and national standards   ☐ ☐ ☐ ☐
-

Throughout the consultation

- Provide structure and undertake in stages, each clearly signposted to the patient   ☐ ☐ ☐ ☐
- Establish rapport and build the relationship   ☐ ☐ ☐ ☐
-

			U B U B U B U B
Self-assessed as at least borderline:	Signature:	Date:	S E S E S E S E
Peer-assessed as ready for tutor assessment:	Signature:	Date:	U B U B U B U B S E S E S E S E
Tutor-assessed as satisfactory:	Signature:	Date:	U B U B U B U B S E S E S E S E

Notes

Suite 2 Procedural skills

Unit 7 Infection control, health, and safety

7.1 Hand washing
7.2 Infection control and surgical scrubbing up
7.3 Personal protective equipment
7.4 Moving and handling, and general health and safety skills

Unit 8 Diagnostic skills

8.1 Vital clinical signs
8.2 Venepuncture
8.3 Electrocardiography: cardiac monitoring and recording a 12-lead ECG
8.4 ECG monitoring and rhythm recognition
8.5 ECG: basic principles and interpretation
8.6 Peak expiratory flow rate meter, inhalers, and nebulizers
8.7 Spirometry
8.8 Urinalysis and pregnancy testing
8.9 Nose, throat, skin wound, and midstream urine sample collection
8.10 Nutritional assessment
8.11 Lumbar puncture
8.12 Arterial blood gas sampling and interpretation

Unit 9 Therapeutic skills

9.1 Oxygen therapy
9.2 Peripheral intravenous cannulation
9.3 Making up drugs for parenteral administration
9.4 Intradermal, subcutaneous, and intramuscular injections
9.5 Blood transfusion
9.6 Urinary catheterization: male and female
9.7 Local anaesthesia
9.8 Surgical suturing
9.9 Nasogastric tube insertion
9.10 Wound care and diabetes foot ulcer management
9.11 Blood glucose monitoring

Unit 7   Infection control, health, and safety

7.1 Hand washing

Background

Healthcare-associated infections affect thousands of patients in UK hospitals every year and result in serious illness, prolonged hospital stays, and even long-term disability and death. Pathogens can be transmitted from patient to patient on the hands of healthcare workers. Scrupulous hand hygiene is the most important single measure to reduce such infections. We have known about this for a long time as the 2009 World Health Organization (WHO) *Guidelines on Hand Hygiene in Health Care* states:

> *In 1847, Ignaz Semmelweis was appointed as a house officer in one of the two obstetric clinics at the University of Vienna … He observed that maternal mortality rates, mostly attributable to puerperal fever, were substantially higher in one clinic compared with the other (16% versus 7%). He also noted that doctors and medical students often went directly to the delivery suite after performing autopsies and had a disagreeable odour on their hands despite hand washing with soap and water before entering the clinic. He hypothesized therefore that 'cadaverous particles' … caused the puerperal fever. … Semmelweis recommended that hands be scrubbed in a chlorinated lime solution before every patient contact and particularly after leaving the autopsy room. Following the implementation of this measure, the mortality rate fell dramatically to 3% in the clinic most affected and remained low thereafter.*

Modern cynics will perhaps be persuaded by the fact that a hospital in UK that had the third highest rate for *Clostridium difficile* ended up in the best quintile after a concerted campaign by the new chief executive and her infection control team. Semmelweis was not so fortunate. His ideas did not gain acceptance – he often denounced prominent European obstetricians as irresponsible murderers – and he died in an asylum at the age of 47. His ideas on antisepsis were only later proven to be correct by Louis Pasteur.

Clinical indications

Wash hands with soap and water when:

- They are visibly dirty or soiled with blood or other body fluids
- Dealing with patients with diarrhoea or vomiting
- Before and after every shift and after visiting the rest room
- Contact with spore-forming bacteria is suspected.

WHO specifically defines '5 Moments' for hand hygiene as an *aide-memoire* to effective infection control:

- *Moment 1*   Before touching a patient
- *Moment 2*   Before a clean/aseptic procedure
- *Moment 3*   After body fluid exposure risk
- *Moment 4*   After touching a patient
- *Moment 5*   After touching patient's surroundings

Alcohol-based hand gel may be used in other circumstances. Hand washing should be undertaken before any patient contact. This includes history taking alone as physical contact; even a hand shake can transmit infection.

Physiological principles

Washing hands with soap and water removes pathogens from the skin mechanically. Alcohol gel kills many types of bacteria, including meticillin-resistant *Staphylococcus aureus* (MRSA), viruses, including influenza and human immunodeficiency virus (HIV), and fungi. However, it is not effective against non-lipid-enveloped viruses such as norovirus, spore-forming bacteria such as *C. difficile*, and protozoa. When such organisms are suspected washing with soap and water is necessary.

Contradictions

Emergency situations: you may not get an opportunity to wash your hands before attending to a cardiac arrest!

Method

Equipment and preparation

Ensure that your arms are bare below the elbows, your nails are short and all jewellery has been removed, although a plain wedding band is usually allowed. False nails or nail varnish are not allowed. Adjust water to a comfortable temperature, wet hands under running water, dispense one dose of soap into cupped hands, and create lather.

Explanation and consent

Although no explanation or consent is needed, it will be useful to have demonstrated hand washing with gel in front of the patient to reinforce that you have done this. This will reassure the patient!

Professionalism

Always adhere scrupulously to local policy and follow the advice of the infection control team to the letter.

Complications

The occupational health department should be contacted if soap or gel causes irritation.

Technique

Hand wash using an accepted technique. The steps in Figure 7.1 are slightly modified from Ayliffe's original technique from 1978. Hand wash using the eight-step technique for 10–15 seconds vigorously and thoroughly. Steps 1–6 consist of five strokes rubbing backwards and forwards; you should follow just these steps when using an alcohol-based gel wash.

Wet hands thoroughly with clean water

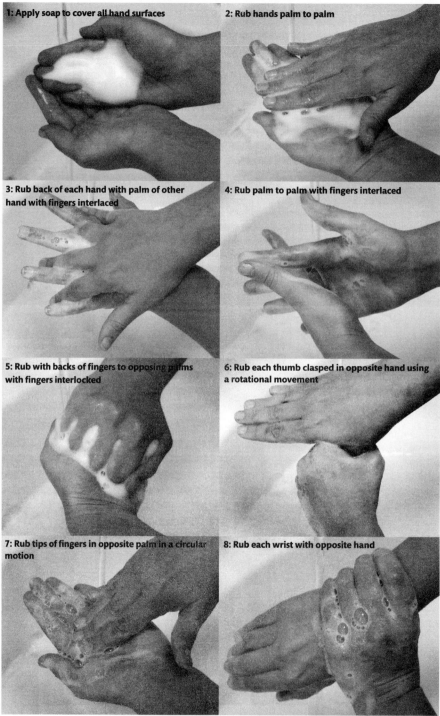

1: Apply soap to cover all hand surfaces

2: Rub hands palm to palm

3: Rub back of each hand with palm of other hand with fingers interlaced

4: Rub palm to palm with fingers interlaced

5: Rub with backs of fingers to opposing palms with fingers interlocked

6: Rub each thumb clasped in opposite hand using a rotational movement

7: Rub tips of fingers in opposite palm in a circular motion

8: Rub each wrist with opposite hand

Rinse hands with water and dry thoroughly with disposable paper towel
Hand washing should take 15-30 seconds

Figure 7.1 Hand washing technique.

Patient safety tip

✔ Patients should be fully aware of the importance of hand hygiene and positively encouraged to check that healthcare workers have washed their hands before physical contact.

Student name:	Medical school:	Year:

Hand washing

Please wash your hands using the eight-step technique.

		Self	Peer	Peer /tutor	Tutor
Explanation and consent	● Can explain why hand hygiene is important	☐	☐	☐	☐
	● Can state when to use soap and water and when to use alcohol gel	☐	☐	☐	☐
	●	☐	☐	☐	☐
Equipment and preparation	● Ensures that arms are bare below the elbows, nails are short, and all jewellery other than a plain wedding band has been removed	☐	☐	☐	☐
	● Adjusts water to a comfortable temperature, wets hands under running water, dispenses one dose of soap into cupped hands, and creates lather	☐	☐	☐	☐
	●	☐	☐	☐	☐
Procedure	*Hand wash using the eight-step technique for 10–15 seconds vigorously and thoroughly:*	☐	☐	☐	☐
	● Right palm over back of left hand and left palm over back of right	☐	☐	☐	☐
	● Palm to palm, fingers interlaced	☐	☐	☐	☐
	● Backs of fingers to opposing palms, fingers interlocked	☐	☐	☐	☐
	● Rotational rubbing of right thumb in left palm and vice versa	☐	☐	☐	☐
	● Rubbing of finger tips of right hand in left palm and vice versa	☐	☐	☐	☐
	● Rubbing of wrists	☐	☐	☐	☐
	● Rinse hands thoroughly under running water	☐	☐	☐	☐
	● Dry hands with a disposable paper towel.	☐	☐	☐	☐
	●	☐	☐	☐	☐
Post-procedure management	● Aware of the need to contact the occupational health department in the event of skin irritation	☐	☐	☐	☐
	●	☐	☐	☐	☐
Professionalism	● Understands the need of communicating the importance of hand hygiene to patients and colleagues	☐	☐	☐	☐
	●	☐	☐	☐	☐

				Self	Peer	Peer /tutor	Tutor
Self-assessed as at least borderline:	Signature:		Date:	U B S E	U B S E	U B S E	U B S E
Peer-assessed as ready for tutor assessment:	Signature:		Date:	U B S E	U B S E	U B S E	U B S E
Tutor-assessed as satisfactory:	Signature:		Date:	U B S E	U B S E	U B S E	U B S E

Notes

Source: World Health Organization (2009) *WHO Guidelines on Hand Hygiene in Health Care. First Global Patient Safety Challenge Clean Care is Safer Care 2009*. Geneva: WHO.

7.2 Infection control and surgical scrubbing up

Background

Infection control is both a process and a state of mind. The clinical environment is one in which many affected individuals can interact with unaffected, susceptible individuals. In other words, patients and clinical staff are both vectors and victims of infections. This is well illustrated by the example of the frequent outbreaks of norovirus with nausea and vomiting affecting staff and patients alike. The control of the spread of infection is a personal and a public health issue. Not only does it protect your patients but it also protects you. This chapter will not only deal with the public health aspects of infection control but will also cover the basics of what you need to be aware of in a ward, clinic, or theatre environment.

Consider disposal and recycling of waste in the most effective manner for reducing carbon dioxide emission and cost control. Clinical waste usually cost 200–400% extra for disposal in comparison to 'domestic waste', most of which can be recycled (paper and cardboard, glass, metal, batteries, etc.). Most hospitals in the UK do not recycle waste.

Infection control

Clinical Indications

To prevent yourself from being part of the chain of infection when working in a clinical environment.

- Assume that the person most likely to spread infection is you. You have the potential to spread infection to every single one of your patients.
- Simple measures can break the chain: hand washing, alcohol gel, gloves, aprons, and safe disposal of contaminated material.
- Attention to detail matters: apply the principles of infection to everything you do, every time you do it.

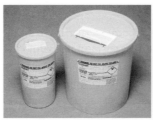 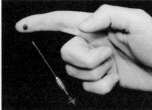 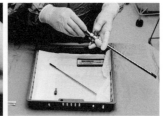

Always, always have a suitable sharps disposable bin handy when needed

An accidental needlestick injury: the anxiety, the fear, usually 100% preventable

Into the human body: Scrubbing up, key to safety

Figure 7.2 Images in infection control and surgical scrubbing up.

Anatomical and physiological principles

Your skin protects you from infection; it is a physical barrier keeping the outside, outside. For most day-to-day situations it is perfectly adapted and quite adequate. However, the hospital environment is not one for which we have specifically evolved so some extra help with our natural defences is required. Several species of commensal bacteria live on our skin; we need these as part of our defence against more serious pathogens. These serious pathogens are concentrated in hospitals, on and in the patients we care for. The chance of gathering them on our own skin is vastly increased and therefore the chance of passing them on to another person is also increased. Unfortunately, while we may be fit and healthy and able to fight off these pathogens, the other people in hospital are more likely to be unwell, immunocompromised, or otherwise unable to resist infection. The main premise of infection control is that it is much easier to prevent infection than to treat it and that it is unethical not to make concerted efforts to prevent infection.

Key principles

1 Prevention is better than cure.

2 Prevention is simple, cheap and reproducible.

3 Prevention is everybody's ethical responsibility.

4 If prevention is not possible, limitation of the spread of infection through timely isolation and intervention is the next step. This isolation can be escalated from a side room, to a ward, to a hospital as required. Intervention usually requires some form of immunological prevention (vaccination) or treatment (antibiotics, antivirals).

5 Sharps and needlestick injuries still happen in all hospitals in UK and are almost 100% preventable with the strictest of attention to good clinical practice.

Contraindications

None. There is never any excuse not to take appropriate infection control measures.

In sensitized individuals, or those with skin conditions such as eczema or dermatitis, the usual ward alcohol gels may not be appropriate but occupational health departments can provide different gel formulations that may be substituted or their use may simply have to be discontinued in favour of hand washing for a few individuals. Alternative soap products and gloves can also be provided.

Procedure

A good understanding of the pathogens you will be encountering is important, as is an appreciation of the ways in which your patients may be more at risk of infection. These ways will differ according to patient groups – respiratory patients will be more at risk of colonization with *Pseudomonas*, surgical patients will have wounds susceptible to *Staphylococcus* or *Streptococcus*, children will be vulnerable to *Haemophilus influenzae*.

Safe disposal of materials that have come from or been in contact with patients should be a priority in order to protect you, those who work alongside you, and other patients. Even if the patient you have just seen is well, transfer of bacteria from them to a more susceptible individual has the potential to be fatal.

Equipment

This is task specific. The general principles involve a few moments thought before you start any task. If you think through from preparation to waste disposal before you start you will have fewer false starts or 'excuse me while I just find ...' moments.

- **Preparation**: what infection control preparation do you need for the task? Will a squirt of alcohol gel suffice or do you need gown and gloves? Is a sharp bin needed?

- **Execution**: what are you about to do? Do you have the correct equipment? Have you a suitable place to carry out the procedure? If you are doing something on the ward, do you need to protect other patients from what you are about to do? Do you need an assistant? Are they protected?

- **Completion**: what are you going to do with any equipment you have used? Do you have a clinical waste bag for soiled disposables or dressings? Do you have a sharps bin? Do you have a trolley to move quantities of equipment safely without risk of dropping, spilling, sloshing, or jabbing something over or into other people? It might seem a pain to find a trolley before that bladder wash-out but you will be glad of it with a litre of blood stained urine in a kidney bowl on your way to the sluice.

- **Specifics**: these are specifics of the pathogen(s) in question and the routes by which it may endanger others.
  - ○ Bronchoscopy for patients with or suspected of having tuberculosis – protect any staff in the room with the correct FFP3 (filtering facepiece) face masks. Protect other patients when moving your at-risk patient from their negative pressure room with a FFP3 face mask.
  - ○ Venepuncture/other exposure prone procedures on individuals with known/suspected blood borne viruses – gloves, apron, eye protection, scrupulous attention to the disposal of sharps.

Professionalism

The GMC guide 'Good Medical Practice' section 43 states:

You must protect patients from risk of harm posed by another colleague's conduct, performance or health. The safety of patients must come first at all times.

You may sometimes think the 8-step guide to hand washing a little tedious, but hand washing saves lives. First do no harm.

Complications

Most of the complications arise from not paying attention to infection control measures with considerable morbidity and mortality.

Surgical hand antisepsis

Background

Hand washing aims to remove the surface contamination from skin prior to procedures to prevent casual contamination or infection. Surgical preparation takes this further. While total decontamination of the skin is not possible, surgical hand antisepsis is a systematized method of skin cleansing designed to minimize the transfer of bacteria into open surgical wounds. However, the stripping of all natural oils and commensal flora from your skin leaves it vulnerable to damage so attention should be paid to regular moisturizing in order to maintain skin health and integrity.

Clinical indications

Any practical procedure requiring a greater level of asepsis than normal. Mostly this means any surgical procedure where the skin will be intentionally broken and includes insertion of lines (central, femoral, Hickman, epidural) which will remain *in situ* and therefore act as foreign bodies for bacterial colonization and potential bacteraemia or sepsis.

Physiological principles

As for hand washing and infection control.

Contraindications

Some skin conditions will prevent a successful surgical hand antisepsis. Brushes, while soft, will tear already damaged skin. Using brushes to 'scrub' hands is no longer advocated. Some units use 'brushes' that are solid foam based. The detergents will aggravate inflammatory conditions and the cracks and fissures in broken skin will prevent successful decontamination. Good skin condition is essential.

Procedure

- **Collect equipment**: put on mask and eye protection. Open a surgical gown pack, only touch the outside of the wrappings. Open a pack of the correct size gloves and tip the inner packet onto the sterile paper without touching it.
- **Prepare for wash**: adjust the temperature of the water before you start. Wet your hands and arms to the elbow; allow the water to pass from fingertips to elbows but not to return.

- **Scrubbing up sequence**: use nail cleaning stick to clean under nails (dispose in sharps bin). Wash nails, fingers, hands, wrists and arms as far as the elbow using detergent. Make sure all the parts of the hand highlighted by the eight-point hand washing technique are thoroughly cleaned. There is evidence to suggest that chlorhexidine is more successful at skin decontamination than iodine-based detergents but use the one that suits your skin better. In general three washes are acceptable to most surgeons but certain procedures require fewer washes. If in doubt, ask your senior clinician.
  - ○ Wash: as above, rinse arms from fingertips to elbows.
  - ○ Wash: apply fresh detergent using elbow dispensers, repeat washing process from fingertip to elbow, stop just short of the point reached with the brush. Rinse.
  - ○ Repeat: dispense detergent into hands and wash along the forearms.
  - ○ Finally, wash your hands according to the eight-point technique. Rinse. Be careful not to allow water to run back towards your hands

- **Drying**: hold the towel in your dominant hand and dry arm from fingers towards the elbow. Fold the towel in half with dominant hand so that the wet side that touched other arm is now covered up. Transfer the towel to your clean and dry hand and dry dominant arm. Dry your dominant hand from fingers towards the elbow. Be careful not to touch your skin with your hand. Some surgical gown packs contain two disposable paper towels, one for each arm.

- **Surgical gowning**: hold gown with the neck uppermost and inner side facing you. Carefully allow gown to unfold until you can put your arms in. Be careful, when pushing your arms in that you do not accidentally de-sterilize yourself by touching anything such as scrub room walls or people. Do not allow your hands to exit the cuffs of the gown. An assistant will tie you into the gown.

- **Gloving**: keeping your hands inside the cuffs, open the inner packet of the sterile gloves. This next step is an art and requires practice. Only touching the folded back inner side of the gloves with the cuffs of the gown, manoeuvre one hand into a glove, trying to get as many fingers in the right place as possible and pulling the gloves over the gown cuffs. With the gloved hand only touching the outside of the other sterile glove, insert other hand similarly. Once the gloves are on and gown cuffs covered, adjust your fingers into glove.

- **Tying gown**: the last stage is to figure out which waist tie you pull out of the card before handing the appropriate end of the card to your assistant. You then turn full circle, wrapping the tie around your waist before carefully pulling the tie from the card and finishing the surgical scrub.

Post procedure

- An assistant will untie your gown. Pull the gown forward and off, this will partially invert the gloves over your hands. Discard it in the correct place (laundry bag if reusable, clinical waste bin if disposable).

- Being careful not to touch your hands with the dirty side of the gloves, remove them and discard in the clinical waste bin.

- Never, ever ball up a surgical swab and discard it inside a thrown away glove. The swab count is an essential part of surgical safety and you will delay closure of the wound or subject the patient to unnecessary irradiation as part of the search for a missing swab.

Professionalism

Once scrubbed, keep your hands together and close to your body until you approach the table. Once at the table, keep your hands on the drapes where they are visible but out of the way of instruments. This allows the surgeon to see that your hands are still sterile and to know where you are without having to look up from the operation. If you think you have de-sterilized yourself or some equipment at any point, do not be afraid to speak up even if you are asked to step back and re-scrub. It happens to everyone at some point and is an essential part of maintaining the sterile operating field.

Patient, healthcare professional, and personal safety tips

✔ **Sharp injury**: hospitals will have specific policies on how to deal with a sharps injury. The commonest reason for this is failure to dispose of a sharp safely and in the correct manner. Needles often end up in a domestic or clinical waste bag with the often-cited needlestick injury to cleaning and other staff. In the event of a sharps injury:

○ **First step**: in all cases wash with running warm water and encourage a little blood loss if sharp has caused bleeding in the first place. Apply dressing.

○ **Risk assessment**: ascertain whether this is a clean sterile sharp or contaminated. Assume contaminated if there is any doubt. Report to the occupational health department and complete an incident form.

○ **If there is penetration of skin or any other tissue or bleeding**: assume clinical contamination and seek occupational health support. In some cases samples may need to be taken from patient (if traced) for viral serology. Consent for the samples and testing will be entirely up to the patient. Specific therapy with antiviral agents may be needed in some cases (e.g. hepatitis or HIV risk).

○ **It is important to realize that the risk is very real but sufficiently low to reduce general anxiety**: 1 in 3 if definite hepatitis B contamination, 1 in 30 for hepatitis C, 1 in 300 for HIV.

✔ **Surgical scrub**: often you will be unsupervised when scrubbing up, pay obsessive attention to the correct technique at all times. If you accidentally touch the taps while rinsing your hands, start again. Touch your elbows when drying them – start again. This is tedious, but do you want to be responsible for a postoperative sepsis or a longstanding prosthesis infection?

Student name:	Medical school:	Year:

Surgical

Demonstrate how you would scrub for an operation.

		Self	Peer	Peer /tutor	Tutor
Equipment and preparation	● Selects the correct gown and size of gloves	☐	☐	☐	☐
	● Opens the surgical gown pack, maintaining the sterility of the contents. Opens the gloves packet in the correct manner and drops them onto the open gown pack	☐	☐	☐	☐
	● Put on facemask (and eye protection if appropriate)	☐	☐	☐	☐
	●	☐	☐	☐	☐
Explanation and consent	● Explains the difference between a simple handwash and a surgical scrub and when each is appropriate	☐	☐	☐	☐
	● Can discuss the reasons for surgical antisepsis especially with regard to foreign bodies (lines, meshes, or prostheses)	☐	☐	☐	☐
	●	☐	☐	☐	☐
Procedure	● Selects a detergent, opens pack, and adjusts water temperature	☐	☐	☐	☐
	● Cleans under fingernails and disposes of the pick in a sharps bin	☐	☐	☐	☐
	● Washes from fingertips to elbows and discards the brush before rinsing in the same direction	☐	☐	☐	☐
	● Repeats the wash with the sponge and extra detergent, discarding the sponge before rinsing	☐	☐	☐	☐
	● Washes hands using fresh detergent and the eight-point hand washing technique extending along the arms. Rinses from fingers to elbows as before	☐	☐	☐	☐
	● Picks up the towel without allowing water to run back down the arms from elbow to hand	☐	☐	☐	☐
	● Dries each hand and arm in turn, taking care not to use the same towel/side of the towel for each arm. Disposes of the towel correctly	☐	☐	☐	☐
	● Picks up and dons the gown correctly, without de-sterilizing on any surfaces and keeping hands inside the cuffs of the gown	☐	☐	☐	☐
	● Puts on the sterile gloves as described	☐	☐	☐	☐
	●	☐	☐	☐	☐
Post-procedure management	● Removes the gown and disposes it correctly	☐	☐	☐	☐
	● Removes gloves without touching the outside of the gloves with bare fingers. Disposes them in clinical waste bag	☐	☐	☐	☐
	●	☐	☐	☐	☐
Professionalism	● Understands the need to remain sterile and keep hands visible once scrubbed	☐	☐	☐	☐
	● Understands the etiquette of theatre and the reasons for the proscribed manners of preparation and behaviour	☐	☐	☐	☐
	● Is aware what to do if they become de-sterilized or if they de-sterilize any equipment during the operation	☐	☐	☐	☐
	●	☐	☐	☐	☐

				Self	Peer	Peer /tutor	Tutor
Self-assessed as at least borderline:	Signature:		Date:	U B S E	U B S E	U B S E	U B S E
Peer-assessed as ready for tutor assessment:	Signature:		Date:	U B S E	U B S E	U B S E	U B S E
Tutor-assessed as satisfactory:	Signature:		Date:	U B S E	U B S E	U B S E	U B S E

Notes

7.3 Personal protective equipment

Background

Personal protective equipment (PPE) is the first line of defence between you and your patient. It consists of simple physical barriers to infection or infestation. In most situations it is used to protect you from your patient and transmitting the infection further afield. In some situations it is used to protect the patient from you, for example, if the patient is neutropenic. Relatively basic PPE measures cost little and save lives.

Clinical indications

PPE is used for:

- **Highly infectious conditions**: PPE must be used for all interactions with these patients (for example: influenza, tuberculosis, *C. difficile,* herpes virus, or scabies infestation)
- **Exposure-prone procedures**: those which put you at risk of exposure to another person's bodily fluids or secretions (for example urinary catheterization, suturing, venepuncture, chest drains, per rectal examination).
- **Patients at risk of infection**: all interactions (for example chemotherapy patients, patients with immune suppression from acquired or congenital immune system deficiencies, transplant patients). This is called 'reverse barrier' infection control.

Anatomical and physiological principles

Intact skin is a very good barrier against most infectious agents but some viruses, bacteria, insects, and airborne pathogens are able to breach it. Different grades of mask can provide a barrier against spreading or being infected by airborne viruses and bacteria. Gloves provide an extra layer between your (susceptible) skin and your patients (infected/infested) skin. You are a powerful vector for the transmission of infection, so PPE protects not just you but all the other patients you will see that day and also your professional, social, and family contacts.

Contraindications

There are no absolute contraindications. Special adjustments may need to be made in relation to latex allergies by using nitrile gloves and using latex-free equipment.

Procedure

Cover all parts of you and your clothing that may come into contact with the patient or their bodily fluids/secretions. This includes your eyes if there is a risk of splashing. Dispose of any contaminated equipment in a safe and timely fashion.

Equipment

This will vary according to the situation but the basics are:

- **Gloves**: latex/nitrile, sterile/non-sterile as appropriate.
- **Apron**: usually plastic but may be colour coded, white for general tasks, red for barrier-nursed patients, yellow for general clinical use.
- **Eye protection**: arguably this should be used for all procedures, practically for any procedure where fluids are likely to be under pressure or in large enough volumes to be splashed. Protective goggles are used for this.
- **Facemask**: when there are airborne pathogens or your patient is at risk from your natural commensal microorganism or infections such as the common cold or influenza.

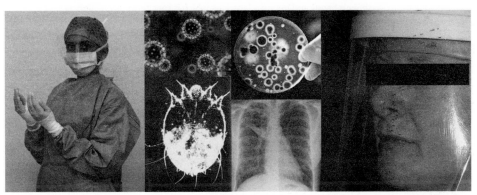

The goggles, mask, gloves and gown: these alone will provide a very high level of protection

Influenza, *Clostridium difficile*, scabies and TB: all controlled effectively by PPE

Many other pieces of equipment will be needed specific to the clinical situation

Figure 7.3 Images in personal protective equipment. Middle images: top left © Sebastian Kaulitzki/iStockphoto; top right © Alexander Raths/iStockphoto

Preparation

- First wash your hands. Hands are the way most infections are passed. Meditate on the phrase 'primum non nocere' (first do no harm).
- Gather your PPE and put it on close to the patient but outside the side room or bed area.
- Carry out your interaction with your patient.

Explanation to patient

Standard aspects of any clinical interaction such as introduction and explanation will apply. It is particularly important to explain to the patient the need for the specific infection control measure for several reasons, which include keeping the patient informed and allaying anxieties in relation to infection procedures.

Post-procedure management

This depends on the specific situation.

- **For airborne pathogens**: take off any gloves, aprons, etc. and dispose of them inside the room, but leave your mask on. Wash your hands inside the room. Exit and then remove your mask.
- **For physically transmitted pathogens**: remove all PPE in the room, wash your hands, and then leave the room.
- **For reverse barrier-nursed patients**: leave the room then remove your PPE. Then wash your hands.

Box 7.1 Typical clinical scenarios: use local guidelines if different

C. difficile

Your patient has had an episode of diarrhoea and has been moved into a side room as a precaution. You are still waiting for stool cultures.

Outside the room, clean your hands and put on gloves and apron. Take the minimum of items into the room (leave the notes and observations file outside). Have the minimum number of people enter the room. When finished, dispose of your apron and gloves in the yellow clinical waste bin in the room. Wash your hands then exit.

Tuberculosis

A patient with confirmed open pulmonary tuberculosis has been moved into a negative pressure side room.

Outside the room, wash your hands and put on a facemask which is specific for protection against tuberculosis. These are often the yellow and white 'duck' masks but this may vary between hospitals. Ensure that the mask fits well with a good seal and you are not breathing in air around the edges of the mask. If you are not about to perform an exposure-prone procedure, the only other PPE you may require is a pair of gloves. After finishing, exit the room closing the door firmly behind you and take off your mask. Dispose it of in a designated clinical waste bin. Wash your hands.

Norovirus

A patient is being nursed on a ward affected by norovirus. The ward is closed to admissions. Some policies will state that only gloves (apron) are needed.

There will be clean scrubs and a clean changing area on or just outside the ward. Change into scrubs and leave all non-essential items in the changing room (this does not include your bleep!). Enter the ward. Before seeing your patient, wash your hands, and put on gloves. Remove your gloves and dispose of in a clinical waste bin. Wash your hands. Leave the ward and go to the dirty changing area. Take off the scrubs and place them in a red dissolvable laundry bag. Wash your hands, then put your clothes back on.

Influenza virus

A patient suspected of having a serious viral illness and swine 'flu (influenza A/H1N1v) has been admitted to your ward.

Influenza virus is spread by inhalation of very small droplets. Surgical masks do not provide sufficient protection against these small droplets. The Health & Safety Executive (HSE) recommends the use of FFP3 masks for any interaction with patients who have or who are suspected of having pandemic influenza if you are likely to come within 1 m of the patient or be involved in a procedure which has a high risk of producing aerosols. Ask for all masks used for infection control, proper fitting of the mask is essential to its effectiveness. All other PPE should be chosen with regard for the task you are intending to perform.

Professionalism: thinking beyond the task

In all situations PPE and any other equipment used should be disposed of carefully and promptly in the correct yellow clinical waste containers. Any fluids should be dealt with appropriately in containers, sluice room, or decontamination facility. All of this should be done by you personally.

You should not put any other person, patient or member or staff, at risk of infection by leaving waste from your actions for someone else to tidy up.

Complications

Always make sure you know if the patient has latex allergy before you start.

Failure of your PPE is the most serious complication. At worst it can ruin your career and leave you with a lifelong health problem of your own. The reality is, while you can make a judgement about the risk a patient may pose to you when they have already had their condition diagnosed and tailor your PPE to the situation, you may be meeting them before a diagnosis has been made and unwittingly put yourself at risk. In order to protect yourself, you should consider all patients a potential source of infection and should always wash your hands before and after any contact.

Don't panic though, for most interactions with infectious patients your own immune system will protect you, but it will pay in the long run to take care of yourself first.

Patient safety tips

✔ **Consider the infectious agent and its mode of transmission**: if you have a patient with an infectious condition which could be transmitted to other patients (such as *C. difficile*, shingles [herpes zoster], MRSA, or scabies) it is advisable to isolate them in a side room where possible. Patients with more serious infections which may pose a threat to the wider public health (tuberculosis, especially multi-drug resistant tuberculosis) should be isolated in a negative pressure room.

✔ **Pressure rooms**: can give added safety in special circumstances

   ○ *Negative pressure* – the inside of the room is kept at a lower pressure than the atmosphere outside which has the effect of pulling the outside air into the room. This keeps the infectious agent inside from getting out (e.g. tuberculosis)

   ○ *Positive pressure* – the inside of the room is kept at a higher pressure than the atmosphere outside which has the effect of pushing the inside air out of the room. This keeps infectious agents from getting in (i.e. for neutropenic patients).

   The distinction seems obvious but is sometimes missed.

✔ **Break the chain of infection**: always be vigilant to infections spreading through a ward. Norovirus is often introduced by a relative or member of staff who thought 'oh, it's just a little bit of vomiting, I'll be ok'. The rules are: if you have any signs of diarrhoea or vomiting you must wait until you are free of all symptoms for 48 hours before returning to the ward. Staff may only suffer a couple of days of misery but your frail, elderly patients with multiple co-morbidities may not survive. Norovirus outbreaks close whole hospitals; and you can break the chain of infection.

PPE and infection control

Describe how you would prepare to examine a patient with confirmed *C. difficile* infection and your post-procedure management.

		Self	Peer	Peer /tutor	Tutor
Equipment and preparation	Considers the infectious agent and its mode of transmission	☐	☐	☐	☐
	Checks if the patient is allergic to latex	☐	☐	☐	☐
	Selects the correct equipment for the task	☐	☐	☐	☐
	Can discuss possible complications and risks of infection to the patient	☐	☐	☐	☐
		☐	☐	☐	☐
Procedure	Washes hands with soap and water or alcohol gel	☐	☐	☐	☐
	Dons the correct PPE – red apron and gloves – outside the patient's room	☐	☐	☐	☐
	Takes the minimum amount of things into the room, particularly leaving the notes outside	☐	☐	☐	☐
		☐	☐	☐	☐
Post-procedure management	Removes all PPE inside the room and disposes of it correctly in the clinical waste bin	☐	☐	☐	☐
	Washes hand with soap and water. Alcohol gel alone is not acceptable.	☐	☐	☐	☐
		☐	☐	☐	☐
Professionalism	Understands the need to dispose of any contaminated materials appropriately and immediately	☐	☐	☐	☐
	Communicates appropriately with nursing staff	☐	☐	☐	☐
		☐	☐	☐	☐
Complications	Understands the wider reasons for personal protection	☐	☐	☐	☐
		☐	☐	☐	☐
Patient safety tips	Infectious patients should be isolated appropriately	☐	☐	☐	☐
	Different infections require different PPE	☐	☐	☐	☐
		☐	☐	☐	☐

	Signature:	Date:	Self	Peer	Peer /tutor	Tutor
Self-assessed as at least borderline:			U B S E	U B S E	U B S E	U B S E
Peer-assessed as ready for tutor assessment:			U B S E	U B S E	U B S E	U B S E
Tutor-assessed as satisfactory:			U B S E	U B S E	U B S E	U B S E

Notes

131

7.4
Moving and
handling, and
general health and
safety skills

7.4 Moving and handling, and general health and safety skills

Background

The National Health Service (NHS) employs approximately 1.5 million people across about 400 organizations and when included with the wider social care sector, this figure rises to 1.7 million workers. It has been estimated that sickness absence costs the NHS alone £1 billion a year and this causes inevitable implications for the effective delivery of health and social care services. A considerable proportion of this is related to musculoskeletal problems secondary to moving and handling patients. It is essential to know how to move and handle patients and objects in general. This is both to avoid any harm to the patient and to ensure that healthcare professionals do not get injured. This section does not have a specific patient safety section as it all about patient and personal safety!

Clinical indications

In clinical care there are multiple different indications for moving and handling – many are in relation to nursing care, clinical examination, and therapeutic reasons. Some common examples are given below.

- **Clinical examination**: sitting up patient at 45° for cardiovascular examination, sitting upright and forward when listening for aortic regurgitation, supporting legs for reflexes, assessing gait.
- **Nursing care**: helping patient mobilize, bath, using the toilet, sitting in chair, helping patient get up after a fall, helping patient transfer from bed to bed, chair to bed, etc.
- **Therapeutic**: sitting patient upright for improved ventilation in a respiratory tract infection, postural drainage in bronchiectasis, positioning for pleural aspiration, lumbar puncture, etc.

Complications of inadequate moving and handling techniques

- **Carers**: the most common injuries that healthcare professionals experience are back injuries and shoulder sprains. It can often be a matters of many weeks or even months before there is full recovery.
- **Patients**: moving, handling, or lifting someone incorrectly can damage fragile skin resulting in bruising or even tears in the skin. Patients have also been reported to develop shoulder and neck injuries, increasing existing breathing difficulties. Incorrect handling increases shear and friction forces on the skin.

Legislative aspects of movement and handling

All healthcare organizations have policies on this topic both to reduce risk to the patient and staff member and to comply with legislation in this field. The main general principles originate from the *Health and Safety at Work etc. Act 1974*. It remains an enabling Act from which regulations, code of practice, and guidance are still made in relation to moving and handling.

Duties of employer: to ensure, so far as reasonably practicable, the health, safety, and welfare of all their employees and others who might be affected by the way they go about their work. The employer does this by:

- Provision and maintenance of systems of work
- Safety in the use, storage and transport of equipment
- Provision of information, instruction, training

- Maintenance of a safe workplace, including access and egress
- Maintenance of a safe and healthy working environment.

Duties of employee: The employee also has distinct responsibilities:

- To take reasonable care of their own health and safety, and those who may be affected by their acts or omissions
- To cooperate with their employer to enable compliance with personal health and safety duties

The Manual Handling Operations Regulations (MHOR) 1992 defined these operations as:

Any transporting or supporting of a load (including the lifting, putting down, pushing, pulling, carrying or moving thereof) by hand or bodily force.

Under the regulations employers must examine their entire manual handling operations in an attempt to reduce the number of manual handling injuries, particularly those affecting the back. The extent of an employer's duty to comply with the regulations is governed by the term 'reasonably practicable' which involves balancing the cost of preventive measures against the likely benefits accrued from their introduction.

Duties of employer

Under the regulations the employer must:

- **Identify** all manual-handling operations performed by their employees
- **Avoid** so far as reasonably practicable any manual handling operations that involve a potential risk of injury. This can be achieved by eliminating, automating, or mechanization
- **Assess** in a suitable and sufficient manner all hazardous manual handling operations that cannot, so far as is reasonably practicable, be avoided
- **Reduce** the risk of injury to their employees arising out of their performance of hazardous manual handling operations, to the lowest levels reasonably practicable
- **Review** and amend as necessary, any risk assessments particularly in relation to reportable injuries.

Duties of employee

Under the regulations, employees, while at work, are required to make full and proper use of any system of work provided for their use by their employer, in compliance with their duty to reduce risks of injuries associated with manual handling operations.

Anatomical and physiological principles

Anatomy of the back

The human spinal column provides support for the head and trunk, encloses and protects the spinal cord and is involved in most movements of the trunk and limbs. Because of these many diverse functions, the back has to be both strong and flexible. This is achieved by virtue of its elaborate arrangement of bones, joints, ligaments and muscles. The vertebral column itself consists of alternating layers of bones (vertebrae) and soft tissue (discs) (Figure 7.4). When viewed from the front or back it appears as a straight structure but from the side it assumes an elongated 'S' shape possessing four distinct regions:

- The cervical region: 7 vertebrae
- The thoracic region: 12 vertebrae
- The lumbar region: 5 vertebrae
- The sacral-coccygeal region: 9 fused vertebrae.

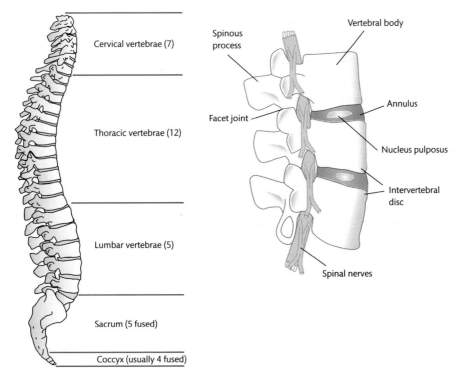

Figure 7.4 The spinal vertebrae.

A spinal segment consists of:

- Two vertebrae and the intervertebral disc between the two vertebrae
- The two nerve roots that leave the spinal cord at each side
- The facet joints, which link the vertebrae, sliding as we bend and twist. They stabilize the spine and protect the discs from excessive bending and twisting movements.

A typical vertebra consists of two functionally distinct parts:

- The vertebral body – which is the main weight-bearing structure
- The neural arch is a bony arch protecting the spinal cord.

The intervertebral disc

These are pads of cartilage linking adjacent vertebral bodies. They provide some shock absorption and allow movement of one vertebra on another. The disc is made up of two parts:

- The **annulus fibrosus**, which is made up of concentric rings of cartilage with fibres running in different directions which help take the strain of movement; it is tough, with the consistency similar to a fingernail
- The **nucleus pulposus**, which is a soft and hydrated jelly-like substance, which moves in response to the pressure exerted on it.

The function of an intervertebral disc is to absorb and dissipate forces transmitted through the spine. The application of a vertical load to the spine causes the disc to flatten and widen as the nuclear fluid is compressed and forced sideways across the disc. In a healthy disc the outer elastic coating of the disc resists these lateral forces. When the load is removed, the fibres of this coating recoil and the disc springs back to its original shape. The strain that the back can safely endure will vary from individual to individual. The ability to regenerate fluid in the discs diminishes with age. Sustained and repetitive loading reduces the volume of water in the intervertebral disc and can cause compression within the annulus. This also leads to increased loading on spinal joints. The ligaments become slacker and are less able to resist bending movements. The disc do not respond favourably to large loads applied in quick succession or those applied over a long period of time. Under these circumstances the recovery of the disc is prevented and it becomes permanently flattened. The disc narrowing is accompanied by a progressive degeneration of the annular fibres with loss of elasticity and consequent loss of the ability to absorb and dissipate future spinal loads decreases. These structural changes can lead to the complete rupture of a disc.

Effect of movement and handling injuries

- **Personal**: pain and suffering to individuals and poor quality of life. In addition to the victim themselves, workplace injuries may also affect their family, friends, and colleagues.
- **Economic**: musculoskeletal disorders (MSDs) are the most common cause of occupational ill health, currently affecting 1.2 million people per year and costing society £5.7 billion. The cost to employers is in the region of £600 million. An estimated 12.3 million working days a year are lost to work-related MSD.
- **Legal**: The legal reasons for preventing accidents in the workplace include the possibility of civil litigation and criminal prosecution.

Avoiding musculoskeletal injuries

- Good/correct posture: traditionally 'good posture' has implied 'erect/straight body position' but if maintained this can impose a greater strain on the body. The ideal posture should be a position of balance where the three vertebral curves are maintained in their ideal, natural 'S' position; requiring minimum effort to maintain but providing maximum mobility and function, maintaining its natural line of gravity. The correct posture in any physical activity is one that:
  ○ Maintains the balance of the body
  ○ Maintains the natural curvature of the spine
  ○ Minimizes the level of spinal stress.

When the spine is in its natural 'S' position it is deemed to be 'safe, strong and secure'. If poor posture is adopted the spine tends to adopt an unsafe 'C' shape where 'care and caution' is needed.

Ergonomics and risk assessment

Ergonomics is a science concerned with the 'fit' between people and their work. It puts people first, taking account of their capabilities and limitations to design safe, effective, and productive work systems. Ergonomics aims to make sure that tasks, equipment, information, and the environment suit each worker, and aspects to consider include:

- The job being done and the demands on the worker
- The equipment used (its size, shape, and how appropriate it is for the task)
- The information used (how it is presented, accessed, and changed)
- The physical environment (temperature, humidity, lighting, noise, vibration)
- The social environment (such as teamwork and supportive management)
- The physical aspects of a person: body size and shape, fitness, and strength
- Posture and the senses, especially vision, hearing, smell and touch
- The stresses and strains on muscles, joints, nerves
- Psychological aspects, such as: mental abilities, personality, knowledge, experience.

Specific examples of health and safety in the working environment

Computer work

- Screen and mouse position, chairs allowing comfort and correct posture.

- Hardware and/or software are not suitable for the task or the person, causing frustration and distress.
- Not enough breaks or changes of activity resulting in mistakes and poor productivity, stress, eye strain, headaches, and other aches or pains.

Manual handling

- The load is too heavy and/or bulky, placing unreasonable demands on the person.
- The load has to be lifted from the floor and/or above the shoulders.
- The task involves frequent repetitive lifting.
- The task requires awkward postures, such as bending or twisting.
- The load cannot be gripped properly.
- The task is performed on uneven, wet, or sloping floor surfaces.
- The task is performed under time pressures and incorporates too few rest breaks.

These problems may result in physical injuries such as low back pain or injury to the arms, hands, or fingers. The problems may also contribute to the risk of slips, trips, and falls.

Work-related stress

- Work demands are too high or too low.
- The employee has little say in how they organize their work.
- Poor support from management and/or colleagues.
- Conflicting demands, e.g. high productivity and quality.

Managing the working day

- Insufficient recovery time between shifts.
- Poor scheduling of shifts.
- Juggling shifts with domestic responsibilities.
- Employees working excessive overtime.

These problems may lead to tiredness or exhaustion, which can increase the likelihood of accidents and ill health. Attention to health and safety can ameliorate most of these problems relatively easily. Risk assessment to identify hazards in the workplace should be done proactively to minimize risks (is something with the potential to cause harm) and risk (the chance, great or small, that someone will be harmed by the hazard).

Safe manual handling

General principles from MHOR include:
- **Avoid** hazardous manual handling operations so far as is reasonably practicable
- **Assess** any hazardous manual handling operations that cannot be avoided
- **Reduce** the risk of injury so far as is reasonably practicable.

Manual handling

An ergonomic approach reduces and controls the risk of injury.

The task

Specific action that occurs during the procedure:
- Posture of carer – avoid stooping
- Ensure load close to trunk

- Avoid twisting or bending the trunk sideways
- Ensure sufficient rest or recovery period
- Involve more people if needed
- Allow enough time and plan task: avoid obstacles
- Ensure safe to progress.

The individual characteristics

Each individual carer is different, consider safety by reflecting on:

- Handling skill and experience
- Familiarity with patient
- Familiarity with handling equipment
- Fitness, strength, height to do task
- Clothing and footwear: ?suitable
- Is the individual pregnant, does he or she have a disability or health problem?

The 'load'

The load is the person or object being moved. Factors to consider are:

- Diagnosis, limitations
- What can they do for themselves?
- Is the patient likely to act unpredictably?
- Weight, height, and shape
- Fatigue
- Physical constraints.

The equipment

Often there are small handling aids such as slide sheet, spinal boards. Mechanical equipment such as hoists is now widely available:

- Ensure that the equipment is fit for purpose and well maintained.
- Only use if you are adequately trained to do so.

The environment

The environment is the area you will perform the task in.

- Ensure there are no space constraints preventing good posture.
- Adjust furniture, e.g. bed for comfort (profile, height to avoid stooping).
- Ensure the floor is safe (not slippery or unstable).
- Ensure there is adequate lighting.
- Ensure there is a comfortable physical environment.

Toolbox of efficient movement and handling principles

Safe manual handling begins at your feet and progresses upwards. There should be an awareness of good posture and movement throughout any handling task. See Figure 7.5.

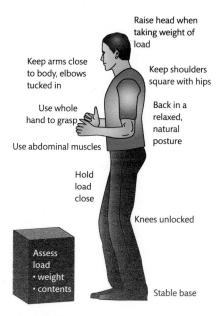

Raise head when taking weight of load

Keep shoulders square with hips

Keep arms close to body, elbows tucked in

Use whole hand to grasp

Back in a relaxed, natural posture

Use abdominal muscles

Hold load close

Knees unlocked

Assess load
• weight
• contents

Stable base

Figure 7.5 Manual handling.

Dynamic stable base

Muscular most efficient when operating on a stable base. Feet to be placed so as to be secure yet adaptable to ensure good balance during movement.

- Keep line of gravity within the base made by the feet: larger base is more stable
- Feet slightly apart with weight evenly distributed with feet free to move as appropriate
- Knees soft to prepare muscles
- Back muscles relaxed
- Movement easy and fluid
- Enables more powerful effort

Movements

Lifting/pushing: one foot placed in front, other foot pointing forward, causing the large tendon at the back of this ankle to be stretched as the body moves forward, so calf muscles contract automatically to produce good thrust.

Moving sideways: the advanced foot should point out in the direction of movement to allow the body to 'follow through' to avoid stiffening of lower limbs and back muscles, knees relaxed to allow the feet to adjust automatically and allow follow through.

Kneeling: soft support (harsh surface can cause muscle stiffening), efficient kneeling involves putting one leg out behind you and lowering the body to kneel on it.

Bed work: height should be adjusted depending on the task. Keep knees/hips soft. If two people of unequal height are working together the bed should be positioned to suit the shorter person.

Natural curves

Back should be in a relaxed, natural posture. Maintain the 'S' shape spine: *strong, safe, secure*. The more erect the back, the easier the load will be on the back.

Soft knees and hips

Shoulders should be level and facing the same direction as the hips. Relaxed knees/hips reduces the risk of top heavy bending.

Box 7.1 Moving and handling – the rules
....

No twisting – frequent bending and twisting action creates high levels of muscle activity and higher resultant spinal loads.

Effective muscle use – relax your muscle first prior to use.

Indirect hold – 'palm hold'. Gripping with the fingers is inefficient and fatiguing. A more diffused palm hold gives greater security. The elastic recoil of the palmar skin and tendons help to sustain the hold. This achieves:

- Comfort for patient/carer: less skin pressure
- Contact made from an extended palm that relaxes on contact to provide a large grip surface area
- Avoids pincer grip, that causes concentration of pressure and tension in hands/forearms.

Chin in/head up – this allows the spine to form natural curves and raises the chest to improve respiration. The shoulders are conditioned to allow more efficient arm action.

Elbows close to body – arms tend be used as levers, so be close to the fulcrum. It is a mistake to make hands and forearms do the work while stretched out from the body (except for pushing/pulling when arms transmit body weight).

Close to load – the risk of damage increases with:

- Weight of load
- Distance of load from the body
- Inclination of the trunk

Breathing

The abdominal muscles are arranged in sheets to protect organs. In inspiration, the diaphragm descends and abdominal muscles contract increasing intra-abdominal pressure, reducing stress on discs by supporting the back.

Use of the body weight

With the use of dynamic stable base, body weight transfer will overcome resistance to movement reducing the amount muscular effort needed.

Forces

Think of the desired direction of movement when applying a force to move a load. Most of the force should be directed in the direction of movement. Keep the chin in to stabilize the shoulders and align spine. Direction should be as horizontal as possible. The load on the disc is greater when pulling than pushing.

Friction

If movement is to be assisted use low friction surfaces (slide sheets). If movement to be resisted, high friction will be used (glide and lock sheets).

Commands and team communication

Establish a team leader, ensure all understand the command and remember to include the patient! Confirm '**Are you ready?**' then the command '**Ready, steady, MOVE (sit, stand, etc**.)'

Summary of lifting technique (Figure 7.6)

- Never lift above shoulder height.
- Make sure your feet are stable.
- Take a firm hold.
- Keep any weight close to your body.
- Keep your back straight and bend your knees.
- Lift as smoothly as possible.

139

7.4
**Moving and
handling, and
general health and
safety skills**

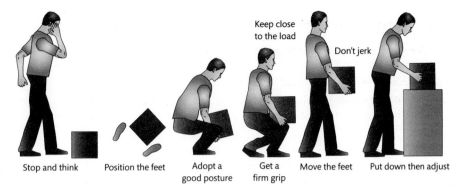

Keep close
to the load

Don't jerk

Stop and think | Position the feet | Adopt a
good posture | Get a
firm grip | Move the feet | Put down then adjust

Figure 7.6 Summary of the lifting technique.

Movement and handling in special circumstances

Bariatric patients

These patients have an assessed weight of 160 kg or more and a body mass index of >40 kg/m^2. Clearly specialized manoeuvres may be required with additional team members. An increasing array of specialized equipment is available, such as hoists integral to a personal bed.

The falling patient

No attempt should be made to catch a falling patient, as this can cause injury to the healthcare professional's spine. If safe to do so, attempt to protect the patient's head during a fall, but not at the risk of injury.

Assisting the fallen patient

To assist a patient from the floor following a fall:

- Assess their physical condition – ?movement may aggravate any new or existing injury.
- If there is no immediate danger for the patient they should be made comfortable.
- Equipment such as hoists, 'manager' inflatable devices, and emergency slide sheets and other helpers should be gathered as necessary
- An immediate rescue should only be conducted in an emergency situation, e.g. danger from fire, flooding or risk of explosion, etc.

Cardiac arrest patient

This patient does not need to be moved to a bed for cardiopulmonary resuscitation (CPR). From a chair, the patient should be lowered to the floor using a safe and suitable manual handling technique. CPR should be carried out on the floor. If there is restricted access, move furniture or slide patient horizontally across the floor (consider sliding sheets). Poor access to patient may result in injury to the rescuer and reduce the mechanical efficiency of CPR.

Student name: Medical school: Year:

Moving and handling

You will be asked some questions in relation to moving and handling in clinical practice. You will also be asked to demonstrate how you would lift a box and move a manikin onto a bed with the help of a colleague.

	Self	Peer	Peer /tutor	Tutor
What are the clinical indications for moving and handling a patient in clinical care? Clinical examination, nursing care, therapeutic	☐	☐	☐	☐
What are the complications of inadequate moving and handling techniques? *Healthcare professional*: back injuries, shoulder sprains. *Patients*: damage fragile skin, shoulder and neck injuries, increase existing breathing difficulties	☐	☐	☐	☐
What are the main duties of the employer in relation to this topic? To ensure the health, safety and welfare of all their employees, by:	☐	☐	☐	☐
● Provision and maintenance of plant and safe systems of work	☐	☐	☐	☐
● Safety in the use, storage and transport of equipment	☐	☐	☐	☐
● Provision of information, instruction, training	☐	☐	☐	☐
● Maintenance of a safe workplace, including access and egress	☐	☐	☐	☐
● Maintenance of a safe and healthy working environment	☐	☐	☐	☐
●	☐	☐	☐	☐
What are the main duties of the employee?	☐	☐	☐	☐
● To take reasonable care of their own health and safety and those who may be affected by their acts or omissions.	☐	☐	☐	☐
● To cooperate with their employer to enable compliance with personal health and safety duties	☐	☐	☐	☐
●	☐	☐	☐	☐
Anatomical and physiological principles	☐	☐	☐	☐
Discuss the anatomy of the back generally and in relation to movement and handling. Arrangement of bones, joints, ligaments, and muscles, cervical region (7 vertebrae), thoracic (12), lumbar (5), sacral-coccygeal (9 fused)	☐	☐	☐	☐
Discuss the function of the vertebral body and intervertebral discs in weight-bearing. Vertebral body, main weight-bearing structure. Neural arch protects spinal cord. Disc, two parts: *annulus fibrosus* (tough rings of cartilage with fibres which take the strain of movement), *nucleus pulposus* (soft jelly, distorts to pressure exerted)	☐	☐	☐	☐
What are the personal, economic, and legal effects of injuries?	☐	☐	☐	☐
What is the ideal posture in avoiding musculo-skeletal injuries? Position of balance with the three vertebral curves are maintained in their ideal, natural 'S' position; requiring minimum effort to maintain but maximum mobility and function	☐	☐	☐	☐
Discuss some of the efficient movement principles that apply to any moving and handling: dynamic stable base, natural curves, soft knees and hips, no twisting, effective muscle use, indirect hold 'palm hold', chin in/head up, elbows close to body, close to load, breathing, use of the body weight	☐	☐	☐	☐
Establish a team leader: ensure all understand the command and remember to include the patient! Confirm 'Are you ready?' then the command *Ready, Steady, MOVE.*	☐	☐	☐	☐
Please can you show how you would lift this box from the ground onto this table which is approximately 70 cm off the ground. Summary of technique: never lift above shoulder height, make sure your feet are stable, take a firm hold, keep weight close to your body, keep your back straight and bend your knees, lift as smoothly as possible.	☐	☐	☐	☐
Please can you help move this patient/manikin further up the bed into a 45° position for ease of breathing: Uses above principles and cooperates with colleague to coordinate the moving of the patient/manikin together	☐	☐	☐	☐

Self-assessed as at least borderline:	Signature:	Date:	U B / S E	U B / S E	U B / S E	U B / S E
Peer-assessed as ready for tutor assessment:	Signature:	Date:	U B / S E	U B / S E	U B / S E	U B / S E
Tutor-assessed as satisfactory:	Signature:	Date:	U B / S E	U B / S E	U B / S E	U B / S E

Notes

Unit 8   Diagnostic skills

8.1 Vital clinical signs

Background

Vital clinical signs are simple bedside observations which can be carried out by medical, nursing and ancillary staff in a short space of time. Very useful clinical information can be obtained from these observations but should always be contextualized to the individual patient and their clinical state and needs. Trends will often be more useful than single readings. Several ways of looking at the observations as a composite exist, which are of particular use in picking up patients who are deteriorating.

The commonest clinical parameters used are:

- **Temperature**: normal range 36.5–37.5 °C
- **Blood pressure**: 90/60 mmHg to 140/90 mmHg
- **Pulse**: 60–100 per minute
- **Respiratory rate**: 12–20 breaths per minute
- **O_2 saturation on room air**: 94–98% usually, 88–92% for COPD patients.

Certain hospitals measure additional information, as routine, in all patients such as urine output, glucose levels, pain, and level of consciousness.

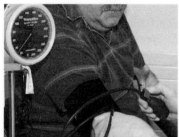

Blood pressure measurement: accurate clinical readings require a high degree of skill

Malaria by numbers...

1,000,000 killed by malaria a year
900,000 of those are young children in sub-Saharan Africa
71% of all deaths are under five
£6.2bn cost to Africa in lost GDP which accounts for 40% of the continent's public health spending
2,000 reported cases of imported malaria in the UK each year

Malaria: worldwide burden is immense, condition often missed in all settings. Characteristic fever is key to diagnosis

Score	3	2	1	0	1	2	3
Resp rate	<9			9-14	15-20	21-29	>29
Heart rate		<41	41-50	51-100	101-110	111-129	>129
Sys BP	<71	71-80	81-89	90-159	160-169	170-199	>199
Temp		<35		35-38.4		>38.4	
AVPU				Alert	Voice	Pain	No response

MEWS score: essential to pick up deteriorating patient early and managing aggressively

Figure 8.1 Images in vital clinical signs.

Physiological principles and techniques

Temperature

The majority of wards now use electronic temperature probes to assess the patient's temperature. The device is simple to use. A disposable tip is inserted over the end of the probe and it is placed into the patient's ear (or axilla). It is held there for 3–5 seconds when a bleep will indicate that the temperature has been read. Mercury thermometers are rarely used in UK clinical practice.

Clinical aspects

- **Fever**: various definitions exist but a temperature rise above the patient's normal temperature by 0.5° or more is useful. In most cases this is a temperature above 37.5 °C. A fever indicates infection, inflammation (e.g. autoimmune conditions such as rheumatoid arthritis, neoplasm, drug reactions, heat stroke, thyrotoxicosis, addisonian crisis)

- **Specific fever types**:
  - ○ **Relapsing fever**: febrile attacks lasting a few days followed by afebrile periods – conditions such as malaria, tuberculosis, brucellosis, Hodgkin's disease, familial Mediterranean fever.
  - ○ **Pel-Ebstein fever**: relapsing fever due to Hodgkin's disease.
  - ○ **Charcot intermittent fever**: rigors, right upper quadrant pain, and jaundice due to intermittent obstruction of the common bile duct.
  - ○ **Malarial fevers**: quotidian (daily fever, due to two distinct groups of *Plasmodium vivax* that sporulate every 48 hours or *P. vivax* and *P. falciparum* together), tertian fever (every 48 hours, typical of *P. vivax*), quartan fever (fever every 72 hours, typical of *P. malariae*), malignant tertian fever (fever and acute cerebral, renal and gastrointestinal manifestations every 48 hours due to *P. falciparum*). More recently, *P. knowlesi* has also been recognized.
  - ○ **Pyrexia of unknown origin** (**PUO**): defined as a fever of at least 38 °C for at least 3 weeks or more without an identifiable cause. With extensive investigation the following are the more common causes: infections (such as: abscess formation, malaria, tuberculosis, human immunodeficiency virus [HIV], endocarditis, fungal infection), neoplasms (such as lymphomas, renal tumours, hepatomas), autoimmune conditions (such as systemic lupus erythematosus, rheumatoid arthritis) and skin conditions (such as drug rashes, psoriasis).

- **Hypothermia**: this is a temperature of less than 35.0 °C. Be aware that some automated thermometers may be less accurate at recording low temperatures. Common causes include poor thermoregulation in elderly patients following exposure to low ambient temperature due to the weather or poor heating, other forms of environmental exposure, severe sepsis, hypothyroidism, adrenal insufficiency, drug or alcohol intoxication.

Blood pressure

Electronic devices are used to record blood pressure in the vast majority of cases. However, there will be instances where electronic devices fail or one is not available. You should therefore be able to record the blood pressure using a manual technique. Mercury sphygmomanometers are being phased out due to the small but distinct risk of mercury intoxication due to spillage and vaporization. Aneroid devices are generally used for manual recording of blood pressure. The procedure below has been adapted from the British Hypertension Society Guidelines 2010.

Method and physiological principles

Explanation, consent, and position

Outline procedure and state that some discomfort may be felt when the cuff is fully inflated but that this will only last a few seconds. Ensure the patient is rested, in a calm, quiet area with feet flat on the floor and back rested or supine. Ideally, there should be a 5-minute rest. The arm should be horizontal and supported at the level of the mid-sternum, rested on a table, chair, or pillow with restrictive clothing removed. An unsupported arm below the mid-sternum will overestimate the systolic and diastolic and vice versa.

Blood pressure cuff

Check size: the bladder component must be at least 80% of the arm circumference at the mid-humeral point. Apply cuff and secure to arm above the antecubital fossa. There should be a mark on the cuff as to where it should be applied in relation to the brachial artery.

- **Brachial artery**: locate by palpation (medial to biceps tendon) and then inflate cuff by pumping the blood pressure bulb after ensuring the seal at the blood pressure bulb is locked.

Inflate cuff to 70 mmHg rapidly then in increments of 10 mmHg until pulse disappears and then reappears during deflation. Note this number (the estimated systolic blood pressure).

- **Auscultation**: apply stethoscope to brachial artery just above the antecubital fossa.

  - Inflate blood pressure cuff until 20 mmHg above the estimated systolic. No sounds should be heard as the higher than systolic cuff pressure should have occluded the brachial artery with no sound from flow possible at the antecubital brachial artery.

- **Systolic**: Deflate the cuff in 2 mmHg decrements per second until repetitive, clear tapping sounds first appear for at least two consecutive beats. At this point the cuff pressure has become just less than the blood pressure. This is known as Korotkoff's first sound and is the systolic pressure.

- **Diastolic**: continue to deflate cuff again. Korotkoff's second and third sound are softer 'swishing' sounds and then become louder as the blood flows into the brachial artery below the now partially occluded cuff. Korotkoff's fourth sounds are distinct muffling sounds that become soft and blowing. When the sounds disappear, this means that there is no obstruction (or turbulence) to blood flow due to the cuff pressure. The cuff pressure at which the Korotkoff's sounds disappear is the diastolic blood pressure (Korotkoff's fifth sound).

- **Blood pressure recoding**: The systolic and diastolic should be recorded, rounded upwards to the nearest even number, e.g. 152/86 mmHg. Be aware of digit preference! These are often guesses that usually end in 5 or 0.

- **Korotkoff's fifth or fourth sound?** In children, pregnancy and sepsis, Korotkoff's fifth sound can often be heard down to 0 mmHg. If this is the case the diastolic should be recorded as the initial muffling of the sounds before they disappear (Korotkoff's fourth sound). Writing the blood pressure as 152/86/8 denotes that the systolic was 152, diastolic as per 4th Korotkoff's sound 86 but that the sounds only disappeared at 8 mmHg.

- **Record blood pressure**: immediately after measurement lest you forget!

Clinical aspects

- **Repeated measurements**: If the blood pressure is elevated for the clinical condition of the patient, then this should be repeated after at least 1 minute. Ideally the patient should not have taken caffeine-based drinks or smoked within the last few hours.

- **Correct cuff size**: at least three distinct sizes are required in children with the standard larger cuff sufficing for most obese people. Using a small cuff (less than 80% of arm circumference) will result in an overestimation of the blood pressure.

- **? Both arms**: The pulse should be palpated in both arms, if there is a difference in quality or character then coarctation of the aorta or even dissection of the aorta should be suspected and blood pressure measured in both arms. Other causes of variation include anatomical variants and the sequelae of surgery such as cardiac catheterization.

- **Cardiac arrhythmias especially atrial fibrillation**: this can lead to a rough measurement only unless taken several times due to the variability in cardiac output.

- **Pregnancy**: sitting position is advocated as the lying position can lead to hypotension due to the mechanical effect of the gravid uterus on the major vasculature. Disappearance of the sounds (Korotkoff's fifth sound) is recommended for measurement of the diastolic blood pressure.

- **Cardiovascular risk profiling**: blood pressure should be measured at least yearly in clinical practice. It is not clearly specified when this should start but several national cardiovascular risk assessments stipulate a full profile including blood pressure, full lipid profile, waist circumference, diabetes screening, assessment of diet, physical activity and smoking status every 5 years starting at the age of 40. Higher risk groups such as the South Asian population and those with a significant family history of cardiovascular disease (CVD) before the age of 60 will start having risk assessment earlier. The British Hypertensive Society has published detailed guidelines on the classification of hypertension (Table 8.1). In clinical practice, hypertension needs to be treated in an individual patient if evidence suggest benefits of treatment.

- **Associated clinical conditions**: the majority (95%) have essential or primary hypertension. Several clinical conditions have hypertension as an associated sign or actually characterizing the condition: type 2 diabetes, thyrotoxicosis, hypothyroidism, Cushing's syndrome, Conn's syndrome, phaeochromocytoma, pre-eclampsia in pregnancy, or even distress or anxiety.
- **Hypotension**: hypotension is often seen in patients with postoperative bleeding, sepsis (due to overwhelming vasodilation), and those who are dehydrated. Early recognition of hypotension is critical for good outcomes with these patients. However, hypotension is often a late presentation of bleeding as the body can compensate with increased sympathetic drive.
- **Pulsus paradoxus**: this is an exaggeration of the normal drop in blood pressure during inspiration in severe respiratory disease such as in a severe asthma attack (>10 mmHg drop in systolic blood pressure in inspiration).
- **Checking for postural hypotension**: 3 minutes lying or sitting then after 1 minute of standing.

Table 8.1 Classification of blood pressure (BP) levels by the British Hypertension Society

BP category	Systolic (mmHg)	Diastolic (mmHg)
Optimal	<120	<80
Normal	<130	<85
High normal	130–139	85–90
Hypertension		
Grade 1: mild	140–159	90–99
Grade 2: moderate	160–179	100–109
Grade 3: severe	≥180	≥110
Isolated systolic hypertension		
Grade 1	140–159	<90
Grade 2	≥160	<90

Pulse

This is one of the easier parameters to measure but is often examined manually so that rate, rhythm, volume, and characteristic can all be assessed. Use fingers, not the thumb.

One of the most accessible pulses is the radial artery, which is felt laterally in the wrist. Pulse is calculated by counting beats for between 10 and 15 seconds and multiplying accordingly by 6 or 4, respectively, for beats per minute (bpm). The character of the pulse is best determined in a major artery, usually the carotid (usually >15 seconds, up to 60 seconds required).

Clinical aspects

- **Tachycardia (>100 bpm)**:Tachycardia can be caused by factors including bleeding, sepsis, respiratory and cardiac failure, uncontrolled arrhythmias, anxiety, thyrotoxicosis and certain drugs such as dihydropyrolidine calcium-channel blockers such as amlodipine or felodipine.
- **Bradycardia (<60 bpm)**: bradycardias are also common and have many causes including heart block and hypothyroidism. It is also commonly seen in patients who are on β-blockers, which suppress the chronotropic effect of the heart (oral agents or even eye drops for glaucoma). Other agents that cause bradycardia include digoxin and diltiazem.

- **Irregular pulses**: the commonest cause of an irregularly irregular pulse is atrial fibrillation. Pulsus bigeminy (normal beat, then ectopic, then compensatory pause), pulsus trigeminy (two normal beats, then ectopic, then compensatory pause) are often missed until the electrocardiogram (ECG) is seen but are easily diagnosed by careful examination of the pulse.

Respiratory rate

This is another simple test to carry out but requires the practitioner to subtly count the breaths without the patient knowing. This prevents any elevated respiratory rates with the patient conscious of their respiratory effort. Ideally this should be carried out during taking the pulse.

Clinical aspects

- **Tachypnoea**: (respiratory rate elevation >20 per minute) is an important parameter as some studies have shown that respiratory rate greater than 27 breaths per minute is an important predictor for cardiac arrests. It is particularly important in early recognition of sepsis as the change in metabolic pH can be compensated by respiration, and excess CO_2 is blown off by raising the respiratory rate.
- **Bradypnoea**: patients who are extremely unwell with central nervous system illness often exhibit bradypnoea (rate less than 10 per minute). Cheyne–Stokes breathing is often seen in dying patients and is characterized by rapid or normal rate breathing that slows to almost or actual apnoea for around 10 seconds and then speeds up with the cycle repeated). Bradypnoea is also seen in patients who have been over-prescribed opiate-based analgesia.

Oxygen saturations

This test is carried out by simple devices placed over the end of the patient's finger, usually the index finger is used. It is one of the most useful non-invasive tests to monitor oxygen saturations. It applies a beam of red light at a frequency between 650 and 805 nm which is absorbed by haemoglobin depending on its O_2 saturation. It can be continually assessed with the probe attached to the patient's finger. However, it does have its limitations, namely false readings when the patient's hands are cold, the device not correctly placed on the finger, or if the patient is wearing nail varnish. The patient's ears and toes can also be used.

Clinical aspects

High oxygen saturation and unwell patient: Do not be reassured by a stable high oxygen saturation alone – a patient with carbon monoxide poisoning can have normal oxygen saturations and be critically ill.

The MEWS system of clinical observations (Table 8.2)

MEWS (modified early warning score) is a system used by many hospitals as a method of identifying patients who have deteriorated or are becoming more unwell. It uses physiological parameters to determine a score which is used to assist doctors and nursing staff in assessing critically ill patients. The basic tenet of the MEWS score is that a patient is more likely to deteriorate and become ill if:

- They are outside of normal limits for clinical parameters such as blood pressure, pulse, temperature
- Several of these parameters are abnormal.

If the parameter is normal, no points are allocated to the risk score. Points are then accrued for each of the clinical parameters if abnormal. The overall score is used to assess risk of further deterioration and an index of the clinical attention that the patient warrants, usually as an emergency.

Table 8.2 MEWS: An example of a modified early warning system for ill or deteriorating patients

Score	3	2	1	0	1	2	3
Heart rate (per minute)	≤30	31–40	40–50	51–100	101–110	111–129	≥130
Systolic blood pressure (mmHg)	<70	71–80	81–100	101–179	180–200	>200	>240
Respiratory rate (per minute)		<9		9–14	15–20	21–29	>30
Temperature (°C)		<35	35.1–36.0	36.1–38.0	38.1–38.5	≥38.6	
Central nervous system response				Alert	Voice	Pain	Unresponsive
Urine output* (ml/kg/h)	Nil	<0.5	<1.0	1.0–1.5	>1.5		

Triggers score may be individualized to patients but scores greater than 5 or any reduction in oxygen saturation to less than 95% would trigger a highly skilled emergency assessment and treatment.
*In the last 4 hours. Local tables should be used.

Improving communication using the SBAR tools

Effective communication, often using parameters and trends from MEWS, is essential in ensuring that the most critically ill patients are given priority by busy clinical staff. It is of little value to an overworked clinician to have just a list of, say, 10 patients who need reviewing without an idea of the urgency of each case.

The **SBAR** tool (**S**ituation, **B**ackground, **A**ssessment, **R**ecommendation) is a basic tool that helps clinicians to remember all the main clinical aspects for the purpose of calling for help and allowing the recipient clinician a better chance of assessing the clinical urgency and further management. This is not dissimilar in concept to the Warwick four-point presentation (general statement, important positive findings, important negative findings, clinical conclusion).

SBAR tool for healthcare communication

Situation

- Name of patient
- Ward, time
- Clinical problem
- Resuscitation status
- ABCDE data
- MEWS score

  Dr Williams, I am calling you about Freda Garrod on Elizabeth Ward. I am concerned about the fact that she has just vomited about half a cupful of blood.

  Her observations are as follows: Airway intact, respiratory rate 12, oxygen sats. 96% on air, BP is lower now at 112/72 with a pulse of 116 sinus rhythm. 1 hour ago the BP was 144/78. Temperature is normal, urine output in the last 4 hours has been 120 mL. Her extremities are warm and well perfused. The patient is alert and orientated. Glucose level is 5.6 mmol/L. MEWS score is now 4.

Background

- Clinical information
- Previous clinical discussion

Freda had injection and banding of oesophageal varices earlier today. She has a background history of liver cirrhosis due to haemochromatosis. There is no other significant past medical history.

Assessment

- What is thought to be happening and why.

I think that this patient is having a bleed from her varices. One of the 3 variceal bands may have dislocated. The blood she is vomiting is fresh bright red.

Recommendation

- Your clear recommendation.

I would like to start an infusion of normal saline 1000 mL over 2 hours. I would also like you to review the patient within the next 30 minutes. I make it 7.45 pm – shall I call you again within 30 minutes if she deteriorates and at 8.15 if you have not been able to come to the ward?

Patient safety tips

- ✔ **Always give deteriorating patients priority** over other tasks and seek senior help early if needed.
- ✔ **Be aware of factors that lead to poor communication** between clinical teams and increase potential for patient harm. This includes: patient related factors such as language barrier or a patient unable to articulate their symptoms, stress due to workload, lack of review of patient due to poor handover of patient to next shift of clinicians, not involving the wider clinical team.
- ✔ **Use MEWS and the SBAR tool regularly**: regular use of these tools will improve communication and give you more confidence in responding appropriate to critically ill or deteriorating patients.
- ✔ MEWS scores are not a substitute for clinical judgement. Patients with long-term conditions, such as COPD, may have high background scores as a result of stable ill health. Therefore, trends in the score may be more important.

Student name:	Medical school:	Year:

Clinical signs, MEWS score, and SBAR

You have been asked to see Dorothy Rivers, age 78. She was recently admitted with confusion and falls. A urinary tract infection (UTI) was thought to be the diagnosis based on symptoms and she has increasing confusion and a change in her vital signs.

	On admission	Now	Self	Peer	Peer /tutor	Tutor
Temperature:	37.8°	38.6°				
Blood pressure:	132/67	108/62				
Pulse:	82	118				
Respiratory rate:	14	22				
O₂ saturation:	96%	91%				
Urine output (weight 80 kg)	60 mL/h	12 mL/h				

		Self	Peer	Peer /tutor	Tutor
What are the main clinical vitals and normal ranges?	• **Temperature**: normal range 36.5–37.5 °C	☐	☐	☐	☐
	• **Blood pressure**: 90/60 to 140/90 mmHg	☐	☐	☐	☐
	• **Pulse**: 60–100 per minute	☐	☐	☐	☐
	• **Respiratory rate**: 12–20 breaths per minute	☐	☐	☐	☐
	• **O₂ saturation**: 94–98%, COPD 88–92%	☐	☐	☐	☐
	• **Urine output**: 1.0–1.5 mL/kg/h	☐	☐	☐	☐
Fever and hypothermia	• Please measure the temperature in this patient/subject	☐	☐	☐	☐
	• State and discuss clinical conditions in which there is fever	☐	☐	☐	☐
	• State and discuss some specific patterns of fever	☐	☐	☐	☐
	• What is hypothermia and how can it arise	☐	☐	☐	☐
Pulse	• Please measure the pulse rate and character in this patient/subject: radial artery for rate and character from major artery, usually the carotid	☐	☐	☐	☐
	• State and discuss conditions which there is tachycardia	☐	☐	☐	☐
	• State and discuss conditions in which there is bradycardia	☐	☐	☐	☐
	• State and discuss common pulse and rhythm abnormalities	☐	☐	☐	☐
Respiratory rate	• Please measure the respiratory rate in this patient/subject:	☐	☐	☐	☐
	• State and discuss conditions in which there is tachypnoea	☐	☐	☐	☐
	• State and discuss conditions in which there is bradypnoea	☐	☐	☐	☐
O₂ saturation	• Please measure oxygen saturations in this patient/subject: uses non-invasive device; ensures optimal conditions for true reading: hands not cold, device correctly placed, no nail varnish	☐	☐	☐	☐
Blood pressure method: please demonstrate using an aneroid device on patient/student	• Explanation, consent and position: ensures subject rested and calm, feet flat on the floor and back rested or supine; arm horizontal and supported	☐	☐	☐	☐
	• Blood pressure cuff: checks size: bladder 80% of arm circumference	☐	☐	☐	☐
	• Correctly places cuff in relation to the brachial artery				
	• Brachial artery location by palpation (medial to biceps tendon): inflates cuff after blood pressure bulb locked, 70 mmHg rapidly then in increments of 10 mmHg until pulse disappears and then reappears during deflation	☐	☐	☐	☐
	• Estimated systolic pressure: the pressure at which brachial pulse returns after deflation	☐	☐	☐	☐
	• Auscultation: applies stethoscope to brachial artery just above the antecubital fossa. Inflates blood pressure cuff until 20 mmHg above the estimated systolic	☐	☐	☐	☐
	• Systolic blood pressure: deflates cuff 2 mmHg per second until repetitive, clear tapping sounds first appear for at least 2 consecutive beats (Korotkoff's first sound)	☐	☐	☐	☐
	• Diastolic blood pressure: deflates cuff again. After Korotkoff's fourth sounds (muffling then soft and blowing) sounds disappear (Korotkoff's fifth sound = Diastolic blood pressure)	☐	☐	☐	☐
	• **Blood pressure recoding**: systolic and diastolic rounded upwards to the nearest even number e.g. 152/86. Writes down blood pressure. Avoids digit preference.	☐	☐	☐	☐
MEWS chart: Use chart from your clinical environment if possible	• For the clinical case above what was the MEWS score on admission?	☐	☐	☐	☐
	• What was the score after deterioration?	☐	☐	☐	☐
SBAR communication: Please use the telephone to tell me about the clinical case above and write out a record for the notes	• **S**ituation	☐	☐	☐	☐
	• **B**ackground	☐	☐	☐	☐
	• **A**ssessment	☐	☐	☐	☐
	• **R**ecommendation	☐	☐	☐	☐

				Self	Peer	Peer /tutor	Tutor
Self-assessed as at least borderline:	Signature:		Date:	U B S E	U B S E	U B S E	U B S E
Peer-assessed as ready for tutor assessment:	Signature:		Date:	U B S E	U B S E	U B S E	U B S E
Tutor-assessed as satisfactory:	Signature:		Date:	U B S E	U B S E	U B S E	U B S E

Notes

8.2 Venepuncture

Background

Venepuncture is the process of entering a vein with a needle in order to obtain one or more blood samples. The two methods are the traditional needle and syringe and needle/vacuum sample bottles. The latter is by far the commonest method of use in UK due to it being safer and faster overall. Butterfly needles can be used in cases of difficulty obtaining venous access.

Clinical indications

Blood samples are used primarily for:

- Diagnostic purposes
- Monitoring levels of blood components.

Anatomical and physiological principles

The veins most commonly used for venepuncture are the upper limb superficial veins at the antecubital fossa. This is because they are easily accessible, easy to palpate, and most numerous. These include the median cubital, cephalic, and basilic vein.

- **Cephalic vein** starts at the radial aspect of the dorsal venous network, and passes upwards along the radial side of the forearm. At the antecubital fossa it gives off the median cubital vein then ascends the lateral border of biceps brachii in the arm, pierces the coracoclavicular fascia and joins the axillary vein just below the clavicle.

- **Basilic vein** starts at the ulnar aspect of the dorsal venous network, moves up the posterior surface of the ulnar side of the forearm. At the antecubital fossa it is joined by the median cubital vein, then ascends the medial border of biceps brachii to the lower border of teres major where it continues as the axillary vein.

- **Median cubital vein** passes obliquely from the cephalic to the basilic vein on the antecubital fossa, and receives a communicating branch from the deep veins of the forearm.

- **Metacarpal veins** on the dorsal aspect of the hand can be used when the necessary; these form a network formed from the unison of the dorsal digital veins. They are easily visualized and palpated, however, they are smaller and thus can be difficult to obtain a blood sample from.

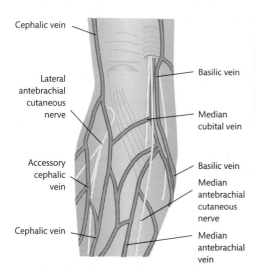

Cephalic vein

Lateral antebrachial cutaneous nerve

Accessory cephalic vein

Cephalic vein

Basilic vein

Median cubital vein

Basilic vein

Median antebrachial cutaneous nerve

Median antebrachial vein

Anatomy of the veins in the antecubital fossa (right arm)

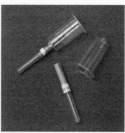

Vacuum sampling device: The sample bottle is only introduced into the needle after venepuncture

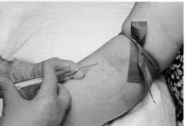

Venepuncture in action: note how the vein has been stabilized

Figure 8.2 Images in venepuncture.

Contraindications

Absolute:

- Fistulae or vascular grafts.

Caution advised:

- Presence of venous fibrosis, haematoma, or oedema
- Localized infection or inflammation
- Other vascular access devices in place such as a cannula
- In post-mastectomy or post-cardiovascular accident patients, the affected side should be avoided as lymphatic drainage may be impaired
- If an intravenous infusion is in progress, use the other arm or stop infusion for at least 5 minutes and ensure this is documented on sample form. Take sample distally if possible.

Procedure

The most common technique for venesection is the vacuum device system. Here the needle is assembled onto an adaptor device, which the blood collecting bottle is then attached to. Blood draws into the bottle due to the vacuum in the sample bottle. The blood bottles can be removed and multiple bottles filled directly from the vein without moving the needle, thus reducing the risk of a needle-stick injury. However, the needle and syringe method or 'butterfly' needle may be easier in more difficult circumstances for venepuncture.

Equipment

- Clean disposable gloves, apron, clean tray and sharps bin, alcohol wipe, tourniquet
- Needle and vacutainer
- Gauze or cotton balls, hypoallergenic tape or sterile plaster as appropriate
- Required blood bottles and request forms

Preparation

- **Wash hands**: before starting the procedure, and after palpating the vein.
- **Locating suitable vein**: when selecting and palpating the vein. Ideally a spongy prominent vein. The following procedures can aid venodilation:
  ○ Hanging the limb by the side of the bed for a few seconds (i.e. below the level of the heart)
  ○ Asking the patient to clench and open their fist several times
  ○ Gently rubbing over the vein with the alcohol wipe when cleaning the site.

Explanation and consent

- **Identify correct patient, introduce yourself, and gain consent from patient**.
- Explain the clinical indication/benefits.
- Explain what the procedure involves in clear straight-forward language.
- Explain the risks/side effects: discomfort from the needle, haematoma, pain, failure to obtain sample, infection.
- Ask whether the patient has a preferred vein to use, as some patients will know which site has worked in the past. Generally use the non-dominant arm.
- Check the patient's understanding and invite questions for clarification.

Procedure

- **Wash hands, wear gloves, and apron**.

- **Apply tourniquet** 5–10 cm above the venepuncture site. Patient may need to clench/ unclench fist to bring out the veins. Tourniquet must not be too tight so as to occlude the arterial circulation!
- **Palpate vein** and put on clean gloves (do not need to be sterile).
- **Clean skin** with a chlorhexidine and alcohol wipe, clean multi-directionally for 30 seconds then allow to dry.
- While waiting for site to dry, **release tourniquet and assemble equipment**.
- **Assemble vacuum device: connect sheathed needle to the plastic sleeve** (the sleeve allows easy insertion of vacuum sample bottles onto needle). Reapply tourniquet. Then remove the needle cover. Warn patient that they will feel a scratch.
- **Introduce needle into vein bevel upwards**: smooth continuous action.
- **Hold needle in vein and plastic sleeve very still**: if necessary steady your hand against the patient's arm. Push the blood bottle into the plastic sleeve device so the grey spike (in the sleeve) pierces the rubber stopper of the sample bottle. The vacuum within the bottle will draw blood into the bottle. If this does not happen, the needle is not in the vein and the needle should be repositioned very slightly only; if there is still no sample, the tourniquet should be released and the needle removed. The venepuncture site is covered with sterile gauze and pressure applied.
- **Continue sampling**: keep hand steady while removing blood sample bottle, and inserting and removing the others, gently mix each sample while waiting for the next to fill.
- **Remove tourniquet** once all the blood samples have been taken (**before** removal of the needle).
- **Remove the needle**: use a piece of sterile gauze to gently press over the venepuncture site *while withdrawing*, and once out press firmly over the site for approximately 2 minutes to avoid blood loss and haematoma formation. Patient should continue to hold the sterile gauze for a further 3–5 minutes.
- **Secure with tape**: or sterile plaster.
- **Thank patient, answer questions**: label samples at bedside and send to laboratory.

Needle and syringe method notes

The steps are similar to above except:

- **Assemble needle and syringe**: use green needle in most cases, a smaller needle is more likely to result in a haemolysed sample. Ensure tops are removed from bottles to fill with blood after the needle has been removed from the syringe. Do **not** fill bottles by pushing needle through the bottletop.
- **Syringe**: use an appropriate size syringe for the volume of blood needed for the sample bottles. Remove the needle cover just before venepuncture.
- **Warn patient and insert needle as above**: withdraw gently on the syringe to check that you are in a vein.
- **Hold needle in vein and syringe very still**: continue to withdraw syringe plunger gently until sufficient blood for the sample has been obtained.
- Other steps as above.

Post-procedure management

- **Dispose of sharps** appropriately.
- **Gently rotate the bottles** to mix the blood and additives and label samples. Remember that labels should not be used for blood cross-match samples. All these bottles must be labelled at the patient's bedside. Identity check should be repeated.

Professionalism: working with colleagues

- Inform key colleagues: nurses, other doctors, carers and family.
- Inform pathology labs if samples are needed more urgently.
- Write clear notes: e.g. venepuncture performed, blood samples sent on (give the date, time and which tests were sent).

Complications

- **Vasovagal syncope** due to pain or sight of blood.
- **Haemolysis** of the blood sample.
- **Haematoma formation** from the venepuncture site. If antecubital vein is used do not ask or let patient flex arm at the elbow. This reduces venous return and increases risk of haematoma.
- **Petechiae** if the tourniquet is applied for too long.
- **Local cellulitis** or septicaemia: uncommon.
- **Infection** directly into the bloodstream.

Patient safety tips

- ✔ **Ensure haemostasis** after finishing procedure, particularly if patient is taking warfarin.
- ✔ **Label bottles at patient's bedside**: to ensure so that there is no risk of mislabelling.

Student name:	Medical school:	Year:

Venepuncture

How would you carry out venesection on a patient? I will ask you some questions, then please demonstrate the procedure.

		Self	Peer	Peer /tutor	Tutor
Background and clinical indications	● Understands indications: diagnostic purposes and monitoring of blood component levels	☐	☐	☐	☐
	● Use of the vacutainer system	☐	☐	☐	☐
	●	☐	☐	☐	☐
Anatomical and physiological principles	● Names of the veins usually used for venesection	☐	☐	☐	☐
	● Pathway of the cephalic vein	☐	☐	☐	☐
	● Pathway of the basilic vein	☐	☐	☐	☐
	● Pathway of the antecubital vein	☐	☐	☐	☐
	●	☐	☐	☐	☐
Cautions and contraindications	● Fistulae or vascular grafts	☐	☐	☐	☐
	● Vascular access devices in-situ	☐	☐	☐	☐
	● Areas of fibrosis, infection, oedema, haematoma	☐	☐	☐	☐
	● Affected sides in patients post-mastectomy/stroke	☐	☐	☐	☐
	●	☐	☐	☐	☐
Procedure	● Hand wash with water and soap and alcohol gel	☐	☐	☐	
	● This is a non-touch technique				
	● Introduction and identifies patient. Informed consent	☐	☐	☐	☐
	● Gives clear explanation: e.g. 'I am going to take a blood sample. We need this to help us diagnose what is wrong.'				
	● Equipment selection: gloves, tray and sharps bin. tourniquet, chlorhexidine/alcohol wipe, vacutainer and needle, sterile gauze and tape	☐	☐	☐	☐
	● Applies tourniquet, palpates the vein, cleans the skin, releases tourniquet, correctly assembles the vacutainer. Re-applies tourniquet and dons gloves	☐	☐	☐	☐
	● Inserts the needle with the bevel facing up at 35–40° into the vein. Attaches the blood bottles to the vacutainer device to take the sample	☐	☐	☐	☐
	● Releases the tourniquet then withdraw the needle. Applies a sterile gauze over the site until haemostasis is achieved				
	● Good communication demonstrated throughout the procedure and encourages patient to ask questions	☐	☐	☐	☐
	● Disposes of sharps/equipment. Washes hands	☐	☐	☐	☐
	●	☐	☐	☐	☐
Post-procedure management	● Labels the blood bottles at the patient's bedside	☐	☐	☐	☐
	● Documents procedure into clinical notes	☐	☐	☐	☐
	● Ensures samples are sent to laboratory	☐	☐	☐	☐
	●				
Professionalism: working with colleagues	● Communicates sensitively, thanks the patient, addresses any questions or concerns, washes hands	☐	☐	☐	☐
	● Completes all documentation legibly and unambiguously	☐	☐	☐	☐
	● Communicates appropriately with nursing staff	☐	☐	☐	☐
	●	☐	☐	☐	☐
Complications	● Syncope	☐	☐	☐	☐
	● Haemolysis	☐	☐	☐	☐
	● Haematoma	☐	☐	☐	☐
	● Petechiae	☐	☐	☐	☐
	● Local cellulitis or septicaemia	☐	☐	☐	☐
	●	☐	☐	☐	☐
Patient safety tips	● Ensures haemostasis	☐	☐	☐	☐
	●	☐	☐	☐	☐
Global assessment	● Would you be happy for this student to be supervised to perform venepuncture in a real patient?	☐	☐	☐	☐
	●	☐	☐	☐	☐

			Self	Peer	Peer /tutor	Tutor
Self-assessed as at least borderline:	Signature:	Date:	U B S E	U B S E	U B S E	U B S E
Peer-assessed as ready for tutor assessment:	Signature:	Date:	U B S E	U B S E	U B S E	U B S E
Tutor-assessed as satisfactory:	Signature:	Date:	U B S E	U B S E	U B S E	U B S E

Notes

8.3 Electrocardiography: cardiac monitoring and recording a 12-lead ECG

Background

Cardiac monitoring and the 12-lead ECG are two of the commonest procedures undertaken in routine clinical care especially in inpatients.

Clinical indications for ECG monitoring

- **Acute coronary syndrome (ACS)**: it is important to rule in or out a cardiac cause early, to refer appropriately and urgently for possible interventions including medical management, angioplasty and revascularization, thrombolysis, or even coronary artery bypass surgery.
- **Other possible cardiac conditions**: patients with chest pain, shortness of breath, history of blackouts, falls, palpitations or syncope, pre-surgery, prior to or during drug treatments (e.g. amiodarone, phenytoin).
- **Potential rhythm problems**: deteriorating patient, patient with electrolyte abnormalities such as hypokalaemia, hyperkalaemia, patients on dialysis (often), certain drugs being given such as amiodarone infusion.
- **Routine monitoring**: during anaesthesia, high-risk obstetrics delivery, intensive care unit (ITU) and coronary care unit (CCU) cases.

Anatomical and physiological principles

The human body consists of a large percentage of water, which is a good conductor of electricity. Surface electrodes will therefore be excellent at picking up the electrical activity (depolarization) of the heart from even the limb leads which can be over a metre from the heart itself and from the precordial leads which may only be less than 2 cm from the cardiac surface. An elegant way to regard the ECG is that it is a graph, plotting cardiac voltage against time. The function of the basic cardiac monitor is to provide information on the rate and rhythm of the heart. The 12-lead ECG (which actually uses only 10 leads) is a record of the electrical activity of the heart from several different angles. This enables both the recognition and identification of heart arrhythmias and damage to the heart in specific anatomical locations, particularly due to ischaemia.

Contraindications

There are no specific contraindications unless there is specific pathological situation such as bullae or burns that can make applications of electrodes to the skin relatively contraindicated.

Three-lead cardiac monitoring

- **Advantages**: easily accessible, quick and easy to apply, does not require a high degree of skill, gives an overview of cardiac cycle/ general information
- **Disadvantages**: information obtained is not specific, unable to analyse ST-T segment changes with accuracy, cannot diagnose ACS (which requires a 12-lead ECG).

Preparation

Wash your hands before starting the procedure. There is always the risk of the clinician contaminating the patient and the equipment.

Explanation and consent

- Identify correct patient, introduce yourself and gain consent from patient.
- Explain the clinical indication/benefits.
- Explain what the procedure involves in clear straight-forward language.
- Explain the risks/side effects: discomfort from the electrode placement pads on removal with hair loss, occasional haematoma with fragile skin.
- Check the patient's understanding and invite questions for clarification.

Procedure and equipment

- **Place leads**: right shoulder (soft tissue, not bony prominence), left shoulder, midaxillary line horizontally around from the apex of the heart. Good skin preparation is essential to ensure a high quality ECG trace. Dry skin if wet. Clean with an alcohol wipe if greasy.
- **Connect leads**: to monitor. It is important that the clinician is familiar with the monitor, its alarms (setting and releasing), and battery life if not connected to the main electricity supply.

Post-procedure management

- **Dispose of waste** appropriately.

Professionalism: working with colleagues

Inform key colleagues: nurses, other doctors, carers and family. Seek senior help if needed. Write clear notes, e.g.:

> *Cardiac monitor in situ: sinus rhythm at 76 per minutes with inverted T waves. Any significant abnormality should be investigated further with a 12-lead ECG.*

12-lead ECG

- **Advantages**: more accurate spatial information acquired, can diagnose ACS and previous ischaemic heart disease with high degree of certainty, can analyse ST-T segments changes, three-dimensional view of the heart, more leads to aid diagnosis of arrhythmias.
- **Disadvantages**: requires more skill to perform, leads must be placed at specific points on patient. If performed incorrectly could be harmful to patient if diagnosis made from imprecise positioning of the electrodes. More time consuming. Need patient cooperation to ensure good quality trace.

Preparation, explanation, and consent

As above.

Procedure and equipment

- **Limb leads placement** (Figure 8.3)
- Place the four limb electrodes: one on the flexor aspect of each wrist, and each ankle. The right ankle lead is a neutral lead and plays no role in the ECG itself. Electrode placement may need to be changed to enable a clear ECG recording, i.e. patients with Parkinson's disease or limb amputation. Ensure that the limb electrodes remain symmetrical.

  ○ Red = right wrist, yellow = left wrist, green = left ankle, black = right ankle

- **Connect leads** to 12-lead ECG recorder. It is important that the clinician is familiar with the machine, especially the paper speed settings and the voltage gain functions.

Anatomical landmarks
Start at the angle of Louis
(Right manubriosternal
angle), the 1st rib space
below this is the 2nd
intercostal space (ICS).

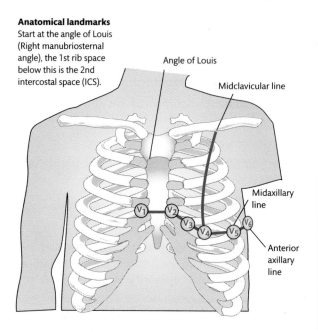

Angle of Louis

Midclavicular line

Midaxillary
line

Anterior
axillary
line

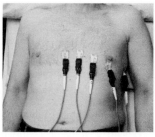

Chest leads placement (V1–V6):

V1: Right 4th ICS, right sternal
border
V2: Left 4th ICS, left sternal border
V3: Sited between V2 and V4
V4: 5th ICS, midclavicular line (left)
V5: Sited between V4 and V6 in the
anterior anxillary line
V6: Midaxillary line, same horizontal
plane as V4

V4, V5, and V6 electrodes should be a
straight line

Figure 8.3 Position of ECG leads: be precise in placing leads in the correct anatomical position.

Post-procedure management

● **Dispose of waste** appropriately. Explanation to patient if needed.

Professionalism: working with colleagues

Inform key colleagues: nurses, other doctors, carers and family. Seek senior help if needed. Write clear notes on what the ECG shows.

Trouble shooting

Problems such as artefacts can often can often be corrected by adopting simple techniques. The 'filter' button is present on most ECG machines and can be used to rule out artefacts. It is recommended that a trace should be performed both with and without the 'filter on', to enable more accurate interpretation. If the filter is used, this should be stated on the ECG trace.

A wandering baseline (Figure 8.4)

This can be due to poor skin contact.

● Use abrasive 'prep' tape

● Make sure the skin is clean and dry

● Ask the patient to briefly hold their breath if possible to reduce interference from breathing.

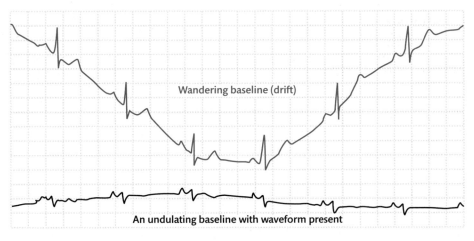

Figure 8.4 A wandering baseline.

Patient safety tips

✔ **Ensure close attention to monitoring especially if the patient is deteriorating**. Print off any strips of the ECG needed for later use such as discussion with senior or monitoring improvement or deterioration.

✔ **Consider using the hands-free** defibrillation pads in patients at high risk of needing defibrillation. These pads will also allow safe defibrillation if needed. These are safer to use in an emergency than standard defibrillation pads. However, if skin contact is inadequate, it could result in arching of electricity when defibrillating. Rhythm recognition will also be less than in a standard monitor.

✔ **12-lead electrode placement**: the placement of electrodes is standardized, with the patient supine on a bed. However, this is not always achievable due to the patient's clinical condition. It is important to write on the trace the position/placement of electrodes if deviated from the standard, as treatment may be dependent on the recording.

Student name:	Medical school:	Year:

Recording a 12-lead electrocardiogram (ECG)

Please can you record a 12-lead ECG on this patient/manikin.

		Self	Peer	Peer /tutor	Tutor
Washes hands	● Wash hands or apply alcohol gel ●	☐	☐	☐	☐
Understands indications and anatomy	● Understands indications for performing an ECG ● Demonstrates a knowledge of the anatomy of the heart, ● electrical conduction, and ECG electrode placement ●	☐	☐	☐	☐
Obtains informed consent; explanation to patient	● Introduces themselves, and identifies patient ● Clearly explains what they are going to do, and why ● Obtains consent from patient ●	☐	☐	☐	☐
Communication skills	● Appropriate communication throughout ● Allows patient to ask questions ● Reassures as required ●	☐	☐	☐	☐
Appropriate preparation	● Ensures that the ECG machine is ready for use, and electrodes are available and in date ● Ask the patient to remove the necessary clothing (assist if required), maintaining their dignity ● Ensures patient is comfortable, in a recumbent position ● Explains to patient that they will need to lay as still as possible during the procedure ●	☐	☐	☐	☐
Technical ability	**Chest lead placement** ● **V1**: Right 4th ICS, right sternal border ● **V2**: Left 4th ICS, left sternal border ● **V3**: Sited between V2 and V4 ● **V4**: 5th ICS, midclavicular line ● **V5**:Sited between V4 and V6, anterior axillary line ● **V6**: 5th ICS, midaxillary line, same horizontal plane as V4 ● **V4, V5, and V6** electrodes should be in a straight line	☐	☐	☐	☐
	Limb lead placement ● One on the flexor aspect of each wrist, and each ankle ● Red = right wrist, Yellow = left wrist, Green = left ankle, Black = right ankle	☐	☐	☐	☐
	● Understands standard settings on ECG machine, and the indication for altering these, and how to do this ● Demonstrates knowledge and understanding regarding the use of the 'filter' button ●	☐	☐	☐	☐
Seeks help as appropriate	● Seeks expert help immediately in the event of the patient ● complaining of chest pain or arrhythmia ●	☐	☐	☐	☐
Post-procedure management	● Removes electrodes ● Ensures patient name and other identification, date and time of recording is documented clearly on the ECG ● Ensures that the ECG machine is ready for use and plugged into the mains supply ●	☐	☐	☐	☐
Professionalism	● Communicates with patient ● Respects the patient's privacy and dignity at all times ●	☐	☐	☐	☐
Overall ability to perform procedure	● Assess globally, would you be happy for this student to be supervised and perform a 12-lead ECG on a real patient? ●	☐	☐	☐	☐

				Self	Peer	Peer/tutor	Tutor
Self-assessed as at least borderline:	Signature:	Date:		U B S E	U B S E	U B S E	U B S E
Peer-assessed as ready for tutor assessment:	Signature:	Date:		U B S E	U B S E	U B S E	U B S E
Tutor-assessed as satisfactory:	Signature:	Date:		U B S E	U B S E	U B S E	U B S E

8.4 ECG monitoring and rhythm recognition

Background

Cardiac monitoring and the 12-lead ECG are easy investigations to request and obtain in clinical practice – the challenge is the accurate and timely interpretation of the ECG record. ECG interpretation represents a major source of anxiety for many junior clinicians but a mastery of the basics of electrocardiophysiology and pathological variants will allow most clinicians to become adept at recognizing well over 90% of common clinical abnormalities and plan appropriate treatment. This section will cover interpreting of arrhythmias and the next will focus on the 12-lead ECG.

Clinical indications for ECG interpretation

- All the reasons for ECG monitoring will apply here. For the full assessment of a patient to rule out an ACS the full 12-lead ECG must be performed.
- ECG interpretation is a vital skill in a cardiac arrest situation to provide emergency care, for example, to defibrillate or not.

Anatomical and physiological principles

The conduction system of the heart (Figure 8.5)

The conduction system of the heart refers to the electrical pathway.

- The electrical impulse starts at the sinoatrial (SA) node (right atrium) and fires at a rate of 60–100 per minute.
- Impulse then passes to the atrioventricular (AV) node.
- After a brief pause, the impulse continues down the bundle of His, the bundle branches (L, R), and then spreads along the Purkinje fibres.
- Bundle of His and Purkinje fibres are specialized high-velocity nerves that transmit the stimulatory impulse to the myocardium for contraction.
- After contraction (depolarization) there is a brief refractory or rest period (repolarization) before the next impulse causes the next contraction and cardiac beat.

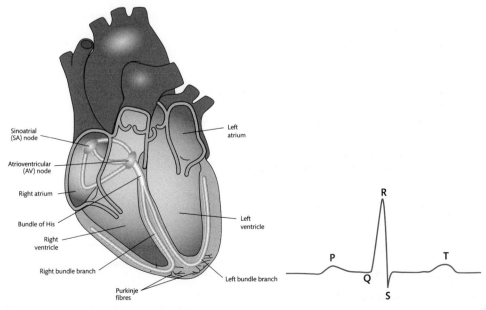

Figure 8.5 The conduction system of the heart.

The ECG complex (Figure 8.6)

Normal values

- *P wave*: base 3 mm, height 2.5 mm
- *PR interval*: (actually PQ interval): 0.12–0.20 seconds, 3–5 mm
- *QRS width*: <0.12 seconds, <3 mm
- *Q – T interval*: <0.42 seconds, <6 mm, usually adjusted for rate

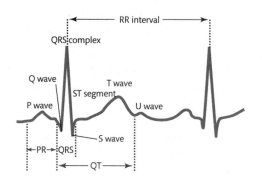 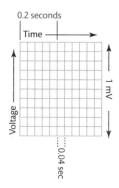

Figure 8.6 The ECG complex.

Definitions to aid diagnosis

- **Sinus**   1 P wave before each QRS complex, normal PR interval
- **Tachycardia**   heart rate >100 complexes/minute
- **Bradycardia**   heart rate <60 complexes/minute
- **Rate**   300 divided by number of 5 mm square (at standard ECG paper rate of 2.5 cm per second)
- **Broad complex**   ventricular rhythm or bundle branch block
- **Narrow complex**   atrial or supraventricular rhythm

In health

- **Normal ECG complex**: consists of P, Q, R, S and T waves.
- **P wave**: represents L and R atrial depolarization and indicates that the SA node electrical impulse has fired.
- **Q wave**: is the first downward dip, below the baseline, represents septal depolarization. May be absent.
- **R wave**: is the first upward peak after the P wave, represents ventricular depolarization.
- **QRS complex**: represents left and right ventricular depolarization towards the electrode. Indicates that the AV node electrical impulse has fired with impulse generated into the His-Purkinje system.
- **S wave**: represents ventricular contraction away from the electrode.
- **T wave**: represents repolarization of the ventricles.
- **U wave**: represents repolarization of the Purkinje fibres. Prominent in electrolyte imbalance (especially hypokalaemia). Some authorities claim it is due to papillary muscle repolarization.

In disease

- **ECG complex**: can be widened, slurred or narrowed.
- **P wave**: p pulmonale is a taller **P**eaked P wave, represents right atrial enlargement. P mitrale is a wider bifid '**M**' wave as in mitral stenosis representing separation of L and R atrial contraction.

- **Q wave**: if there is non-viable myocardium immediately behind the electrode, then viable myocardial in the septum or right ventricle will contract away from this electrode causing a deeper, slurred Q wave. Q waves are therefore a sign of a recent or old myocardial infarct. Q waves are pathological if they are ≥25% of the height of the partner R wave or greater than 0.04 seconds in width or greater than 2 mm in depth.

- **R wave**: smaller R waves are seen in pericardial effusions, pericarditis, emphysema, and previous infarction. Typically <10 mm in height in all V leads would indicate 'poor R wave progression' and pathology.

- **QRS complex**: widened in bundle branch block. A slur on the upstroke of the R wave (delta wave) and a shortened PR interval is seen in Wolff–Parkinson–White (WPW) syndrome.

- **R+S wave**: in the V leads, if the tallest R wave and deepest S wave add up to greater than 35 mm, then this is consistent with left ventricular hypertrophy by voltage criteria.

- **Bundle branch block (BBB)**: in right BBB (RBBB) the complexes are widened with an RSR[1] pattern in V1 and a QRS pattern in V6. In LBBB the complexes are also widened with a QRS pattern in V1 and RSR[1] pattern in V6.

- **ST elevation**: may indicate myocardial infarction. Concave upwards elevation is seen in pericarditis. There is persisting elevation in old myocardial infarction with an aneurysmal or flabby myocardium *in situ*.

- **U wave**: prominent in hypokalaemia. May indicate papillary muscle or septal repolarization.

Paper speed and calibration

The ECG plots voltage against time onto a graph. The standard voltage is set to 10 mm/mV and the speed 25 mm/second. Calibration of the machine is indicated by the square wave at the end of a rhythm strip (1 mV is equivalent to 10 mm height).

Basic rhythm analysis

Asking the following questions using a systematic approach will enable basic interpretation.

This staged approach can be used to describe and diagnose most common arrhythmias and help appropriate action and treatment. This was first advocated by the Resuscitation Council UK (website accessed December 2010).

Reading a rhythm strip: six-stage approach

- **How is the patient?** The first and most important question before the six-stage approach.

- **Do they have a pulse?** What is your initial assessment of this patient? ABCDE assessment: airway, breathing, circulation, disability, exposure.

1 **Is there electrical activity?** Is the patient attached properly, is there a problem with the leads, check pulse.

2 **What is the ventricular (QRS) rate?** In adults usually 60–100 bpm, other rates can be normal: resting, exercising, stress, emotions, coffee.

3 **Is the QRS rhythm regular or irregular?** Is it atrial fibrillation? Measure the RR intervals.

4 **Is the QRS width normal or prolonged?** Measure QRS. Is it related to pre-excitation, ST elevation myocardial infarction, BBB?

5 **Is atrial activity present?** Is there a P wave before QRS complexes? Usually there should be one with a normal PR interval.

6 **How is atrial activity related to ventricular activity?** This will determine whether ? atrial flutter, ? short PR in WPW, first-, second-, or third degree heart block.

Please note if there is no pulse with any electrical rhythm that you would expect to have a cardiac output, the rhythm is called **pulseless electrical activity (PEA)** and full advanced life support cardiopulmonary resuscitation (CPR) is started. BBBs (Figure 8.7) can make interpretation of ECG rhythms difficult, new left BBB (LBBB) often indicates myocardial infarction in a suitable clinical context. Always ask the question: does the patient need a 12-lead ECG?

Left bundle branch block characteristics

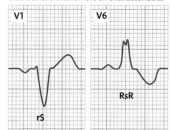

Right bundle branch block characteristics

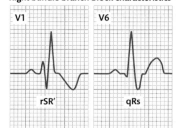

LBBB: V6 is normally the best lead to pick up LV activity. In LBBB, the small RV component is picked up as the first notch in the V6 R wave and then only later is the delayed LV activity picked up as the second notch.

RBBB: V1 is normally the best lead to pick up RV activity. In RBBB, the small LV component is picked up first (r) and then only later is the delayed RV activity picked up as R.

Figure 8.7 Patterns of complexes in bundle branch block. The complexes are broad, >0.12 seconds, as left and right ventricular contractions are not synchronous.

Common ECG rhythms and interpretation

How is the patient? If no pulse, then rhythm is pulseless electrical activity

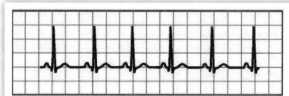

Sinus rhythm: normal rate

Electrical activity: Yes

QRS rate: 100

QRS width: Normal (<3 mm)

QRS ?regular: Yes

Atrial activity: Clear P waves

Atrial & QRS relation: 1 P per QRS, Normal PR

From SAN (P wave), depolarization follows normal conduction pathway. Contains all normal components of cardiac cycle, correct morphology, correct association. Normal rate limit 60-100bpm.

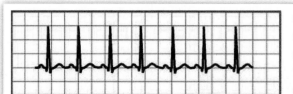

Sinus rhythm: tachycardia

Electrical activity: Yes

QRS rate: (300/2.3)

Tachycardia, 130 bpm

QRS width: Normal (<3 mm)

QRS ?regular: Yes

Atrial activity: Clear P waves

Atrial & QRS relation: 1 P per QRS, Normal PR

Sinus Tachycardia: from SAN (P wave), but tachycardia >100 bpm. If perfusion needs to increase, ie exercise, autonomic nervous system increases rate of SAN discharge. *Causes:* anxiety, caffeine, drugs, heart failure

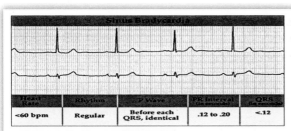

Sinus rhythm: bradycardia

Electrical activity: Yes

QRS rate: (300/5.7)

Bradycardia, 53

QRS width: Normal (<3 mm)

QRS ?regular: Yes

Atrial activity: Clear P waves

Atrial & QRS relation: 1 P per QRS, Normal PR

Sinus Bradycardia: from SAN (P wave), but bradycardia <60 bpm. If perfusion requirements are reduced, i.e. during sleep/rest, autonomic nervous system slows rate of SAN discharge. **Causes:** ischaemia, fibrosis, drugs, physical fitness

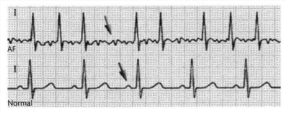

Atrial fibrillation

Electrical activity: Yes

QRS rate: Fast/slow

QRS width: Normal (<3 mm)

QRS ?regular: irregular

Atrial activity: Yes, but no true P waves (compare normal)

Atrial & QRS relation: Irregular transfer of atrial activity to ventricles

Common with. Irregularly irregular. Atria quiver instead of co-ordinated contraction → loss of cardiac output & failure. Fibrillation waves vary in shape, duration, amplitude and direction. QRS may be narrow or broad. Atrial rate commonly 300-600bpm

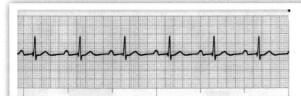

Atrial Flutter:

Electrical activity: Yes

QRS rate: (300/2.3)

Tachycardia: 130

QRS width: Normal (<3 mm)

QRS ?regular: regular

Atrial activity: Yes, but atrial flutter waves, no true P waves

Atrial & QRS relation: Yes occasionally, only 1 QRS per 3–4 atrial flutter waves

Saw tooth flutter waves. Degree of heart block present as not all atrial flutter waves produce a QRS (can denote as 3 to1 block etc) . Atrial rate commonly 300bpm. Rapid and regular contractions.

1ˢᵗ Degree Heart Block

Electrical activity: Yes

QRS rate: (300/5) = 60

QRS width: Normal (<3 mm)

QRS ?regular: regular

Atrial activity: P waves, but PR prolonged, >3 mm (0.12 seconds)

Atrial & QRS relation: Yes, but entry delayed at AVN

1ˢᵗ Degree Heart Block: Common, especially after inferior MI as right coronary artery supplies the AVN. Can deteriorate into higher degrees of block.

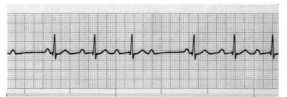

Also known as Wenckebach's phenomenon. ***PR prolongs, prolongs drops: cycle restarts***. Localized to the AVN and not associated with increased morbidity unless heart disease present such as MI or abnormality in His-Purkinje system.

2nd Degree Heart Block: Mobitz Type I

Electrical activity: Yes

QRS rate: Normal <100

QRS width: Normal (<3 mm)

QRS ?regular: irregular

Atrial activity: Yes, P waves. But PR gets longer and longer until QRS dropped

Atrial & QRS relation: Yes, with above pattern

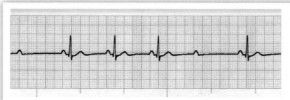

2nd Degree Heart Block: Mobitz Type II: Normal PR when QRS does happen. Not all P waves produce a QRS. Carries high risk of progression to complete heart block and risk of increased mortality.

2nd Degree Heart Block: Mobitz Type II

Electrical activity: Yes

QRS rate: bradycardia

QRS width: Normal (<3 mm)

QRS ?regular: Regular then irregular

Atrial activity: Yes, P waves with normal PR when QRS occurs. But not all P waves lead to a QRS complex

Atrial & QRS relation: Yes, with above pattern

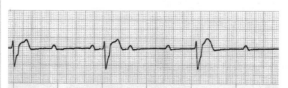

3rd Degree Heart Block: The atrial (P waves) and ventricles (QRS) contract independently. The bradycardia rate is set by a non-His-Purkinje ventricular pacemaker. Hence the prolonged QRS as initial contraction is through the slower myocardium. High risk pacing needed.

3rd Degree Heart Block:

Electrical activity: Yes

QRS rate: bradycardia

QRS width: Prolonged (>3 mm)

QRS ?regular: QRS independently regular no relation to regular P waves

Atrial activity: Yes, P waves but there is no link to QRS

Atrial & QRS relation: None

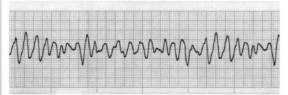

Electrical activity present, but bizarre QRS complexes do not result in co-ordinated contractions to sustain cardiac output. There is no output. **Urgent CPR & defibrillation required**.

Ventricular Fibrillation

Electrical activity: Yes

QRS rate: Variable bizarre

QRS width: Prolonged (>3 mm)

QRS ?regular: Very irregular

Atrial activity: Not seen on trace

Atrial & QRS relation: None

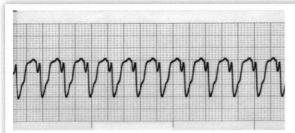

Electrical activity present, but output may be reduced or absent. Broad complex therefore ventricular origin or bundle-branch block. If there is no output. **Urgent CPR & defibrillation required**.

Ventricular Tachycardia

Electrical activity: Yes

QRS rate: Tachycardia

QRS width: Prolonged: (>3 mm)

QRS ?regular: regular

Atrial activity: Difficult to see clearly

Atrial & QRS relation: Difficult to establish

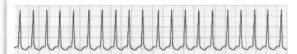

No electrical activity present. No output. Exclude treatable causes. Occasional electrical complexes may be seen such as odd P wave or QRS complexes as part of agonal rhythm. **Urgent ALS CPR**

Asystole

Electrical activity: No

QRS rate:

QRS width:

QRS ?regular:

Atrial activity:

Atrial & QRS relation:

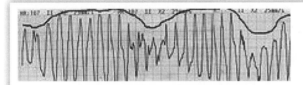

Supraventricular tachycardia: SVT a rhythm where **ventricular depolarization (QRS)** is normal but that the exact mechanism of dysfunction within the atria cannot be identified due to the tachycardia. Often **paroxysmal and self-terminating. Rhythms include:** Atrial tachycardia, atrial flutter, atrial fibrillation, re-entry tachycardia (with accessory pathway), AV nodal re-entry and Wolff-Parkinson-White syndrome (AV by-pass tract)

Torsades de pointes: polymorphic VT with a characteristic twist of the QRS complex around the isoelectric baseline. Can degenerate into VF. Associated with long QT syndrome. An R-on-T can initiate torsades.

ECG rhythm recognition

This assessment is based around a discussion of the main components of the ECG complex and their physiological and pathological correlates.

Use at least a few ECG rhythm traces from your own clinical work areas to allow additional questions to be undertaken in the same format as suggested.

	Self	Peer	Peer/tutor	Tutor

What are the clinical indications for an ECG or ECG monitoring?
●

In relation to the conduction system of the heart: please discuss the pathway of the normal cardiac impulse using the diagram of the ECG complex below and specific reference to SA and AV nodes, bundle of His and Purkinje fibres
●

Discuss each of the following in physiology and pathology
● P wave and PR interval
● Q wave
● R wave
● S wave
● QRS complex
● T wave and ST segment
● L and R Bundle branch Block
●

Using the method outlined in this chapter: use the RCUK six-stage approach to determine what each the following rhythms is: briefly discuss management
●

What is the very first consideration in interpreting a rhythm strip? What is the condition of the patient: undertake ABCDE assessment.
●

Rhythms: Determine electrical activity, QRS rate, QRS width, ?regular, atrial activity, atrial and QRS relation and final diagnosis for each rhythm

1

2

3

4

5

6

Do you consider this student to be competent in ECG rhythm recognition?
●

	Signature:	Date:	Self	Peer	Peer/tutor	Tutor
Self-assessed as at least borderline:			U B S E	U B S E	U B S E	U B S E
Peer-assessed as ready for tutor assessment:			U B S E	U B S E	U B S E	U B S E
Tutor-assessed as satisfactory:			U B S E	U B S E	U B S E	U B S E

Notes

8.5 ECG: basic principles and interpretation

Background

The 12-lead ECG is carried on the vast majority of patients who are admitted for routine and emergency surgery or as a medical emergency. There is a common misconception that it is very difficult to become proficient in ECG interpretation. In reality, a stepwise approach based on physiological, anatomical, and pathological findings allows the ECG to become a valuable assessment of cardiac function and disease. The very detailed nuances of ECG interpretation will not be covered here as the main focus will be on correctly diagnosing important clinical emergencies and presentation of basic findings.

Basic physiological, anatomical, and pathological principles

The standard 12-lead ECG is basically a representation of the heart's electrical activity recorded from electrodes on the body surface.

The ECG records electrical potentials as they travel through the myocardium. In order for this to occur an electrical circuit is required to relay these signals back to the machine. The circuit must consist of three poles, positive (+ve), negative (−ve), and earth. One of the basic principles of electrocardiography is that:

- An electrical force moving towards a lead will always produce a positive deflection
- An electrical force moving away from a lead will always produce a negative deflection.

Other principles

- **The 12-lead ECG** provides spatial information about the heart's electrical activity in three orthogonal directions: right ↔ left; superior ↔ inferior; anterior ↔ posterior.
- **Each of the 12 leads** represents a particular orientation in space, as indicated in Figures 8.8 and 8.9. 12-lead refers to the 12 positions of cardiac electrical activity recorded (I, II, III, aVR, aVL, aVF, V_1, V_2, V_3, V_4, V_5, V_6) from the 10 electrical leads placed on the patient.
- **The rhythm strip**: usually recorded from lead 2 and placed at the bottom of the 12-lead ECG. A calibration notch is usually placed in all ECGs to denote 1 mV (milli volt).
- **1 mV** of electrical activity causes a 10 mm deflection vertically.
- **ECG speed is usually 25 mm per second**. Each 25 mm length is therefore 1 second, 5 mm is 0.2 seconds, 1 mm is 0.04 seconds
- **Sensitivity of the ECG** in terms of mV/10 mm or speed may be changed if there is a marked increase in electrical activity as in severe left ventricular hypertrophy. A tachycardia may be easier to interpret if the ECG speed is increased.
- **The left ventricle is electrically dominant in ECG terms**: the left ventricular muscle mass is larger than the mass of the right ventricle. This produces a deep S wave in V1 as the main direction of force is away from that lead and a tall R wave in V6 as the main electrical force is travelling toward that lead. The QRS complexes in the chest leads therefore, predominantly, reflect left ventricular activity.

Frontal plane limb recordings

Bipolar limb leads

Measure the potential difference between two limbs (L: left, R: right, A: arm, L: leg).

- **Lead I**   LA (+) to RA (−). In health: predominantly +ve deflection.

- **Lead II** LL (+) to RA (–). In health: predominantly +ve deflection
- **Lead III** LL (+) to LA (–). In health: predominantly +ve deflection but can be –ve as normal variant.

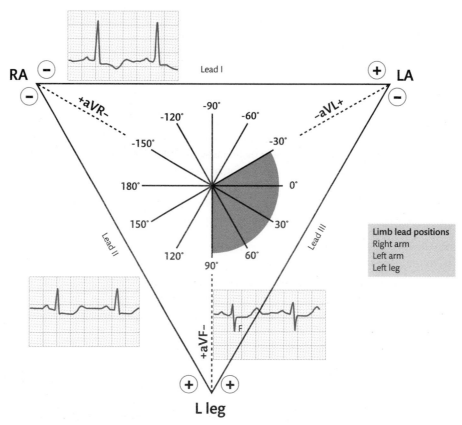

Figure 8.8 Frontal plane limb recordings. Einthoven's triangle

Augmented unipolar limb leads

Modified central terminal augments voltage by 50%, measures the difference between one limb lead (+) and the average of potentials at other two.

- **Lead aVR** RA (+) to (LA and LL), rightward. In health: a –ve deflection is recorded.
- **Lead aVL** LA (+) to (RA and LL), leftward. In health: usually +ve but can be –ve or equiphasic.
- **Lead AVF** LF (+) to (RA and LA), inferior. In health: usually +ve.

Six chest leads (anterior or precordial leads)

These record the passage of electrical potentials through the myocardium in the horizontal plane. The R wave height gradually increases from V1 to V6 with V5 generally being the tallest point. The ventricular septum is first depolarized from left to right. This tends to produce a small r wave in V1 and a small q wave in V6.

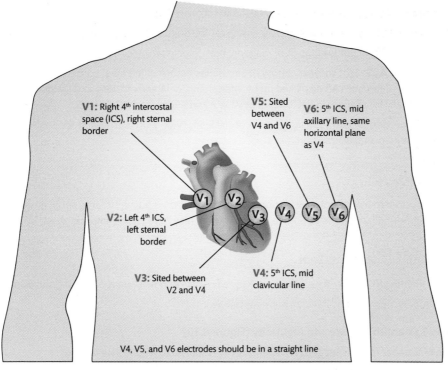

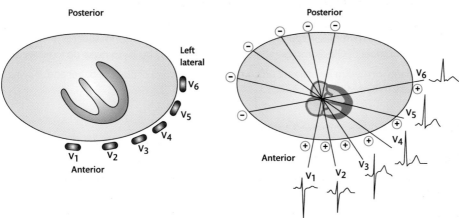

Figure 8.9 Chest leads.

Anatomical correlates of the ECG leads

I Lateral	**aVR**	**V1** Anterior	**V4** Anterior
II Inferior	**aVL** Lateral	**V2** Anterior septal	**V5** Anterior
III Inferior	**aVF** Inferior	**V3** Anterior septal	**V6** Anterior lateral

- **Anterior ACS**: left anterior descending (LAD) coronary artery
- **Inferior ACS**: right coronary artery (usually, can be branch of LAD)
- **Lateral ACS**: circumflex branch or diagonal branch of left main coronary artery.
- **Posterior ACS**: right coronary artery or circumflex branch of left main coronary artery. A posterior infarction can be picked up by inferior and/or lateral changes, and by looking specifically for changes in tall R waves in V1–V2 and ST depression in V1–V3.
- **RV infarction**: ST elevation in right precordial leads (V3R, V4R) is usually in conjunction with inferior myocardial infarction.

Interpretation

It is important to have a systematic approach to ECG interpretation in order to avoid missing subtle abnormalities on the ECG trace, some of which may have clinical importance.

Six-step ECG analysis tool

'Rate, Rhythm, ST, ABC' – [1]Rate, [2]Rhythm-PQR, [3]ST, [4]Axis, [5]Bundle Branch, [6]Clinical Conclusion (The superscript numbers indicate the steps below.)

Step 1 Establish the rate and regularity (Figure 8.10)

The ECG paper speed is set at 25 mm per second as standard. To calculate the rate:

- **Method 1**: If the rhythm is regular count the number of large (5 mm) squares between each QRS complex. Divide 300 by this.
- **Method 2**: If the rhythm is irregular count out 6 seconds (30 large 5 mm squares of ECG) – count the number of QRS complexes that occur and multiply by 10, to make up to 60 seconds

Check regularity of rhythm by marking off complexes on an edge of piece of paper and moving along to check if rhythm is regular or not.

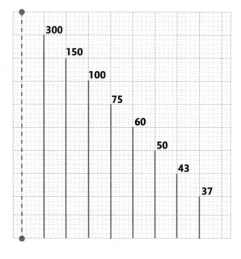

300
150
100
75
60
50
43
37

Figure 8.10 ECG length between complexes and heart rate per minute. ?bradycardia <60, ? tachycardia >100.

Step 2 Rhythm-PQR

- ? normal sinus rhythm ? atrial activity before each QRS complex?
- Presence of P waves before each QRS or absence of any atrial activity?
- Normal P wave morphology, amplitude and duration?
- Presence of fibrillation or flutter waves (atrial fibrillation/ flutter)?
- How is atrial activity related to ventricular activity ?
- PR interval, is it normal (0.12–0.20 seconds/3–5 small squares)?

- Prolonged PR could indicate heart block (first- , second- , third-degree)
- Is there evidence of pre-excitation?

Pre-excitation is the early activation of ventricular tissue by an atrial impulse. In WPW syndrome, an accessory pathway connects the atria to the ventricles. Typical ECG features are: short PR interval (≤0.12 seconds/3 small squares); delta waves (initial slurring of QRS complex); widened QRS complexes; ST-T changes; possible axis deviation.

Step 3 ST-segment

Especially for ACS or previous IHD. Always exclude: ST elevation myocardial infarction, non-ST elevation myocardial infarction, unstable angina, old myocardial infarction, ischaemic changes (Figure 8.11), new LBBB.

Look for:

- **ST segment depression or elevation or T-wave inversion**: all are classic signs of ACS. ST segment should be level with base line – elevation/depression of more than 1 mm is significant in limb leads ; 2 mm in chest leads (V leads).
- **Q waves** indicate previous ischaemia.
- **R wave** progression: should increase from V1 to V6.
- **? evidence of LVH**: R waves in any V leads should not exceed 27 mm in height and S waves do not exceed 30 mm. R wave amplitude in limb leads should be <20 mm. LVH (by ECG voltage criteria) any R wave and any S wave in V leads having a combined voltage >3.5 mV (35 mm).
- **Low voltage QRS complexes** could be as a result of obesity, pericardial effusion, chronic obstructive airways disease, ischaemic heart disease
- **T wave** should be concordant with the preceding QRS complex (i.e. both positive or both negative). T wave amplitude rarely exceeds 10 mm in chest leads or 5 mm in limb leads.

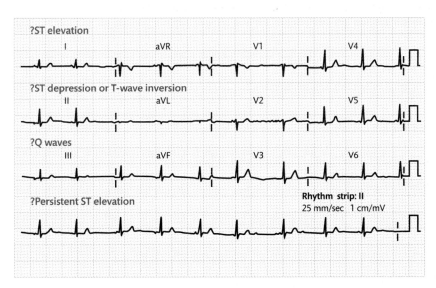

Figure 8.11 Look for ischaemic changes on ECG: the above ECG does not show ischaemia.

Step 4 Axis (Figure 8.12)

? normal, left, right

Frontal plane QRS axis equates to the mean direction of electrical forces within the ventricles. In a normal heart the impulse travels from sinus node to apex (11–5 o'clock) direction – normal QRS axis usually lies –30° to +90°.

Simple method for QRS determination:

	Normal axis (–30° to +90°)	Right axis (+90° to 180°)	Left axis (–30° to –90°)
Lead 1	+ve	-ve	+ve
Lead 11	+ve	Either	–ve
Lead 111	either	+ve	–ve

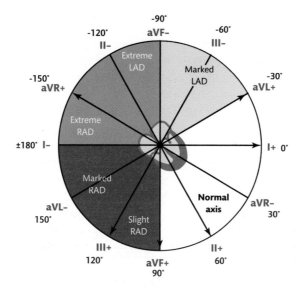

Figure 8.12 Determining the cardiac axis: using limb leads only, the axis will be aligned to the tallest R wave, opposite the deepest S wave and 90° to the isoelectric lead.

Step 5 Bundle branch block: ? left, ? right

Damage to the bundle branches could result from infarction or ischaemia and will delay depolarization of the affected chamber, causing a significant widening of the QRS complex. Look for development of new LBBB, this usually indicates infarction.

Typical features of LBBB and RBBB: recall William Morrow (1843–1929), an incorporator of the American Red Cross.

- **LBBB**
  - ○ Widened QRS *(V1-'W' , V6 'M'), this recalls 'W' ILLIA 'M'*
  - ○ Deep wide S wave V1–V3
  - ○ May see loss of septal Q wave V6
  - ○ ST depression and T wave inversion in V4– V6 , I and AVL
  - ○ ST elevation V1–V3 (resemble STEMI)
- **RBBB**
  - ○ Widened QRS *(V1-'M' , V6 'W'), this recalls 'M' ORRO 'W'*
  - ○ Slurred S wave V6
  - ○ Dominant R wave V1 (r SR or q R complex)
  - ○ ST depression and T wave inversion V1–V3

Step 6 Clinical conclusion

Does what you find, fit with the patient's clinical picture? For example, does the patient with ST elevation also have chest pain or symptoms suggestive of an ACS? If an arrhythmia is present, is this compromising the patient, is it a rhythm they will tolerate? Does the patient have a pacemaker and is this why the ECG is abnormal? Look at the patient's history, signs and ECG and plan management according to findings- often urgent! Use a clear template to present findings. Consider using the four-point presentation (general, important positive findings, important negative findings, clinical conclusion), for example:

> *"This is a 12-lead ECG on a 57-year-old man who came in with a 4-hour history of severe chest pain. The rate is 56 per minute and sinus rhythm. The main abnormal finding is the presence of ST elevation in leads II, III and aVF. There is no evidence of axis deviation or bundle branch block or left ventricular hypertrophy. In conclusion, this ECG is consistent with a ST elevation acute myocardial infarction. The leads affected suggests that this is an inferior myocardial infarction. The right coronary artery is likely to be involved as evidenced by the bradycardia. This patient needs senior review and urgent preparation for emergency angioplasty and/or thrombolysis."*

Patient safety tips

✔ **Interpret ECG findings** with the full clinical history and examination and investigations such as troponin T. Changes of myocardial infarction can also be seen in: right and left ventricular hypertrophy, pericarditis, LBBB, hypertrophic obstructive cardiomyopathy, dilated cardiomyopathy, cardiac contusion, cardiac tumours, pulmonary embolism, pneumothorax, hyperkalaemia, intracranial haemorrhage (trauma, stroke, or subarachnoid haemorrhage).

✔ **Critical window of opportunity for angioplasty and/or thrombolysis** is a few hours only. The earlier the patient is referred for expert cardiological intervention the better the likelihood of survival and greater proportion of myocardium preserved. Seek help from seniors early if you think an ACS should be considered on the basis of the ECG.

✔ **Pericarditis**: there is a distinctly different type of ST elevation that is concave upwards rather than the flatter ST elevation seen in acute myocardial infarction. Many ECG leads will be involved or the pericarditis may be anatomically delineated. Thrombolysis is potentially harmful.

✔ **Initial ECG** in an ACS patient may be normal or show hyperacute peaked T waves only. Changes evolve over hours, so repeat several ECGs if there is a high index of suspicion.

✔ **Think pulmonary embolism**: the classically described ECG changes (S1, Q3, T3, tachycardia, right axis deviation) are actually rare even when the pulmonary embolism has been confirmed by computed tomography angiography. Be sure never to miss pulmonary embolism clinically or on an ECG though.

✔ **Tall, tented T waves** are associated with hyperkalaemia. Urea and electrolytes should always be known in any ACS or arrhythmia. Refractory arrhythmias may be due to calcium or magnesium deficiencies.

✔ **Severe hyperkalaemia (>7 mmol/L)**: can lead to all the acute ST segment changes consistent with ACS. Correct K^+ levels before considering angiography/angioplasty.

The ECG: basic principles and interpretation

Review and translate findings/discuss basic principles of this ECG.
The student is shown an ECG from the clinical environment.

		Self	Peer	Peer /tutor	Tutor
Washes hands	● Washes hands or applies alcohol gel between handling of patient equipment/property	☐	☐	☐	☐
	●	☐	☐	☐	☐
Understands indications and anatomy	● Demonstrates a knowledge of the anatomy of the heart, electrical conduction, and ECG 12-lead placement	☐	☐	☐	☐
	●	☐	☐	☐	☐
Obtains informed consent	● Identifies that the correct patient details (name, date of birth, gender, and hospital number) are documented on the ECG	☐	☐	☐	☐
	●	☐	☐	☐	☐
Explanation to patient	● Explains to patient that ECG will be reviewed and results discussed	☐	☐	☐	☐
	●	☐	☐	☐	☐
Communication skills	● Appropriate communication throughout	☐	☐	☐	☐
	● Allows patient to ask any questions about findings on ECG	☐	☐	☐	☐
	● Discusses implications of results and gives reassurance as required	☐	☐	☐	☐
	●	☐	☐	☐	☐
Appropriate preparation	● Clarifies that **right** ECG belongs to **right** patient and notes time and date of recording. Patient details are documented on ECG (as above). Checks to see if any other detail is documented which may impact on interpretation (i.e. patient sitting up). Obtains patient notes to identify any previous ECGs for comparison. Identifies appropriate area to review ECG and prevent distraction	☐	☐	☐	☐
	● Scans **chest and limb leads**, checks the voltage on vertical axis is 10 mm/mV	☐	☐	☐	☐
	●	☐	☐	☐	☐
Technical ability	Uses a systematic approach for 12-lead ECG interpretation:				
	● **Rate**: Establishes the **rate and regularity of rhythm** using the rhythm strip running along bottom section of ECG (lead II) and viewing all other leads	☐	☐	☐	☐
	● **Rhythm analysis (PQR)**: looks for **evidence of atrial activity (P waves)**; measures PR interval and establishes relationship between atria and ventricles	☐	☐	☐	☐
	● **ST segment changes**: abnormal findings communicated, in particular ST-T wave segment changes in ACS and ischaemic heart disease	☐	☐	☐	☐
	● **Axis**: calculates based on QRS complexes in limb leads, defines normal axis, left axis, right axis	☐	☐	☐	☐
	● **Bundle branch block**: ? Is there evidence of right or left BBB, demonstrates knowledge of specific features of bundle branch block	☐	☐	☐	☐
	● **Clinical conclusion**: relates ECG findings to patient's clinical condition and presenting symptoms into a meaningful conclusion	☐	☐	☐	☐
	●	☐	☐	☐	☐
Patient safety tips	● Seeks expert help immediately if unable to interpret ECG; shows awareness of limitations in own expertise. On discovering a problem on ECG seeks help early to institute treatment	☐	☐	☐	☐
	● Establishes if there is **evidence of acute event, e.g. acute coronary syndromes**				
Post-procedure management	● Documents ECG findings in patients notes and files ECG in correct notes	☐	☐	☐	☐
	●	☐	☐	☐	☐
Professionalism	● Communicates with patient; respects the patients' privacy and dignity at all times	☐	☐	☐	☐
	●	☐	☐	☐	☐

				Self	Peer	Peer /tutor	Tutor
Self-assessed as at least borderline:	Signature:	Date:		U B S E	U B S E	U B S E	U B S E
Peer-assessed as ready for tutor assessment:	Signature:	Date:		U B S E	U B S E	U B S E	U B S E
Tutor-assessed as satisfactory:	Signature:	Date:		U B S E	U B S E	U B S E	U B S E

Notes

Further information
See the Resuscitation Council UK website (www.resus.org.uk) and http://library.med.utah.edu/kw/ecg/ecg_outline.

175

8.6
**Peak expiratory
flow rate meter,
inhalers, and
nebulizers**

8.6 Peak expiratory flow rate meter, inhalers, and nebulizers

Background

The peak expiratory flow rate (PEFR) can be determined at the bedside, and provides a basic measure of lung function that can be used to monitor current function and sequentially to see if there is improvement or deterioration. It is defined as the best of three forced expiratory blows from the total lung capacity with a maximum pause of 2 seconds before blowing. It reflects the diameter of the bronchial tree and represents the high volume and speed of expiratory airflow that occurs in the first 10 milliseconds of forced expiration. It is measured in litres per minute.

Clinical indications

The PEFR has a role in both diagnosis and monitoring of asthma. Spirometry has superseded PEFR measurement in many settings, but PEFR still has a useful role to play in diagnosis and monitoring of patients with asthma as it is easy and quick to teach. In chronic obstructive pulmonary disease (COPD), use of PEFR is not part of the definition for diagnosis but may be useful for domiciliary monitoring or to document diurnal variation to differentiate from asthma. However, in severe COPD, the PEFR will tend to seriously underestimate the severity of airflow obstruction. PEFR depends on effort and technique and the normal ranges are wide. Current tables do not encompass ethnic diversity.

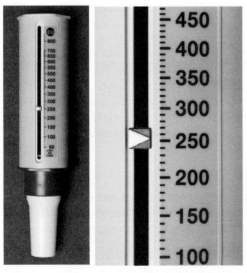
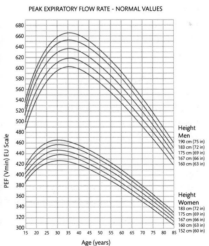

Standard peak flow meter: measures from 0 to 800 L/min

Point and calibration gauge: 10 L/min per notch

PEFR normal values by height and gender; separate tables exist for children

Figure 8.13 Images in PEFR.

Asthma diagnosis

- **Detection and measure of severity**: of airway obstruction acutely.
- **Assisting diagnosis of asthma**: variability of PEFR (morning and evening) in a diary over 2 weeks. PEFR variability is expressed as the difference between the highest and lowest PEFR as

a percentage of the highest PEFR. The upper limit of normal is around 20%. In COPD the peak flow is reduced, but there is little variability.

- **Diagnosing occupational asthma**: looking at peak flow readings at work and away from work.
- **Identifying reversibility**: pre and post treatment in asthma diagnosis. A significant increase in PEFR (>15% or >60 L/min)) indicates reversible airflow obstruction and suggests a positive response to inhaled corticosteroids.

Asthma monitoring

- **In established asthma**, however, symptom-based monitoring is adequate in the majority of patients.
- **Identification of severity of exacerbation of asthma**: a change in peak flow is more useful than the actual value.
- **Limitations**: the diagnosis of asthma is a clinical one: there are no standardized findings on investigation. Tests of airflow obstruction may provide support for a diagnosis of asthma. However, normal results on tests, especially when asymptomatic, do not exclude the diagnosis. Serial measures of PEFR show poor concordance with disease activity and do not reliably rule the diagnosis of asthma in or out. Restrictive deficits cannot be detected with PEFR reliably. The various causes of airflow obstruction cannot be differentiated by PEFR. Indeed PEFR does not discriminate between patients with established airflow limitation due to asthma from those whose airflow obstruction is due to other conditions. Patients may have more than one cause of airflow obstruction; in particular, asthma and COPD commonly coexist.

Physiological and professional principles

Predicted normal reference values

Peak flow varies by age, sex, height, and even ethnicity. Specialized tables and charts exist to identify what an individual's predicted peak flow rate is. In men values up to 100 L/min lower than predicted are considered within normal limits, for women the equivalent figure is 85 L/min. In men peak flow is maximal around age 35, whereas in women it peaks around age 30. A peak flow more than 40 L/min lower than expected suggests a problem with effort or technique. In normal subjects there is some variability in PEFR. The reading is often slightly higher in the evening compared to the morning, although in people with asthma this variability is much greater (usually >20% of maximal PEFR).

Assessment of severity of asthma

An indication of the severity of an asthma attack in an individual patient can be gauged from the in-attack PEFR as a percentage of the patient's usual best PEFR (British Thoracic Society (BTS)/Scottish Intercollegiate Guidelines Network (SIGN) guidelines) (BTS website, accessed December 2010).

- **Moderate asthma attack**: PEFR <75% of best or predicted.
- **Severe asthma attack**: PEFR <50% of best or predicted.
- **Life-threatening asthma attack**: <33% of best or predicted
- Reduction in peak flow to 50–75% of predicted or best is a moderate exacerbation, 33–50% represents a severe exacerbation, <33% suggests a life-threatening exacerbation (BTS/SIGN guidelines).

Peak flow meters

These are now available on prescription and supplied with peak flow diary charts. Since 2004 all peak flow meters have been standardized to a new EU scale. Some meters, but not all, will identify the scale the meter uses on the meter itself. The newer EU scale meters have a higher degree of accuracy and should now be used instead of older meters. You must ensure that the predicted values chart is for the meter scale you are using. The most commonly used peak flow meter brand is Mini Wright. In this brand the EU scale is shown as blue text on a yellow background.

Normal range meters can measure flow within the ranges 0–800 L/min, low range meters go from 0 to 400 L/min. For most adults and children, normal range meters are used. Only in individuals with severe airways disease are low range meters used – where predicted or best peak flow is less than 250 L/min.

Children

Measuring lung function in children younger than 5 years of age is difficult and requires techniques which are not widely available. Above 5 years of age, conventional lung function testing is possible in most children in most settings. Peak flow values in children correlate best with height. The difference between sexes increases with age.

Contraindications

Clearly a patient who cannot adequately follow the instructions for use due to reasons of age, learning disability or other incapacity may not be able to have PEFR measurements. The results may be useless for clinical management in these patients.

Possible errors

- Not taking full inspiration or delay from full inspiration to performing test >2 seconds.
- Blocking the mouthpiece with tongue or teeth or fingers blocking pointer.
- Poor mouth seal: may be due to loose fitting false teeth or facial palsy.
- Not blowing with maximal force: instead blowing for maximal duration.
- Poor technique: coughing or spitting.

Sequence

Equipment and preparation
- EU scale (EN 13826 standard) PEFR with integral one-way valve
- Corresponding predicted value chart (EU scale)
- Disposable mouthpiece

Explanation and consent
Describe the method of performing peak flow to the patient. In particular emphasize:
- Full inspiration prior to blowing, and not to hold it
- Blow out as hard and fast as possible, *not* as long as possible
- Good seal around the mouthpiece and their tongue/teeth do not obstruct the blow
- Hold the peak flow meter horizontally – fingers not obstructing the pointer
- Inform patient that it will be the best of three
- Warn them that the process may make them cough.

Procedure
- Stand (preferably) or sit, positioning the pointer to zero.
- Hold the meter horizontally and ensure fingers are not obstructing the pointer.
- Instruct patient to take a full breath in and immediately seal lips around mouthpiece.

- Within 2 seconds of the full inspiration blow out as hard and fast as possible.
- Note the reading. Repeat twice more and take *highest* figure as peak flow rate.
- Compare this figure to the predicted value (or patient's own best reading) and express it as a percentage of that value.

Professionalism

Since a large amount of the work done in respiratory care and monitoring is performed by specialist nurses, it is imperative that the predicted and actual peak flow readings are recorded in the patient's notes. This provides information for annual reviews and also background information for comparison by other professionals who may see the patient at a time when they are less well. It is also important to make a comment on the peak flow technique: if a reading is low but technique is good, it provides useful context for interpretation of results.

Making the patient aware of their predicted peak flow and encouraging them to remember their usual individual normal peak flow is invaluable.

Patient safety tips

✔ **Infection control**: always follow the manufacturer's guidance on infection control. Most meters used in hospitals or primary care settings are fitted with an integral one-way valve that prevents inhalation of any of the previous patients' breath that could remain in the meter. Meters without this are considered to be single patient use. However, if a patient is suspected of having a serious communicable disease it is safer to dispose of the meter. Disposable mouthpieces should be used, or plastic mouthpieces should be sterilized between patients. The peak flow meters themselves can also be disinfected in accordance with manufacturer's guidance.

Despite the theoretical risk, literature reviews have found there is little evidence of cross-infection from lung function equipment.

Inhalers and nebulizers

An inhaler is a medical device that aims to deliver medication directly via the airways in the lungs. The medication can then act therapeutically on the airways to cause bronchodilatation, reduction in inflammation or dry secretions. The optimum therapeutic benefit from an inhaler is highly dependent on individual technique.

A nebulizer is a machine that vaporizes liquid medication into a fine respirable mist to be inhaled into the lungs via a mouthpiece or mask. The use of a nebulizer does not require the patient to use a specific technique for its therapeutic use and in most cases, the maximal therapeutic benefits are obtained just through normal breathing during the duration of the nebulizer treatment. Nebulizers can be pressure driven by compressed air or oxygen and it is important in type 2 respiratory failure due to COPD that air is used, however, in asthma it should be oxygen driven.

There are also ultrasonic nebulizers.

Metered dose inhaled pressurized aerosol

Metered dose inhalers (MDIs) contains a pressurized inactive gas that propels a dose of drug in each 'puff'. Each dose is released by pressing the top of the inhaler. An alternative to the standard MDI is the breath activated MDI. With these the patient does not have to push the canister to release a dose but the dose is triggered by the patient's own deep inspiration.

Historically, the propellant gas in MDI inhalers was CFC (chlorofluorocarbon, capable of damaging the ozone) but all new generation inhalers are CFC free.

Correct technique for inhaler use:

1 Shake the inhaler and hold upright.

2 Breathe out and immediately close lips around mouthpiece.

3 Depress plunger at start of *slow* inspiration.

4 Inspire as much as possible to total lung capacity.

5 Hold breathe for 10 seconds.

6 Breathe out slowly.

MDI with spacer

Spacers are placed between the inhaler and the mouth and acts as a reservoir which holds the drug when the inhaler is pressed. A valve exists at the mouth end and ensures that the drug is kept within the spacer. During inspiration the valve opens and the drug is delivered, during expiration the valve closes. Spacer devices probably allow the most effective method for inhaler deposition of particles within the lung and are less dependent on technique.

Correct technique for MDI use:

1 Shake the inhaler and hold MDI upright and spacer in correct position for device.

2 Keep lips on mouthpiece.

3 Breathe one to five moderate breaths in and out.

4 Be sure valve is operating.

5 Keep spacer clean and dry.

Dry powder inhalers

These inhalers instead of gas propellant for drug delivery contain the drug in powder form that is inhaled.

Correct technique for dry powder inhalers:

1 Follow instruction for preparation of device.

2 Breathe out.

3 Place lips firmly around mouthpiece.

4 Breathe in rapidly and deeply.

5 Hold breath for 10 seconds.

Types of inhaler by pharmacological class

β_2-agonists

- **Short-acting relievers**: salbutamol, terbutaline
- **Long-acting**: salmeterol, formoterol

Anticholinergic bronchodilators

- **Short-acting relievers**: ipratropium bromide
- **Long-acting**: tiotropium

Steroid preventive inhalers

- Corticosteroids: beclometasone, budesonide, fluticasone

Some inhaler combinations

- Combivent: salbutamol and ipratropium bromide
- Seretide: combination of fluticasone and salmeterol
- Symbicort: combination of budesonide and formoterol
- Fostair: combination of beclometasone and formoterol

Types of nebulizer solution

- Salbutamol: short-acting β_2-agonist
- Ipratropium bromide: anticholinergic bronchodilator
- Normal saline

Nebulizer correct technique

- Follow instruction for preparation of device.
- Normal breathing though mouthpiece or facemask.
- Breathe continuously until mist no longer produced by nebulizer.

Patient safety tips

✔ Peak flow meters: if used correctly and a diary of PEFR values kept, this can help the earlier diagnosis of a potential exacerbation. The patient can then augment treatment and seek help from healthcare professionals if needed. This can often result in community management rather than in-patient care.

✔ Inhaler technique: it is critical to evaluate inhaler technique in all patients. Errors in administration will result in ineffective delivery of the drugs and potentially lead to other drugs being used with significantly more side-effects (e.g. oral steroids).

✔ Nebulizers: the same applies for nebulizers as well.

✔ Infection: theoretical risk; use disposable devices where possible.

Table 8.3 Advantages and disadvantages of inhaler-types and nebulizers

Advantages	Disadvantages
MDI inhalers	
Small and portable	Perfect technique absolutely essential
Cheap	Unsuitable for the very young, elderly, confused,
Quick to use	arthritic, other disabilities
	Cold jet may irritate throat
MDI with spacers	
Coordination unimportant	Bulky but usually left at home for morning and
Can be used by almost all patients, including children	evening doses only
May reduce systemic absorption of corticosteroids	Valves sometimes stick or become incompetent
Dry powder inhalers	
Coordination unimportant	Relatively expensive
Can be used by almost all patients	Require rapid inspiration and higher inspiratory
Small and portable	flow
No CFCs	Preparing device requires a little skill
Nebulizers	
Coordination unimportant	Cumbersome, noisy equipment (compressor)
Can be used for all ages	Expensive
	No more effective than other devices at same dosage
	Treatment takes a long time (5–10 minutes)

Student name:	Medical school:	Year:

PFER meter, inhalers, and nebulizers

This assessment will consist of questions and demonstration of three clinical skills in this subject area. The assessor will act as a simulated patient for PEFR measurement and the inhaler technique. A manikin or the assessor will be used for demonstration of nebulizer use.

		Self	Peer	Peer/tutor	Tutor
What are the clinical indications for PEFR measurement		☐	☐	☐	☐
Specifically in relation to asthma what is the role of PEFR in diagnosis		☐	☐	☐	☐
Specifically in relation to asthma what is the role of PEFR in monitoring		☐	☐	☐	☐
What are the limitations of PEFR measurement?		☐	☐	☐	☐
What are the predicted normal reference values and how are they affected throughout the day?		☐	☐	☐	☐
Assessment of severity of asthma: how are following defined?	● **Moderate asthma attack**: PEFR <x % of best or predicted ● **Severe asthma attack**: PEFR <y % of best or predicted ● **Life-threatening asthma attack**: <z% of best or predicted	☐ ☐ ☐	☐ ☐ ☐	☐ ☐ ☐	☐ ☐ ☐
What are the contraindications to PEFR measurement?		☐	☐	☐	☐
What are possible errors in PEFR measurement?		☐	☐	☐	☐
Please carry out PEFR measurement in this subject?		☐	☐	☐	☐
Equipment and preparation	● PEFR meter and chart, disposable mouthpiece	☐	☐	☐	☐
Explanation and consent	1 Emphasizes full inspiration prior to blowing, and not to hold it, blow out as hard and fast as possible, *not* as long as possible, good seal around the mouthpiece 2 Holds the peak flow meter horizontally – fingers not obstructing the pointer 3 Inform patient that it will be the best of three 4 Warn them that the process may make them cough	☐ ☐ ☐ ☐	☐ ☐ ☐ ☐	☐ ☐ ☐ ☐	☐ ☐ ☐ ☐
Procedure	1 Stands (preferably) or sits, positions the pointer to zero 2 Holds the meter horizontally and ensure fingers are not obstructing the pointer 3 Instructs patient to take a full breath in and immediately seal lips around mouthpiece 4 Instructs patient to blow out as hard and fast as possible within 2 seconds of the full inspiration 5 Notes the reading. Repeats twice more and take *highest* figure as peak flow rate 6 Compares this figure to the predicted value (or patient's own best reading) and expresses it as a percentage of that value	☐ ☐ ☐ ☐ ☐	☐ ☐ ☐ ☐ ☐	☐ ☐ ☐ ☐ ☐	☐ ☐ ☐ ☐ ☐
Professionalism	● Records in patient's notes. Involves other healthcare professionals as needed. Explains results to patient, mentions consider updating patient's own peak flow diary	☐	☐	☐	☐
Inhalers and nebulizers: discusses indications; instructs patient or subject on how to use an inhaler and checks done correctly	Instructs patient to: ● Shake the inhaler and hold upright ● Breathe out and immediately close lips around mouthpiece ● Depress plunger at start of *slow* inspiration ● Inspire as much as possible to total lung capacity ● Hold breath for 10 seconds and breathe out slowly	☐ ☐ ☐ ☐ ☐	☐ ☐ ☐ ☐ ☐	☐ ☐ ☐ ☐ ☐	☐ ☐ ☐ ☐ ☐
Drugs used in inhalers or nebulizers by pharmacological class	● State commonly used β_2-agonists and their side effects ● States commonly used anticholinergic bronchodilators and their side effects ● States commonly used steroid inhalers and their side effects	☐ ☐ ☐	☐ ☐ ☐	☐ ☐ ☐	☐ ☐ ☐
Please set up this nebulizer for use in this manikin/subject. The 'drug' used will be 5 mL normal saline for injection	● Explanation to 'subject' ● Prepares and assembles equipment and places exactly 5 mL of normal saline into reservoir ● Places nebulizer mask onto 'subject' ● Uses air or oxygen to drive the nebulizer after switching device on ● Appreciates: nebulizers can be pressure driven by compressed air or oxygen.(In type 2 respiratory failure due to COPD air is used. In asthma it should be oxygen driven)	☐ ☐ ☐ ☐ ☐	☐ ☐ ☐ ☐ ☐	☐ ☐ ☐ ☐ ☐	☐ ☐ ☐ ☐ ☐
Patient safety tips	● Discusses infection control, disposable mouthpieces, disposable meter ● Ensure patient education for optimal monitoring and drug efficacy	☐ ☐	☐ ☐	☐ ☐	☐ ☐

			Self	Peer	Peer/tutor	Tutor
Self-assessed as at least borderline:	Signature:	Date:	U B S E	U B S E	U B S E	U B S E
Peer-assessed as ready for tutor assessment:	Signature:	Date:	U B S E	U B S E	U B S E	U B S E
Tutor-assessed as satisfactory:	Signature:	Date:	U B S E	U B S E	U B S E	U B S E

Notes

8.7 Spirometry

Background

Spirometry is an extremely useful but easy to conduct test that should be used in the investigation of all respiratory causes of breathlessness. It is preferable to PEFR in diagnosis because it allows clearer identification of airflow obstruction and the results are less dependent on effort. It is the preferred initial test to assess the presence and severity of airflow obstruction. Spirometry is able to accurately identify airflow obstruction, differentiate between obstructive and restrictive problems and provide an estimate of severity. It is better than peak flow at detecting mild obstruction and is less likely to underestimate severity of obstruction in more severe disease.

Clinical indications

- **Non-acute assessment of shortness of breath**: detection of obstructive or restrictive lung deficits, or mixed. This may include respiratory, cardiac, or systemic causes.
- **Assessment of severity of airway obstruction or lung restriction**: forced expiratory volume in 1 second (FEV_1) is an indicator of maximal exercise capacity and FEV_1% predicted is strongly correlated with disability in chronic respiratory diseases. FEV_1% predicted is used to quantify severity.
- **Reversibility testing**: a significant increase in FEV_1 (>12% from baseline or 400 mL) following trial of treatment indicates reversible airways obstruction.
- **Prognosis**: FEV_1 % predicted is closely related to prognosis in COPD.
- **Monitoring**: progression of disease especially COPD and emphysema.

Physiological and professional principles

Spirometry typically measures relaxed vital capacity, forced vital capacity (FVC), FEV_1 and the ratio of FEV_1 to FVC.

FEV1% predicted determines the degree of severity and is closely related to prognosis in COPD. FEV_1 is largely independent of effort and is highly repeatable. Predicted normal ranges are based on age, sex, height, and ethnicity. Normal ranges are widely available and robust. The full set of physiological measures are show in Figure 8.14. The FVC and FEV_1 are specific standardized measures of the vital capacity.

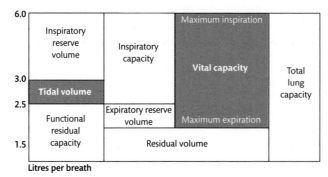

Figure 8.14 Respiratory physiological normal values.

Definitions

- **Forced vital capacity** (**FVC**): after breathing out to full expiration, the patient is instructed to breathe in with a maximal effort and then exhale as forcefully and rapidly as possible. The FVC is the volume of air, in litres, that is expelled into the spirometer following a maximum inhalation effort.
- **Forced expiratory volume** (**FEV**): at the start of the FVC measurement, the volume of air delivered through the mouthpiece at timed intervals of 0.5, 1.0, 2.0, and 3.0 seconds is recorded. The integrated sum of these is usually over 95% of the FVC. FEV_1, is the volume of air, in litres, that is exhaled into the mouthpiece in the first second. It should be at least 70% of the FVC.
- **Relaxed vital capacity** (**RVC**): is the total volume of air, in litres, expelled in a relaxed expiration, starting from full inspiration. It can also be measured as the maximum volume of air inspired into the lungs in a relaxed inspiration from a position of maximal expiration. Its main purpose is to permit more reliable estimation of vital capacity in individuals with significant airway collapse (and thus trapping of air) when expiration is forced. It removes the dynamic compression of airways that occurs with forcible exhalation, which can artificially reduce vital capacity.
- **FEV_1:FVC** is expressed as a ratio or a percentage. Increasingly FEV_6 is being shown as being a valid alternative to FVC.

Obstructive deficits

These are due to narrowing of the airways, which prevents the air exiting the lungs as quickly as possible. Total lung volume is generally not affected (except in severe chronic disease) and thus the vital capacity is usually normal. However, because the rate of expiration of air is less than normal, the volume of air expelled in 1 second will be less than 80% of that predicted. A reduced FEV_1 with a normal FVC will result in an FEV_1/FVC ratio being <70% and determines whether there is obstruction. Where predicted range is not available a ratio of less than 70% is the ratio used to determine obstruction. However, it is the FEV_1% predicted which determines the degree of severity of obstruction and is closely related to prognosis in COPD. FEV_1 is largely independent of effort and is highly repeatable.

Restrictive deficits

These are due to a reduction in the absolute volume of the lungs. As the total volume of the lungs is reduced, it can be expected that the volume expired in 1 second would also be reduced. As a result both FVC and FEV_1 are reduced, with the greater effect being on FVC. The FEV_1/FVC ratio is therefore preserved, or sometimes increased in comparison with predicted normal.

Spirometry will also typically produce a flow/volume curve and a volume/time trace. These traces will aid in the diagnosis of upper airways obstruction as, for example, with a goitre that is causing tracheal obstruction. The carbon monoxide diffusion capacity (DLCO) is used to measure gas transfer across the alveolar-blood capillary membranes. This is reduced in interstitial lung disease and emphysema.

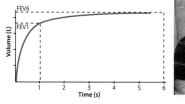
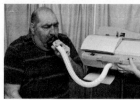
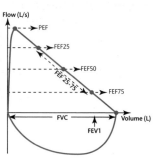

Spirometry: forced breath out; the FEV1 (first second) and FVC at 6 seconds

Spirometry machine and trace

Flow volume loop: the main 'boat' is inspiration and 'sail' expiration

Figure 8.15 Images in spirometry.

Normal

FEV_1 >80% predicted, FVC >80% predicted, FEV_1/FVC ratio ≥0.7.

Obstructive pattern

FEV_1: <80% predicted, FVC >80% predicted, FEV_1/FVC ratio <70%. For COPD severity use (Gold 2010)

- Mild: FEV_1/FVC <0.7, FEV_1 ≥80% predicted
- Moderate: FEV_1/FVC <0.7, FEV_1 50–79% predicted
- Severe: FEV_1/FVC <0.7, FEV_1 30–49% predicted
- Very severe: FEV_1/FVC <0.7, FEV_1 <30% predicted.

TLC increased or normal, residual volume increased:

- Asthma, COPD, emphysema
- Bronchitis, bronchiectasis, inhaled foreign body
- Obliterative bronchiolitis, large airway stenosis
- Intraluminal lung cancer.

Restrictive pattern

FEV_1: normal or mildly reduced, FVC <80% predicted, FEV_1/FVC ratio >0.7.

TLC decreased, residual volume decreased:

- Intrinsic lung disease: pulmonary fibrosis, connective tissue disease, sarcoidosis, drug-induced lung disease, pulmonary oedema.
- Extrinsic lung disease: chest wall, pleura and neuromuscular disorders, e.g. pleural effusion/fibrosis, mesothelioma, kyphoscoliosis, ankylosing spondylitis, myasthenia gravis, motor neurone disease, multiple sclerosis.

Definition of reversibility for diagnosis of asthma or reversible COPD:

- **Bronchodilator reversibility**: Spirometry 15–20 minutes after inhalation of β-agonist (four puffs salbutamol via MDI or 2.5 mg salbutamol via nebulizer) or 30–45 minutes after inhalation of anticholinergic (four puffs ipratropium via MDI or 250 µg via nebulizer).
- **Corticosteroid reversibility**: Before and following 30 mg prednisolone once daily for 2 weeks, or 6–12 week trial of high dose inhaled corticosteroid (e.g. 500 µg beclometasone twice daily).

Contraindications to spirometry

- **Children less than 5 years of age**: as with peak flow, measurements in very young children are unlikely to be successful.
- **Acute illness**: because of the considerable breathing control required to perform spirometry correctly, the patient should not be experiencing a considerable exacerbation of their symptoms at the time of testing.
- Note that a normal result when a patient has no symptoms does not exclude a diagnosis of airways disease, particularly asthma.

Sequence

Equipment and preparation

Patients should be asked to avoid:

- Taking a short-acting bronchodilator within 2–4 hours of the test
- Taking a long-acting β-agonist within 12 hours of the test
- Taking a long-acting inhaled anticholinergic or sustained-release theophylline within 24 h of the test
- Vigorous exercise within 30 minutes of the test
- Eating a substantial meal within 2 hours of the test
- Wearing restrictive clothing. Bladder should be empty ideally for comfort
- Ideally, smoking within 24 hours of test
- Alcohol within 4 hours of test.

Explanation and consent

- Sit the patient comfortably. Sitting is preferred to standing in spirometry because the repeated blowing can cause light-headedness. Sitting is thus safer.
- Explain to the patient that different instructions will be given at different times and to listen carefully to instruction. There will be repeated forced expiration, a minimum of three times.
- Demonstration of technique along with explanation will help achievement of technically satisfactory results.
- Emphasize to patient that the tongue should not occlude the mouthpiece and teeth should be placed around the outside of the mouthpiece.

Procedure

- Measure height without shoes and record age, gender, and ethnicity.

First measure relaxed vital capacity:

- Nose clip may be required, or the patient can pinch the nose.
- Advise patient to breathe in as deeply as possible.
- Expiration at a sustained and comfortable speed until no further air can be exhaled. This should not be done forcibly. It should be like a deep sigh.
- Repeat at least twice.

Then measure forced exhalation:

- Nose clip not usually required.
- Advise patient to breathe in as deeply as possible.
- Forced expiration as fast and hard as possible until no further air can be exhaled.
- Encourage patient to continue to blow as hard as possible throughout procedure.
- Repeat for a minimum of three readings.
- A minimum of 30 seconds should be left between blows to allow the patient time to recover.

- May be repeated up to eight times in a single session.
- The test is stopped if less than 0.05 L has been expired over 2 seconds or duration of exhalation exceeds 15 seconds. Patients with airflow obstruction may take around 10 seconds to complete.

Ensure results are technically satisfactory. This is demonstrated by:

- Smooth tracings: irregularities suggest coughing or variable effort.
- Almost vertical rise in flow-volume curve to a peak: slow rise suggests suboptimal effort.
- Volume/time trace must rise directly from baseline: S shape indicates slow start to exhalation.
- Time to peak flow <300 ms.
- Full blow: flow/volume returns smoothly to axis, volume/time reaches plateau.
- The FEV_1 and FVC readings must be less than 100 mL/5% different between the best two blows.

Complications

- Dizziness from hyperventilation
- Excessive coughing
- Distress caused by prolonged expiration/difficulty performing the test

Patient safety tips

✔ **Infection control**: Disposable mouthpieces should be used, or plastic mouthpieces should be sterilized between patients.

✔ Adjust normal values for ethnicity, values in South-Asians are around 10% lower than in white caucasians.

✔ Use low resistance barrier filter to minimize infection and protect equipment from exhaled respiratory secretions.

Student name:	Medical school:	Year:

Spirometry

Please can you perform basic spirometry on this patient?
Student is asked to perform spirometry on a patient or the assessor

		Self	Peer	Peer /tutor	Tutor
Washes hands	● Hand wash with water and soap or alcohol gel	☐	☐	☐	☐
Understands indications and anatomy	● States need for investigation and monitoring of	☐	☐	☐	☐
	● respiratory function, e.g. diagnosis of obstructive airways disease, assessment of severity of lung restriction	☐	☐	☐	☐
	● States definitions and normal ranges of FEV and FVC	☐	☐	☐	☐
	●	☐	☐	☐	☐
Obtains informed consent	● Introduction and identifies patient	☐	☐	☐	☐
	● Gains informed consent – clear explanation, e.g. 'I am	☐	☐	☐	☐
Explanation to patient, often including complications	● going to carry out a test of your lung function.'	☐	☐	☐	☐
	● Explains and demonstrates to patient how to perform the test	☐	☐	☐	☐
	●	☐	☐	☐	☐
Communication skills	● Assessment throughout the procedure, allows patient to ask questions, provides clear explanation of how to perform the test to the patient	☐	☐	☐	☐
	●	☐	☐	☐	☐
Appropriate preparation	● Configures spirometer by measuring and inputting correct information: height, gender, age, ethnicity	☐	☐	☐	☐
	● Recognizes that expected values are typically pre-programmed into spirometer	☐	☐	☐	☐
	●	☐	☐	☐	☐
Technical ability especially with any special equipment and sharps	● Ensures patient is sitting comfortably and loose clothing is removed	☐	☐	☐	☐
	● Applies nose clip if needed	☐	☐	☐	☐
	● Asks patient to take a deep breath in, seal lips around mouthpiece and breathe out in a relaxed manner, as in a deep sigh	☐	☐	☐	☐
	● Repeats test, allowing time for patient to recover between blows. Asks the patient to breathe in deeply, seal lips around the mouthpiece and breathe out as hard, fast and fully as possible, giving encouragement during procedure	☐	☐	☐	☐
	● Repeats test twice more, allowing time for patient to recover between blows	☐	☐	☐	☐
	● Assesses patient technique throughout and ensure that data are technologically sound	☐	☐	☐	☐
	●	☐	☐	☐	☐
Aseptic technique	● Use new disposable mouthpiece per patient	☐	☐	☐	☐
	● Asks patient to dispose of the mouthpiece in yellow bag or wears gloves to dispose of mouthpiece and then washes hands	☐	☐	☐	☐
	●	☐	☐	☐	☐
Seeks help as appropriate	● Discusses finding with senior as appropriate	☐	☐	☐	☐
	●	☐	☐	☐	☐
Post-procedure management	● Is able to print out results and files in notes	☐	☐	☐	☐
	● Interprets data correctly	☐	☐	☐	☐
	●	☐	☐	☐	☐
Professionalism	● Explains results to the patient and allows patient opportunity to ask questions	☐	☐	☐	☐
	● Thanks patient	☐	☐	☐	☐
	●	☐	☐	☐	☐
Overall ability to perform procedure	● Assess globally, would you be happy for this student to be supervised to conduct respiratory function tests on a real patient?	☐	☐	☐	☐
	●	☐	☐	☐	☐
Patient safety tips	● Use correct reference ranges for the ethnicity of the patient	☐	☐	☐	☐
	● Disposable mouthpieces for infection control	☐	☐	☐	☐
		☐	☐	☐	☐

				Self	Peer	Peer/tutor	Tutor
Self-assessed as at least borderline:	Signature:		Date:	U B S E	U B S E	U B S E	U B S E
Peer-assessed as ready for tutor assessment:	Signature:		Date:	U B S E	U B S E	U B S E	U B S E
Tutor-assessed as satisfactory:	Signature:		Date:	U B S E	U B S E	U B S E	U B S E

Notes

8.8 Urinalysis and pregnancy testing

Background

The urine dip is a quick and easy test that is performed 'at the bed side'. It is widely used in screening for renal tract problems, especially checking for an urinary tract infection. The 'Multi-stix' or similar analysis also offers useful information in many other clinical conditions.

The test strip contains reagents within each coloured square that will undergo a chemical reaction with a certain constituent in the urine. The reaction and colour produced is proportional to the amount of constituent present. The dipstick container usually has timing guidance, i.e. how long after dipping the most accurate colour/level is shown – some may take up to 2 minutes, many are seconds only.

Positive results on a urine dip should prompt further investigations such as with midstream urine (MSU) culture and sensitivity, blood biochemistry, and imaging as appropriate to the clinical scenario. The result should be clearly documented in the patient's notes as there will usually be no other record such as the laboratory report as for most other investigations. Pregnancy testing is a specific urine test, separate from the 'Multi-stix' urinalysis, but will be covered in this section as well.

Clinical indications

- **Pre-screening and preoperative assessment**
- **All patients on admission to hospital**: as soon as clinically indicated or within 24 hours
- **Urinary tract infection (UTI) clinical signs/symptoms**: e.g. confusion, incontinence, burning sensation, offensive smelling odour, pain, pyrexia, cloudy urine
- **Other renal tract disease suspected**: e.g. stones, nephropathy, malignancy.
- **Diabetic ketoacidosis**: diagnosis and monitoring
- **Dehydration**: visually dark urine on inspection
- **Jaundice**.

Contraindications

There are no specific contraindications to this test. Clearly clinical judgement is needed to ascertain whether a particular specimen of urine is of clinical value – those contaminated by soiling, non-fresh specimen or obviously very bloody will be less useful. The test is non-invasive, rapid, cheap, and does not require specialist knowledge to perform.

As with all investigations it should be performed and interpreted within the clinical context.

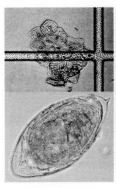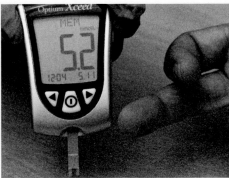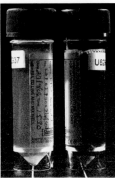

Direct microscopy of the urine can be revealing: epilthelial cells secondary to an UTI, and a schistosomiasis cyst are shown.

Follow up any glycosuria with an initial finger-prick blood glucose level and consider diabetes mellitus–often missed!

Urine dipstick essentially as part of preoperative preparation–do not miss urinary tract infection, diabetes or jaundice. Exclude pregnancy when needed.

Figure 8.16 Images in urinalysis and pregnancy testing.

Sequence

Ideally an MSU sample should be obtained, therefore if a positive result is found it can immediately be sent for other analysis such as urine culture.

The sample should be taken into a sterile container. This must not contain boric acid initially (usually a red-topped bottle used for sending MSU for culture), as this will affect the result.

Inspection of the urine

While not advocating an elaborate detailed inspection the following clinical points are important:

- **Smell**: if there an ammonia smell, an infection with nitrite-splitting bacteria such as *Proteus* is possible.
- **Appearance**: Several possibilities to consider here:
  ○ **Port-wine colour**: haematuria
  ○ **Port-wine urine with clots of blood**: severe haematuria!
  ○ **Dark urine**: dehydration
  ○ **Normal** straw-coloured, lager-colour urine
  ○ **Light coloured urine**: well-hydrated, diuresis phase post-renal failure, ?diabetes insipidus
  ○ **Cloudy urine**: proteinuria, infection
  ○ **Green urine**: *Pseudomonas* infection
  ○ **Blue urine**: certain over-the-counter treatments
  ○ **Intensely dark urine**: 'black water fever' seen in severe malaria
  ○ **Bright orange urine**: rifampicin treatment – warn patient!

The reagent stick must be carefully used according to the exact instructions of the manufacturer especially in relation to the timing of when a test result can be recorded.

Patient safety and clinical governance tips

Any and all investigations should be performed for a purpose and interpreted appropriately. If, for example, the dipstick is positive for protein (greater than trace), it would be appropriate to send urine for albumin/creatinine ratio. Not to do so, particularly in a patient with diabetes, would not be good practice.

Urine dipstick using a multi-reagent stick

Bilirubin **Range: Negative, Trace, +, ++, +++,**

This is *not* a normal finding in the urine. If present it indicates biliary obstruction. NB: *un*conjugated bilirubin is water- *in*soluble, once conjugated by enzymes in the hepatocytes it is excreted into the biliary system- if this cannot pass into the gut (due to obstruction) and be degraded by bacteria, no urobilinogen is produced and the water-soluble conjugated bilirubin is filtered by the kidneys and excreted.

Blood **Range: Negative, Non-haemolysed (Trace or ++), Haemolysed (Trace or +, ++, +++)**

Haematuria results from bleeding somewhere along the urinary tract (kidneys, ureters, bladder or urethra). Infections may cause microscopic haematuria. Other causes to consider include renal stones, anticoagulant therapy, microemboli (numerous causes), tumours (malignant and benign of any part of tract), prostate disease and trauma.

An MSU should always be sent for microscopy to confirm presence of red cells.

NB: Patients over the age of 50 with unexplained microscopic haematuria warrant urgent specialist referral- ensure haematuria and suspected cause documented and followed up by GP to ensure this has resolved after treatment (to avoid missing bladder/renal cancers). Menstrual blood loss is a common cause of a positive result- ask the patient!

Glucose **Range: Negative, Trace, +, ++, +++, ++++**

An abnormal finding due to high blood sugar levels, or leakage of glucose during the filtration process. A positive result should always prompt blood tests for diabetes mellitus. Renal glycosuria can occur in healthy kidneys (pregnancy, but investigate for gestational diabetes), or in renal disease (e.g. glomerulonephritis).

Ketones **Range: Negative, Trace, +, ++, +++, ++++**

Found in dehydration, starvation and diabetic ketoacidosis. For DKA, glucose should also be present on the dip stick.

Ketones are formed from fatty acid breakdown and provide energy to the heart and brain when glucose is not available, hence their production when insufficient insulin is present to allow cells to utilize glucose from the circulation. Ketone molecules are acids hence increased levels result in a drop in blood pH.

Leukocyte esterase **Range: Negative, Trace, +, ++, +++**

This enzyme is produced by white blood cells as a sign of inflammation. When detected in the urine it typically indicates infection. If *only* leukocytes are present without nitrites/blood/protein the sample is probably contaminated (e.g. by vaginal secretions). The test should be repeated with a fresh sample.

N-acetyl-glucosaminidase **Range: Negative, Trace, +**

This is a renal tubular enzyme. Its presence indicates tubular damage and may be positive in pyrexia.

Nitrites **Range: Negative, Positive**

A positive result indicates infection. Gram negative bacteria in the urine reduce nitrates to nitrites. A test may return negative if the bladder was recently voided as the pathogen needs time for the reaction to occur- ideally 4-8 hours should have passed prior to the sample being obtained.

The normal level in the urine is zero, hence any colour change on the stick is considered positive.

In combination with leukocytes the test has a sensitivity of 87% and of specificity 67%.

pH **Range: 5.0, 6.0, 6.5, 7.0, 7.5, 8.0, 8.5**

Normal pH varies between 4.5 and 8.0. Testing is useful in patients with renal stones as the urine pH is lower when uric acid is elevated making stone formation more likely. Altering the pH (i.e. urinary alkalinization with potassium citrate or acetazolamide) can reduce stone formation.

Protein **Range: Negative, Trace, +, ++, +++, ++++**

Small amounts of protein may be physiological, e.g. orthostatic /after heavy exercise/ pyrexia/ sexual activity (male)/simple UTI.

However, as a rule, a normally functioning kidney should not allow protein to filter through the glomerular apparatus. The presence of protein strongly suggests renal disease. 24 hour urine collection for assessment should be carried out. Diabetic and hypertensive nephropathies are common causes of chronic kidney disease with progressive proteinuria (these patients should be assessed with Albumin: Creatinine ratio). Other causes include pre-eclampsia, vasculitis, connective tissue disorders and glomerulonephritis.

Specific gravity **Range: 1.000, 1.005, 1.010, 1.015, 1.020, 1.025, 1.030**

Not accurate nor reliable- use clinical judgement! The specific gravity is an indication of urine concentration i.e. the patient's hydration status. Note: specific gravity decreases with age.

Urobilinogen **Range (mg/dl): 0.2, 1, 2, 4, 8 or more**

This is a normal finding in the urine as part of the excretion process from bilirubin degradation. Increased levels indicate hepato-cellular dysfunction or increased bilirubin production. A lack of urobilinogen indicates intrahepatic obstruction.

Pregnancy testing

Background

Pregnancy tests are widely used both by the public and by healthcare professionals. All urine tests depend on the measurement of human chorionic gonadotrophin (hCG) by immunoassay.

Physiological principles

hCG is a pregnancy-specific hormone and is produced by the trophoblast. It is released in large quantities from the villous syncytiotrophoblast into the maternal blood. Currently and historically there have been many different methods of detecting hCG to confirm pregnancy. These include: direct haemagglutination, haemagglutination inhibition, latex agglutination inhibition, radioimmunoassay (RIA), radio receptor assay, and enzyme immunoassay (EIA).

The higher sensitivity of RIA was until recently still called for in the early and accurate diagnosis of early ectopic pregnancy. Currently, in general testing, EIA is the commonest method used. The qualitative detection of hCG in serum or urine using EIA is reported to be as sensitive as RIA. Preference for EIA over RIA methods is based on the advantages of greater shelf-life, lack of radioactive hazards, and no need for specialized disposal.

Timing of the test

Initially hCG is secreted by the implanting blastocyst. It appears in maternal blood around 6–8 days following fertilization; the levels rise rapidly to reach a peak at 7–10 weeks. With most current pregnancy test kits (sensitivity 25 units/L) urine may reveal positive results 3–4 days after implantation; 98% will be positive by 7 days (the time of the expected period). A negative result 7–10 days after the missed period virtually ensures that the woman is not pregnant. With the present generation of test kits, false-positive results due to interfering materials are extremely unlikely. Current pregnancy tests have high sensitivity and specificity which is unlikely to be surpassed either by better tests or alternative technology in the near future.

Procedure

- There are several reliable EIA pregnancy testing on the market. The instructions must be read specifically for the test used. Interpretation of the positive signal will differ in design and colour from test to test.
- Ensure that the pregnancy device is not past its expiry date and that it has been stored in the circumstances advised.
- Test results should be correlated with specific patient and clinical findings, and patients with negative or equivocal results should be retested a few days later if the diagnosis is critical to immediate clinical care.
- hCG levels for pregnancy testing has several limitations, including substantial daily variation in hCG levels in individual women, difficulty in interpreting whether a single value is normal for gestational age, and the length of the biological half-life of intact hCG.

Special circumstances

- **Ectopic pregnancy**: The rate of increase of hCG is most easily determined from two samples drawn 48 hours apart. The difference between the two hCG values obtained is expressed as a percentage of the initial value, and should be 66% or greater for this sampling interval.
- **Miscarriage**: this is associated with falling levels of hCG. Stable or increasing values in a threatened abortion would suggest continued viability of the pregnancy.
- **Extrauterine production**: hCG is also secreted by cancerous human tissues, particularly in the intestinal, urinary, and respiratory tracts, and in the fallopian tubes. In germ cell tumours of the testis, hCG is a useful marker in about half of the patients, and in many non-trophoblastic cancers, β-hCG is a strong and independent prognostic marker.
- **Fetal trisomy 21**: maternal serum levels are usually elevated.

Patient safety

- ✔ In a female with acute abdominal pain, quantification of hCG may be useful in diagnosing ectopic pregnancy.
- ✔ Consider pregnancy testing prior to specific radiological investigations, e.g. CT abdomen.

Student name:		Medical school:		Year:			

Urinalysis 1

Please test this patient's urine.

		Self	Peer	Peer /tutor	Tutor
Washes hands	● Hand wash with water and soap using the Ayliffe technique ●	☐	☐	☐	☐
Understands indications	● Pre-screening and preoperative assessment ● All patients admitted to hospital within 24 hours of arrival ● On recognition of any or all of the following clinical signs/symptoms, i.e. UTI symptoms – burning sensation, offensive smelling odour, pain, pyrexia, cloudy urine ●	☐	☐	☐	☐
Obtains informed consent	● Introduces themselves ● Gains informed consent ●	☐	☐	☐	☐
Explanation to patient	● Clear explanation of procedure ●	☐	☐	☐	☐
Communication skills	● Assessment throughout the procedure and allows patient to ask questions ●	☐	☐	☐	☐
Appropriate preparation	● Places receptacle on toilet/commode or provides a clean disposable urinal. ● Ask patient to urinate into receptacle and provide a minimum of 10 mL ● Prepares patient and maintains privacy and dignity ●	☐	☐	☐	☐
Collection of sample	● Dons clean pair of gloves and apron in accordance with standard infection control precautions ● Covers the receptacle and remove from the toilet; carefully transfers to the sluice area ● Tests sample immediately after voiding to avoid contamination and confusion ●	☐	☐	☐	☐
Collection of urinalysis reagent strips	● Checks the expiry date of the strips on the bottle label and ensures the strips have been stored in a cool dry place (not refrigerated) ●	☐	☐	☐	☐
Tests the urine	● Immerses the entire reagent testing strip in to the urine sample, ensuring all reagent areas are covered. Remove excess urine by running the edge of the strip against the rim of the receptacle ●	☐	☐	☐	☐
Getting the correct result	● Rest the strip on the rim of the receptacle for the required time stated by the manufacturers. Understands time is important as changes in the pad follow a 'colour reaction curve' reading the strip too early will lead to inaccurate results ● Hold the strip vertically and compare test areas closely with the colour chart on the bottle label (without touching the label) ●	☐	☐	☐	☐
Post-procedure management	● Waste disposal in accordance with trust guideline ● Documents time, date, clinical reason, any problems ● Accurately interprets results ● Report abnormal findings as appropriate ●	☐	☐	☐	☐
Professionalism	● Communicates to team members ● Thanks staff ● Thanks patient and informs them of result where appropriate ●	☐	☐	☐	☐
Overall ability to perform procedure	● Assess globally, would you be happy for this student to be supervised to perform a urinalysis ●	☐	☐	☐	☐

				Self	Peer	Peer/tutor	Tutor
Self-assessed as at least borderline:	Signature:		Date:	U B S E	U B S E	U B S E	U B S E
Peer-assessed as ready for tutor assessment:	Signature:		Date:	U B S E	U B S E	U B S E	U B S E
Tutor-assessed as satisfactory:	Signature:		Date:	U B S E	U B S E	U B S E	U B S E

Notes

Student name:	Medical school:	Year:

Urinalysis data interpretation

Ann-Marie Winter, age 19, has come into the emergency department with severe lower abdominal discomfort and urinary frequency. Her last period was 8 weeks ago. She is haemodynamically stable. A urine dip and urinary hCG is performed. She is not on any regular medication and has no known allergies.

		Self	Peer	Peer/tutor	Tutor
Urine dip: Nitrites positive, leucocytes +2, blood +2, protein +3, pH 6.5, glucose negative, ketones +1, bilirubin negative, urobilinogen 1, specific gravity 1.020, N-A-G negative	● Nitrites – indicate bacteria present in urine, i.e. UTI	☐	☐	☐	☐
	● Leucocytes/blood/protein– consistent with infection	☐	☐	☐	☐
	● pH – normal result	☐	☐	☐	☐
	● Glucose – no indication of diabetes mellitus	☐	☐	☐	☐
	● Ketones – likely mild dehydration	☐	☐	☐	☐
	● Bilirubin/urobilinogen – normal result	☐	☐	☐	☐
	● Specific gravity – higher end of scale would fit with mild dehydration	☐	☐	☐	☐
	● N-A-G – normal result	☐	☐	☐	☐
	●	☐	☐	☐	☐
hCG: positive	● hCG indicates pregnancy consistent with no period for 8 weeks	☐	☐	☐	☐
	● Need to consider an ectopic pregnancy. Urinary hCG gives no specific quantity – serial blood hCG may be useful particularly in early stages when an ultrasound may not be able to identify an interuterine pregnancy with certainty. NB: hCG should typically double every 48 hours, slow increase or remaining constant implies ectopic	☐	☐	☐	☐
	●	☐	☐	☐	☐
Other tests to perform and why?	● Blood hCG – confirmation and also sensible to get level especially if suspecting an ectopic as may need to monitor	☐	☐	☐	☐
	● Ultrasound scan of the pelvis – confirmation of interuterine or ectopic pregnancy due to severe pain	☐	☐	☐	☐
	● Group and save – if suspecting an ectopic always required (plus check if anti-D required)	☐	☐	☐	☐
	●	☐	☐	☐	☐
Seeks help as appropriate	● Discuss case with senior/on-call gynaecology to get urgent scan and specialist input	☐	☐	☐	☐
	● Consideration of antibiotics at this stage important. Note: trimethoprim is an anti-folate drug, *not* appropriate in early pregnancy. Always check hospital guidelines/*BNF*/discuss drug of choice with senior before prescribing	☐	☐	☐	☐
	●	☐	☐	☐	☐
Post-procedure management	● Documents abnormal results, produces management plan, and plans follow-up, e.g. of MSU for sensitivities	☐	☐	☐	☐
	●	☐	☐	☐	☐
Professionalism	●		☐	☐	☐
Explanation to patient	● Explains result to patient as appropriate and explains management plan; allows patient opportunity to questions	☐	☐	☐	☐
	●	☐	☐	☐	☐

	Signature:	Date:	Self	Peer	Peer/tutor	Tutor
Self-assessed as at least borderline:	Signature:	Date:	U B S E	U B S E	U B S E	U B S E
Peer-assessed as ready for tutor assessment:	Signature:	Date:	U B S E	U B S E	U B S E	U B S E
Tutor-assessed as satisfactory:	Signature:	Date:	U B S E	U B S E	U B S E	U B S E

Notes

8.9 Nose, throat, skin wound, and midstream urine sample collection

Background

Effective treatment of infection relies upon identification of the causative organism as well as appropriate prescription of antibiotics to treat the infection. By taking a sample from the infected area, microbiology laboratories are able to identify microorganisms and assess antibiotic sensitivity. It is the clinician's responsibility to select the correct site from where to take a sample and to collect material using strictly aseptic technique. Aseptic technique is particularly important when collecting samples to minimize contamination from commensal flora and to prevent introduction of new bacteria thereby causing further infection.

Clinical indications

Nose swabs

Collected to detect:

● Carriage of meticillin-resistant *Staphylococcus aureus* (MRSA)

● Pathogens causing respiratory infection.

Throat swabs

Indicated when an acute sore throat is likely to be caused by bacterial infection. The likelihood of bacterial infection is increased in the presence of three or four of the following: tonsillar exudates, tender anterior cervical lymph nodes, absence of cough or history of fever.

Wound swabs

Only wounds that are associated with a clinical diagnosis of infection should be swabbed. Symptoms include: swelling, pain, erythema, increased temperature, increased exudates, foul odour. If left untreated, the wound infection may become systemic. Infection of chronic wounds is more difficult to detect, but may have delayed wound healing, atrophy of granulation tissue and excess exudate.

MSU sample

Indicated for:

● Men and young children presenting with symptoms of UTI

● Women with recurrent UTI

● Asymptomatic pregnant women

● Symptomatic diabetic and immunosuppressed patients

195

8.9
Nose, throat,
skin wound, and
midstream urine
sample collection

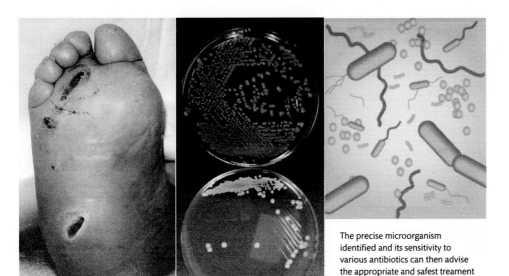

The precise microorganism
identified and its sensitivity to
various antibiotics can then advise
the appropriate and safest treatment

Diabetes foot ulcer: secondary
infection may prevent or reduce rate
of healing

Appropriate swabs are often essential
to a microbiological diagnosis

Figure 8.17 Images in microbiological sample collection. Middle and right © Ford, *Medical Microbiology* (OUP, 2010).

Anatomical and physiological principles

- The nose, throat, and skin are sites of normal flora, therefore pathogenic and non-pathogenic bacteria will be present in the swab samples.

- The bladder is a normally sterile site, but urine must pass through the non-sterile distal urethra and the sample can easily become contaminated by urethral and perineal organisms.

Assessing the patient's clinical picture is important for interpreting the microbiological findings. Certain medical conditions and epidemiological factors can affect the types of microorganism that proliferate (Table 8.4) and the consequent clinical condition.

- High glucose levels in the tissue of a diabetes patient provides a suitable environment for bacterial proliferation:

    ○ Areas that are especially prone to infection are the urinary tract and skin wounds

    ○ Foot ulcers are a concern in the diabetes patient as complex infection, including osteomyelitis, can result.

- Patients who are immunocompromised are susceptible to infection from microorganisms which are normally less harmful.

- Diabetes and immunocompromised patients are particularly sensitive to urinary tract infections and require a lower threshold of suspicion for collection of an MSU sample.

Table 8.4 Common pathogenic microorganisms found in the nose, throat, skin and urine

Urine

Escherichia coli, Proteus mirabilis, Staphylococcus saprophyticus, Klebsiella spp., *Pseudomonas aeruginosa, Enterococcus* spp.

Nose

Staphylococcus aureus including *MRSA, Haemophilus influenzae*

Throat

Group A β-haemolytic streptococcus, Group C and G β-haemolytic streptococcus, *Neisseria meningitidis, Chlamydia, Mycoplasma*

Skin or wound

Staphylococcus aureus including MRSA, β-haemolytic streptococci, enterococci, *Enterobacter* sp., *E. coli, Klebsiella* sp., *Proteus* sp., *Bacteroides* spp., *Clostridium*

Contraindications

Nose

None specifically, certainly do not insert swab any distance into nostril if a cerebrospinal fluid (CSF) leak is suspected.

Throat

Suspected acute epiglottitis.

Skin

Routine, repetitive swabbing to accompany changes of wound dressing is not advantageous. In the absence of clinical signs of infection swabbing should not be performed.

MSU

Sample collection is not usually necessary for non-pregnant women with uncomplicated UTI

Sequence

Nasal swab

- Equipment and preparation:
  - Personal protective equipment (PPE): gloves, disposable apron (where required)
  - Kidney bowl
  - Swab and transport medium, patient labels.
  - Put on gloves, apron, and any other protective equipment then lay out the equipment on the trolley and assess nostrils.
- Explanation and consent:
  - Ask patient to confirm their name and date of birth
  - Introduce yourself and clarify your position in the medical team
  - Explain the rationale for taking this sample and what the results may show
  - Obtain verbal informed consent, no need for written consent.
- Procedure
  - A sterile, moistened swab should be inserted into the nostril

○ The patient's head should be tilted back to visualize the nostril in case a polyp is obstructing the passage of the swab

○ Place the swabs in the transport medium and break the shaft off the swab to allow closure of the container (if needed).

● Post-procedure management

○ Explain to the patient where the samples will go and what may need to occur following the result

○ All samples to be sent to the microbiology laboratory should have patient name and NHS or hospital number clearly annotated. Location and clinician should be included.

○ Date and site of sample collection should also be marked

○ Samples for urgent processing should be marked as such

○ To avoid rejection of the sample, the request forms should be fully completed.

● Professionalism

○ Ensure the patient understands what is happening and maintain dignity of the patient. Inform key colleagues and write up clinical notes.

Throat swab

● Equipment and preparation:

○ PPE if required

○ Equipment as for taking a nasal swab

○ Tongue spatula.

● Explanation and consent:

○ As per nasal swab, specifically for throat swab.

● Procedure:

○ Collect necessary equipment and organize workspace

○ Ask patient to open their mouth and stick their tongue out, then use a tongue spatula to depress the tongue

○ Use a sterile cotton swab to swab both of the tonsillar arches and the posterior naso-pharynx, without touching the sides of the mouth

○ Insert swab into transport tube.

● Post-procedure management and professionalism

○ As per nasal swab.

Skin wound swab

Swabbing techniques demonstrate huge variation according to wound preparation, area sampled, duration of sampling, and even the swab type used.

● Equipment and preparation:

○ Barrier nursing equipment: gloves, apron, mask, cap if required

○ Sterile swabs and gauze

○ Sterile saline solution

○ Transport medium.

● Explanation and consent

○ As per nasal swab, specifically for skin wound swab.

● Procedure:

○ Irrigate the wound with sterile saline solution to remove any exudate, detritus, or commensal bacteria

○ Remove this solution using suction, if needed, and dry gently with sterile gauze

○ Moisten a swab and retract the edges of the wound gently and track through the wound in a zig-zag fashion, avoiding contacting the adjacent skin

○ The neck of the swab should be rotated between the fingers so as to increase coverage of the swab tip. Use separate swabs for multiple areas within a large wound and record this in the notes

○ Insert swab into transport tube and label appropriately

○ Date and time of sample collected should be recorded also

○ The site of specimen collected, as well as the type of tissue from which it was collected (e.g. granulation tissue) should be recorded.

● Post-procedure management and professionalism

○ As per nasal swab.

MSU sample

● Equipment and preparation:

○ To avoid any contamination by commensal or skin flora, the patient should be asked to clean their genital area before the sample is collected. Clean the superficial urethral area first

○ Female patients should be asked whether they are menstruating so as not to confuse menses with haematuria during the sample collection.

● Explanation and consent:

○ As per nasal swab, specifically for MSU collection.

● Procedure:

○ After cleaning their genital area, the patient should begin urinating. A collection cup should be brought into the urine stream mid-urination, then the rest of the urine voided. This is known as the 'clean-catch method'.

○ The urine can be analysed using a reagent dipstick test. This will detect the following: red blood cells, leucocytes, protein, ketones, pH, bilirubin, nitrites.

● Post-procedure management and professionalism

○ As per nasal swab.

Complications

● **Wound swab**: contamination of a wound.

● **MSU**: nil for the patient apart from contamination of the urine sample if either the stream is not collected properly or the urethral opening is not cleaned sufficiently.

Patient safety tips

✔ **Barrier nursing**: The importance of barrier nursing should be stressed with gloves, apron, and masks used where appropriate. This is to protect both the patient and the caregiver from acquisition of infection. Also this technique helps to prevent contamination of the wound swab with non-pathogenic bacteria, which would give a false-positive result.

✔ **Microbiology results**: It is important to act on the result of the microbiological work (Figure 8.18) both to protect the patient from infection and avoid inappropriate antibiotic use.

Student name:	Medical school:	Year:

Nasal swab collection and microbiology sampling

Please can you take a nasal swab from this patient/manikin/student? Also complete the relevant request form and prepare sample for transit to microbiology laboratory.

		Self	Peer	Peer /tutor	Tutor
Understands indications	• Equipment and preparation	☐	☐	☐	☐
	• PPE: gloves, disposable apron	☐	☐	☐	☐
Procedure: obtaining a nasal swab	• Kidney bowl, swab and transport medium, patient labels	☐	☐	☐	☐
	• Dons gloves, apron, lays out equipment on the trolley	☐	☐	☐	☐
	• Explanation and consent	☐	☐	☐	☐
	• Ask patient to confirm their name and date of birth	☐	☐	☐	☐
	• Introduce yourself and clarify your position in the medical team	☐	☐	☐	☐
	• Explain the rationale for taking this sample and what the results may show	☐	☐	☐	☐
	• Obtain verbal informed consent, no need for written consent	☐	☐	☐	☐
	• Procedure	☐	☐	☐	☐
	• Inserts a sterile, moistened swab into the nostril	☐	☐	☐	☐
	• Head tilted back to visualize the nostril to exclude polyp	☐	☐	☐	☐
	• Places swabs in the transport medium and break the shaft off the swab to allow closure of the container (if needed)	☐	☐	☐	☐
	• Post-procedure management	☐	☐	☐	☐
	• Explain to the patient where the samples will go and what may need to occur following the result	☐	☐	☐	☐
	• All samples to be sent to the microbiology laboratory should have patient name and NHS or hospital number clearly annotated	☐	☐	☐	☐
	• Date and site of sample collection should also be marked	☐	☐	☐	☐
	• Samples for urgent processing should be marked as such	☐	☐	☐	☐
	• Request forms should be fully completed	☐	☐	☐	☐
	• Professionalism	☐	☐	☐	☐
	• Ensures the patient understands what is happening and maintains dignity of the patient; inform key colleagues and writes up clinical notes	☐	☐	☐	☐
	•	☐	☐	☐	☐

General Microbiology requests

Please use the form to have a discussion on the indication for each test and a hypothetical patient in whom the test may be needed

Urine samples

Respiratory samples

swabs: genitourinary medicine, general others

Serology

Faeces

Mycology

Hosp No./NHS No.		Consultant / GP	Signature
Surname		Ward / Surgery	
Forename		GP Address	NHS ☐
D.O.B.	Sex: M / F		PP ☐
Address			Cat II ☐
Post code		Copy to:	

Please give relevant information
Date & time collected ..../......../.......... ..../......../..........
Blood takers signature

URINE	RESPIRATORY	SWABS	VIROLOGY
MSU	CULTURE ☐	HVS / LVS ☐	HELICOBACTER PYLORI ☐
CSU	TB ☐	CERVICAL ☐	SYPHILIS ☐
PREGNANCY TEST	FLUID ☐	URETHRAL ☐	HIV ☐
	Please state type	PENILE ☐	HEPATITIS Infection screen
FAECES / **MYCOLOGY**		CHLAMYDIA ☐	HEPATITIS A ☐
CULTURE	Please state site	EYE ☐	HEPATITIS B ☐
OTHER please state ☐	_____ ☐	EAR ☐	HEPATITIS C ☐
		NOSE / THROAT ☐	IMMUNITY SCREEN ☐
Other tests:		SKIN ☐	Please state test _____
		OTHER _____ ☐	
		MRSA ☐	ATYPICAL SEROLOGY ☐
		Please state site _____	GENTAMICIN ☐
		ESBL SCREEN ☐	VANCOMYCIN ☐
		Please state site _____	

☐ ☐ ☐ ☐

☐ ☐ ☐ ☐

				Self	Peer	Peer/tutor	Tutor
Self-assessed as at least borderline:	Signature:	Date:		U B S E	U B S E	U B S E	U B S E
Peer-assessed as ready for tutor assessment:	Signature:	Date:		U B S E	U B S E	U B S E	U B S E
Tutor-assessed as satisfactory:	Signature:	Date:		U B S E	U B S E	U B S E	U B S E

Notes

8.10 Nutritional assessment

Background

This is an important skill in assessing patients in almost all clinical encounters, particularly when admitted to hospital as an emergency case or when planning a surgical procedure. Optimizing nutrition in these groups of patients has been shown to improve mortality and reduce morbidity. It is a sad indictment of human global human affairs that the human population has millions suffering from under-nutrition, with 50 million pre-school children in Africa alone having protein energy malnutrition (PEM). On the other hand there are in excess of 200 million cases of type 2 diabetes in whom obesity has played a major aetiological factor.

Physiological principles

Water

Water forms 50–60% of the lean body weight in men and 45–50% in women. This equates to approximately 45 L in a 75 kg man. Water balance is maintained by the thirst mechanism and the urine concentrating and diluting functions. At least 1 L/day is needed; in reality, 2–4 L are usually drunk with the excess excreted. The three main 'water' compartments are:

- Intracellular: 30 L (one-third of body weight)
- Extracellular: 10 L (one-eighth of body weight)
- Plasma: 5 L (4–5%).

Sodium and potassium

With respect to sodium, the reference nutrient intake (RNI) is only 70 mmol or 1.6 g. The range varies widely and around 5 g on average in UK. There is considerable evidence of the link between high sodium chloride intake and hypertension. Potassium requirements are similar around 70–100 mmol/L per day.

Energy

This will vary from patient to patient depending on the basal metabolic rate, physical activity, and the need for thermogenesis. The daily calorific intake for a 55-year-old man is usually 2500 calories/day (and 2000 calories/day for a similar female). Any excess of calories will result in weight gain. In the vast majority of patients the only way to lose weight is consume fewer calories than required on a daily basis for metabolism.

Protein

The RNI is 0.75 g/kg body weight. In hospital patients approximately 0.9–1.6 g protein/kg body weight is needed per day. Clearly catabolic states such as sepsis and burns will require considerably more protein in relation to clinically stable patients. It is important for vegetarians to eat a wide array of allowable protein choices to allow sufficient amounts of the essential amino acids to be made available (histidine, isoleucine, lysine, leucine, methionine, phenylalanine, threonine, tryptophan, valine).

Fat

Overall intake of fat should be less than 30% of the total calorie intake. Saturated fat should only comprise one-third (10%), polyunsaturates 12% and mono-unsaturates 6%. There are four essential polyunsaturated fatty acids: linoleic and α-linolenic (diet only), eicosapentaenoic and docosahexaenoic (partly made in body).

Carbohydrates

Approximately 60% of calorie intake should be from polysaccharides (starch), disaccharides (e.g. sucrose, lactose) and monosaccharides (glucose, fructose); 30 g of dietary fibre (cellulose, pectins, gums, hemicelluloses) is recommended via the minimum five fruits and vegetables daily consumption.

Micronutrients: vitamins and minerals

Deficiencies are not as rare as we may think, indeed deficiencies are often missed in clinical practice.

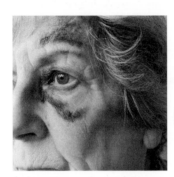

Bruising: usually due to skin fragility, do consider vitamin C deficiency

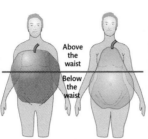

An increased waist:hip ratio is strongly associated with type 2 diabetes mellitus and increased CVD risk: pear good, apple bad!

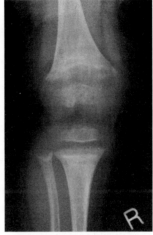

Rickets is caused by vitamin D deficiency. The symptoms include fractures, myopathy, and fatigue.

Figure 8.18 Images in nutrition. Left © Mary Hope/iStockphoto; right © Dr Wade H. Gaved

Nutritional assessment

Nutrition support should be considered in all patients who are malnourished or at risk of malnutrition This section draws on the National Institute for Health and Clinical Excellence guidance on nutrition (2006). The autonomy of the patient must remain paramount at all times with opportunity given to allow the patient to make informed decisions about their care and treatment. In many cases the patient's family and other carers will also be involved. Treatment should be supported by evidence-based written information tailored to the patient's needs and culturally sensitive. Additional needs due to, for example, physical, sensory or learning disabilities should be addressed.

All hospital inpatients on admission and all outpatients at their first clinic appointment should be screened. People in care homes should be screened on admission and when there is clinical concern. Oral, enteral, or parenteral nutrition support may be need. Swallowing problems should be taken into account.

Definitions

- **Body mass index** (**BMI**) is weight in kilograms divided by height in metres squared (Table 8.5).
- **Malnourished**: any of:
  - ○ BMI of less than 18.5 kg/m^2
  - ○ Unintentional weight loss greater than 10% within the last 3–6 months

Table 8.5 Body mass index definitions

BMI (kg/m²)	Classification
<18.5	Underweight
18.5 to 24.99	Normal range
25.00 to 29.99	Overweight
30.00 to 34.99	Obesity
35.00 to 39.99	Very obese
≥40	Morbid obesity

There are some ethnicity specific adjustments: South-Asian ethnicity overweight category starts at a BMI of 23.00.
For type 2 diabetes or cardiovascular disease risk the waist circumference is a more specific indicator of risk than BMI.

- ○ BMI of less than 20 kg/m² and unintentional weight loss greater than 5% within the last 3–6 months.
- **Risk of malnutrition**: any of:
  - ○ Have eaten little or nothing for more than 5 days and/or are likely to eat little or nothing for the next 5 days or longer
  - ○ Have a poor absorptive capacity, and/or have high nutrient losses and/or have increased nutritional needs from causes such as catabolism.

Nutritional red flags: any of the following:

- Unintentional weight loss, fragile skin, poor wound healing, apathy
- Wasted muscles, poor appetite, altered taste sensation
- Impaired swallowing, altered bowel habit
- Loose-fitting clothes, or prolonged intercurrent illness.

All acute hospital trusts should have a multidisciplinary nutrition support team. This could include dietitians, gastroenterologist, gastrointestinal surgeons, nutrition nurse, pharmacists, caterers, biochemistry staff, speech and language therapists, clinicians such as anaesthetists and radiologists to insert specialist feeding ports such as percutaneous endoscopic gastrostomy (PEG) tubes, central venous cannulae.

Ethical and legal issues

When starting or stopping nutrition support:

- Obtain consent and, as always, act in the patient's best interest
- Provision of nutrition support may not be always be appropriate. Clinical decisions on withholding or withdrawing of nutritional support require a consideration of both ethical and legal principles (in the UK – common law and statutes, including the Human Rights Act 1998).

Assess for dysphagia

Patients with acute and chronic neurological conditions and those who have undergone surgery or radiotherapy to the upper respiratory or upper gastrointestinal tract are at high risk of dysphagia. In clinical practice the sip test is easy to perform; however, there needs to be early recourse to a more definitive assessment in many cases by a speech and language therapist.

Classic signs and symptoms

- Coughing or choking before, during or after swallowing
- Difficult, painful chewing or swallowing
- Regurgitation of undigested food
- Difficulty controlling food or liquid in mouth
- Drooling
- Hoarse voice
- Globus sensation
- Nasal regurgitation
- Feeling of obstruction
- Unintentional weight loss – for example, in people with dementia

More difficult signs and symptoms

- Change in respiration pattern
- Unexplained temperature spikes
- Wet voice quality
- Tongue fasciculation (? motor neurone disease)
- Xerostomia
- Heartburn
- Change in eating – for example, eating slowly or avoiding social occasions
- Frequent throat clearing
- Recurrent chest infections
- Atypical chest pain

If dysphagia present

- Feed via a tube into the stomach unless there is upper gastrointestinal dysfunction.
- In people with upper gastrointestinal dysfunction (or an inaccessible upper gastrointestinal tract) consider post-pyloric (duodenal or jejunal) feeding.
- Consider gastrostomy for long-term (4 weeks or more) enteral tube feeding.
- Percutaneous endoscopic gastrostomy (PEG) tubes can be used 4 hours after insertion.

Post surgery

If no signs of nausea or vomiting.

- In post-abdominal surgical patients consider postoperative oral intake within 24 hours of surgery.
- In post-caesarean or gynaecological surgical patients consider postoperative oral intake within 24 hours of surgery.

Parenteral nutrition

Access

- In hospital, parenteral nutrition can be given via a dedicated peripherally inserted central catheter.
  - A free dedicated lumen in a multi-lumen centrally placed catheter may also be used.
- For short-term feeding (less than 14 days) consider feeding via a peripheral venous catheter for patients who have no need for central access. Take care in choosing catheters. Pay

attention to pH, tonicity and long-term compatibility of the parenteral nutrition mixture in order to avoid administration or stability problems.

● Tunnelling subclavian lines are recommended for long-term use (more than 30 days).

Nutritional treatment prescription (see also Tables 8.6 and 8.7)

● Ensure total intake of prescribed nutrition support accounts for:

  ○ Energy, protein, fluid, electrolyte, mineral, micronutrients and fibre needs

  ○ Activity levels and the underlying clinical condition (e.g. catabolism, pyrexia)

  ○ Gastrointestinal tolerance, metabolic instability, and risk of refeeding problems.

● For people who are not severely ill or injured, nor at risk of refeeding problems, nutritional prescription should usually provide:

  ○ 25–35 kcal/kg/day total energy

  ○ 0.8–1.5 g protein (0.13–0.24 g nitrogen)/kg/day

  ○ 30–35 ml fluid/kg

  ○ Adequate electrolytes, minerals, micronutrients, and fibre, if appropriate.

Table 8.6 Vitamins

Vitamin	Dietary source and treatment (Rx)	Deficiency disease/symptoms/signs
A – retinol	Liver, diary foods, eggs, fish oils, carrot, broccoli (plant β-carotene) **Rx: retinol orally or intramuscularly**	**Xerophthalmia, keratomalacia, bitot spots, night blindness, increased sensitivity to infection, follicular keratosis**
B_1 – thiamine	Cereals, beans, nuts, pork **Rx: thiamine intravenous/ intramuscularly then orally**	Alcoholic diet or starvation (hyperemesis, carcinoma of the stomach, anorexia nervosa) → Wernicke–Korsakoff syndrome with confusion, ataxia, nystagmus, dementia, psychosis Beriberi: polyneuropathy (dry), oedema, pleural effusions, ascites (wet)
B_2 –riboflavin	All plants and animal cells especially: diary, leafy vegetables **Rx: riboflavin orally**	Rare: angular stomatitis, red tongue, seborrhoeic dermatitis
B_3 – niacin	All plants, meat, fish, eggs, diary **Rx: nicotinamide orally**	Pellagra: rare triad of dermatitis, diarrhoea, dementia. Tuberculosis treatment with isoniazid causes B_6 deficiency, which reduces niacin synthesis. Also in phaeochromocytoma and carcinoid
Pantothenic acid and biotin	All plant and animal cells **Rx: oral biotin**	Extremely rare → dermatitis
B_6 – pyridoxine	All plants and animal cells **Rx: pyridoxine orally**	Alcoholic diet or isoniazid Rx → polyneuropathy
B_{12}	Meat, fish, eggs, diary, bacteria, not in plants **Rx: intramuscular B in most cases or high dose orally**	Vegetarians and those on metformin high risk → pernicious anaemia, glossitis/ angular stomatitis, tiredness, neuropathy, posterior and lateral column loss (sub-acute combined degeneration of the cord), dementia

Table 8.6 *(Continued.)*

Vitamin	Dietary source and treatment (Rx)	Deficiency disease/symptoms/signs
Folate	Green vegetables esp. spinach and broccoli, enriched cereals **Rx: folic acid 5 mg orally**. All in preconception and first trimester. All gestational diabetes or on any anticonvulsants	Anaemia, glossitis Neural tube defects more likely if deficiency in first trimester pregnancy. Diabetes reduces folate, anticonvulsants induce enzymes → low folate
C – ascorbic acid	Fresh fruit and vegetables especially citrus fruits, potatoes **Rx: ascorbic acid orally**	Elderly frail eat very little fresh fruits and vegetables → scurvy: weakness, myalgia, keratosis of hair (corkscrew-like), perifollicular haemorrhage (petechial), hyperplasia of gums, increased bruising, anaemia, poor wound healing
D	Skin photo-activation to produce cholecalciferol → liver to 25-OH vitamin D → kidney to 1,25-OH vitamin D, diary **Rx: 800 IU vitamin D with calcium or 1,25-OH vitamin D in renal disease**	Osteomalacia in adults: bone pain, tiredness, proximal muscle weakness, low back pain Rickets in children: skeletal deformities (frontal bossing, tibial bowing, genu valgum/varum), costochondral junction overgrowth (rachitic rosary)
E – tocopherols and tocotrienoles	Vegetables and especially seed oils, nuts, **Rx: α-tocopherol**	Neuropathy with ataxia, ? related to cardiovascular disease and dementia Mental and neurological abnormalities if not replaced in $\alpha\beta$-lipoproteinaemia
K	(K_1) leafy vegetables, diary, soya and rape oils, (K_2) intestinal bacteria **Rx: phytomenadione intramuscular or oral** All neonates at delivery to prevent haemorrhagic disease of newborn	Inadequate synthesis of clotting factors → bruising with increased INR and prothrombin time

Seriously ill or injured people

Introduce enteral or parenteral nutrition cautiously in seriously ill or injured people. Start at no more than 50% of the estimated target energy and protein needs and build up to meet full needs over the first 24–48 hours. Provide full requirements of fluid, electrolytes, vitamins, and minerals from the outset.

Monitoring

Review the indications, route, risks, benefits and goals of nutrition support at regular intervals.

- **Nutritional**: assess intake from oral, enteral or parenteral nutrition initially daily then less often dependent on clinical state. Use fluid balance charts.
- **Anthropometric parameters**: weight, BMI, mid-arm circumference or triceps skin thickness, usually monthly, if weight cannot be measured
- **Gastrointestinal function**: nausea/vomiting, diarrhoea, constipation, abdominal distension
- **Nasogastric tube**: see Unit 9. check position with pH paper etc
- **Gastrostomy or jejunostomy**: check stoma site and tube position daily visually.
- **PEG tubes** have to be rotated to prevention the flange becoming stuck firmly into the gastric wall (buried bumper syndrome).
- **Parenteral nutrition** catheter sites to minimize infection and thrombophlebitis.

Table 8.7 Nutritional mineral elements

	Dietary source and treatment (Rx)	Deficiency
Fe (iron)	Meat, fish, leafy green vegetables, diary **Rx: iron supplementation orally**	Deficiency leads to anaemia Fe overload to endocrine dysfunction: diabetes, adrenal insufficiency
Calcium	Diary, meat **Rx: calcium with vitamin D**	Deficiency leads to osteoporosis, tetany, perioral paraesthesia, proximal myopathy
Copper	Legumes, seafood, cereals, nuts **Rx: trace mineral supplement**	Anaemia, neuropathy. Rare genetic condition with malabsorption (Menkes' kinky hair syndrome with growth failure, mental retardation, brittle bones) Copper overload: Wilson's disease with cirrhosis, dysarthria (basal ganglia involvement), Kayser–Fleischer ring in eye, dementia
Zinc	Meat, fish and most plants **Rx: trace mineral supplement**	Malabsorption disorder: acrodermatitis enteropathica with scaling dermatitis and diarrhoea; increased infections, poor wound healing, hair loss
Iodine	Seafood, diary, meat **Rx: iodinated salt**	Goitre in deficiency areas with hypothyroidism
Fluoride	Seafood, tea, fluoridated water	Deficiency or non-use of fluoridated water → dental caries Excess: fluorosis of tooth enamel (discoloration, ridging, pitting))
Phosphate	Most foods	Deficiency risk in total parenteral nutrition (TPN) patients (refeeding syndrome) leads to weakness and anorexia
Magnesium	Most foods	Deficiency risk in TPN patients

Other essential minerals include: selenium (deficiency → cardiomyopathy), chromium → pancreatic insufficiency especially diabetes, cobalt → anaemia, manganese → dermatitis. Role of cadmium, vanadium, molybdenum, nickel unclear.

- **Laboratory monitoring**:
  - Baseline: urea and electrolytes (U&Es), glucose, magnesium, phosphate, liver function tests (LFTs), international normalized ratio (INR) if any bleeding or if any intervention needed, including passage of NG tube, calcium, albumin, total protein, full blood count (FBC) if anaemic.
  - Vitamin B_{12}/folate, iron usually taken at baseline. Ferritin may be useful to work out meaning of abnormal Fe level.
  - C-reactive protein (CRP) may be useful to monitor acuteness of case to adjust nutritional requirements.
  - Consider zinc, copper, selenium, manganese, 25-OH vitamin D. These are usually not needed as supplementation takes place as part of most feeding regimens.
  - Vitamins A, D, E, and K are fat-soluble and can be affected in a variety of malabsorption states such cholestatic jaundice. The other vitamins are water soluble.

Patient safety tips

✔ Thorough clinical history taking and examination is crucial – it is amazing how many times nutritional deficiency is picked up in clinical practice. Many people, sadly, suffer from malnutrition in developed countries.

✔ The key aspect of patient safety in relation to nutrition is that a basic nutritional assessment must be carried out on all patients. There are several screening tools and a brief synopsis of the Malnutrition Universal Screening Tool (MUST) tool is presented here. The precise scoring tables are available on the British Association for Parenteral and Enteral Nutrition (BAPEN) website.

✔ Consider the refeeding syndrome. This is the onset of metabolic disturbances such as hypophosphataemia and hypokalaemia after the restoration of normal nutritional requirement in a severely malnourished individual. The syndrome can result in confusing cardiac failure, paralysis and paralytic ileus.

Malnutrition Universal Screening Tool

MUST is a screening tool for malnutrition developed by BAPEN based on the following steps:

1 Calculation of the patient's BMI.

2 Note patient's percentage unplanned weight loss (converted to score).

3 Establishing the acute disease effect and score.

4 Overall risk of malnutrition calculated from the above.

5 Use management plan to treat patient:

   ○ **Low risk**: screening repeated at specified intervals. In hospitals this is weekly.

   ○ **Medium risk**: document dietary intake for 3 days if hospital. If clinical concern increase nutritional support and consider dietetic advice.

   ○ **High risk**: refer to dietitian and/or hospital nutrition support team.

Student name:　　　　　　　　Medical school:　　　　　　　　Year:

Nutritional assessment

Please carry out a nutritional assessment on this (simulated) patient. Some questions will be asked in relation to important clinical aspects of nutrition as well.

		Self	Peer	Peer /tutor	Tutor
Which are the important categories of patients that should be considered for more urgent nutritional assessment ?	• Those admitted to hospital as an emergency case • Planning a surgical procedure (improves mortality and reduces morbidity) •	☐ ☐ ☐	☐ ☐ ☐	☐ ☐ ☐	☐ ☐ ☐
Water: name the three main water compartment and their water content	• Approximately 45 L in a 75 kg man. • Intracellular 30 L • Extracellular 10 L • Plasma 5 L •	☐ ☐ ☐ ☐ ☐	☐ ☐ ☐ ☐ ☐	☐ ☐ ☐ ☐ ☐	☐ ☐ ☐ ☐ ☐
Sodium and potassium: state daily amount needed and consequences of excess	• RNI is only 70 mmol or 1.6 g. High sodium chloride intake and hypertension are linked. Potassium requirement are similar (70–100 mmol/L) •	☐ ☐	☐ ☐	☐ ☐	☐ ☐
Energy: state daily requirements	• Daily calorific intake for a 55-year-old man is approx. 2500 calories per day and it is 2000 calories for a similarly aged woman •	☐ ☐	☐ ☐	☐ ☐	☐ ☐
Protein: state the RNI and clinical condition in which requirements are increased	• RNI is 0.75 g/kg body weight. Hospitals patients need approx. 0.9–1.6 g protein/kg bodyweight. Catabolic states such as sepsis and burns will require considerably more protein in relation to clinically stable patients •	☐ ☐	☐ ☐	☐ ☐	☐ ☐
Fat: state daily fat intake advice in terms of total calorie intake and name the four essential fatty acids	• Intake of fat should <30% of total calories. Essential polyunsaturated fatty acids: linoleic and α-linolenic (diet only), eicosapentaenoic and docosahexaenoic (partly made in body) •	☐ ☐	☐ ☐	☐ ☐	☐ ☐
Carbohydrates (CHO): state forms of CHO in diet and overall calorie proportion	• Approx. 60% of calorie intake from polysaccharides (starch), disaccharides (e.g. sucrose, lactose) and monosaccharides (glucose, fructose) •	☐ ☐	☐ ☐	☐ ☐	☐ ☐
Vitamins: what are the consequences of vitamin C deficiency? Vitamin B_{12} deficiency? How is treatment given?	•	☐	☐	☐	☐
Minerals: what would be the consequences of a low calcium or low iron level. How is treatment given?	•	☐	☐	☐	☐
How is the BMI calculated and what are the units?	• Weight in kilograms divided by height in metres squared • What is the BMI of a person who weighs 104 kg and has a height of 172 cm? • What do the following BMI indicate in terms of the obesity classification? • 42.1 = morbid obesity, 21.8 = normal, 32.5 = obesity, South Asian 24.1 = overweight. •	☐ ☐ ☐ ☐ ☐	☐ ☐ ☐ ☐ ☐	☐ ☐ ☐ ☐ ☐	☐ ☐ ☐ ☐ ☐
Define malnourished state	Any of: • BMI of <18.5 or unintentional weight loss >10% within last 3–6 months or BMI <20 and unintentional weight loss >5% within last 3–6 months •	☐ ☐	☐ ☐	☐ ☐	☐ ☐
Nutritional red flags: name some that may be apparent on clinical history or examination	• Unintentional weight loss, fragile skin, poor wound healing, apathy, wasted muscles, poor appetite, altered taste sensation, impaired swallowing, altered bowel habit, loose fitting clothes, or prolonged intercurrent illness •	☐ ☐	☐ ☐	☐ ☐	☐ ☐

Ethical and legal issues: discuss in relation to a dying patient	• Obtain consent and, as always, act in the patient's best interest	☐	☐	☐	☐
	• Provision of nutrition support may not be appropriate	☐	☐	☐	☐
	•	☐	☐	☐	☐
Name some signs of dysphagia that may be apparent on clinical examination	• Coughing or choking, painful chewing or swallowing, regurgitation of undigested food, difficulty controlling food or liquid in mouth, drooling, hoarse voice, globus sensation, nasal regurgitation, feeling of obstruction, unintentional weight loss	☐	☐	☐	☐
		☐	☐	☐	☐
Parenteral nutrition: how can this be given?	• Via a dedicated peripherally inserted central catheter or via a peripheral venous catheter	☐	☐	☐	☐
	•	☐	☐	☐	☐
Nutritional treatment prescription: what would be prescribed for a day?	• 25–35 kcal/kg/day total energy, 0.8–1.5 g protein kg/day, 30–35 ml fluid/kg	☐	☐	☐	☐
	•	☐	☐	☐	☐
Monitoring: what are the key aspects?	• **Nutritional**: assess intake from oral, enteral, or parenteral nutrition	☐	☐	☐	☐
	• **Anthropometric parameters**: weight, BMI, mid-arm circumference or triceps	☐	☐	☐	☐
	• **Gastrointestinal function**: nausea/vomiting, diarrhoea, constipation, abdominal distension	☐	☐	☐	☐
	• **Gastrostomy or jejunostomy or PEG**: check daily	☐	☐	☐	☐
	• **Laboratory monitoring. Consider**: U&Es, glucose, magnesium, phosphate, LFTs, INR, calcium, albumin, total protein, FBC, B_{12}/folate, iron	☐	☐	☐	☐
	•	☐	☐	☐	☐
Malnutrition Universal Screening Tool (MUST): what key parameters are used in the MUST nutritional assessment tool? How is high risk patient treated?	• BMI, % unplanned weight loss (converted to score), acute disease effect	☐	☐	☐	☐
	• **High risk**: refer to dietitian and/or hospital nutrition support team	☐	☐	☐	☐
	•	☐	☐	☐	☐

			U B S E	U B S E	U B S E	U B S E
Self-assessed as at least borderline:	Signature:	Date:				
Peer-assessed as ready for tutor assessment:	Signature:	Date:				
Tutor-assessed as satisfactory:	Signature:	Date:				

Notes

8.11 Lumbar puncture

Background

A lumbar puncture is performed for diagnostic and therapeutic reasons (Table 8.8). This procedure gives access to the CSF, which can be analysed biochemically, microbiologically, and histologically. The main biochemical analysis is for protein and glucose. It is possible to culture the CSF fluid for bacteria and conduct a polymerase chain reaction (PCR) on it, if indicated, to look for causes of viral meningitis and encephalitis. This includes herpes simplex, cytomegalovirus, and influenza.

Table 8.8 CSF analysis in different clinical states

Clinical disease	Protein	Glucose	Cell count	CSF pressure
Bacterial meningitis (*Neisseria meningitides, streptococcus pneumonia*)	raised	Low	More than 50 polymorphs	Raised
Viral meningitis, measles, chickenpox	Normal or slightly elevated	Normal	Lymphocytes	Normal
Tuberculosis meningitis (*Mycobacterium tuberculosis*)	Moderately raised	Low	Lymphocytes	Raised or normal
Cryptococcus meningitis	Normal or slightly elevated	Normal or low	Lymphocytes	Raised or normal
Malignant meningitis leukaemia	Moderately raised or normal	Normal	Malignant cells or reactive cells	Raised or normal
Encephalitis	Normal or slightly elevated	Normal	lymphocytes	Raised or normal
Subarachnoid haemorrhage	Raised	Normal	Red cells raised	Raised or normal
Idiopathic intracranial hypertension	Normal	Normal	Normal	Raised often v high
Guillain–Barré syndrome	Normal then raised	Normal	Raised lymphocytes	Normal
Multiple sclerosis	Slightly elevated oligoclonal bands	Normal	Raised lymphocytes	Normal
Spinal cord compression or spinal tumours	Very raised	Normal	Reactive or normal	Low often

Normal CSF findings: appearance clear and colourless

Appearance	Colourless, crystal-clear
Manometer pressure	7-18 cm (H$_2$O) CSF height in lumbar puncture position
Protein	0.20–0.60 g/L
Glucose	3.0–4.5 mmol/L (or ≥66% of blood level)
Cell count	0–5 mononuclear cell per mm^3, no polymorphs
Red cells or xanthochromia	Nil and absent
Oligoclonal bands	Absent
Immunoglobulin G	<15% of CSF protein

Clinical indications

Diagnostic

- Meningitis: bacterial, viral or fungal.
- Subarachnoid haemorrhage, fresh red blood cells acutely with xanthochromia persisting for up to 7 days.
- Neurological conditions: multiple sclerosis, Guillain–Barré syndrome, subacute sclerosing panencephalitis, prion disease.
- Central nervous system (CNS) leukaemia.

Therapeutic

- Draining off CSF in idiopathic intracranial hypertension.
- Intrathecal drugs: only if specifically trained.
- Spinal anaesthesia for abdominal, pelvic or lower limb surgery.

Anatomical and physiological principles

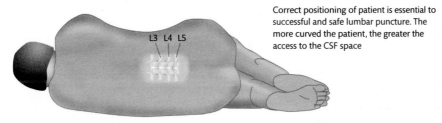

Correct positioning of patient is essential to successful and safe lumbar puncture. The more curved the patient, the greater the access to the CSF space

L3 L4 L5

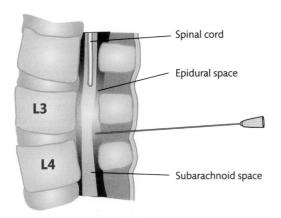

Spinal cord

Epidural space

L3

L4

Subarachnoid space

Needle track: skin, supraspinous ligament, between two spinous processes, interspinous ligament, ligamentum flavum, dura and arachnoid, CSF space

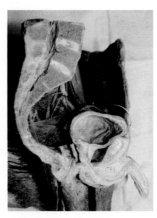

Section through lower vertebral column showing L4, L5, S1

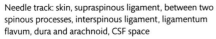

Figure 8.19 Images in lumbar puncture.

Anatomical principles

- The spinal cord ends at L1/L2 and splits into the cauda equina.
- The CSF space is best accessed at L4–5 or L3–4.
- The needle is inserted into the midline between two spinous processes.
- After penetrating the skin, the first line of resistance is the interspinous ligament and then the ligamentum flavum.
- Once the ligamentum flavum is transverse there is a small give and needle travels in more easily as it goes into the liquid CSF space (subarachnoid space).

Contraindications

- Raised intracranial pressure: papilloedema, vomiting, drowsiness, bradycardia, hypertension
- Bleeding diathesis: low platelets, INR raised, disseminated intravascular coagulation
- Local infection
- Spinal tumour: neoplasm or abscess

Procedure

The procedure described is the one specifically for the commonest indication, which is to diagnose meningitis or subarachnoid haemorrhage. The needle is inserted in the L4–5 interspace, through the skin, subcutaneous fat, supraspinous ligament, interspinous ligament, ligamentum flavum, and into the CSF space. A sample is taken as per the clinical indication.

Equipment and preparation

Select correct equipment:

- Apron, gloves, face mask, sterile pack, antiseptic solution, sterile gauze dressing, or film dressing.
- 10 mL lidocaine 1% injection for topical anaesthesia, orange and green needles, 10 mL syringes
- Lumbar puncture (spinal needle) 22 or 24 or 25 gauge usually. Incidence of headaches least with the small diameter 25 gauge needle.
- Three sterile sample bottles (label 1, 2, 3) and a glucose bottle.
- Culture bottles (usually blood culture).
- Lumbar puncture manometer with three-way tap with 40 cm of tube length at least.

Preparation

- Lay out equipment on trolley and assemble manometer.

Explanation and consent

Gain consent from patient. Main points to emphasize:

- State purpose of the investigation and specific reason in this patient
- State main steps
- State main risks and an idea of the prevalence
- Explain that you will ask the patient about pain and other potential problems throughout
- Obtain verbal consent, some hospitals may have a written consent policy for lumbar puncture.

Procedure

- **Position the flexed patient on their left side**: arms flexed, spine flexed, and legs flexed. This is the fetal position in effect. Ask the patient to hold onto their knees to open up the supra-spinous process even more. An obsession with correct positioning of the patient is extremely important to success.
- **Identify the right anterior superior iliac spine**: vertical line from here to the bed will cross the L3–4 interspinous space in the midline posteriorly. Identify L4–5 interspace as the one immediately below the L3–4 interspace.
- **Identify the L4–5 interspinous space**: feel and mark it with a pen or an indentation using blunt plastic, e.g. clean specimen bottle top.
- **Wash hands and put on sterile gloves**: standard technique.
- **Check assembly of equipment**.
- **Check lumbar puncture needle**: stylus able to ride in and out of needle.

- **Clean skin and apply drapes**: with antiseptic agent (usually 2% chlorhexidine or iodine-based solution), second thorough re-clean at intended site of lumbar puncture.
- **Local anaesthesia with 1% lidocaine**: At lumbar puncture site inject a very small amount (0.25 mL) and create an intradermal wheal, orange small gauge needle.
- **Swap to green needle and infiltrate lidocaine down towards the CSF space**: draw back on the syringe repeatedly to ensure that a blood vessel or the CSF space has not been encountered. A standard size venepuncture needle is used at this stage therefore infiltration into the CSF space is very unlikely. Allow at least 2 minutes for the local anaesthetic to take effect.
- **Introduce spinal needle at the lumbar puncture site**: almost perfectly perpendicularly in all planes with a slight shift towards the umbilicus of 20°.
- **Advance needle through the two ligaments and into the CSF space**: this will be around 4–7 cm in most cases. As you progress through the ligamentum flavum and dura, a little sudden give or click is encountered when the needle passes in to the CSF space.
- **If bone is encountered**: withdraw needle and re-position.
- Once the CSF space is encountered, withdraw the stylus from the needle and CSF should come out gently. Be ready to put the stylus back in immediately a few drops have been seen.
- **The manometer**: (closed to the needle) is brought, ready assembled, adjacent to the spinal needle and stylus removed. The manometer is placed on immediately. The CSF pressure is measured by turning the three-way tap to connect the spinal needle to the manometer. CSF pressure measurement is undertaken.
- **Biochemistry sample bottles 1, 2, 3**: The manometer three-way tap is then closed to the spinal needle and CSF in the manometer tube put into the first biochemistry bottle.
- **Adjust three-way tap to close to manometer and open to connect CSF space to sample bottle 2**: Collect around 10 drops, further 10 drops into sample bottle 3. Collect further samples as needed, e.g. 10 drops for microbiology, 10 drops for cytology, 10 drops glucose bottle
- **Withdraw the needle slowly**: and put a dressing on the lumbar puncture site.
- **Discard all unnecessary and used clinical equipment safely**.

Post-procedure management

The patient must lie flat on their back for 1 full hour at least; some authorities recommend 4 hours. A moderate headache is very likely after a lumbar puncture. The classic post-lumbar puncture headache is described as dull, constant, and occipital. It is relieved by lying still and flat. Meningism can be present. Paracetamol with or without codeine will be effective analgesia in most cases. Adequate hydration will also help.

Working with colleagues

Write clear notes, e.g.:

'Lumbar puncture to check for subarachnoid haemorrhage. Explanation to patient and verbal consent obtained.

Aseptic technique:

- Skin cleaned with chlorhexidine solution
- 0.25 mL intradermal 1% lidocaine followed by 9 mL using green needle
- 25 gauge spinal needle used
- First attempt not successful. patient re-positioned.
- New needle used, 24 gauge

Clear CSF encountered:

- Pressure 16 cm of CSF fluid

- 3 serial samples taken for biochemistry including xanthochromia
- Microbiology sample taken
- Glucose sample taken

Patient advised re lying flat for 1 hours and advice re headaches given to patient and nurses.'

Complications

- Headaches
- Coning: extremely rare if no space-occupying lesion and no papilloedema. The patient will become drowsy and comatose. Cardiorespiratory compromise will ensue. Emergency management for coning: tilt head down, high-flow oxygen to create cerebral vasoconstriction, mannitol.

Patient safety tips

- ✔ **Exclude space-occupying lesion by urgent computed tomography (CT) scan of the head**.
- ✔ Never do lumbar puncture in a patient with papilloedema unless CT head is normal.
- ✔ Clear at least 30 minutes to do this procedure, do not feel rushed.
- ✔ Always consider the anatomy of the route that the spinal needle has to take.
- ✔ If you fail, do rotate the needle a little just in case the needle is adjacent to a cauda equina nerve.
- ✔ A persistent headache post lumbar puncture requires expert opinion; occasionally 25 mL of the patient's own blood can used to seal up the CSF at the site lumbar puncture by a clinician experienced in this technique

Lumbar puncture

Please perform a lumbar puncture on this manikin: you are have been asked to perform this procedure because of a suspected diagnosis of subarachnoid haemorrhage. A CT scan has been found to be normal with no evidence of a space-occupying lesion.

		Self	Peer	Peer /tutor	Tutor
Wash hands	•	☐	☐	☐	☐
Clinical indications	• **Diagnostic**: meningitis, subarachnoid haemorrhage, multiple sclerosis, Guillain–Barré syndrome, central nervous system leukaemia	☐	☐	☐	☐
	• **Therapeutic**: Draining CSF in idiopathic intracranial hypertension, intrathecal drugs: only if specifically trained; spinal anaesthesia for abdominal, pelvic, or lower limb surgery	☐	☐	☐	☐
	•	☐	☐	☐	☐
Anatomical and physiological principles	• CSF space is best accessed at L4–5 or L3–4	☐	☐	☐	☐
	• Use of L3–L4 by indentifying anterior superior iliac spines	☐	☐	☐	☐
	•	☐	☐	☐	☐
Contraindications	• Raised intracranial pressure: papilloedema, vomiting, drowsiness, bradycardia, hypertension	☐	☐	☐	☐
	• Bleeding diathesis: low platelets, INR raised, disseminated intravascular coagulation	☐	☐	☐	☐
	• Local infection or spinal tumour: neoplasm or abscess	☐	☐	☐	☐
	•	☐	☐	☐	☐
Equipment and preparation	**Selects correct equipment**:				
	• Apron, gloves, face mask, sterile pack, antiseptic solution, dressing	☐	☐	☐	☐
	• 10 mL 1% lidocaine, orange and green needles, 10 mL syringes	☐	☐	☐	☐
	• Lumbar puncture (spinal needle) 24 or 25 gauge usually	☐	☐	☐	☐
	• Three sterile sample bottles (label 1, 2, 3) and a glucose bottle; culture bottles	☐	☐	☐	☐
	• Lumbar puncture manometer with three-way tap with 40 cm of tube length	☐	☐	☐	☐
	Preparation:				
	• Lay out equipment on trolley and assemble manometer.	☐	☐	☐	☐
	•	☐	☐	☐	☐
Explanation and consent	Gains consent from patient main points to emphasis:				
	• States purpose of the investigation and specific reason in this patient	☐	☐	☐	☐
	• States main steps, main risks, and an idea of the prevalence	☐	☐	☐	☐
	• Obtains consent	☐	☐	☐	☐
	•	☐	☐	☐	☐
Procedure	• **Positions the flexed patient on their left side**	☐	☐	☐	☐
	• **Identifies the right anterior superior iliac spine**: vertical line from here to the bed will cross the L3–4 interspinous space in the midline posteriorly	☐	☐	☐	☐
	• **Identifies the L4–5 interspinous space**: feel and mark it with a pen or an indentation using blunt plastic, e.g. clean specimen bottle top	☐	☐	☐	☐
	• **Washes hands and put on sterile gloves**	☐	☐	☐	☐
	• **Checks lumbar puncture needle**: patent and stylus able to ride in and out of needle	☐	☐	☐	☐
	• **Applies drapes and cleans skin**: with antiseptic agent, second thorough re-clean at intended site of lumbar puncture	☐	☐	☐	☐
	• **Local anaesthesia with 1% lidocaine**: At lumbar puncture site inject a very small amount (0.25 ml) and create an intradermal wheal with narrow gauge needle.	☐	☐	☐	☐
	• **Swap to green needle and infiltrate lidocaine down towards the CSF space**: draw back on the syringe repeatedly to ensure that a blood vessel or the CSF space has not been encountered. Allow at least 2 minutes for the LA to take effect	☐	☐	☐	☐
	• **Introduce spinal needle at the LP site**: almost perfectly perpendicularly in all planes with a slight shift towards the umbilicus of 20 degrees	☐	☐	☐	☐
	• **Advance needle through the two ligaments and into the CSF space**: states a little sudden give or click may be encountered when the needle passes into CSF.	☐	☐	☐	☐
	• **If bone is encountered**: withdraw needle and re-position	☐	☐	☐	☐
	• Once the CSF space is encountered, withdraw the stylus from the needle and CSF should come out gently.				
	• **The manometer**: (closed to the needle) is placed on correctly. CSF pressure is measured by turning the 3 way tap to connect the spinal needle to the manometer.	☐	☐	☐	☐
	• **Biochemistry sample bottles 1, 2, 3**: The manometer 3 way tap is then closed to the spinal needle and CSF in the manometer tube put into the first bottle.	☐	☐	☐	☐
	• **Adjust 3 way tap to close to manometer and open to connect CSF space to sample bottle 2**: Collect around 10 drops into bottle 2 and 3. Collect further samples as needed, e.g. 10 drops each for microbiology, cytology, glucose.	☐	☐	☐	☐
	• **Withdraw the needle slowly**: and put a dressing on the LP puncture site	☐	☐	☐	☐
	•	☐	☐	☐	☐

Post-procedure management	● Patient must lie flat on their back for 1 full hour	☐	☐	☐	☐
	● Post-lumbar puncture headache: relieved by lying still and flat. Meningism can be present	☐	☐	☐	☐
	● Treatment: paracetamol ± codeine and adequate hydration will also help	☐	☐	☐	☐
	●	☐	☐	☐	☐
Working with colleagues	● Writes clear notes	☐	☐	☐	☐
	●	☐	☐	☐	☐
Complications	● Coning: extremely rare if no space-occupying lesion and no papilloedema	☐	☐	☐	☐
	● Emergency management for coning: tilt head down, high-flow oxygen to create cerebral vasoconstriction	☐	☐	☐	☐
	●	☐	☐	☐	☐
Patient safety tips	● **Exclude space-occupying lesion by urgent CT head**	☐	☐	☐	☐
	● Clear at least 30 minutes to do this procedure, do not feel rushed	☐	☐	☐	☐
	● Always consider the anatomy of the route that the spinal needle has to take	☐	☐	☐	☐
	●	☐	☐	☐	☐

			U B S E	U B S E	U B S E	U B S E
Self-assessed as at least borderline:	Signature:	Date:				
Peer-assessed as ready for tutor assessment:	Signature:	Date:				
Tutor-assessed as satisfactory:	Signature:	Date:				

Notes

8.12 Arterial blood gas sampling and interpretation

Background

Arterial blood gas (ABG) and acid–base analysis is undertaken on an arterial sample obtained directly from a peripheral artery, most commonly the radial artery at the wrist. The femoral artery, or more rarely, the brachial artery can also be used for arterial blood sampling. Blood is drawn via a single percutaneous needle puncture. ABG is frequently used in the assessment and monitoring of the critically ill patient to determine oxygenation, gas exchange in the lungs, and acid-base levels. Most ABG analysers also provide information on electrolyte balance and haemoglobin.

Clinical indications

- Evaluation of ventilation, oxygenation, and acid–base status:
  - Diagnostic evaluation of the critically ill patient in conditions, such as: respiratory failure, cardiac failure, hepatic failure, renal failure, multi-organ failure, sepsis, trauma, burns, diabetic ketoacidosis.
- Evaluation of the patient's response to therapeutic intervention:
  - Oxygen therapy, mechanical ventilation, fluid management.
- Patient monitoring during procedures or investigations:
  - Abdominal surgery, cardiopulmonary surgery, sleep studies, exercise testing

Anatomical and physiological principles

The artery is identified by palpation of the pulse at a site where it runs subcutaneously. No tourniquet is required. The accessible sites for arterial puncture are the radial artery at the wrist, the brachial artery in the antecubital fossa, and the femoral artery in the groin. Arteries in the foot are rarely used for sampling but can be useful for arterial cannulation. The most commonly used site is the radial artery at the wrist. The oxygen concentration that the patient is receiving at the time of the sample, should ideally, have been consistent for at least 15 minutes prior to the procedure.

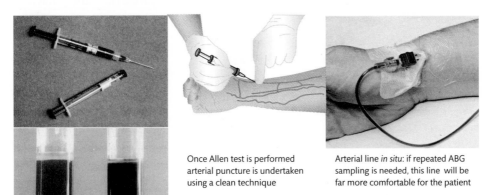

Once Allen test is performed arterial puncture is undertaken using a clean technique

Arterial line *in situ*: if repeated ABG sampling is needed, this line will be far more comfortable for the patient

Syringes commonly used in ABG sampling
Note bright red colour of normal arterial blood on left and dark venous looking arterial blood in methaemoglobinaemia

Figure 8.20 Images in arterial blood gas sampling.

Contraindications

- Any pre-existing lesion or infection at the puncture site.
- Presence of a surgical shunt (e.g. in dialysis patient) at the site or proximal to the site.
- History of peripheral vascular disease in the extremity selected for sampling.
- Coagulopathy or high-dose anticoagulation therapy (relative contraindication).
- Inadequate collateral circulation confirmed by a negative Allen's test (see below).

Procedure

The skin is punctured and the needle advanced until the syringe starts filling with arterial blood. Suction is then applied to the syringe to withdraw the arterial sample for analysis. Initial hand wash.

Equipment

- Gloves, antiseptic skin cleanser, 21 gauge or smaller needle, heparinized blood gas syringe.
- Sterile gauze and dressing.

Preparation

If the radial artery is to be sampled, Allen's test should be performed. This ensures that the collateral blood supply is intact and that in the event of damage to the radial artery, there will be no long-term sequelae due to ischaemia of the hand. **If the test is negative then another extremity should be selected for arterial puncture**.

Allen's test (after finding radial and ulnar arteries at the wrist; Figure 8.22)

- **Stage 1**: the patient makes a fist and elevates the hand for approximately 15–30 seconds. Explain that this can often be uncomfortable. Simultaneously apply pressure to both the radial and ulnar arteries. Ask the patient to open their hand. The palm of their hand will appear pale due to the blood supply via the radial and ulnar arteries being occluded.
- **Stage 2**: Release the pressure on the ulnar artery while maintaining pressure on the radial artery. Refill should occur in 6 seconds. This is a **positive Allen's test and normal**. The palm will return to normal colour and you may proceed with sampling.
- **Stage 3**: If the colour does not return within 5–10 seconds, the ulnar arterial supply to the hand is not sufficient and the ABG sample should not be taken from the radial artery. This is a **negative Allen's test**.

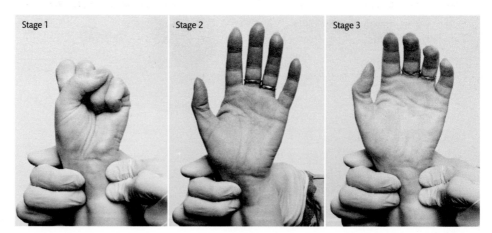

Figure 8.21 Allen's test.

Explanation and consent

Gain verbal consent from the patient.

- State the purpose of the test and the reasons for doing the test in this patient.
- Outline the main steps of the procedure.
- Warn the patient about the risk of bleeding, haematoma, infection, and arterial occlusion.
- Arterial puncture is a painful procedure and local anaesthetic may be used. A small intra-dermal bleb with a track towards the artery with 1% lidocaine is usually sufficient.

Procedure

- **Wash hands and put on clean gloves**.
- **Stabilize the wrist using a towel or pillow**: slightly extend wrist to move radial artery superiorly slightly in relation to extensor tendons
- **Locate the artery**: by pulsation just proximal to the wrist crease. Assess diameter and depth of artery in relation to the skin. Find point of maximal pulsation. Leave fingers proximal to the point of intended sampling. Consider fixing the artery by pulling skin taut either side of the artery with the non-dominant hand.
- Clean with chlorhexidine/alcohol swab in multiple directions over the arterial sample site. Do not repalpate site after cleaning.
- **Angle the needle to 45° and warn patient that they will feel a sharp scratch**: the needle is angled opposite to the direction of blood flow.
- **Advance the needle slowly into the artery**: until a flashing pulsation of blood is seen in the bottom of the attached syringe. Apply suction on syringe once blood is seen.
- There are two methods that are used to enter the artery with the needle:
  - The needle can be inserted with suction applied. When the needle enters the artery it will fill automatically (preferred method).
  - The needle can be inserted through the artery and withdrawn slowly until it enters the artery and the syringe fills (more painful, but may be needed in difficulty, do not use unless advised by senior experienced clinician)
- **Re-directing the needle**: If needed, withdraw almost to the skin surface, before re-directing.
- **Sample**: withdraw 1.5–2 mL of blood.
- **Remove the needle and immediately apply immediate and firm pressure** to the puncture site with sterile gauze for 2–5 minutes. Increase compression time for patients with coagulation disorders or on high-dose anticoagulation therapy. Another colleague may help with this while the sample is processed by the sampler.
- **Expel any air bubbles**: from the sample immediately. Invert sample gently several times to mix in the heparin.
- **Discard all unnecessary and used clinical equipment safely**.

Working with colleagues

- Label the sample and lab request form accurately at the bedside.
- Inform the lab of the pending delivery of the sample and send it immediately, on ice (blood is a living tissue and will continue to consume oxygen and produce carbon dioxide).
- Document a record of the procedure in the healthcare records.

Complications

- Painful procedure and infection risk to patient
- Artery may not be palpable (arteriospasm)
- Needle stick injury risk to clinician

- Thrombosis, distal embolization, and ischaemia
- Haemorrhage, haematoma or vasovagal response
- Anaphylaxis from local anaesthetic (where used)
- Accidental venous puncture obtaining a venous sample
- Analytical error: the ABG only reflects the patient's condition at the time of sampling.

Interpreting the ABG result

The pH is maintained within the normal range by compensatory intracellular and extracellular buffers and also by the buffer mechanisms of the lungs and kidneys. By far the most important buffer in the body is the carbonic acid-bicarbonate system.

$$H_2O + CO_2 \leftrightarrow H_2CO_3 \leftrightarrow HCO_3^- + H^+$$

The components of the carbonic acid-bicarbonate buffer system can be varied independently of each other. The concentration of CO_2 may be adjusted by changes in ventilation. The kidneys regulate secretion of H^+ in urine.

Hypoxaemia (low PaO_2) is defined as a partial pressure of oxygen less than 8 kPa. **Hypercapnia** (high $PaCO_2$) defines whether it is type I or type II respiratory failure. Type I respiratory failure is characterized by hypoxaemia and normocapnia while type II respiratory failure is characterized by hypoxia and hypercapnia.

Compensatory mechanisms

If either kidneys or lungs are overwhelmed in regulating acid-base homeostasis, the other can help to compensate. Respiratory compensation for metabolic acidosis is fast, the lungs respond quickly by increasing ventilation and blowing off CO_2. In situations of metabolic alkalosis, the lungs respond quickly to decrease ventilation and retain CO_2. In contrast, renal compensatory mechanisms for respiratory disorders work more slowly. Kidneys regulate pH by controlling the secretion of H^+ and the reabsorption of bicarbonate in addition to HCO_3^- production.

Base excess

The base excess or deficit refers to the amount of base present in the arterial blood gas sample.

It is defined as the amount of strong acid that must be added to each litre of fully oxygenated blood, at 37 °C and normal $PaCO_2$ to return the pH to 7.40. The actual base excess is the unadjusted amount that is present in the sample. The standard base excess value is one that is adjusted to a haemoglobin of 5 g/dL and gives a better indication of the base excess of the entire extracellular fluid compartments.

Anion gap

Measuring the anion gap is important in conditions of metabolic acidosis, in order to narrow down the possible causes. Body fluids contain a variety of ions. The total number of the anions and cations must be equal. Blood tests tend to measure most cations but fewer anions. Therefore, there are a number of unmeasured anions, in particular, negatively charged proteins and organic acids. This is termed the 'anion gap', which may be raised or decreased. A raised anion gap is caused by excess acid, whereas metabolic acidosis with a normal anion gap is usually caused by a loss of base.

Interpreting the ABG result (Tables 8.9 and 8.10)

221

8.12
Arterial blood
gas sampling and
interpretation

Table 8.9 ABG: normal range and interpretation

	ABG parameters normal values	
Acidosis: pH is low	pH 7 .45–7.35	Alkalosis: pH is high
Acidosis: H^+ is high	H^+ 35–45 nmol/l	Alkalosis: H^+ is low
Hypoxaemia (PaO_2 <8 kPa) With normal $PaCO_2$ Type I respiratory failure	PaO_2 10.5–13.5 kPa	Hypoxia (PaO_2 <8 kPa) With $PaCO_2$ >6.0 kPa Type II respiratory failure
Respiratory acidosis: $PaCO_2$ >6.0	$PaCO_2$ 4.7–6.0 kPa	Respiratory alkalosis: $PaCO_2$ <4.7
Metabolic acidosis: HCO_3^- <22	HCO_3^- 22–28 mmol/L	Metabolic alkalosis: HCO_3^- >28
Metabolic acidosis: Less than –2	Base excess ± 2	Metabolic alkalosis: More than +2 (base excess)
	O_2 saturation >95%	
Hypoxia, sepsis, shock usually high	Lactate ≤2.0 mmol/L	Raised in lactic acidosis, diabetic ketoacidosis (DKA), alcohol abuse, renal failure
	Anion gap 12–16 mmol/L	

Step-by-step guide to interpreting the ABG result: ? Type I or II respiratory failure
1: pH ? acidosis or alkalosis →
2: $PaCO_2$? high, respiratory acidosis, ? low, respiratory alkalosis →
3: HCO_3^- ? high, metabolic alkalosis. ? low, metabolic acidosis →
4: Cross check $PaCO_2$ and HCO_3^- to see if there is a respiratory or metabolic cause with or without compensation
5: If acidosis check anion gap. Always remember glucose, K^+, lactate, haemoglobin levels.

Table 8.10 The four primary acid–base disorders with clinical examples

Respiratory acidosis: (due to ineffective ventilation)	**pH: low**	**$PaCO_2$: high**	**HCO_3^-: low, normal or high**
Acute respiratory distress (e.g. asthma attack, airway obstruction) Chronic (e.g. chronic obstructive pulmonary disease) CNS depression: opiates, sedation, stroke, raised intracranial pressure Myasthenia gravis, Guillain–Barré syndrome			
Metabolic acidosis: (increased acid or anaerobic tissue respiration)	**pH: low**	**$PaCO_2$: low-normal**	**HCO_3^-: low**
Lactic acidosis type A from anaerobic metabolism (e.g. shock, sepsis, ischaemia) Lactic acidosis type B from reduced lactate metabolism (e.g. liver failure) Diabetic ketoacidosis Gastrointestinal loss of bicarbonate (e.g. from diarrhoea, colitis) Ingestion of exogenous acid (e.g. salicylate) Poisoning (tricyclic antidepressants, methanol or ethylene glycol) Renal loss of bicarbonate (e.g. conditions of renal tubular acidosis, Addison's)			
Respiratory alkalosis: (due to hyperventilation)	**pH: high**	**$PaCO_2$: low**	**HCO_3^-: normal-low**
Respiratory: pneumothorax, pulmonary embolism, pneumonia, early asthma attack CNS induced: subarachnoid haemorrhage, stroke, meningitis General causes of hyperventilation: pain, panic attacks, thyrotoxicosis, fever			
Metabolic alkalosis: (excess H^+ loss, base load or dehydration)	**pH: high**	**$PaCO_2$: normal-high**	**HCO_3^-: high**
Prolonged vomiting: hyperemesis gravidarum, pyloric stenosis, anorexia nervosa Hypokalaemia or dehydration or chloride loss associated with use of diuretics			

Examples

Here are some worked examples of different acid–base disturbances.

pH (7.45–7.35)	PaO$_2$ (10.5–13.5 kPa)	PaCO$_2$ (4.7–6.0 kPa)	HCO$_3^-$ (22–28 mmol/L)	Clinical case
pH 7.29	PaO$_2$ 8.0	PaCO$_2$ 8.6	HCO$_3^-$ 30.9	1: A 68-year-old man admitted with worsening shortness of breath and a history of chronic obstructive pulmonary disease (COPD). His ABG on air is shown

Respiratory acidosis: the patient is hypoxic (low PaO$_2$) and has acidosis (low pH). PaCO$_2$ is high. Standard bicarbonate is high (expected to be low), reflecting a degree of metabolic compensation, usually secondary to chronic hypercapnia in patients with COPD
Management: medically with nebulizers, steroids, and antibiotics. Non-invasive ventilation may be needed

pH 7.54	PaO$_2$ 23.5	PaCO$_2$ 3.8	HCO$_3^-$ 24.1	2: A tall 23-year-old woman is seen in A&E with a 24-hour history of shortness of breath. A chest X-ray shows a moderately sized pneumothorax. ABGs on air are shown

Respiratory alkalosis: the patient has alkalosis (high pH). PaCO$_2$ is low. Standard bicarbonate is normal. This is respiratory alkalosis. The patient has developed a spontaneous pneumothorax. She is hyperventilating, achieving good oxygenation, but blowing off CO$_2$
Management: chest drain, emergency release of tension pneumothorax if indicated by rapid deterioration

pH 7.19	PaO$_2$ 16.4	PaCO$_2$ 2.1	HCO$_3^-$ 6.2	3: A 37-year-old woman with type 1 diabetes is admitted via A&E with a 2-day history of abdominal pain, urinary frequency, nausea, vomiting, and general malaise

Metabolic acidosis: acidosis (low pH) and hypocapnia (low PaCO$_2$) with low bicarbonate, indicating a metabolic acidosis. Most likely DKA due to urinary tract infection. Check urine for ketones
Management: correction of dehydration and hyperglycaemia with intravenous crystalloid and insulin infusion. Close monitoring: glucose, K$^+$, renal function, HCO$_3^-$

pH 7.51	PaO$_2$ 14.2	PaCO$_2$ 6.0	HCO$_3^-$ 35.0	4: A 59-year-old man with previous peptic ulcer disease is admitted to the surgical team with persistent vomiting and dehydration. Na$^+$ 140, K$^+$ 2.5, Cl$^-$ 86 (all mmol/L)

Metabolic alkalosis: Alkalosis (high pH) with a normal PaCO$_2$ and high HCO$_3^-$. This is a hypokalaemic hypochloraemic alkalosis due to K$^+$ and Cl$^-$ loss from persistent vomiting secondary to pyloric stenosis.
Management: intravenous fluid replacement with NaCl 0.9% and K$^+$ then ? surgery for pyloric stenosis.

Patient safety tips

✔ Choose the site for arterial puncture with the easiest access. The femoral site should only be used if radial sampling is difficult due to the need for monitoring the puncture site for an extended period.

✔ Warn the patient that the procedure may be painful, especially at the wrist. Offer local anaesthetic where appropriate, but this involves a second needle puncture.

✔ Delay in running the sample will affect the results: O$_2$ consumption continues as well as CO$_2$ production.

✔ Suspect you have a venous sample if the pO$_2$ or O$_2$ saturation is significantly lower than expected. Re-draw the sample.

✔ **Always consider the ABG results in light of the clinical picture – do they fit with the clinical picture?**

Student name:	Medical school:	Year:

ABG sampling

Please can you take an ABG from this patient/manikin and interpret the result?

		Self	Peer	Peer /tutor	Tutor
Washes hands	● Hand wash with water and soap or alcohol gel using the Ayliffe technique	☐	☐	☐	☐
	●	☐	☐	☐	☐
Understands indications and anatomy	● Understands when it is appropriate to request that an ABG is performed	☐	☐	☐	☐
	● Able to explain location of veins, arteries, and nerves. Performs Allen's test	☐	☐	☐	☐
	● Understands the risks associated with ABG sampling	☐	☐	☐	☐
	●	☐	☐	☐	☐
Obtains informed consent	● Introduction and ensures they have the correct patient by checking both verbally and against wrist band	☐	☐	☐	☐
Explanation to patient, often including complications	● Consent: Clear explanation, e.g. 'I am going to take a sample of blood to test. I will need to fill one syringe. You will feel a sharp scratch from the needle'	☐	☐	☐	☐
	●	☐	☐	☐	☐
Communication skills	● Assessment throughout the procedure and allows patient to ask questions	☐	☐	☐	☐
	●	☐	☐	☐	☐
Appropriate preparation	● Selects equipment and checks expiry dates and seals	☐	☐	☐	☐
	● Blood gas syringe and needle, gloves, alcohol gel, sterile gauze swabs, 2% chlorhexidine/70% alcohol swabs, sterile plaster, blood test request form, sharps bin, and tray	☐	☐	☐	☐
	●	☐	☐	☐	☐
Appropriate analgesia	● Considers use of local analgesia	☐	☐	☐	☐
	●	☐	☐	☐	☐
Technical ability especially with any special equipment and sharps	● Selects appropriate artery (radial, brachial, femoral)	☐	☐	☐	☐
	● Cleans artery area for 30 seconds with chlorhexidine/alcohol swab and allows to dry	☐	☐	☐	☐
	● Prepares needle and blood gas syringe	☐	☐	☐	☐
	● Alcohol gel on hands and applies gloves	☐	☐	☐	☐
	● Warns patient of sharp scratch and performs arterial puncture	☐	☐	☐	☐
	● Once 1.5–2 mL of blood obtained removes needle, applies cap and applies adequate pressure with sterile gauze swab for 5 minutes	☐	☐	☐	☐
	● Disposes of sharps safely	☐	☐	☐	☐
	● Ensures bleeding has stopped and applies sterile plaster	☐	☐	☐	☐
	●	☐	☐	☐	☐
Aseptic technique	● Appropriate cleansing of site	☐	☐	☐	☐
	● Understands need for disposal of sharps and risk of potential infections	☐	☐	☐	☐
	●	☐	☐	☐	☐
Seeks help as appropriate	● Discuss complications, e.g. failure to obtain sample, haematoma, bleeding	☐	☐	☐	☐
	●	☐	☐	☐	☐
Post-procedure management	● Labels syringe and blood test form at the patients bedside, aware of biohazard labels and when to use	☐	☐	☐	☐
	● Communicates with laboratory	☐	☐	☐	☐
	● Documents in patient's notes that test taken	☐	☐	☐	☐
	● Knows normal ABG values	☐	☐	☐	☐
	●	☐	☐	☐	☐
Professionalism	● Communicate to patient re: procedure and need for test	☐	☐	☐	☐
	● Allows patient opportunity to ask questions	☐	☐	☐	☐
	● Thanks patient	☐	☐	☐	☐
	●	☐	☐	☐	☐
Overall ability to perform procedure	● Assess globally, would you be happy for this student to be supervised to take an arterial blood sample on a real patient?	☐	☐	☐	☐
	●	☐	☐	☐	☐

			Self	Peer	Peer /tutor	Tutor
Self-assessed as at least borderline:	Signature:	Date:	U B S E	U B S E	U B S E	U B S E
Peer-assessed as ready for tutor assessment:	Signature:	Date:	U B S E	U B S E	U B S E	U B S E
Tutor-assessed as satisfactory:	Signature:	Date:	U B S E	U B S E	U B S E	U B S E

Notes

Unit 9   Therapeutic skills

9.1 Oxygen therapy

Background

Oxygen is commonly used as a therapeutic agent in clinical practice. Although it clear that it is a drug, it is rarely specifically prescribed or closely monitored. It is also perceived as a panacea for breathlessness. Its specific indication, however, is as a treatment for hypoxaemia. Oxygen has not been shown to benefit non-hypoxaemic dyspnoeic patients. When used appropriately, it is life-saving. There is also the very real potential for harm and even apnoea when given to a patient with a hypoxic drive.

The aim of the treatment with oxygen should be directed by a patient-specific target oxygen saturation and the goal should be a normal or near-normal oxygen saturation without risk of hypercapnia. There are numerous indications requiring varying concentrations of oxygen prescription, especially in emergency situations, depending on severity of illness of patient. The main physiological principles have been covered in Unit 8, Section 8.12.

Note: The British Thoracic Society guidelines have been used extensively in this section.

Clinical indications

Emergency prescription of oxygen is required in any of the following clinical conditions.

- Critical illness
  - Cardiac arrest, post-cardiac arrest, resuscitation, sepsis, shock, major trauma, anaphylaxis, near-drowning, pulmonary haemorrhage, head injury
  - Carbon monoxide poisoning (in this case disregard high saturations on oximetry as saturation monitors are unable to distinguish between oxyhaemoglobin and carboxyhae-moglobin and even PaO_2 will be normal as well, but tissue hypoxia persists).
- Serious illness
  - Acute hypoxia (cause not known yet), acute asthma, pneumonia, lung cancer, acute heart failure, pulmonary embolism, pleural effusion, pneumothorax, severe anaemia, sickle cell crisis, worsening lung fibrosis, postoperative dyspnoea.
- Chronic obstructive pulmonary disease (COPD) and other illness requiring controlled oxygen: cystic fibrosis, chronic neuromuscular disorders, chest wall disorders, morbid obesity.
- Conditions requiring close monitoring but not oxygen unless hypoxaemia:
  - myocardial infarction and acute coronary syndrome (ACS), cerebrovascular accident, pregnancy and obstetric emergencies, most poisoning and drug overdoses (except carbon monoxide poisoning) metabolic and renal disorders, hyperventilation and dysfunctional breathing.
- COPD and other respiratory condition requiring long-term oxygen therapy.

Please ensure you refer to local policy before undertaking any procedure.

Critical illness

Any patient with critical illness should have a full assessment and a protocol similar to below:

- **A prompt clinical and laboratory assessment**: of the patient should be conducted by including history, examination, record of vital signs, venous blood tests and arterial blood gas (ABG) sampling. A normal pulse oximetry saturations *does not* exclude need for ABG sampling as it does not reflect hypercapnia. Therefore ABG sampling and a full blood count (FBC)/urea and electrolytes (U&Es) should be done as early as possible.

- **Initial oxygen therapy**: is via a reservoir mask with 15 L/min oxygen. Once stable, reduce oxygen and aim for O_2 saturation 94–98%. If oximetry is unavailable, continue reservoir mask until definitive treatment is available.

- **Patients with COPD or other diseases with risk of hypercapnia**: who are critically ill should have initially same strategy as for other critically ill patients until ABG analysis is available and subsequent reassessment for oxygen requirements. Aims for O_2 saturations of 88–92%.

- **Record oxygen saturations, concentration of inspired oxygen and other vital signs**.

- **Oxygen should be prescribed**: by trained clinical staff with target saturations on the drug chart.

- **Target saturations**: 94–98% in most acutely ill patients, 88–92% in those with risk of hypercapnia.

- Most non-hypoxic dyspnoeic patients do not benefit from oxygen but a drop of 3% or more in target saturations should prompt re-assessment of oxygen needs.

Serious illness

Any patient with serious illness should have a full assessment and a protocol similar to below:

- **Initial oxygen therapy**: nasal cannula at 2–6 L/min oxygen or simple face mask at 5–10 L/min oxygen. Obtain oximetry and or ABG sampling according to clinical state of patient.

- **For patients not at risk of hypercapnia and O_2 saturation <85%**: switch over to reservoir mask with 10–15 L/min.

- **Record oxygen saturations, concentration of inspired oxygen and other vital signs**.

- **Oxygen should be prescribed**: by trained clinical staff with target saturations on the drug chart.

- **Target saturations**: 94–98% in most acutely ill patients, 88–92% in those with risk of hypercapnia. If target not reached with nasal cannula or face mask, assess patient/senior help and switch over to reservoir bag. Adjust O_2 saturation to 94–98% if PaO_2 is normal (unless there is past history of type 2 respiratory failure requiring non-invasive ventilation [NIV] or invasive positive pressure support [IPPV]) and recheck ABGs in 30–60 minutes.

COPD and other illness requiring controlled oxygen

In patients with COPD and other risk factors of hypercapnia, who are not critically ill, should have a full assessment and a protocol similar to below:

- **If ABGs are not available**: use 28% Venturi mask at 4 L/min and aim for O_2 saturations of 88–92% for patients with risk of hypercapnia but no previous acidosis.

- **Adjust O_2 saturation target range to 94–98%**: if $PaCO_2$ is normal on ABGs (if no past history of NIV/IPPV) and recheck ABGs in 30–60 minutes.

- **In patients with previous history of respiratory acidosis**: aim at prespecified saturations (these patients may have an oxygen alert card and their own Venturi masks with them).

- **If diagnosis is unknown**: patient is >50 years old, long-term smoker, history of chronic dyspnoea on minor exertion (on walking level ground) and no other obvious cause of dyspnoea, should be considered and managed as COPD. In such cases, forced expiratory volume in 1 second (FEV_1)/FVC should be measured on arrival to hospital and pre-discharge as well.

- **ABG sampling should be repeated**: in such cases after 30–60 minutes or sooner if clinical deterioration prompts. If $PaCO_2$ is raised but pH is ≥7.35 or H^+ ≤45 nmol/L, this suggests that patient has probably long-standing hypercapnia and aim for targets saturations of 88–92%. If patient is hypercapnic ($PaCO_2$ ≥6 kPa) and has acidosis (pH <7.35 or H^+ >45 nmol/L), consider NIV, especially if acidosis has persisted for more than 30 minutes despite treatment.

Conditions requiring close monitoring but not oxygen unless hypoxaemia

In certain clinical conditions patients usually do not require oxygen unless specifically indicated. In such circumstances patients should have a full assessment and a protocol similar to below:

- **If hypoxaemic**: the initial oxygen therapy is nasal cannula at 2–6 L/min oxygen or simple face mask at 5–10 L/min oxygen. If saturations are less than 85% use reservoir bag (if not at risk of hypercapnia).
- Recommended O_2 saturation targets are 94–98% unless stated otherwise.
- **If oximetry is not available**: use oxygen as above until oximetry or ABG sampling is available.
- **In patients with COPD or risk of type 2 respiratory failure**: treat as COPD until ABG results are available, then act accordingly.

Long-term oxygen therapy in COPD

Long-term oxygen therapy (LTOT) has been shown to improve survival in COPD patients. It is indicated in patients with PaO_2 <7.3 kPa when stable, or 7.3–8 kPa when stable and one of the following: secondary polycythaemia, nocturnal hypoxaemia, peripheral oedema, or pulmonary hypertension. Blood gases should be performed on two occasions, 3 weeks apart.

- Patients should breathe supplemental oxygen for at least 15 hours a day.

Assess the need for oxygen therapy in patients with:

- Severe airflow obstruction (FEV_1 less than 30% predicted)
- Cyanosis or polycythaemia
- Peripheral oedema
- Raised JVP or O_2 saturations ≤92% (breathing air).
- Consider assessment for patients with moderate airflow obstruction (FEV_1 30–49% predicted).

Practices should have a pulse oximeter to ensure all patients needing LTOT are identified.

Oxygen concentrators should be used to provide the fixed supply at home for LTOT. Ambulatory oxygen should be prescribed for patients already on LTOT who want to continue with therapy outside the home. Short-burst oxygen therapy should only be considered for episodes of severe breathlessness not relieved by other treatments.

Oxygen therapy in pregnancy

Pregnant women with major trauma, sepsis, shock, or other acute illness, should receive same oxygen therapy as any other seriously ill patient with a target saturation of 94–98%.

A similar strategy should be planned for women with hypoxaemia due to acute complications of pregnancy (collapse due to amniotic fluid embolism, eclampsia, antepartum or postpartum haemorrhage).

Equipment for oxygen therapy

The following equipment is normally available in any area where oxygen is administered (Figures 9.1–9.3).

Non-rebreathing mask (NRB)

In clinical practice this is usually referred to as the reservoir bag (Figure 9.1). To prime the bag it is run through with 100% oxygen (15 L/min) for a few seconds and left at least two-thirds full of its maximum capacity. The patient will inhale around half of the residual oxygen in the reservoir bag which is then replaced from the 100% oxygen source. A one-way valve in the NRB allowed exhaled air to be diverted away from the reservoir bag and into the atmosphere. Therefore there is no mixing of the exhaled and inhaled air which would reduce the inhaled oxygen to less than the estimated 100%. In reality the NRB allows oxygen to be delivered at around 75–90%.

Venturi mask

Delivers a precise, specified concentration of oxygen to the patient regardless of ventilator rate, tidal volume and oxygen flow rate. The minimum suggested flow rate for each mask is shown on each Venturi device. They are suitable for patients requiring controlled oxygen therapy (e.g. COPD). They are available in 24, 28, 35, 40 and 60% oxygen concentrations (Figure 9.2).

Nasal cannulae

Nasal cannulae (Figure 9.3) can be used to deliver low and medium dose oxygen concentrations. The concentration of oxygen delivered is highly dependent on the patient's respiratory rate, tidal volume and oxygen flow rate. However, the device is inexpensive, comfortable for the patient and allows the patient to eat, drink and talk.

Simple face mask (Hudson mask)

The simple face mask can provide medium (40–60%) concentrations of oxygen. The device is suitable for those with hypoxaemic respiratory failure (Type 1). The oxygen flow rate, patient's tidal volume and respiratory rate determines the actual concentration of oxygen delivered. Usual flow rate is between 5-10 L/min providing 40–60% oxygen concentration.

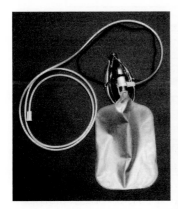

Figure 9.1 Reservoir bag.

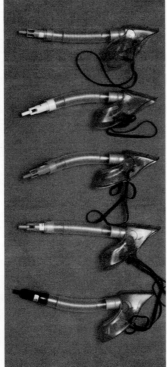

24% Oxygen venturi mask (blue)

28% Oxygen venturi mask (white)

35% Oxygen mask (yellow)

40% Oxygen mask (red)

60% Oxygen mask (green)

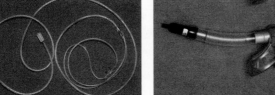

Figure 9.3 Nasal cannula.

Figure 9.2 Oxygen masks. (See picture suite for colour version.)

Patient safety tips

✔ **Remember that too little oxygen is dangerous, as is too much oxygen**. It will be only by close clinical monitoring of vital signs and, particularly, ABG sampling and measurement of O_2 saturations that the optimal oxygen therapy for an individual patient can be prescribed.

✔ **Oxygen therapy is often not given**: even when intended. As a drug it must be properly prescribed with its dose, method of administration and duration of treatment, and any special requirements such as monitoring (Figure 9.4).

✔ Set target O_2 saturations for each patient.

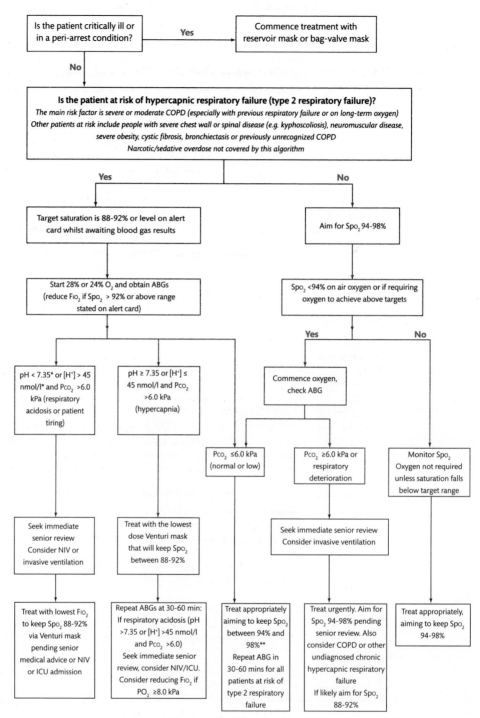

Is the patient critically ill or in a peri-arrest condition? — **Yes** → Commence treatment with reservoir mask or bag-valve mask

No

Is the patient at risk of hypercapnic respiratory failure (type 2 respiratory failure)?
The main risk factor is severe or moderate COPD (especially with previous respiratory failure or on long-term oxygen)
Other patients at risk include people with severe chest wall or spinal disease (e.g. kyphoscoliosis), neuromuscular disease, severe obesity, cystic fibrosis, bronchiectasis or previously unrecognized COPD
Narcotic/sedative overdose not covered by this algorithm

Yes

Target saturation is 88-92% or level on alert card whilst awaiting blood gas results

Start 28% or 24% O_2 and obtain ABGs (reduce F_{IO_2} if Spo_2 > 92% or above range stated on alert card)

pH < 7.35* or [H⁺] > 45 nmol/l* and Pco_2 >6.0 kPa (respiratory acidosis or patient tiring)

pH ≥ 7.35 or [H⁺] ≤ 45 nmol/l and Pco_2 >6.0 kPa (hypercapnia)

Seek immediate senior review Consider NIV or invasive ventilation

Treat with the lowest dose Venturi mask that will keep Spo_2 between 88-92%

Treat with lowest F_{IO_2} to keep Spo_2 88-92% via Venturi mask pending senior medical advice or NIV or ICU admission

Repeat ABGs at 30-60 min: If respiratory acidosis (pH >7.35 or [H⁺] >45 nmol/l and Pco_2 >6.0) Seek immediate senior review, consider NIV/ICU. Consider reducing F_{IO_2} if PO_2 ≥8.0 kPa

No

Aim for Spo_2 94-98%

Spo_2 <94% on air oxygen or if requiring oxygen to achieve above targets

Yes

No

Commence oxygen, check ABG

Pco_2 ≤6.0 kPa (normal or low)

Pco_2 ≥6.0 kPa or respiratory deterioration

Monitor Spo_2 Oxygen not required unless saturation falls below target range

Seek immediate senior review Consider invasive ventilation

Treat appropriately aiming to keep Spo_2 between 94% and 98%** Repeat ABG in 30-60 mins for all patients at risk of type 2 respiratory failure

Treat urgently. Aim for Spo_2 94-98% pending senior review. Also consider COPD or other undiagnosed chronic hypercapnic respiratory failure If likely aim for Spo_2 88-92%

Treat appropriately, aiming to keep Spo_2 94-98%

Any increase in F_{IO_2} must be followed by repeat ABGs in 1h (or sooner if conscious level deteriorates)
*If pH is <7.35 ([H⁺] >45 nmol/l) with normal or low $Paco_2$, investigate and treat for metabolic acidosis and keep Spo_2 94-98%
**Patients previously requiring NIV or IPPV should have a target range of 88-92%, even if the initial $Paco_2$ is normal.

ABG   arterial blood gas
COPD   chronic obstructive pulmonary disease
F_{IO_2} fraction of inspired oxygen
ICU   intensive care unit
NIV   non-invasive ventilation
Pco_2 carbon dioxide tension
Spo_2 arterial oxygen saturation measured by pulse oximetry

Figure 9.4 British Thoracic Society algorithm from guidelines for emergency use of oxygen.

Student name:	Medical school:	Year:

Oxygen therapy

Emergency prescription of oxygen is required in the management of many clinical conditions.

	Self	Peer	Peer /tutor	Tutor
Please state some conditions for each of the highlighted categories:				
• **Critical illness:** Cardiac arrest, post-cardiac arrest, resuscitation, sepsis, shock, major trauma, anaphylaxis, near-drowning, pulmonary haemorrhage, head injury	☐	☐	☐	☐
• **Serious illness:** acute hypoxia (cause not known yet), acute asthma, pneumonia, lung cancer, acute heart failure, pulmonary embolism, pleural effusion, pneumothorax, severe anaemia, sickle cell crisis, worsening lung fibrosis, postoperative dyspnoea	☐	☐	☐	☐
• **COPD and other illness requiring controlled oxygen:** COPD, cystic fibrosis, chronic neuromuscular disorders, chest wall disorders, morbid obesity.	☐	☐	☐	☐
• **Conditions requiring close monitoring but not oxygen unless hypoxaemia:** myocardial infarction and ACS, cerebrovascular accident, pregnancy and obstetric emergencies, most poisoning and drug overdoses (except carbon monoxide poisoning) metabolic and renal disorders, hyperventilation and dysfunctional breathing	☐	☐	☐	☐
• **LTOT: COPD and other respiratory conditions**	☐	☐	☐	☐
•	☐	☐	☐	☐
What are the special considerations that must be addressed in relation to CO poisoning?				
• High saturations on oximetry must be disregarded as monitors do not distinguish between oxyhaemoglobin and carboxyhaemoglobin. Even PaO_2 may be normal	☐	☐	☐	☐
•	☐	☐	☐	☐

How would you specific manage the following categories of patients?
Critical illness:
Serious illness:
COPD and other illness requiring controlled oxygen

Critical illness:

	Self	Peer	Peer /tutor	Tutor
• **A prompt clinical and laboratory assessment:** including history O_2 saturations and ABG sampling	☐	☐	☐	☐
• **Initial oxygen therapy:** reservoir mask with 15 L/min oxygen. Once stable, reduce oxygen and aim for O_2 saturations 94–98%.	☐	☐	☐	☐
• **Patients with COPD or other diseases with risk of hypercapnia:** who are critically ill should have initially same strategy as for other critically ill patients until ABG analysis is available and subsequent reassessment for oxygen requirements	☐	☐	☐	☐
• **Target saturations:** 94–98% in most acutely ill patients, 88–92% in those with risk of hypercapnia	☐	☐	☐	☐

Serious illness:

	Self	Peer	Peer /tutor	Tutor
• **Initial oxygen therapy:** nasal cannula at 2–6 L/min oxygen or simple facemask at 5–10 L/min oxygen. Obtain oximetry and or ABG sampling	☐	☐	☐	☐
• **For patients not at risk of hypercapnia and O_2 saturations <85%:** switch over to reservoir mask with 10–15 L/min	☐	☐	☐	☐
• **Record oxygen saturations, concentration of inspired oxygen and other vital signs**	☐	☐	☐	☐
• **Target saturations:** 94–98% in most acutely ill patients, 88–92% in those with risk of hypercapnia	☐	☐	☐	☐
• **If target not reached:** with nasal cannula or face mask, assess patient/senior help and switch over to reservoir bag. Adjust O_2 saturation to 94–98% if PaO_2 is normal (unless there is past history of type 2 respiratory failure requiring NIV or IPPV) and recheck ABGs in 30–60 minutes	☐	☐	☐	☐

COPD and other illness requiring controlled oxygen: In patients with COPD and other risk factors of hypercapnia, who are not critically ill.

	Self	Peer	Peer /tutor	Tutor
• **If ABGs are not available:** use 28% Venturi mask at 4 L/min and aim for O_2 saturations of 88–92% for patients with risk of hypercapnia but no previous acidosis	☐	☐	☐	☐
• **Adjust O_2 saturation target range to 94–98%:** if $PaCO_2$ is normal on ABGs (if no past history of NIV/IPPV) and recheck ABGs in 30–60 minutes	☐	☐	☐	☐
• **In patients with previous history of respiratory acidosis:** aim at prespecified saturations (these patients may have an oxygen alert card and their own Venturi masks with them).	☐	☐	☐	☐
• *ABG sampling should be repeated:* in such cases after 30–60 minutes or sooner if clinical deterioration prompts. If $PaCO_2$ is raised but pH is ≥7.35 or H^+ ≤45 nmol/L, this suggests that patient has probably long standing hypercapnia and aim for targets saturations of 88–92%. If patient is hypercapnic ($PaCO_2$ ≥6 kPa) and has acidosis (pH <7.35 or H^+ >45 nmol/L), consider NIV, especially if acidosis has persisted for more than 30 minutes despite treatment	☐	☐	☐	☐
•	☐	☐	☐	☐

Long-term oxygen therapy in COPD: What are the indications?	• Patients with PaO₂ <7.3 kPa when stable		☐	☐	☐	☐
	• PaO₂ 7.3–8 kPa when stable and one of the following: polycythaemia, nocturnal hypoxaemia, peripheral oedema, or pulmonary hypertension		☐	☐	☐	☐
	•		☐	☐	☐	☐

Long-term oxygen therapy in COPD: What are the indications?

- Patients with PaO_2 <7.3 kPa when stable
- PaO_2 7.3–8 kPa when stable and one of the following: polycythaemia, nocturnal hypoxaemia, peripheral oedema, or pulmonary hypertension
-

☐ ☐ ☐ ☐
☐ ☐ ☐ ☐
☐ ☐ ☐ ☐

Please discuss the following pieces of equipment in relation to oxygen therapy and place them ready for use on the manikin:

Blue   Red

☐ ☐ ☐ ☐

Patient safety: what are the main considerations in relation to oxygen therapy?

- **Remembers that too little oxygen is dangerous, as is too much oxygen**
- **Oxygen therapy must be prescribed**
-

☐ ☐ ☐ ☐
☐ ☐ ☐ ☐
☐ ☐ ☐ ☐

Self-assessed as at least borderline:	Signature:	Date:	U B S E U B S E U B S E U B S E
Peer-assessed as ready for tutor assessment:	Signature:	Date:	U B S E U B S E U B S E U B S E
Tutor-assessed as satisfactory:	Signature:	Date:	U B S E U B S E U B S E U B S E

Notes

9.2 Peripheral intravenous cannulation

Background

A cannula is a flexible tube that is inserted into a peripheral vein. Cannulae are usually placed in the peripheral veins in the lower arm but may occasionally also be placed in the veins of the foot if there are no other sites available. Veins of the lower extremities should not be routinely used in adults due to the risk of embolism, thrombophlebitis, and difficulty of visual access to look for complications.

Clinical indications

Intravenous (IV) cannulation is indicated in numerous clinical scenarios:

- Clinical emergencies for the provision of IV therapeutic including fluids, antibiotics, cardiac resuscitation drugs. In many cases, IV cannulation is undertaken to ensure access if needed in the event of the patient developing more serious illness.
- Transfusion of blood fluids and/or blood products.
- Antibiotics when the oral route is not effective.

Anatomical and physiological principles

Anatomically superficial veins are the veins are not paired with an artery. Deep veins are usually paired with an artery.

Upper limbs

- Antecubital fossa (medial cubital vein), basilic vein (ulnar side), cephalic vein (radial side) and metacarpal veins, dorsal venous arch.

Lower limbs

- Dorsal venous arch, plantar veins

Physiologically the speed of IV fluid depends on several factors including size of cannula, different types of giving sets and the delivery mechanisms including pump and mechanical. The size of cannula influences the speed of fluid delivery. The choice of cannula is dependent on the clinical setting and the indication of use. Please note the flow rates may differ slightly depending on the manufacturer.

Contraindications

Absolute

- Arteriovenous (AV) fistula, patient refusal, ipsilateral mastectomy, trauma of the extremity.

Relative

- Overlying skin abnormality (cellulitis, burns, active background skin condition).

Equipment

- Personal protective equipment: apron, non-sterile gloves, sharps bin and tray.
- Tourniquet (ideally disposable), alcohol swab/chlorhexidine wash.
- Cannulae (correct size), transparent occlusive cannula dressing, 10 mL syringe with sterile normal saline flush, gauze. Loosen cap of cannula, remove and leave on tray to retrieve later.

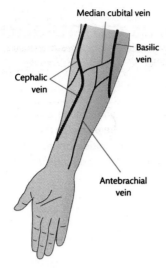

Veins of the anterior forearm
The site of location of the intravenous (IV) cannula will depend on the clinical indication, size of the IV cannula desired, size of the vein in the patient, and patient comfort. The back of the hand is commonly used (dorsal venous arch). In the foot, the greater and lesser saphenous veins and the dorsal venous arch can be cannulated.

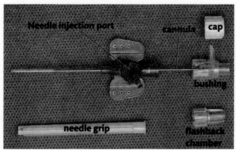

Generally a pink or green IV cannula is used.

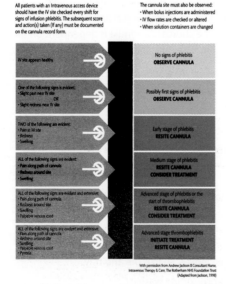

Several versions of checklists for screening for complications of IV cannulation exists: advice must be followed to reduce risk complications, particularly sepsis and extravasation of IV fluids or drugs administered.

Figure 9.5 Images in peripheral IV cannulation. Left © Andrew Jackson, Consultant Nurse, Intravenous Therapy & Care.

Table 9.1 Summary of size and function of different cannulae

Colour	Size	Flow rate (mL/min)	Clinical indication and use
Blue	22G	30	**Small fragile vein**: used in elderly and paediatric patients. usually used in chronic setting.
Pink	20G	60	**Routine standard**: use for IV drugs and fluids and blood
Green	18G	90	**Emergency standard:** infusion of blood component required at a quicker rate. IV fluids in a more acute setting
Grey	16G	200	**Emergency resuscitation situations:** ideally inserted in large vein in antecubital fossa, especially large volume infusions
Brown/orange	14G	340	**Emergency/theatre situations:** for rapid transfusions including whole blood, blood components or viscous fluids

Explanation and consent

Introduce yourself and gain consent from patient. Main points to emphasize are:

- State: purpose of cannula, specific reason, how long cannula *in situ*.
- Explain the procedure, state the main steps, show cannula.
- Allow the patient to ask any questions.
- Make sure patient is sitting or lying comfortably with limb supported.
- If the vein to be cannulated is lower than the heart it will be far more prominent and easier to access.

Procedure

A cannula is inserted into an appropriate superficial vein. In certain patients, children or those with needle phobia, topical analgesic gel can be used. This usually has to be applied a minimum of an hour prior to cannulation and wiped off before cannula is inserted.

- **Wash hands and put on clean non-sterile gloves**.
- **Assess venous anatomy and find suitable vein**: ideally use the non-dominant arm or hand. Pay attention to depth of vein, avoid venous valves (checked by direction of flow). The vein site should feel full and spongy.
- **Apply tourniquet**: ask patient to clench and unclench hand to encourage venous filling. The vein may be lightly tapped to encourage vasodilation by inducing histamine release.
- **Palpate vein site and clean skin**: use appropriate swab (usually chlorhexidine/alcohol). Do not re-palpate the vein once it is clean. A cleansed site should now not come in contact with any non-sterile item (non-touch technique).
- **Immobilize vein** and hold steady with the non-dominant hand (index finger and thumb), ('tethering and anchoring').
- **Angle the needle to 20–30° and warn patient that they will feel a sharp scratch**: the needle is angled to the direction of blood flow. Ensure steady grip using the needle grip (and flashback chamber with practice).
- **Advance the cannula and needle slowly into the vein**: until a flashback is seen in the bushing at the point where the plastic cannula ends at the flashback chamber.
- **Release tourniquet**: otherwise copious venous blood will leave the cannula.

- **Withdraw the needle and immediately place cap onto the flashback chamber**: if needed, clean up any blood with clean gauze or tissue.
- **Secure the cannula**: with special adhesive dressing.
- **Flush with 10 mL sterile normal saline**: remembering to check the expiry date.
- **Discard all unnecessary and used clinical equipment safely**: special attention to all sharps
- **Record the site of cannulation, any failed attempts, complications and planned removal date**: also, date the cannula if sticker provided and place appropriately on the cannula adhesive dressing.

Post-procedure management

- Inspect the cannula site daily and look for signs of inflammation.
- Replace cannula every 72 hours.

Professionalism: working with colleagues

- Try a maximum of two or three attempts with expert referral if unsuccessful.
- Discuss complication with senior colleague, e.g. failure to cannulate, haematoma.
- Make nursing staff aware of cannulation, so for example, drugs can now be given or an IVI set up.

Complications

- **Localized phlebitis**: ensure the site is checked daily. If there are any signs of infection, remove and re-site the cannula. See Table 9.2.
- **Cellulitis**: common complication, especially if the patient has diabetes.
- **Bleeding from site**: this can be due to the venous wall not closing firmly around the cannula. Re-siting may be needed, raise arm to reduce venous engorgement or apply pressure to distal veins to reduce venous flow to cannula. This may correct problem in a few minutes.
- **Air embolism, catheter fracture, and embolism**: rare if care taken as in above steps.

Table 9.2 The grades of phlebitis and action needed (adapted from Jackson, 1998)

Visual infusion phlebitis score (VIP)	Appearance	Diagnosis	Action Always assess need
0	IV site appears clean and healthy	No signs of phlebitis	Observe cannula
1	Slight pain or redness near cannula site	Possible signs of phlebitis	Observe cannula
2	Two of the following: Pain, erythema, swelling	Early phlebitis	Remove cannula
3	All of the following: Pain, erythema, swelling	Medium stage phlebitis	Remove cannula
4	All of the following: Pain, erythema, swelling Venous cord(s) palpable	Advanced stage phlebitis or start of thrombophlebitis	Remove cannula
5	All below, widespread: Pain, erythema, swelling Venous cords palpable Pyrexia	Advanced thrombophlebitis	Re-site cannula and start treatment ? antibiotics

Always assess need for IV cannula before re-siting. Phlebitis will often be associated with cellulitis. In case of cellulitis consider antibiotics against *Streptococcus* and *Staphylococcus*

Patient safety tips

✔ **Never re-insert the metal needle**: once removed as there is increased risk of damage to the plastic cannula (and possible embolization if broken off) and risk of needle stick injury. Newer cannula mechanism with needle protectors will not allow this. It is always better to explain to the patient and try another site.

✔ **Explanation**: explain any restriction in mobility and try to emphasize the importance to protect the cannula site.

✔ **Daily inspection and review of cannula need**: Assess needs such as continuing IV infusion or IV drugs such as antibiotics.

✔ **Haematomas**: these can result after repeated venepuncture, and often lead to a reduced choice of suitable veins to access. So upon removal of a cannula ensure digital pressure is applied for approximately 3 minutes after removal with elevation of the arm. Note apply pressure for longer in patients on warfarin.

✔ **Vein rolling**: this may occur during insertion so it is important to maintain skin tension through insertion which can be aided by holding the vein proximally and distally to the insertion site with thumb and index finger of the non-dominant hand. This is known as 'anchoring'.

Student name: Medical school: Year:

Peripheral IV cannulation

You have been asked to see a patient who is due to have surgery soon for an elective knee replacement. Please insert a peripheral venous cannula in this manikin/patient.
I will ask some questions before and during the procedure.

		Self	Peer	Peer /tutor	Tutor
What are the clinical indications for IV cannulation?	• IV fluids including blood transfusion, drugs	☐	☐	☐	☐
What are suitable sites for IV cannulation?	• **Upper limbs:** antecubital fossa (medial cubital vein), basilic vein (ulnar side), cephalic vein (radial side) and metacarpal veins, dorsal venous arch	☐	☐	☐	☐
	• **Lower limbs:** dorsal venous arch, plantar veins	☐	☐	☐	☐
Point to and name the main parts of this IV cannula:	• Needle, cannula, bushing, injection port, needle grip, flashback chamber, cap	☐	☐	☐	☐
	• Discusses use of the different colour cannulae shown using facts from Table 9.1.	☐	☐	☐	☐
What are the contraindications to IV cannulation?	• **Absolute:** AV fistula, patient refusal, ipsilateral mastectomy, trauma of the extremity	☐	☐	☐	☐
	• **Relative:** Overlying skin abnormality (cellulitis, burns, skin disease)	☐	☐	☐	☐
Prepares equipment	• Personal protective equipment: apron, non-sterile gloves, sharps bin and tray	☐	☐	☐	☐
	• Tourniquet, cleaning swab, cannulae (correct size), cannula dressing, 10 mL syringe with sterile normal saline flush, gauze	☐	☐	☐	☐
Explanation and consent	• Introduction, consent from patient	☐	☐	☐	☐
	• Explanation: purpose of cannula, specific reason, how long cannula *in situ*, explains procedure, shows cannula	☐	☐	☐	☐
	• Allows the patient to ask any questions	☐	☐	☐	☐
	• Patient is sitting or lying comfortably with limb supported	☐	☐	☐	☐
Procedure	• **Washes hands and put on clean non-sterile gloves**	☐	☐	☐	☐
	• **Assesses venous anatomy and finds suitable vein:**	☐	☐	☐	☐
	• **Applies tourniquet:** asks patient to clench and unclench hand if needed	☐	☐	☐	☐
	• **Palpates vein site and clean skin:** do not re-palpate the vein once it is clean.	☐	☐	☐	☐
	• **Immobilizes vein** and holds steady with the non-dominant hand	☐	☐	☐	☐
	• **Angles the needle to 20–30° and warns patient that they will feel a sharp scratch**	☐	☐	☐	☐
	• **Advances the cannula and needle slowly into the vein:** until a flashback is seen	☐	☐	☐	☐
	• **Releases tourniquet:** otherwise copious venous blood will leave the cannula	☐	☐	☐	☐
	• **Withdraws the needle and immediately place cap onto the flashback chamber:** if needed, cleans up any blood with clean gauze or tissue	☐	☐	☐	☐
	• **Secures the cannula:** with special adhesive dressing.	☐	☐	☐	☐
	• *Flush with 10* mL *sterile normal saline:* checks expiry date.	☐	☐	☐	☐
	• *Discard all unnecessary and used clinical equipment safely:*	☐	☐	☐	☐
	• *Record the site of cannulation, any failed attempts, complications and planned removal date:* Also, date and place cannula sticker	☐	☐	☐	☐
Post-procedure management: what should be done?	• Inspection of the cannula site daily and looks for signs of inflammation	☐	☐	☐	☐
	• Replaces cannula every 72 hours	☐	☐	☐	☐
Professionalism: working with colleagues	• Maximum of two or three attempts then expert referral. Discusses complications with senior.	☐	☐	☐	☐
	• Makes nursing staff aware of cannulation: so treatment can be given	☐	☐	☐	☐
Complications: what are the main complications?	• Localized phlebitis and or cellulitis	☐	☐	☐	☐
	• Bleeding from site	☐	☐	☐	☐
	• Air embolism, catheter fracture and embolism: rare if care taken as in above steps	☐	☐	☐	☐
	• Understands use of VIP score and actions needed	☐	☐	☐	☐
Patient safety tips	• Never re-insert the metal needle	☐	☐	☐	☐
	• Daily inspection and review of cannula need	☐	☐	☐	☐
	• Avoiding haematomas: especially after repeated venepuncture or removal of cannula. Ensures digital pressure for around 3 minutes with arm elevation	☐	☐	☐	☐

				Self	Peer	Peer /tutor	Tutor
Self-assessed as at least borderline:	Signature:		Date:	U B S E	U B S E	U B S E	U B S E
Peer-assessed as ready for tutor assessment:	Signature:		Date:	U B S E	U B S E	U B S E	U B S E
Tutor-assessed as satisfactory:	Signature:		Date:	U B S E	U B S E	U B S E	U B S E

Notes

9.3 Making up drugs for parenteral administration

Background

This is a relatively common task for a junior doctor and other clinicians such as pharmacist and nurses. There is considerable potential for error which can be virtually eliminated with close attention to basic principles of prescribing and safe administration. This section will concentrate on preparation of drugs for IV administration. Non-IV injections are covered elsewhere.

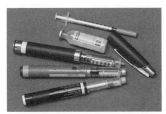

IV Insulin must always be measured out very carefully: ± 2 units can result in hyperglycaemia or hypoglycaemia, respectively.

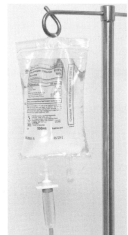

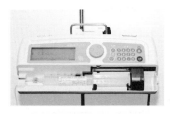

The GIK regimen is commonly used in surgery in patients with diabetes mellitus: most specific clinical outcomes are improved such as infection rates.

If more than one infusion is given into a single intravenous cannula it is particularly important to check for drug(s)/infusion(s) compatibility.

Figure 9.6 Images in making up drugs for parenteral administration.

Clinical indications

Certain drugs need to be added to standard IV fluids such as 0.9% normal saline for injection or 5% dextrose. This is usually because the dose of the drug is most accurately given after it has been diluted or the agent itself causes a local reaction at the site of infusion unless it is diluted by an infusing fluid. Common examples in clinical practice are:

- Insulin as in the glucose-insulin-K^+ (GIK regimen) during surgery to stabilize glucose levels
- Antibiotics such as gentamicin and vancomycin
- Agents such as amiodarone in cardiac arrhythmias (usually given via a central line).

Anatomical and physiological principles

The main parenteral (non-gastrointestinal tract) routes are as follows:

- **Intravenous**: insulin, antibiotics, furosemide, hydrocortisone
- **Intramuscular**: metoclopramide, insulin if no IV access
- **Subcutaneous**: heparin, diamorphine, haloperidol
- **Intradermal**: lidocaine, Bacillus Calmette Guerin vaccine (BCG; tuberculosis vaccine)
- **Intrathecal**: **only under expert supervision**, with two clinicians involved throughout to check procedure

- Topical (dermal), nasal, inhalational, conjunctival, aural, sublingual, vaginal, intraurethral, intra-osseus, intra-coronary via catheter, interpleural, peritoneal, bladder, intrauterine.

Contraindications

A detailed clinical history should be undertaken to exclude allergies. Any potential drug reaction and contraindications should also be determined.

Preparing a GIK regimen

- Use 500 mL 10% glucose (dextrose) containing 10 mmol K^+ (therefore K^+ 20 mmol/L) unmodified (soluble, regular).
- Add insulin 16 Units of soluble insulin.
- Infused at 80 mL/h using an infusion pump

Equipment

- IV infusion set, IV infusion stand, infusion device
- Soluble insulin, standard preparation as 100 Units/mL and infusion bag (500 mL of 10% glucose with 10 K^+ mmol), insulin syringe marked in single units for accuracy.
- Non-sterile gloves (not essential with insulin).

Preparation

Wash hands. As for any prescription check and specifically for parenteral medication, check:

- Correct drug prescription for the correct patient at the correct time.
- Correct dose, correct route of administration. Do not confuse oral dose with IV, IV dose with intrathecal dose. The dose will be different and can result in fatal errors.
- Correct expiry date.
- Colleague to check above with you if needed.

Explanation and consent

- Introduce yourself and gain consent from the patient.
- State purpose of the parenteral medication/infusion.
- State how long the treatment will take to deliver.
- State main side-effects and what patients should look out for.

Procedure

In the example below, the clinician has been asked to prepare a bag of IV fluid with insulin as part of preparation for surgery in a patient with type 2 diabetes mellitus whose glucose levels are usually in between 8 and 14 mmol/L. General principle not specific to the exact task will also be covered.

- **Prepare all equipment** onto work surface or trolley.
- **Recheck drug**.
- **Draw up medication**: in the example 16 Units of soluble insulin using an insulin syringe
- **Inject insulin into sterile port of infusion bag**: after removing sterile cap. If the insulin needle is too short to do this, take off needle and use longer narrowest needle that will work.
- **Mix well by inverting bag at least six times**: do not shake bag and create air bubbles.

- **Administration set preparation (as for IV infusion)**:
  - ○ **Close flow clamp** on administration set
  - ○ **Remove protective cap** from the spike of the administration set.
  - ○ **Insert spike into the infusion bag**: push and twist the spike in fully.
  - ○ **Hang the fluid on the 'drip stand'**: squeeze bag to allow 50% drip chamber to fill.
  - ○ **Slowly open the roller clamp and prime the administration set**: allow fluid to run through leaving the set 'primed'. The roller clamps is again closed.
  - ○ **Attach prepared infusate with drug into an infusion device**.
  - ○ **Have ready the cannula connection end of the administration set**: remove the protective cap from the IV cannula and quickly connect the administration set.
  - ○ **Tape IV the line in position**: Use a 'belay' to reduce complications and pain.
  - ○ **Open roller clamp to allow infusion device to take over rate of infusion**.
  - ○ **Monitor to assess fluid flow**.
- **Discard all unnecessary and used clinical equipment safely**: Special attention to sharps if generated. Discard all unnecessary packaging appropriately
- **IV prescription completion**: Record that infusion has been given (see Table 9.3).

Table 9.3 Infusion rates for 1000 mL intravenous fluid

Hours per 1000 mL IV according to prescription	Infusion device rate		Manual infusion rate Drops/min*
	mL/h	mL/min	
1 hour	1000	16.7	320
2 hours	500	8.3	160
4 hours	250	4.2	80
6 hours	166	2.8	60
8 hours	125	2.1	40
12 hours	83	1.4	30

*Assuming there are 20 drops in 1 mL.

Post-procedure management

- Ensure patient is comfortable
- Record the time the infusion commenced (sometimes batch numbers are also required to be documented on IV rota proforma).

Professionalism: working with colleagues

- Communicate with the patient regarding procedure
- Allow patient to ask questions
- Consider discussing particular side effects with staff on ward: e.g. allergic reaction to antibiotics, ototoxicity due to gentamicin, hypoglycaemia due to insulin.

Complications

Risks with IV drugs can be immediate and severe, reversal can be difficult:

- **Anaphylaxis**: ensure the patient's allergies are known to you.

- **Fluid and drug incompatibility**: ensure that the infusate and drug are compatible. Check compatibility with clinical pharmacist or senior if unsure.

- **Localized phlebitis and or cellulitis**: ensure the site is checked throughout the infusion for any signs of phlebitis and corrective action taken.

- **Extravasation and infiltration**: the drug and infusate enters the subcutaneous tissue. Consider checking IV cannula patent by injecting a few millilitres of sterile normal saline.

- **Fluid overload**: Lookout for the symptoms and physical signs of fluid overload. This should be especially checked in cardiac failure patients.

- **Systemic infection**: An IV infusion will always be a potential source of infection. Monitor vital signs and the insertion site.

Patient safety tips

These will be the same as for IV infusions generally:

✔ **Fluid balance**: always consider the amount of fluid given to the patient and the indication.

✔ **Monitor electrolytes**: IV fluids can precipitate electrolyte imbalance therefore should always be checked *before* prescribing.

✔ **Check vital signs**: these should be done before, during and after fluid infusion. When prescribing fluids always observe vital signs.

✔ **High risk patients when administrating any IV fluids**: Cardiac failure, any renal failure, diabetic ketoacidosis or hyperosmolar hyperglycaemia syndrome, any liver disease, hyponatraemia.

✔ **Safe use of the infusion device**: make sure that the device has been correctly set up with appropriate alarms in place.

Making up drugs for parenteral administration

Please prepare an infusion of Pabrinex (IV B vitamins) in 5% dextrose for the following patient:

Mr Winston Smith (Fox Covert, 36 Oceania Drive, Eastport, EB8 4GO; date of birth 24 July 1948, hospital number GE9087589, Orwell Ward) has been admitted because of confusion, imbalance, and vomiting. He has around 12 units of alcohol on a daily basis and smokes 25 cigarettes a day (and has done since the age of 18). On examination he has a Mini-Mental Test score of 4/10, ataxia, and nystagmus)

		Self	Peer	Peer /tutor	Tutor
Sodium 139 mmol/L	Potassium 3.6 mmol/L	Urea 3.2 mmol/L			
Creatinine 106 µmol/L	Hb 9.3 g/dL	ECG: Normal			
Interprets clinical data correctly	• What condition is this patient developing or at very high risk of: Wernicke–Korsakoff syndrome	☐	☐	☐	☐
	• How do you calculate pack years of smoking?	☐	☐	☐	☐
	• How many in this patient?	☐	☐	☐	☐
	• What could the possible causes of anaemia be in this patient?	☐	☐	☐	☐
States indications and need for parenteral (IV) drug administration	• Patient at risk of full-blown of Wernicke–Korsakoff syndrome which is thiamine responsive	☐	☐	☐	☐
	• Above syndrome is the triad of cognitive changes (confusion, confabulation, stupor, coma), Ataxia (broad-based gait, cerebellar signs), nystagmus (other eyes such as lateral rectus palsy, fixed pupils) delirium tremens, hypotension and hypothermia are additional features	☐	☐	☐	☐
Equipment	• IV infusion set, IV infusion stand, gloves, infusion device	☐	☐	☐	☐
Legal prescription requirements, specifics for parenteral administration	• Full name and address of the patient, age or date of birth	☐	☐	☐	☐
	• Text: printed or written legibly in black ink (with correct spelling)	☐	☐	☐	☐
	• Dated and signed by the prescriber, prescriber's name under signature (ideally)	☐	☐	☐	☐
	• Checks correct drug and dose is being injected with name checked	☐	☐	☐	☐
	• Checks route of administration is correct; does not confuse oral dose with IV, IV dose with intrathecal dose. The dose will be different and can result in fatal errors	☐	☐	☐	☐
	• Checks correct expiry date, colleague to check above with you	☐	☐	☐	☐
Explanation and consent	• Introduction and gains consent from the patient	☐	☐	☐	☐
	• States purpose of the parenteral medication/infusion	☐	☐	☐	☐
	• States how long the treatment will take to deliver	☐	☐	☐	☐
	• States main side effects and what patients should look out for	☐	☐	☐	☐
Procedure (check order)	• Prepares all equipment onto work surface or trolley	☐	☐	☐	☐
	• Draws up medication and inject into sterile port	☐	☐	☐	☐
	• Mixes well by inverting bag at least six times, does not shake bag and create air bubbles	☐	☐	☐	☐
	• Closes valve on giving set and inserts sharp giving set end into the infusion bag outlet	☐	☐	☐	☐
	• Hangs infusion bag, squeezes drip chamber several times until it is 50% full	☐	☐	☐	☐
	• Prime tubing. Clears any bubbles by tapping or flicking the tubing	☐	☐	☐	☐
	• Attaches to IV cannula and adjust drip rate using the infusion device or manually	☐	☐	☐	☐
	• Tapes the infusion line in a 'belay'	☐	☐	☐	☐
Post-procedure Management	• Sign that you have completed the giving of the prescription	☐	☐	☐	☐
Professionalism	• Informs key colleagues, especially in relation to monitoring of the infusion and side-effects such as worsening shortness of breath due to cardiac failure or an allergic reaction	☐	☐	☐	☐
Complications	• Allergic reaction	☐	☐	☐	☐
Patient safety tips	• Correct drug, correct dose, correct route, correct patient	☐	☐	☐	☐
	• Uses an infusion device, far more accurate than a manual setting	☐	☐	☐	☐
	• **Adds tips on** the infusion device from nursing staff: alarms, power loss, etc.	☐	☐	☐	☐
	• **Seeks help as appropriate** (**BNF, clinical guidelines, clinical pharmacist, other suitable colleague**)	☐	☐	☐	☐
	•	☐	☐	☐	☐

				Self	Peer	Peer/tutor	Tutor
Self-assessed as at least borderline:	Signature:	Date:		U B S E	U B S E	U B S E	U B S E
Peer-assessed as ready for tutor assessment:	Signature:	Date:		U B S E	U B S E	U B S E	U B S E
Tutor-assessed as satisfactory:	Signature:	Date:		U B S E	U B S E	U B S E	U B S E

Notes

9.4 Intradermal, subcutaneous, and intramuscular injections

Background

Injection involves the administration of a substance into the body by puncturing the skin, using a hollow needle and syringe. There are several routes of injection, depending on the layer where the substance is injected: intradermal (id), subcutaneous (sc) and intramuscular (im).

Clinical indications

The subcutaneous and intramuscular routes are generally used if:

- The drug will be destroyed by intestinal secretions
- The drug is not absorbed by the alimentary tract
- The patient is unable to take the drug orally
- The drug is unavailable in oral form.

Intradermal

- Allergy testing
- Immunological tests (tuberculin skin test, Mantoux's test)
- Administration of local anaesthetics.

Subcutaneous

- Drugs which require slow absorption, e.g. diamorphine or enoxaparin
- Drugs which require frequent injection, e.g. insulin
- Administration of fluids if the patient has no venous access. However, absorption is slow (e.g. 1000 mL over 12 hours). Only 0.9% normal saline can be given reliably and without significant irritation.

Intramuscular

- To deliver drugs that require quick absorption and release, especially in some emergencies e.g. adrenaline and morphine.

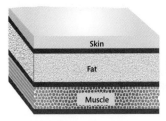
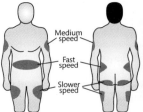
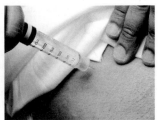

Intradermal injection: into the skin only, the needle is angled at 10-20 °
Subcutaneous injection: into the fat layer, the needle is angled at 90 °
Intramuscular injection: needle is at least 20mm long to reach muscle.

Insulin injection sites: the precise rate of absorption of insulin is dependent on where it is injected.

Modern insulin pens: are engineered to very high specifications and can deliver insulin accurately to 0.5 of a unit if needed and relatively painlessly due to the fine sharp needle.

Figure 9.7 Images in intradermal, subcutaneous and intramuscular injections

243

9.4
**Intradermal,
subcutaneous,
and intramuscular
injections**

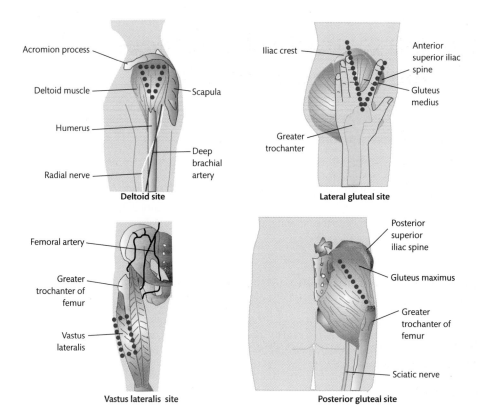

Figure 9.8 Sites of intramuscular injection

Anatomical and physiological principles

- **Epidermis and dermis**: these are the two layers of the skin. In an intradermal injection the substance is injected into the layers of the skin. Only a small volume can be given intradermally, 0.5 mL or less.

- **Subcutaneous tissue or the superficial fascia**: is between the skin and deep tissues, such as muscle and bone. It has variable thickness and fat content. In a subcutaneous injection the substance is administered into the subcutaneous tissue or superficial fascia. These tissues have a low volume blood supply and absorption is slow. The amount of drug that can be given by this route is limited to 0.5–2 mL. It can be used if the drug is highly soluble and unlikely to irritate the subcutaneous layer.

- **Muscles**: are surrounded by a thin layer of fibrous tissue called the deep fascia. In an intramuscular injection the substance is administered into the muscle (Figure 9.8). This has a good blood supply allowing the drug to be absorbed rapidly. The amount of drug is limited to 1–4 mL depending on the size of the muscle (deltoid 1 mL, gluteal 4 mL). Compared with IV injection, onset of action is slower.

Contraindications to intradermal, subcutaneous, and intramuscular injections

- Cellulitis, allergy to drug, coagulopathy or thrombocytopenia.

Equipment

- Non-sterile gloves. Basic equipment tray is useful. Sharps disposal bin.
- Intradermal, subcutaneous, or an intramuscular injection
- Appropriate needles and syringes
- Prescription chart to check drug dose and route and identify correct patient.

Intradermal

- The needle sizes used for intradermal injection are usually 26G brown.

Subcutaneous

- The needle sizes used for subcutaneous injection are:
  - 29G (insulin syringe needles)
  - 26G brown/25G (subcutaneous needles).

Intramuscular

- The needle sizes used for intramuscular injection are usually 23G blue/21G green.
- The needle length should be selected according to weight to ensure the medication is administered correctly into the intramuscular layer. General guidance:
  - 2.5 cm needle (31.5–40 kg)
  - 5–7.5 cm needle (40.5–90 kg)
  - 10–15 cm needle (above 90 kg).

One needle should be used for drawing up the medication, and a new needle should be used to administer the medication. This is in case the needle gets damaged or blunted, and reduces the chance of infection. It is important to follow the recommendations regarding route of administration of each specific drug.

Preparation

- Standard precautions such as correct hand washing, and non-sterile gloves. Skin cleansing prior to injection will depend on local policy.
- Visible dirty skin should be cleaned with soap and water.
- Use 2% chlorhexidine/70% alcohol products to clean skin prior to administering the injection (depends on local policy).
- Using alcohol-based products to clean the skin is not recommended for patients administering insulin as it hardens the skin.
- For enoxaparin (Clexane), only physically clean skin is required.

Explanation and consent

Introduce yourself and gain consent from patient. Main points to emphasize are:

- State: purpose of injection, main steps
- Allow the patient to ask any questions
- Identify suitable site for the injection and ensure privacy.

Procedure

Intradermal, subcutaneous or intramuscular injection is given as prescribed to the correct patient. The prescription would have been checked and the patient would be assessed as safe to have the treatment especially in relation to clinical state and allergies.

Intradermal

- For allergy testing the flexor surface of the non-dominant forearm is used.
- Intradermal injections are given at 10° into skin with the needle bevel upwards.
- Warn patient of impending injection, can be very painful.
- A bleb appears on the skin surface if the needle is in the correct position (a *peau d'orange* appearance).

Subcutaneous

- Subcutaneous injections are given in the following areas: the abdomen, deltoid area, and the top of the thigh.
- Insulin or enoxaparin syringes are now given at 90° into a pinched up skinfold using short needles.
- Brown or orange needles can be used at 45–90° depending on the size of the patient and the depth of their subcutaneous layer.
- Injection sites should be rotated when drugs are being repeatedly administered via the subcutaneous route to prevent damage to the site.
- Once the needle has been inserted, pull back on the syringe piston to ensure a vein has not been entered. If blood is aspirated the needle must be removed. Blood in the syringe indicates that the drug may have been administered IV or even into an artery rather than subcutaneously.
- Warn patient of impending injection, can be painful.

Intramuscular

- Intramuscular injections are given in the following areas: deltoid, ventrogluteal, dorsal gluteal, or vastus lateralis site.
- The skin is pulled taut to one side and then once the injection has been administered and the needle withdrawn, the tissue is released to cover the entry site and keep the drug within the injection site (modified Z track technique).
- Intramuscular injections are given at an angle of 90° to the skin.
- Once the needle has been inserted, pull back on the syringe piston to ensure a vein has not been entered. If blood is aspirated the needle must be removed. Blood in the syringe indicates that the drug may have been administered IV or even into an artery rather than intramuscularly.
- If blood is aspirated, withdraw needle, repeat procedure with a new needle at a different site.
- Injection sites should be rotated when drugs are being repeatedly administered via the intramuscular route to prevent damage to the site.

Post-procedure management

If area is bleeding consider sterile dressing, e.g. sterile plaster.

Professionalism

- Communicate with the patient to explain the procedure and need for injection.
- Allow the patient an opportunity to ask questions.
- Write clear notes, document or sign drug given. Discuss, inform colleagues if needed.

Complications

General

- Infection – ensure correct use of standard precautions and ensure the site is visibly clean before use
- Sterile abscesses – rotate injection sites
- Oedematous sites – drugs will not be absorbed
- Anaphylaxis – check allergies before giving drugs
- Bleeding – check for bleeding disorders
- Lipohypertrophy/lipoatrophy – rotate injection sites
- Inadvertent IV injection – aspirate before injection

Intramuscular injection

- Haemorrhage – intramuscular injection contraindicated in anticoagulated patients
- Nerve damage – ensure the correct site is used
- Embolus – aspirate prior to administering the drug

Patient safety tips

✔ As with drugs ensure: right patient, right medicine, right route, right dose, right site, right time.

✔ Ensure patient is not allergic to drug.

✔ Avoid sites of infection, inflammation, swelling or skin lesions.

✔ Beware of anticoagulant treatment or bleeding disorders.

✔ Know your anatomy (sciatic nerve)

Student name: Medical school: Year:

Intradermal/subcutaneous/intramuscular injection

Please demonstrate how you would give this manikin an intradermal/subcutaneous/intramuscular injection. I will ask for answers based around some clinical headings and to carry out the procedure.

Columns: Self | Peer | Peer/tutor | Tutor

Background

Understands indications:
- intradermal – allergy diagnosis, immunological test ☐ ☐ ☐ ☐
- intramuscular/subcutaneous – oral administration of drug not possible because of drug or patient factors ☐ ☐ ☐ ☐
- ☐ ☐ ☐ ☐

Anatomical and physiological principles
- Layers: epidermis, dermis, subcutaneous tissue, deep fascia, muscle ☐ ☐ ☐ ☐
- Intradermal: injection goes into skin ☐ ☐ ☐ ☐
- Subcutaneous: injection goes into subcutaneous tissue ☐ ☐ ☐ ☐
- Intramuscular: injection goes into muscle ☐ ☐ ☐ ☐
- Absorption is fastest in muscle because of good blood supply ☐ ☐ ☐ ☐
- ☐ ☐ ☐ ☐

Contraindications
- Infection of injection site ☐ ☐ ☐ ☐
- Allergy to drug ☐ ☐ ☐ ☐
- Coagulopathy (intramuscular injection) ☐ ☐ ☐ ☐
- ☐ ☐ ☐ ☐

Procedure
- Handwash with water and soap or alcohol gel ☐ ☐ ☐ ☐
- Introduction and identifies patient ☐ ☐ ☐ ☐
- Clear explanation: e.g. 'I am going to inject this medication into your skin/under your skin/into your muscle. You may feel some discomfort as I insert the needle and then inject the medication.' ☐ ☐ ☐ ☐
- Obtains informed consent ☐ ☐ ☐ ☐
- Checks medication: name, dose, timing, and expiry date ☐ ☐ ☐ ☐
- Checks for patient allergies ☐ ☐ ☐ ☐
- Uses one needle to prepare the medication and a new needle to administer medication ☐ ☐ ☐ ☐
- Expels any air in syringe ☐ ☐ ☐ ☐
- Apron, gloves, sharps bin and tray, sterile gauze ☐ ☐ ☐ ☐
- Selects correct needle for injection: ☐ ☐ ☐ ☐
  ○ Intradermal: 26G brown
  ○ Subcutaneous: 29G, 26G brown or 25G
  ○ Intramuscular: 23G blue or 21G green, needle length according to weight
- Selects appropriate site ☐ ☐ ☐ ☐
  ○ Intradermal: e.g. anterior forearm
  ○ Subcutaneous: e.g. abdomen, thigh or arm
  ○ Intramuscular: e.g. deltoid, ventrogluteal, dorsogluteal or vastus lateralis site
- Cleanses site ☐ ☐ ☐ ☐
- Gently pinches up (intradermal/subcutaneous) or stretches (intramuscular) skin between thumb and index finger ☐ ☐ ☐ ☐
- Warns patient of sharp scratch ☐ ☐ ☐ ☐
- Holds needle and syringe correctly ☐ ☐ ☐ ☐
  ○ Intradermal: 10° angle to skin and inserts the needle just into the skin
  ○ Subcutaneous: 45° or 90° angle to the skin and inserts below skin
  ○ Intramuscular: 90° angle to the skin and inserts two-thirds of needle
- Aspirates to check for blood for 5–10 seconds (intramuscular ?) ☐ ☐ ☐ ☐
- Administers drug slowly ☐ ☐ ☐ ☐
- Removes needle from the skin and disposes of needle and syringe into the sharps bin ☐ ☐ ☐ ☐
- Applies pressure to the site with sterile gauze if required ☐ ☐ ☐ ☐
- Good communication demonstrated throughout the procedure and allows patient to ask questions. ☐ ☐ ☐ ☐
- ☐ ☐ ☐ ☐

Post-procedure management
- Documents administration of medication ☐ ☐ ☐ ☐
- ☐ ☐ ☐ ☐

Professionalism: working with colleagues
- Communicates sensitively, thanks the patient, addresses any questions or concerns, washes hands ☐ ☐ ☐ ☐
- Completes all documentation legibly and unambiguously ☐ ☐ ☐ ☐
- ☐ ☐ ☐ ☐

Complications		U B S E	U B S E	U B S E	U B S E
	• Anaphylaxis	☐	☐	☐	☐
	• Infection	☐	☐	☐	☐
	• Sterile abscess	☐	☐	☐	☐
	• Non-absorption in oedematous site	☐	☐	☐	☐
	• Haemorrhage (intramuscular)	☐	☐	☐	☐
	• Nerve damage (intramuscular)	☐	☐	☐	☐
	• Embolus (intramuscular)	☐	☐	☐	☐
	•	☐	☐	☐	☐
Patient safety tips	• Ensure patient is not allergic to drug	☐	☐	☐	☐
	• Avoid sites of infection, inflammation, swelling and skin lesions	☐	☐	☐	☐
	• Beware of anticoagulation and bleeding disorders	☐	☐	☐	☐
	•	☐	☐	☐	☐
Global assessment	• Would you be happy for this student to administer an intradermal/subcutaneous/ intramuscular injection into a real patient?	Yes/No/Unsure			
	•	☐	☐	☐	☐

			U B S E	U B S E	U B S E	U B S E
Self-assessed as at least borderline:	Signature:	Date:				
Peer-assessed as ready for tutor assessment:	Signature:	Date:				
Tutor-assessed as satisfactory:	Signature:	Date:				

Notes

9.5 Blood transfusion

Background

When current policies are followed and all associated precautions taken blood transfusion is relatively safe. However, the chain of events from taking the sample for cross-matching to administration of the blood component is long: error at any stage can result in adverse events which may be serious or even fatal. Serious Hazards of Transfusion (SHOT) scheme data contain many examples of this. It is the responsibility of all those involved in blood transfusion to be fully aware of all national and local policies and guidelines.

One of the greatest risks, according to SHOT reports, is *Incorrect Blood Component Transfused (IBCT)*. This is defined as all reported episodes where a patient was transfused with a component which did not meet appropriate requirements or which was intended for someone else. This includes 'wrong blood' incidents and pre-transfusion testing errors. A disproportionate number of IBCT events occur between 8.00 pm and 8.00 am. Patients should only be transfused at night if there is an urgent clinical indication. IBCT and other specific adverse events should be reported to SHOT.

Clinical indications (Table 9.4)

Whole blood – blood in its unprocessed state – is now used only in very rare circumstances. For routine use it is separated into components, of which the most commonly used are red blood cells (RBCs), platelets, and fresh frozen plasma (FFP).

Table 9.4 Clinical indications and the components used

Component	Clinical indication
Red blood cells	Anaemia Haemorrhage
Platelets	Thrombocytopenia: acute, chronic or chemotherapy induced
Fresh frozen plasma	Massive haemorrhage Coagulation factor deficiency May be used for the immediate reversal of warfarin effect in the presence of bleeding

Physiological principles

The purpose of cross-matching is to ensure that the recipient's serum contains no antibodies against antigens on the donor red blood cells. In an emergency uncross-matched O Rhesus-negative blood can be given if the life-saving need of a transfusion outweighs the risk of an antibody-mediated transfusion reaction. All blood components are tested for infections, including hepatitis B and C, human immunodeficiency virus (HIV), and cytomegalovirus. If cytomegalovirus-negative blood is required it must be specifically requested since not all units are cytomegalovirus negative.

Contraindications

There are no absolute contraindications to transfusion apart from patient refusal; however, the benefits of the procedure must be weighed against the possible hazards. Alternatives should always be considered such as Vitamin K and prothrombin complex concentrate (PCC) to reverse warfarin effect, intravenous iron for iron-deficiency anaemia, and cell salvage for blood loss in surgical procedures.

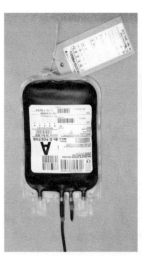

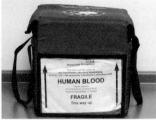

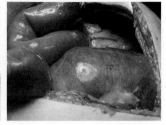

Blood transfusion administration set:
a special blood filter chamber is
incorporated.

Blood transfusion: commonest
hazards are in relation to errors in
patient identity and mislabelling of
samples.

Figure 9.9 Images in blood transfusion.

Equipment and preparation

Equipment for venepuncture, correct blood sample tube, transfusion request form, IV infusion rota form. If a suitable IV cannula is not already *in situ* one should be inserted before the blood is brought to the clinical area.

Explanation and consent

- The patient should give informed – but not written – consent. Clearly state the indication for blood transfusion, its benefits, and possible side-effects and risks. This discussion should be documented in the patient's records.
- Information leaflets are available.
- Should the patient refuse transfusion, for example on grounds of religious or ethical belief, refer to local policy and ensure consultant involvement.

Procedure

Exact procedures may vary slightly between hospitals: check your local blood transfusion policy. However, most units will follow policies similar to these.

- **Cross-matching and patient identity check:** ensure you have the right patient. Ask the patient, if possible, to state their surname, first name, and date of birth and check the wristband. If the patient is not capable of a response, check with a relative or a member of staff.
- **Request form:** this must be completed as fully as possible although in an emergency situation the Hospital Transfusion Laboratory (HTL) will be aware that not all the information may be available. Some local policies may require that the form be handwritten.
- **Patient's details and request form:** full name, date of birth, hospital and/or NHS number *must* be provided, also the name, signature, and contact number of the person requesting the blood. The reason for request, current haemoglobin level (except in an emergency), blood product, and number of units required must be stated.
- **Urgent request:** if blood is required urgently HTL must be informed by telephone.
- **Labelling of blood sample tubes:** this must be completed at the bedside, the details on the sample tube must be *handwritten,* and the details on the sample tube, request form, and wristband must be identical.
- **Blood prescription:** for adults blood and components are prescribed in *units* on an IV infusion rota. Red blood cells can be stored in a blood fridge for up to 35 days after donation. Each unit is labelled with an expiry date: once removed from controlled storage it must

be transfused within 4 hours. Therefore, in a stable adult patient red blood cells should be prescribed as 1 unit over 3–3.5 hours maximum, not 4 hours.

- **FFP and platelets**: these have a short 'shelf-life' and in most adults should be transfused as soon as possible after removal from controlled storage: the expiry time will be stated on the label.
- **Furosemide:** if furosemide is to be administered during transfusion it must be prescribed on the medicine chart, *not* on the IV infusion rota.
- **Positively identify the patient prior to transfusion:** ask the patient, if possible, to state their surname, first name, and date of birth and check the wristband.
- **The patient's details on the blood pack and the wristband must be identical.** If there is a discrepancy make every effort to identify the patient correctly and withhold the transfusion if the clinical situation permits.
- **Use specialized blood administration set and connect to a suitable IV cannula.**
- **For most transfusions use an IV infusion device:** this ensures accuracy of flow rate and alarms can be set to trigger when the infusion finishes or becomes blocked.

Post-procedure management

During a transfusion the patient should be monitored closely and the observations recorded by the nursing staff. The required frequency of observations varies according to local policy but we recommend:

- **Pre-transfusion:** temperature, pulse, and blood pressure.
- **Transfusion commences:** The nurse should stay with the patient for the first 15 minutes of the transfusion.
- **Temperature, pulse, and blood pressure after 15 minutes and hourly thereafter**: depending on the patient's condition.
- **Repeat above:** with every unit transfused.
- **Continuing observations:** temperature, pulse, and blood pressure 4-hourly for 24 hours post-transfusion.
- **Advise patient to report any symptoms during transfusion.**

Professionalism

Communicate sensitively, thank the patient, address any questions or concerns, wash hands, document the procedure fully and accurately, and communicate appropriately with the nursing staff.

Complications

Signs and symptoms of a transfusion reaction include:

- Urticaria, rash, dyspnoea, rigor
- Loin pain
- Headache
- Hypo- or hypertension
- Pyrexia, tachycardia, anaphylaxis (rare).

When informed of a suspected transfusion reaction, tell the nursing staff to *stop* the transfusion immediately. Then:

- Assess the patient and phone HTL
- Complete the *Request for Investigation of an Apparent Blood Transfusion Reaction* form and send to HTL

- Send unused blood to HTL
- Send specimens to Microbiology and HTL.

Serious complications of blood transfusion are very rare but include:

- Acute haemolytic transfusion reaction (Figure 9.10)
- Reaction to infusion of a bacterially contaminated unit
- Transfusion-related acute lung injury (TRALI)
- Acute fluid overload
- Severe allergic reaction or anaphylaxis.

Patient safety tips

✔ Be absolutely sure you have identified the patient accurately.

✔ Never transfuse unnecessarily and always consider alternatives to transfusion.

✔ Except in urgent clinical situations, avoid transfusion between 8.00 pm and 8.00 am.

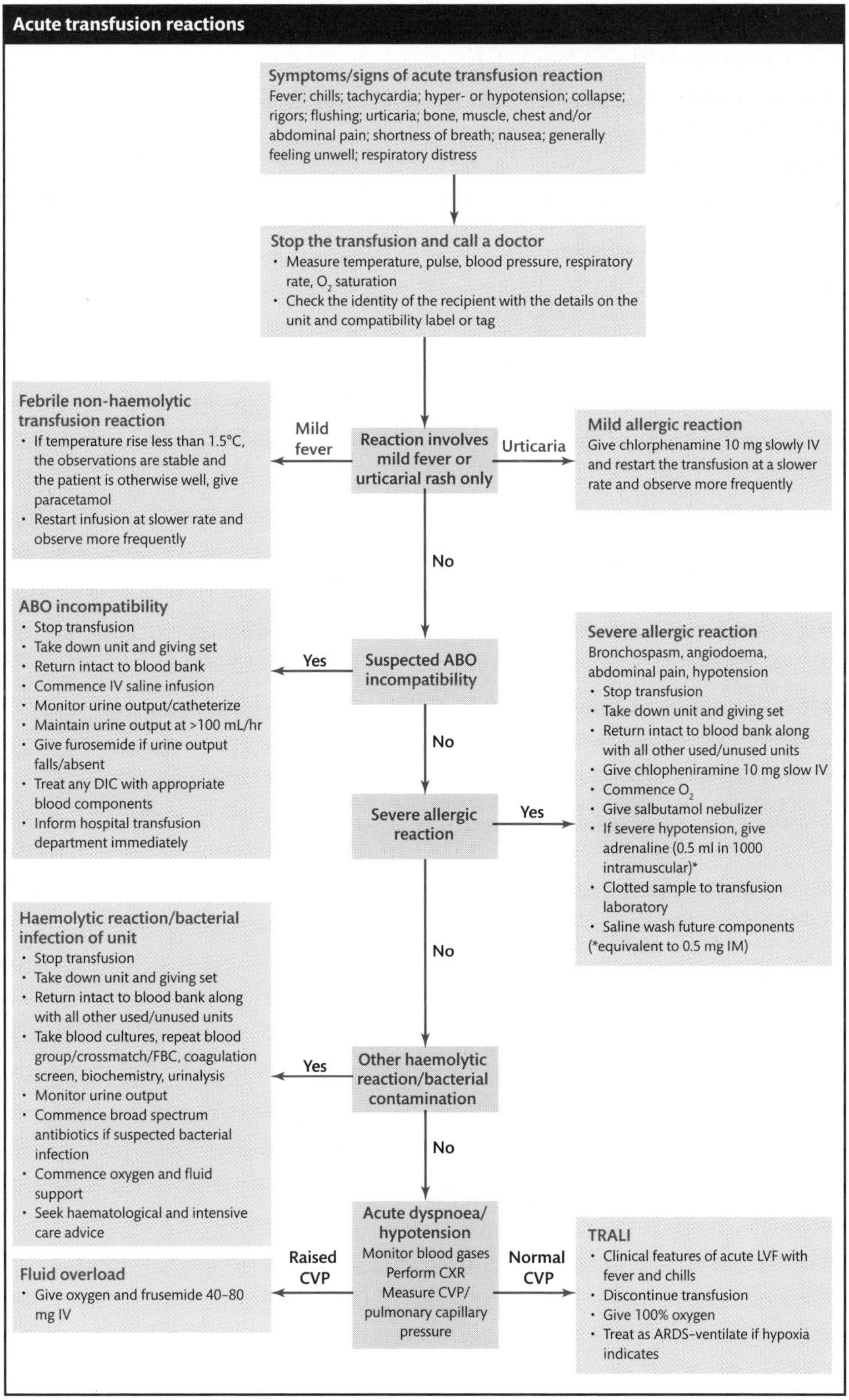

Acute transfusion reactions

Symptoms/signs of acute transfusion reaction
Fever; chills; tachycardia; hyper- or hypotension; collapse;
rigors; flushing; urticaria; bone, muscle, chest and/or
abdominal pain; shortness of breath; nausea; generally
feeling unwell; respiratory distress

↓

Stop the transfusion and call a doctor
- Measure temperature, pulse, blood pressure, respiratory
  rate, O$_2$ saturation
- Check the identity of the recipient with the details on the
  unit and compatibility label or tag

↓

**Febrile non-haemolytic
transfusion reaction**
- If temperature rise less than 1.5°C,
  the observations are stable and
  the patient is otherwise well, give
  paracetamol
- Restart infusion at slower rate and
  observe more frequently

← Mild fever — **Reaction involves
mild fever or
urticarial rash only** — Urticaria →

Mild allergic reaction
Give chlorphenamine 10 mg slowly IV
and restart the transfusion at a slower
rate and observe more frequently

↓ No

ABO incompatibility
- Stop transfusion
- Take down unit and giving set
- Return intact to blood bank
- Commence IV saline infusion
- Monitor urine output/catheterize
- Maintain urine output at >100 mL/hr
- Give furosemide if urine output
  falls/absent
- Treat any DIC with appropriate
  blood components
- Inform hospital transfusion
  department immediately

← Yes — **Suspected ABO
incompatibility**

↓ No

Severe allergic reaction
Bronchospasm, angiodoema,
abdominal pain, hypotension
- Stop transfusion
- Take down unit and giving set
- Return intact to blood bank along
  with all other used/unused units
- Give chlopheniramine 10 mg slow IV
- Commence O$_2$
- Give salbutamol nebulizer
- If severe hypotension, give
  adrenaline (0.5 ml in 1000
  intramuscular)*
- Clotted sample to transfusion
  laboratory
- Saline wash future components
(*equivalent to 0.5 mg IM)

**Severe allergic
reaction** — Yes →

↓ No

**Haemolytic reaction/bacterial
infection of unit**
- Stop transfusion
- Take down unit and giving set
- Return intact to blood bank along
  with all other used/unused units
- Take blood cultures, repeat blood
  group/crossmatch/FBC, coagulation
  screen, biochemistry, urinalysis
- Monitor urine output
- Commence broad spectrum
  antibiotics if suspected bacterial
  infection
- Commence oxygen and fluid
  support
- Seek haematological and intensive
  care advice

← Yes — **Other haemolytic
reaction/bacterial
contamination**

↓ No

Fluid overload
- Give oxygen and frusemide 40–80
  mg IV

← Raised CVP — **Acute dyspnoea/
hypotension**
Monitor blood gases
Perform CXR
Measure CVP/
pulmonary capillary
pressure — Normal CVP →

TRALI
- Clinical features of acute LVF with
  fever and chills
- Discontinue transfusion
- Give 100% oxygen
- Treat as ARDS–ventilate if hypoxia
  indicates

Figure 9.10 Acute transfusion reactions

Student name:	Medical school:	Year:

Blood transfusion

Describe how you would prepare a patient for blood transfusion, take blood for cross-matching, and your post-procedure management.

		Self	Peer	Peer /tutor	Tutor
Equipment and preparation	● Selects the correct equipment	☐	☐	☐	☐
	● Records the reason for transfusion in the patient's records	☐	☐	☐	☐
	● Documents the correct component, the number of units required and the appropriate time when the component is needed	☐	☐	☐	☐
	●	☐	☐	☐	☐
Explanation and consent	● Washes hands with alcohol gel or soap and water	☐	☐	☐	☐
	● Positively identifies the correct patient by surname, first name, date of birth, and wristband	☐	☐	☐	☐
	● Explains the reasons for transfusion and the procedure to the patient, and obtains verbal consent	☐	☐	☐	☐
	● Can discuss possible complications and risks of transfusion to the patient	☐	☐	☐	☐
	● Is aware of need to report adverse events due to blood transfusion to SHOT	☐	☐	☐	☐
	● Documents informed consent in the patient's records	☐	☐	☐	☐
	●	☐	☐	☐	☐
Procedure	● Identifies the correct request form for cross-match	☐	☐	☐	☐
	● Completes the form in full or minimum dataset required by HTL	☐	☐	☐	☐
	● Correctly takes blood sample	☐	☐	☐	☐
	● Completes the sample tube label in full and in handwriting at the bedside	☐	☐	☐	☐
	● Is aware that there must be verbal communication with HTL for urgent requests	☐	☐	☐	☐
	● Prescribes blood and components on IV infusion rota with signature and date	☐	☐	☐	☐
	● Clearly and individually prescribes component and number and rate of units	☐	☐	☐	☐
	● Prescribes medications to be given concurrently (e.g. furosemide) on medication chart with signature and date	☐	☐	☐	☐
	●	☐	☐	☐	☐
Post-procedure management	● Understands what monitoring is required during transfusion	☐	☐	☐	☐
	● Can discuss what to do in the case of a suspected transfusion reaction	☐	☐	☐	☐
	●	☐	☐	☐	☐
Professionalism	● Communicates sensitively, thanks the patient, addresses any questions or concerns, washes hands	☐	☐	☐	☐
	● Completes all documentation legibly and unambiguously	☐	☐	☐	☐
	● Communicates appropriately with nursing staff	☐	☐	☐	☐
	●	☐	☐	☐	☐

Self-assessed as at least borderline:	Signature:	Date:	U B S E	U B S E	U B S E	U B S E
Peer-assessed as ready for tutor assessment:	Signature:	Date:	U B S E	U B S E	U B S E	U B S E
Tutor-assessed as satisfactory:	Signature:	Date:	U B S E	U B S E	U B S E	U B S E

Notes

9.6 Urinary catheterization: male and female

255

9.6
Urinary
catheterization:
male and
female

Background

Urinary catheterization is the aseptic insertion of a sterile tube (catheter) into the urinary bladder for the purpose of instilling or draining fluid. Catheters are usually inserted urethrally, however if this is not possible due to blockage or for reasons of patient choice the suprapubic route may be used. In this case the catheter is inserted through the abdominal wall and into the bladder. This is probably the most complicated of all procedures that a junior clinician is expected to undertake.

Clinical indications

- To monitor urine output for fluid balance and indication of renal function post operatively
- To drain the bladder in urine retention
- To monitor urine output (fluid balance and renal function) in critically ill patients
- To empty the bladder prior to surgery or labour
- To instil fluid, irrigation, or cytotoxic drugs
- To perform bladder function tests (urodynamics)
- As a last resort for incontinence if all other methods fail (long-term 'in-dwelling' catheter).
- Long-term 'in-dwelling' suprapubic catheter (changed every 3 months) for chronic causes of complete lower urinary tract obstruction/dysfunction.

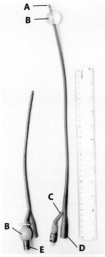

Urinary catheter:

A Scalloped Catheter eye (luminal exit x2)

B balloon

C bifurcation

D main lumen connects to drainage tube

E water port with colour-coded collar

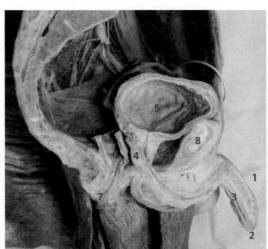

10F	12F	14F	16F	18F
3.3 mm	4 mm	4.7 mm	5.3 mm	6 mm

The external diameter is measured in Charrière French gauge (3 F = 1mm, therefore 14 F is 4.7mm diameter)

Sagittal section of the male pelvis:
1 penis
2 external urethral meatus
3 urethra
4 prostate
5 bladder
6 rectum
7 anus
8 pubic symphysis

Figure 9.11 Images in bladder catheterization.

Anatomical and physiological principles

Male

Male urethra: extends from the bladder neck to the external urethral meatus at the tip of the glans penis. There are three parts, the *prostatic* urethra (3 cm), *membranous* urethra (1.25–2 cm) and *cavernous* (penile/spongy) urethra (15 cm). At the base of the bladder is the autonomic (involuntary) internal urethral sphincter (IUS), and below the prostate gland, the membranous urethra (which perforates the urogenital diaphragm, or pelvic floor) is completely surrounded by circular muscle fibres of the external urethral sphincter (EUS), under voluntary control. Even if the bladder is full, the micturition reflex can be inhibited by maintaining voluntary contraction of the EUS, until convenient to void. Therefore, the prostate gland separates the two urethral sphincters that control bladder outflow. You should mentally visualize and feel where the tip of the catheter is as you advance and know the structures you are negotiating. Catheterization in a male is potentially technically difficult for various anatomical (or pathological) reasons:

- **Longer course**: (relative to the female) and S-shape (particularly through the relatively inflexible passage of the bulbar and prostatic regions).

- **Length of the urethra**: (particularly after transurethral resection of the prostrate [TURP]) means a standard two-way catheter is only just into the bladder when the bifurcation has reached the glans. Always ensure the bifurcation is at the glans when filling the balloon.

- **Prostatic region**: resistance often encountered as the rubbery balloon-covered area of the catheter shaft passes through the prostate, particularly if there is benign prostatic hyperplasia or malignancy. Usually the resistance is easily overcome by maintaining firm but gentle pressure and keeping the catheter moving smoothly inward. **Clinical tips**:
  - Hold the penis vertically with gentle traction (initially 90° then reduce to 60°).
  - Ensure copious lubricating gel (with local anaesthetic usually lidocaine) – always apply some to the balloon area and tip.
  - A larger gauge catheter is relatively stiffer and stronger and will usually pass more easily provided the meatus is accommodating. Silicone catheters can be easier to insert.
  - PTFE-latex catheters are softer and more pliable than silicone so may be worth trying a stiffer-feeling catheter.

- **External urethral sphincter**: Spasm of the sphincter is felt as a springy resistance that is not easily overcome by pressure. Often a problem in young males, particularly if the patient is anxious (inability to voluntarily relax). **Clinical tips**:
  - Try more gel to anaesthetize the membranous urethra
  - Consider a slightly larger gauge catheter to reduced tip kinking (normally size 12, large size if large prostate gland).

- **Pathological reasons for technical difficulty in catheterization**:
  - **Phimosis**: chronic inflammation and scarring of the prepuce (foreskin) leading to a scarred inelastic constricted opening in the prepuce, so the foreskin cannot be retracted, e.g. balanitis xerotica obliterans (BXO).
  - **Meatal stenosis/stricturing/'pinhole meatus'** males post circumcision, BXO, congenital – seek urological expertise.
  - **Urethral strictures**: congenital, scarring from previous surgery/stricturoplasty, can occur at any region of the urethra.
  - **Previous TURP**: this sometimes facilitates catheterization, but can lead to a cavernous prostatic urethra, with a high bladder neck, and tendency for the catheter tip to find or create false passages into the prostate, or not pass over the bladder neck. Can be overcome by straightening the penis, holding vertically until the catheter is advanced into the prostatic urethra, then pulling the penile shaft down horizontally and taut (glans caudally) thus allowing the catheter tip to flick up and over the bladder neck.
  - **Hypospadias** – occasionally difficulty identifying the orifice.

○ **Gross penile dependent oedema –** difficulty identifying the orifice if buried under oedematous foreskin. Firm manual compression will help, holding the penis in a closed fist with gauze soaked in 10–20% dextrose usually works (and for reducing most paraphimoses).

Female

The female urethra is short (up to 4 cm), and technically very easy to negotiate. Be absolutely sure that the urethral orifice has been correctly identified as superior to the vaginal opening. The instil gel can be applied directly to the level of the EUS ensuring it is relaxed before administering gel into the urethra. Occasionally there may be a stricture, and the patient may well regularly perform intermittent self-catheterization. In this case, try a smaller gauge catheter e.g. 8–10, and/or seek urological expertise.

Contraindications

Relative contraindications

- **Suspected male urethral injury or transection** (classic sign of blood at the urethral meatus) following major blunt or penetrating pelvic trauma and urological expertise should be immediately sought. Supra-pubic catheterization or specialist urethral catheterization or surgical reconstruction may be needed.
- **Recent prostatectomy** (<6 months), **recent TURBT** (transurethral resection of bladder tumour) (<6 weeks), **recent TURP** (<12 weeks).

Caution advised

- Known urethral/meatal stricture/stenosis.
- Retention following history of frank haematuria, or recent admission with frank haematuria (may need three-way catheterization and irrigation).
- Recent failed catheterization or one or more failed attempts at this presentation, or traumatic catheterization (bleeding)
- Previous TURP, radical prostatectomy.
- Latex allergy – check carefully the composition of catheter you select (use silicone catheter if allergy).

Equipment

- Personal protective equipment: apron, sterile gloves (two pairs), consider protective eyewear.
- Clean hands and prepare cleanly wiped trolley.
- Appropriate catheter type and size: normally French gauge 12 *female*, 12 *male* – ensure correctly specified *male* or *female* label. Length: male 40–45 cm, female 20–26 cm.
- Sterile gel with local anaesthetic (for Instillagel 11 mL for male, 6 mL for female), alcohol rub, 10 mL syringe, 10 mL sterile water, catheter bag, sterile or antiseptic solution, pre-sealed catheterization pack (usually includes trays, sterile drape, waste bag, sterile gauze, catheter bag).

Explanation and consent

Valid informed consent is essential. Currently accepted practice for urinary catheterization is to document 'verbal consent obtained' in the notes.

- **Introduce yourself, build rapport**
- **Explain the clinical indication/benefits**: stress importance to care and no alternative exists. Explain the benefits of monitoring urine output/renal function and for appropriate fluid resuscitation/balance, or to relieve bladder outflow obstruction, and prevent obstructive nephropathy. Explain how long it is likely to remain *in situ*.

- **Explain what the procedure involves**: in clear straight-forward language take the patient through each step in advance. Showing the tube to the patient can be reassuring. Part of the explanation could be:

  The catheter is about 4 or 5 mm diameter rubber or soft plastic tube. After waiting a few minutes for the anaesthetic gel to work, the catheter is gently inserted into your penis/urethra and on into your bladder. Once urine is seen, a small balloon at the tip of the catheter is inflated with sterile water to stop the tube falling out, and the tube is connected to the drainage bag. It is very important that you not pull the catheter. It can be very painful and result in a lot of bleeding.

Consider drawing a sketch of the anatomy and passage of the tube.

- **Explain the risks/side effects**: mention risk of urinary tract infection and minor trauma to the urethra and bleeding. Reassure patient that this is a safe, straightforward routine procedure that is performed every day. State that there may be some discomfort or stinging but not painful as local anaesthetic gel is used.
- **Check the patient's understanding and invite any questions for clarification**.
- **Obtain and document valid consent**: Fill in the written consent form, if needed, summarizing the procedure, indication, benefits, risks, and invite them to sign the form. In most cases verbal informed consent is adequate but must be documented in the patient's notes and clinical indication stated. If informed consent could not be obtained, document the reason and that the procedure would be performed in the patient's best interests, stating the clinical indication. In most cases a bladder scan should be performed first.

Procedure for both sexes

- Ensure chaperone is present, irrespective of gender of patient or doctor.
- Prepare the patient maintaining privacy and dignity, and communicate with patient throughout:
  - ○ Patient lies supine, ensure comfortable.
  - ○ Wash hands and apply apron.
  - ○ Open catheter pack carefully to not desterilize inner surface and contents.
  - ○ Gel wash hands. Don sterile gloves. Ask the assistant (chaperone) to open onto tray the 10 mL syringe, local anaesthetic gel, and to open the vial of 10 mL sterile water, hold it inverted so you can draw it into 10 mL syringe, maintaining sterility. Ask the assistant to help prepare the antiseptic solution. Hand the waste bag (in the pack) to the assistant and ask them to attach it to the edge of the trolley. All the above can be done as a single person procedure.

Male urinary catheterization

- **Draping**: such that the patient has just the genital area exposed (use drape with hole in the middle). Clean the surface of the flaccid penis, foreskin and upper scrotum with sterile or antiseptic solution.
- **Cleaning the penis**: take white gauze (8 × 8 cm), unfold and refold lengthways to create a strip (16 × 4 cm). With the gauze, on the dorsum retract the foreskin, using left index and middle fingers opposing thumb. Expose the glans and corona, thoroughly clean particularly the junction of foreskin and corona with gauze. Hold the penis up vertically and cleanse the ventral penis and meatus with a third soaked cotton ball. Keep holding the penis vertically under traction, with the left hand.
- **Local anaesthetic**: explain that gel will sting a little initially. Apply over the meatus to allow good anaesthesia of the meatal labia and then instil the remaining gel directly into the urethra. Occlude the urethra at the base of the glans to ensure LA does not flow out. Wait 3 minutes for the LA gel to take effect, explain this and that it will take an hour to wear off.

- **Open catheterization pack, rewash hands and don new gloves**: Carefully open the catheter onto the tray. There may be the 10 mL syringe pre-filled in the same package as the catheter. There are also packs with the catheter pre-connected to the drainage bag ensuring complete asepsis. Some packs have the balloon pre-filled.

- **Insertion**: Some clinicians prefer completely removing the catheter from the sterile sleeve or insert the catheter grasping the part-torn sleeve whilst simultaneously removing it. The latter is better for asepsis as the catheter is not touched directly. In practice this is very difficult but an assistant with sterile gloves will be very useful. Keep the catheter bifurcation in a kidney dish (to keep it sterile and catch the urine).

  ○ Hold penis vertically with the left hand using a fresh strip of gauze, and begin inserting the catheter (tell the patient you are about to do this). It usually slides easily until it reaches the membranous urethra. Maintain constant gentle pressure and smooth movement. If well anaesthetized it should pass the EUS with this technique. If there is springy resistance at this point the EUS is probably in spasm. Try steady pressure.

  ○ If no progress, you may have to try a larger catheter (e.g. 16G instead of 12G) after repeat cleansing and more LA gel (20 mL is safe for normal weight adult males otherwise use sterile simple lubricating jelly).

  ○ Once past the EUS, you may feel a steady level of resistance as it passes through the prostate, before clear urine gushes out into the kidney dish.

  ○ At this point move swiftly, push the catheter well in, so bifurcation is at the glans (hold in using left hand), connect the drainage bag, and inflate the balloon with 10 mL sterile water.

  ○ Draw foreskin forward to cover the glans and remove drape by tearing. Mop up any spilled urine and clean and dry the patient. Avoid touching the catheter more than necessary.

Female urinary catheterization

- As for male initial steps – explanation and consent, preserve dignity

- **Draping**: position patient supine, ask patient (may need assistance) to flex knees keeping ankles together then allow knees to flop apart to give access to perineum. Drape accordingly.

- **Cleaning the external urethral orifice**: explain throughout. With index and middle fingers of left hand (elbow towards head end of patient and dorsal surface of your hand facing you), gently part the labia majora to identify the urethral orifice. This can be difficult in older women, as it appears to migrate up into the vaginal vault on the anterior wall. Use sterile or antiseptic solution to cleanse just the external urethral orifice. Paint from top downwards towards the perineum with a single pass. Do not take the swab back up to the meatus again.

- **Local anaesthetic**: As for males, explain it will sting a little initially, squirt 6 mL of LA gel onto the external urethral orifice, and the remainder into the urethra. (The majority will shoot straight into the bladder given the short length of the urethra!). Wait for at least 3 minutes to allow the LA gel to take effect; explain it will take an hour to wear off.

- **Open catheterization pack, rewash hands and don new gloves**: carefully open the catheter onto the tray.

- **Insertion (female)**

  ○ In females it is easier to leave the catheter in the torn plastic sleeve. Place the catheter in sterile kidney dish and transfer placing on drape or bed just below the patient, keeping the catheter and sleeve sterile.

  ○ Explain you are now going to insert the catheter. Expose the external urethral orifice as before with the left hand.

  ○ Insert the catheter smoothly until urine begins to drain. Swiftly but carefully remove the remaining sleeve, pass the catheter up to bifurcation point, attach the drainage tubing and inflate the balloon.

  ○ Do not inflate balloon unless urine drains.

  ○ Gently draw back on the catheter until the springy resistance indicates the balloon is at the bladder neck, remove the drape, and clean up as above.

259

9.6
Urinary
catheterization:
male and
female

Post-procedure management

- Place drainage bag below level of bed and attach securely to suitable catheter stand or rack with bedside hook. Ensure no tension on catheter.
- Take note of the residual volume of urine (important if indication was retention): <800 mL acute retention, >1000–1200 mL chronic retention.
- Document procedure in the notes, including name of chaperone.

Professionalism

Inform key colleagues. Communicate clearly, calmly, and politely throughout the procedure with both the patient and your assistant. This will help to reassure the patient and increase the likelihood of successful uncomplicated catheterization, and you are more likely to have a positive and helpful assistant.

Document the procedure in the notes remembering the following points:

- Verbal/written informed consent obtained
- Chaperone present (e.g. 'RGN L Smith')
- Aseptic technique throughout
- Prepared with sterile or antiseptic solution, draped
- LA gel: 11 mL male, 6 ml female
- 12G PTFE-latex Foley catheter inserted, expiry date (affix label for batch details, expiry date). Foreskin drawn forward to re-cover glans
- 'Atraumatic, patient comfortable, passed easily' (or, e.g. 'passed with some resistance, mild discomfort, no complications/haemorrhage')
- Clear urine seen
- Balloon inflated with 10 mL sterile water
- Residual volume: 600 mL, urine appearance – clear/turbid/rosé/dark red/clots/frank blood
- Your signature, print name, date, time.

Complications

- **Infections and trauma**: High risk of urinary tract infection, so only catheterize for good clinical indications. In the USA, estimates suggest overall incidence of bacteriuria of 8%. Insertion can also cause bruising and trauma to the urethral mucosa which then acts as entry points for microorganisms into the blood and lymphatic system. Scar tissue is also easily formed as a result of trauma.
- **Haemorrhage**: particularly if the patient has benign prostatic hypertrophy (BPH) or previous TURP. Fresh red blood may appear at the lumen of the catheter, or blood bypassing the catheter. This may be from direct abrasion of the advancing catheter. Do not pull out the catheter, particularly if you have already drained clear urine. Ask for prompt review from a surgical or urology colleague. If you are sure you have not entered the bladder consider withdrawal but if it is a small amount of blood and only slowly oozing it will probably stop and the catheter *in situ* will help to tamponade. It is better to ask for a surgical or urology review before just pulling out the catheter. If you are not sure you are in the bladder, and have not seen urine *do not inflate the balloon*, as this will often cause pain and haemorrhage. Bear in mind the patient who has had previous TURP, as the sometimes cavernous prostate may accommodate a loop of catheter and even if some urine drains, the balloon may still be in the prostatic urethra, which may cause haemorrhage if you inflate.
- **Reactive haemorrhage** follows drainage for chronic (often asymptomatic/painless) retention. The chronically distended bladder with overstretched wall and trabeculae will have distended submucosal veins. Once decompressed by draining clear urine, the urine can

turn rose or frank haematuria as the veins bleed with loss of the tamponade effect of the full bladder.

- **False passages** through the prostatic urethra, particularly if the patient has previously had TURP. This usually leads to haemorrhage, rarely serious sequelae, but more a technical challenge to the urology team, and may require a cystoscopy. If you find resistance at the level of the prostate and cannot find the bladder with the techniques described, do not continue repeated advances; remove the catheter and seek specialist help.

- **Paraphimosis** is where the prepuce slides back and gets trapped behind the corona of the glans. Likely to occur if the foreskin was tight before catheterization e.g. BXO. Paraphimosis should be anticipated in such cases, and either choose not to try to retract the foreskin to catheterize, or take extra care to ensure it has slid forward fully afterwards, with regular review. It is quite possible to catheterize without retracting the foreskin, it is just conventional to do so, to ensure the coronal area is well cleansed and one has a good view of the external urethral meatus, but this is not essential if experienced. Once the foreskin meatal skin is trapped behind the glans, the skin and mucosa behind it swells with oedema, so the whole foreskin becomes quite distorted in appearance and may appear to be partially or even completely covering the glans. However, the tight band of the leading edge of the foreskin needs to be released from behind the corona to resolve the paraphimosis.

Resolving a paraphimosis

- Soak some gauze in 20% or 50% dextrose solution, and take a pair of sterile gloves.
- Obtain verbal consent, explaining to the patient what has happened and what you need to do. With a chaperone present, wrap the penis in the soaked gauze.
- Grasp the penis (particularly around the foreskin and glans) with a closed fist and apply a firm squeezing compression. Ensure there is not too much discomfort.
- Maintain the compression for 5 minutes or so, then try to draw the foreskin forward, ideally without changing your hand position.
- If not immediately successful: inspect; the oedema should have reduced significantly so the band may be more obvious and you may be able to manipulate it past the corona (use one or both hands and try pushing with gloved finger tips radially placed behind the band). For this it may be worthwhile using some LA gel for anaesthesia and lubrication.
- If not, repeat the compression for a few more minutes with fresh soaked gauze and try to reduce. If you cannot resolve the phimosis surgical help (? needs surgical intervention, e.g. dorsal slit under LA or formal circumcision).

Patient safety tips

- ✔ **Never use a female catheter in a male patient!** There are several cases of fatal haemorrhage reported due to inflation of the balloon in a male urethra and traumatic haemorrhage. Some hospitals have now stopped stocking female catheters. Male catheters can be used in females. Male catheters must be 40–45 cm in length.
- ✔ **Consider the individual patient's anatomy**, evident pathology, e.g. previous history of TURP/prostatectomy as you can take these into account when you perform the procedure and adapt your technique.
- ✔ **Always stop if the patient develops significant discomfort or pain**, keep talking to the patient and assess how significant it is.
  - ○ Otherwise remove the catheter, keep communicating with the patient to reassure, try to relieve anxiety.
  - ○ Consider whether you should ask a more experienced clinician to perform the procedure.
  - ○ Think about using analgesia with an anxiolytic effect such as morphine with antiemetic. Morphine will also reduce EUS spasm.

○ After TURP you may get some drainage of urine with the tip into the bladder neck, but the catheter shaft with balloon still at the level of the prostate. Do not inflate the balloon unless the catheter has gone into the bifurcation and feels like it is well into the bladder. Inflating the balloon in a post-TURP prostatic urethra does not usually do much harm, but if it were pulled back out it could cause some trauma through the urethra distally.

✔ **Meticulous hygiene and catheter care is essential**. Advise the patient to avoid handling or touching the catheter, ensure it remains visibly clean, and nurses should take a catheter specimen of urine (CSU) using aseptic technique. Leave a catheter *in situ* only as long as it is absolutely necessary, however replacing one earlier than the lifespan of the catheter type is of no value at all if the patient is asymptomatic and it is draining well. All urinary bladders will develop bacterial colonization if there is a long-term catheter *in situ*. Only give antibiotics or replace the catheter if symptoms/signs of urinary tract infection.

✔ Consider a larger size urinary catheter if debris, haematuria, or benign enlarged prostate gland.

Student name:	Medical school:	Year:

Urinary catheterization

Please insert a urinary catheter into this male manikin's bladder.

		Self	Peer	Peer /tutor	Tutor
Washes hands	• Handwash with water and soap, alcohol gel alone not sufficient for aseptic technique	☐	☐	☐	☐
	•	☐	☐	☐	☐
Understands indications and anatomy	• Urinary retention/pre-op/critically unwell	☐	☐	☐	☐
	• Aware of different positioning and angles that may be required to pass catheter through urethra	☐	☐	☐	☐
	• Aware of length of urethra and position of prostate	☐	☐	☐	☐
Obtains informed consent	• Introduces themselves	☐	☐	☐	☐
	• Gains informed consent	☐	☐	☐	☐
Explanation to patient, often including complications	• Clear explanation of procedure, e.g. 'I am going to pass a tube into your bladder, it will go into the bladder via the penis to allow the urine to drain out'	☐	☐	☐	☐
	• Explains risks and asks about latex allergy	☐	☐	☐	☐
Communication skills	• Assessment throughout the procedure and encourages patient to ask questions	☐	☐	☐	☐
Appropriate preparation	• Cleans trolley correctly, places equipment on bottom shelf	☐	☐	☐	☐
	• Selection of equipment: trolley, appropriate catheter type and size, LA gel 11 mL (males), sterile gloves × 2 pairs, apron, alcohol rub,10 mL syringe, catheter bag, sterile water 10 mL, sterile or antiseptic solution, waste bag, sterile gauze and catheterization pack	☐	☐	☐	☐
	• Prepares patient and maintains privacy and dignity	☐	☐	☐	☐
	•	☐	☐	☐	☐
Appropriate analgesia	• Ensures use of 11 mL LA gel for men, aware the gel may cause stinging sensation on initial administration	☐	☐	☐	☐
	•	☐	☐	☐	☐
Technical ability especially with any special equipment and sharps	• Use aseptic technique throughout	☐	☐	☐	☐
	• Applies sterile gloves retracts the foreskin and cleans shaft, glans and urethral meatus using Normasol solution	☐	☐	☐	☐
	• Arranges sterile drape, administers LA gel 11 mL, maintains penile position upright and meatus closed for 3–5 minutes to allow to take effect	☐	☐	☐	☐
	• Washes hands and applies new pair of gloves, opens catheter, slowly inserts catheter smoothly until urine begins to drain and then passes catheter up to bifurcation point	☐	☐	☐	☐
	• Attaches bag and inflates balloon	☐	☐	☐	☐
	• Repositions foreskin	☐	☐	☐	☐
	•	☐	☐	☐	☐
Aseptic technique	• Cleaning of trolley, placing of equipment on bottom shelf, opening packets correctly and aseptic technique throughout	☐	☐	☐	☐
	•	☐	☐	☐	☐
Seeks help as appropriate	• Reasons for failure to catheterize: e.g. stricture, spasm	☐	☐	☐	☐
	• Discusses complications, e.g. haematuria, paraphimosis	☐	☐	☐	☐
	• Discusses what to do if no urine drains	☐	☐	☐	☐
	•	☐	☐	☐	☐
Post-procedure management	• Waste disposal	☐	☐	☐	☐
	• Explain that LA gel will take an hour to wear off	☐	☐	☐	☐
	• Documents time, date, clinical reason, aseptic technique, Instillagel, catheter size, type and expiry date, any problems, amount of urine drained and colour	☐	☐	☐	☐
	•	☐	☐	☐	☐
Professionalism	• Communicates to team members; thanks staff; thanks patient and ensures they are dry and comfortable	☐	☐	☐	☐
	•	☐	☐	☐	☐
Overall ability to perform procedure	• Assess globally, would you be happy for this student to be supervised to insert a catheter on a real patient?	☐	☐	☐	☐
	•	☐	☐	☐	☐

			Self	Peer	Peer /tutor	Tutor
Self-assessed as at least borderline:	Signature:	Date:	U B S E	U B S E	U B S E	U B S E
Peer-assessed as ready for tutor assessment:	Signature:	Date:	U B S E	U B S E	U B S E	U B S E
Tutor-assessed as satisfactory:	Signature:	Date:	U B S E	U B S E	U B S E	U B S E

Notes

9.7 Local anaesthesia

Background

Local anaesthesia is the abolition of sensation in a body part without affecting consciousness or the impairment of central control of vital function. It involves the injection or application of an anaesthetic drug to a specific area of the body. The main advantage is that the complexity and potential for complications of general anaesthesia is avoided. For centuries natives of Peru and Bolivia had chewed the leaves of a shrub, *Erythroxylum coca*, which lessened fatigue and numbed the tongue. These effects were due to the principal alkaloid, cocaine, contained in the plant. In 1860, cocaine was isolated by Niemann, and in 1884, Karl Kohler, a Viennese physician, noted its analgesic effect in the eye and published his results. Lidocaine and benzocaine are the most commonly used local anaesthetics.

Clinical indications

Local anaesthesia allows patients to undergo surgical procedures without pain and distress.

Uses in surgery and dentistry

- Outpatient minor surgery, such as skin biopsies
- Skin suturing
- Caesarean section
- Surgeries on the arms, hands, legs, or feet
- Ophthalmic surgery especially cataracts
- Surgeries involving the urinary tract or sexual organs such as vasectomy

Uses in acute pain

- Labour pain (epidural anaesthesia)
- Postoperative pain (peripheral nerve blocks, epidural anaesthesia)
- Trauma (peripheral nerve blocks, IV regional anaesthesia, epidural anaesthesia)
- Use in chronic pain: including joint injections with steroids

Surface anaesthesia also facilitates some endoscopic procedures such as bronchoscopy or cystoscopy. Spinal anaesthesia is often preferable than general anaesthesia in patients with multiple co-morbidities.

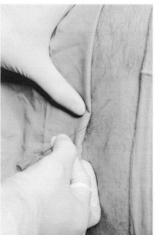

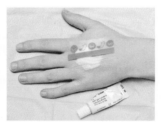

Topical local anaesthesia (LA) prior to venous cannulation in needle phobia or children

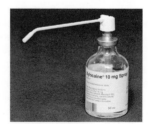

Topical LA spray: used at the back of the throat for upper gastro-intestinal endoscopy

Spinal anaesthesia: many pelvic and lower abdominal surgeries are possible; and especially useful for patients in whom general anaesthesia would be hazardous

Figure 9.12 Images in local anaesthesia.

Anatomical and physiological principles

Local anaesthesia can block almost every nerve between the peripheral nerve endings and the central nervous system. Starting centrally and working peripherally, local anaesthetic solutions may produce following types of anaesthesia

Spinal block

A local anaesthetic is injected into the subarachnoid space where it acts on spinal nerve roots and part of the spinal cord. The resulting anaesthesia usually extends from the legs to the abdomen or chest.

Epidural block

A local anaesthetic is injected into the epidural space where it acts primarily on the spinal nerve roots. Depending on the site and volume injected, the anaesthetized area varies from limited areas of the abdomen or chest to large regions of the body.

Nerve plexus block

Where the injection is made in the vicinity of a nerve plexus, e.g. brachial plexus. The anaesthetic effect extends to the innervation areas of several or all nerves from the plexus.

Peripheral nerve block

Where the injection is made into a single nerve trunk causing anaesthesia over the area of innervations by the nerve, e.g. ring block.

Local infiltration

Where the injection is made into the tissue to be anesthetized, e.g. subcutaneous tissue. The area anaesthetized is limited to the site of injection.

Intravenous regional anaesthesia (IVRA, Bier's block)

This is where the injection is made into a vein of a limb whose circulation is occluded by a tourniquet. The drug fills the limb's venous system and diffuses into tissues where peripheral nerves and nerve endings are anaesthetized. The anaesthetic effect is limited to the area that is excluded from blood circulation and resolves quickly once circulation is restored.

Surface anaesthesia

Where the drug is applied to skin or mucous membrane in the form of spray (e.g. for endoscopy), gel solution (e.g. urinary catheterization) or cream, e.g. EMLA cream. The latter is used especially in children for venepuncture or IV cannulation insertion. The effect is short lasting and is limited to the area of contact.

Field block

Where injection is made in such a manner as to numb the region distal to the injection, e.g. subcutaneous infiltration of the proximal portion of the volar surface of the forearm results in an extensive area of cutaneous anaesthesia that starts 2–3 cm distal to the site of injection.

Mechanism of action of local anaesthetics

Nerve conduction involves the propagation of an electrical signal generated by the rapid movement of ionic species, especially sodium and potassium across the nerve cell membrane.

Depolarization is preceded by a sudden increase in permeability of the cell to sodium ions. This is interfered by local anaesthetic drugs so that depolarization is prevented and nerve fibre block occurs. As the concentration of LA increases, the rate of rise of action potential and maximum depolarization decreases causing slowing of conduction. Finally local depolarization fails to reach the threshold potential and conduction block ensues.

LAs have no or minimal local irritant action and block sensory nerve endings, nerve trunks, neuromuscular junction, ganglionic synapse, and receptors. They also reduce release of acetylcholine from motor nerve endings. Injected around mixed nerve they cause anaesthesia of skin, and paralysis of voluntary muscle supplied by that nerve.

Sensory and motor fibres are inherently equally sensitive. The sensitivity is determined by the diameter of fibres as well as fibre type. In general smaller fibres are more sensitive than larger fibres and non-myelinated are blocked more easily than myelinated fibres. Smaller sensory fibres are more susceptible since they generate high-frequency, longer-lasting action potentials than the motor fibres. Autonomic fibres are more susceptible than somatic fibres. Among the somatic fibres order of blockade of the senses is: pain, then temperature, then touch, then deep pressure.

Addition of a vasoconstrictor, e.g. adrenaline (epinephrine), prolongs duration of action of LA by reducing their rate of removal from the local site into the circulation. They also reduce systemic toxicity and provide a more bloodless field for surgery.

Anaesthetics may be administered with another drug, such as adrenaline, which decreases bleeding by vasoconstriction, and sodium bicarbonate to decrease the acidity of a drug so that it will work faster. In addition, drugs may be administered to help a patient remain calm and more comfortable or to make them sleepy.

Side-effects of local anaesthetics

Toxic effects of local anaesthetics commonly occur because of:

- Excessive dosage
- Direct intravascular injection
- Use of agent in inflamed or vascular area
- Absorption that is too rapid
- Elimination that is too slow
- Idiopathic reaction to anaesthetic agent.

Systemic effects include stimulation of the central nervous system (CNS) followed by depression. In heart they are cardiac depressants and at high concentrations can cause prolongation of cQT interval and can stimulate arrhythmias. They can cause fall in blood pressure due to sympathetic blockade and direct relaxation of smooth muscle.

Clinical feature include:

- **Neurological**: unease, anxiety, euphoria, irritability, perioral tingling, tinnitus, convulsions, or coma
- **Respiratory failure**: due to central and peripheral actions
- **Cardiovascular collapse**: bradycardia, vasodilation, anaphylactic shock
- **Local effects**: pain, delay in wound healing, and necrosis.

LA with adrenaline can specifically result in delayed wound healing by reducing oxygen supply and may increase blood pressure and promote arrhythmias.

Contraindications for LA

- Absolute contraindications for local anaesthesia include a documented local anaesthetic allergy.
- Patients unable to cooperative fully during the procedure.
- LA injection is relatively contraindicated in the presence of inflammation or infection at the injection site.
- Epinephrine is contraindicated when injecting areas with end vessels including digits, pinna, and penis. Also relatively contraindicated in hyperthyroid patients, and dose should be kept to a minimum with tricyclic antidepressants use, due to dysrhythmias.

- Spinal anaesthesia is contraindicated in patients with hypotension, hypovolaemia, vertebral anomalies, and sepsis at the injection site.
- Relative contraindications include large target areas requiring large doses of anaesthetic, liver disease, pseudocholinesterase deficiency, and seizure disorder.
- Prilocaine may be contraindicated in patients with methaemoglobinaemia, sickle cell anaemia, anaemia, or symptoms of hypoxia as it can elevate methaemoglobin levels.

Equipment

- Personal protective equipment (gloves, face shield, apron).
- Antiseptic solution (chlorhexidine or povidone-iodine).
- Syringe (5–10 mL, depending on amount of anaesthesia required).
- One 18 or 20G and one 25 to 30G needle. The large-bore needle is first used to draw the anaesthetic solution from the vial. The small needle is used for infiltration to minimize patient discomfort and reduce tissue trauma. A long needle may be needed and has the advantage of allowing a greater area of infiltration with a single injection site.
- LA solution: 1% lidocaine (Xylocaine) is commonly used.

Explanation and consent

- **Introduce yourself and gain consent from patient**: state purpose of the procedure and the use of LA. Use simple diagram or drawing if necessary.
- **Explain procedure to patient**: inform them that there may be some discomfort on injection, and that, although the anaesthetic should eliminate pain, it will not eliminate all sensation, and pressure and tugging may still be felt when subsequent procedures are performed. Position patient comfortably.
- **Enquire about medical history**: allergies, past reactions in patient and family, relevant systemic illness, such as heart disease, liver disease, peripheral vascular disease, or seizure disorder
- **State main benefits and potential risks**.

Procedure

Injection or topical application of LA is given into the skin to numb the tissues that will be treated by cutting, suturing, injection, biopsy, and other procedures. The main purpose is to reduce pain due to the planned clinical procedure. The steps outlined can be generalized to many situations such as LA for lumbar puncture, removal of skin lesion, etc.

- **Wash hands**:
- **Clean and prepare the skin**: using povidone-iodine or chlorhexidine solution.
- **Create a skin wheal**: by insert the small needle just under the epidermis, aspirate the syringe (by pulling back on the plunger) to confirm the needle is not intravascular and inject a small amount of LA (around 0.5 mL).
- **If blood seen**: withdraw and redirect the needle and repeat aspiration.
- **Inject through the wheal**: slowly inject 0.5 mL LA. Using the same injection point, the needle can be withdrawn and redirected as necessary to reach more tissue. Always start the new injection point in anesthetized tissues if possible
- **Wait for anaesthetic to take effect**: to decrease likelihood of unnecessarily injecting more anaesthetic. Lidocaine requires approximately 1 minute to take effect, whereas bupivacaine may require up to 5 minutes.
- **Test for adequacy of anaesthesia**: by using a pin prick or gentle pinch from forceps. Additional anaesthetic may be required to achieve adequate anaesthesia.

- **Complete the procedure**.
- **Dispose all waste and sharps safely**.

Post-procedure care

- Explain to patient and carers what you have done and how the procedure was conducted. State problems if any.
- Once the LA has worn off, further appropriate analgesia may be required.
- As with most invasive procedures, watch for signs of neurovascular compromise or infection.
- Patients should be alerted to seek clinical attention should signs or symptoms of a complication develop.
- Appropriate plans for follow-up must be made, e.g. removal of sutures.

Professionalism: working with colleagues

Inform key colleagues? Nurses, doctors, carers, and family.

Write clear notes, e.g.:

'Local anaesthesia for suturing of skin cut to left forearm (3 cm)

- Indication: cut to skin following accident.
- Procedure: 1% lidocaine 5 mL. Standard procedure. 4 stitches using 4/0 non-absorbent material after cleaning wound. No complications and patient comfortable.
- Post procedure: patient will return in 5 days for removal of sutures. Advise on infection, opening of wound given. If problems to return to A&E or see GP.

'Staff nurse informed re procedure, discharge and follow-up.'

Patient safety tips

- ✔ **Reassure the patient during anaesthetic injection**: if appropriate, use distraction techniques such as light conversation, during the procedure.
- ✔ **Care with adrenaline-containing solutions**: these are usually labelled in red for easy visibility and should not be used in areas with end vessels.
- ✔ **Lidocaine (Xylocaine)**: is the most commonly used LA (0.5%, 1%, and 2%). The 1% solution is sufficient for most indications. The 0.5% solution can be useful to decrease the risk of systemic toxicity when injecting large volumes. The 2% solution can be used for dental procedures when minimal volumes are preferable.
- ✔ **Maximum dose of lidocaine**: this is 4 mg/kg in a healthy adult. By adding adrenaline (1:100 000), the maximum allowable dose can be increased to 7 mg/kg (0.7 mL/kg if using a 1% solution).
- ✔ **Bupivacaine**: is longer acting than lidocaine and is useful for longer procedures or for anticipated prolonged post-procedure pain. It is four times as potent as lidocaine and therefore is prepared at concentrations one fourth that of lidocaine, 0.25% and 0.5%. The maximum allowable dose for bupivacaine is 2.0 mg/kg, and for bupivacaine plus adrenaline it is 3.0 mg/kg.

Student name: Medical school: Year:

Local anaesthesia

Please demonstrate how you would use local anaesthesia (LA) to numb the skin prior to lumbar puncture. Use this simulated skin device and the equipment provided.

I will also ask you some questions before and during the procedure.

		Self	Peer	Peer/tutor	Tutor
What are the clinical indications for LA	• **Uses in surgery and dentistry:** minor surgery (e.g. skin biopsies, sutures)	☐	☐	☐	☐
	• **Uses in acute pain:** labour pain (epidural anaesthesia), postoperative pain (peripheral nerve blocks, epidural anaesthesia), trauma (peripheral nerve blocks, IV regional anaesthesia, epidural anaesthesia)	☐	☐	☐	☐
	• **Use in chronic pain**: including joint injections with steroids.	☐	☐	☐	☐
Please name specific LA procedures and their anatomical site of action	• **Spinal block:** subarachnoid space acts on spinal nerve roots and cord (legs, abdomen)	☐	☐	☐	☐
	• **Epidural block:** epidural space acts primarily on the spinal nerve roots.	☐	☐	☐	☐
	• **Nerve plexus block:** e.g. brachial plexus for arm surgery	☐	☐	☐	☐
	• **Peripheral nerve block:** single nerve trunk, e.g. finger ring block	☐	☐	☐	☐
	• **Local Infiltration:** e.g. subcutaneous tissue for biopsy	☐	☐	☐	☐
	• **Intravenous regional anaesthesia:** e.g. Bier's block for arm manipulation and surgery	☐	☐	☐	☐
	• **Surface anaesthesia:** to skin or mucus membrane in the form of spray (e.g. endoscopy)	☐	☐	☐	☐
	• **Field block:** to numb region distal to the injection (e.g. forearm)	☐	☐	☐	☐
What is the mechanism of action of a LA?	• LA interferes with the rapid influx of sodium ions into nerve cells, thereby reducing or eliminating depolarization of the nerve	☐	☐	☐	☐
What are the common side effects of LA?	• **Neurological:** anxiety, euphoria, irritability, perioral tingling, tinnitus, convulsions	☐	☐	☐	☐
	• **Respiratory failure:** due to central and peripheral actions				
	• **Cardiovascular collapse:** bradycardia, vasodilation, anaphylactic shock	☐	☐	☐	☐
	• **Local effects:** pain, delay in wound healing, and necrosis	☐	☐	☐	☐
		☐	☐	☐	☐
What are the contraindications for LA	• Allergy, patients unable to cooperate fully during the procedure	☐	☐	☐	☐
	• Inflammation or infection at the injection site	☐	☐	☐	☐
	• Adrenaline contraindicated in areas with end vessels including digits, pinna, and penis	☐	☐	☐	☐
Equipment	• Personal protective equipment (gloves, face shield, apron), antiseptic solution, syringe, one 18 or 20G and one 25 to 30G needle. LA solution	☐	☐	☐	☐
Explanation and consent	• Obtain consent for procedures: written or verbal according to procedure	☐	☐	☐	☐
	• Position the patient supine, or sitting comfortably in bed if this is not possible	☐	☐	☐	☐
	• **Introduce yourself and gain consent from patient**	☐	☐	☐	☐
	• **Explain procedure to patient:** what may be felt during the procedure	☐	☐	☐	☐
	• **Enquire about medical history:** especially allergies, past reactions, and illnesses	☐	☐	☐	☐
Procedure	• **Wash hands, clean and prepare the skin:** using povidone-iodine or chlorhexidine	☐	☐	☐	☐
	• **Create a skin wheal:** with small needle, aspirate syringe to exclude being intravascular	☐	☐	☐	☐
	• **Inject through the wheal:** slowly inject 0.5 mL LA. Redirect to reach more tissue	☐	☐	☐	☐
	• **Wait for anaesthetic to take effect:** lidocaine (1 min), bupivacaine (5 min)	☐	☐	☐	☐
	• **Test for adequacy of anaesthesia:** by using a pin prick or gentle pinch from forceps.	☐	☐	☐	☐
	• **Complete the procedure and dispose of waste and all sharps safely**	☐	☐	☐	☐
Post-procedure care	• Explain to patient and carers. State problems if any	☐	☐	☐	☐
	• Patients alerted to seek clinical attention if complication develops	☐	☐	☐	☐
	• Appropriate plans for follow-up made, e.g. removal of sutures	☐	☐	☐	☐
Professionalism: working with colleagues	• Where relevant inform key colleagues: nurses, doctors carers and family	☐	☐	☐	☐
Patient safety tips	• **Reassure the patient during anaesthetic injection:** use distraction such as conversation	☐	☐	☐	☐
	• **Care with adrenaline-containing solutions:** usually labelled in red for easy visibility	☐	☐	☐	☐
	• **Maximum dose of lidocaine:** 4 mg/kg in a healthy adult; 7 mg/kg with adrenaline	☐	☐	☐	☐
	•	☐	☐	☐	☐

				Self	Peer	Peer/tutor	Tutor
Self-assessed as at least borderline:	Signature:		Date:	U B S E	U B S E	U B S E	U B S E
Peer-assessed as ready for tutor assessment:	Signature:		Date:	U B S E	U B S E	U B S E	U B S E
Tutor-assessed as satisfactory:	Signature:		Date:	U B S E	U B S E	U B S E	U B S E

Notes

9.8 Surgical suturing

Background

The surgical art of suturing can be traced to *circa* 3000BC as evidenced in Edwin Smith's *Surgical Papyrus*. A case described in this manuscript reads: 'Thou shouldst draw together for him his gash with stitching', thereby substantiating the use of this procedure in antiquity. The materials and techniques have changed over the thousands of years; however, promotion of wound healing remains its primary aim.

Suturing is defined as a method of wound closure which realigns tissue planes and apposes edges together, providing support, eliminating dead space, and promoting healing by primary intention. Suturing, like any other clinical skill, is perfected only with practice, and is based on two simple principles: proper technique and gentle tissue handling. The aim of any suturing is clear from this quote:

> *'A good suture heals without complications and leaves without a trace.'*

> Anon

Clinical indications

Sutures are primarily used during operative procedures:

● To join tissues together, such as skin wounds/laceration and operative incisions

● To tie off vessels such as arteries and ducts

● To join tubular structures together, such as blood vessels or bowel anastomoses

● To close defects and holes and reinforce tissues.

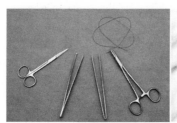 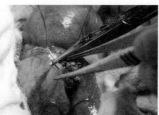 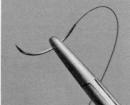

Suture pack contents: needle holder, toothed forceps, scissors, gauze, plastic container for cleaning fluid.

Suturing: key skill in surgery–meticulous attention to detail and technique needed!

A curved tapered needle: safer than the curved cutting needle as less likely to lacerate nerves and vessels.

Figure 9.13 Images in suturing.

Contraindications

There is no absolute contraindication to suturing. The following can be taken as relative contraindications:

● If excessive tension is required to close a wound, an alternative to suturing may be preferred, as excess tension impedes on the final cosmetic appearance of the wound (e.g. in skin flaps or skin grafts).

● Pus or discharge round the site of injury – indicates an infection. And treating of the local infection must take precedence over suturing.

- Puncture wounds or animal bites are mostly not amenable to suturing because of contamination
- Consider alternatives to suturing: stapling, adhesives, adhesive tapes.

The following factors also need to be considered before suturing:

- **Time lapse**: if more than 12 hours from time of injury to presentation, this may not be amenable to suturing (discretion and judgement has to be used in such instances)
- **Site and size of a wound**: dictates the size of suture material needed for the closure and the need or otherwise for tetanus prophylaxis.
- **Depth of wound**: deeper wounds may have associated injury to nerves, blood vessels and tendons. These must be assessed for repair before skin closure.
- **Persistent bleeding**: must be treated in preference to suturing of the wound.

Anatomical and physiological principles

The skin functions as a protective barrier that interfaces with the external environment. It consists of three anatomically distinct layers:

- **Epidermis**: stratified squamous epithelium with ridges. The thickness varies in different types of skin. On the eyelids it is only 0.05 mm thick, while on the palms and soles it is 1.5 mm. The epidermis contains five layers (stratum basale, stratum spinosum, stratum granulosum, stratum lucidum, stratum corneum). The stratum basale, has columnar cells which divide and push already formed cells into higher layers. As the cells move into the higher layers, they flatten and eventually die. The stratum corneum, is made of dead, flat skin cells that shed about every 2 weeks. The specialized cells of the epidermis includes the melanocyte (produces melanin) and the Langerhans cell (immune system).
- **Dermis**: also varies in thickness, it is 0.3 mm on the eyelid and 3.0 mm on the back. Three types of tissue that are present throughout: collagen, elastic tissue, and reticular fibres. The two layers of the dermis are the papillary (blood vessels, lymphatics, nerve cells, fine collagen, and elastin fibres) and reticular layer (vascular plexus, lymph cells, nerve cell, sweat glands, hair follicles, thicker elastic fibres, and more dense specialized nerve cells called Meissner's and Vater-Pacini corpuscles, which transmit the sensations of touch and pressure are also present).
- **Subcutaneous tissue**: a layer of fat and connective tissue that embeds larger blood vessels and nerves. This layer is important in thermoregulation.

The physiology of wound healing

The process of wound healing is usually described as series of steps; in reality there is considerable temporal overlap between all the stages.

- **Vascular and inflammatory phase**: initial phase of vasoconstriction and vasospasm, lasting about 5 minutes, which reduces the loss of blood. Platelets activated by tissue damage, exposure of subendothelial factors and collagen all react to form a platelet plug. Platelets also activate the clotting cascade leading to clot formation. Chemotactic factors lead to vasodilation, and recruitment of inflammatory cells (neutrophils, monocytes, and macrophages). The role of these cells is in the phagocytosis of contaminant bacteria and tissue debridement. They also release additional chemotactic factors leading to fibroblast and endothelial cells activation.
- **Granulation tissue formation**: this matrix contains all the cells required for wound healing: inflammatory cells, fibroblasts and new vasculature. It commences about 3–5 days after the wound. Fibroblasts produce collagen, elastin, fibronectin, and collagenases for tissue remodelling.
- **Re-epithelization**: epidermal cells from the wound margins migrate to cover up the wound. Initially migration occurs without proliferation. Later on epithelial proliferation occurs (maximal at 48–72 hours). Keratinocytes assist by producing matrix components for epithelial adhesion and proteases that debride devitalized tissue.

- **Matrix and collagen remodelling**: Remodelling continues for months after re-epithelization has occurred. Remodelling increases the tensile strength around the wound, reduces erythema, scar tissue, and normalizes the final appearance of the skin. Type III collagen (random formation) is replaced by type I collagen (fibres orientated parallel to skin). Some ethnic groupings have excessive keratinization or reduced remodelling leading to keloid formation.

Local and systemic factors affecting wound healing

Local factors:

- **Infection**: is the most common local cause for delayed healing. All open wounds are essentially contaminated postoperatively by resident bacterial flora
- **Surgical technique**: rough handling of tissue or inappropriate instrumentation can damage skin edges and lead an increased inflammatory reaction
- **Haematoma formation**: excessive bleeding of wound site can lead to formation of a haematoma which delays healing and can act as a nidus for bacterial growth
- **Foreign body reaction**: this can lead to the generation of a prolonged inflammatory response, significantly slowing down wound repair
- **Tissue ischaemia**: disruption of blood flow can lead to tissue ischaemia which results in poor healing or necrosis.

Systemic factors:

- **Deficiency states**: for example vitamin A, C, and K deficiencies all can prolong wound healing
- **Age**: elderly patients have delayed healing
- **Disease states**: such as chronic renal failure, diabetes mellitus, Cushing's syndrome, and hyperthyroidism
- **Medications**: glucocorticoids, anticoagulants, antineoplastic drugs, colchicine, and ciclosporin A.

Suturing equipment notes

- **Curved cutting needle**: has sharp tip and edges, which permits easy advancement through skin. However, its sharp edges can be traumatic to deeper structures such as vessels or nerves.
- **Curved tapered needle**: has a sharp tip but smooth edges, causes less tissue trauma. Preferentially used in suturing deeper structures such as blood vessels. Due to their blunt edges, tapered needles are not good for skin suturing.
- **Straight needles**: can be used without a needle holder. This technique is often preferred in certain surgical areas such as the neck.
- **Suture material**: comes in different sizes and composition (Table 9.5).
    - **Size**: The size and location of a wound dictates the sizes of suture material required. For example: face 6/0 (diameter of suture 0.07 mm), limbs 4/0 (0.15 mm), scalp 2/0 (0.3 mm).
    - **Absorbable or non-absorbable**: Absorbable sutures are dissolved by the tissues and do not require external removal. Non-absorbable sutures remain in place until they are removed. They are less tissue reactive and leave less pronounced scarring as they are removed.
    - **Braided or non-braided**: Non-braided sutures are monofilaments which are preferred for closing skin wounds. Braided sutures are made up of several filaments twisted together. They are easier to knot and have less memory, making them an easier choice in terms of ease of use. However, the intersections of the braided sutures can provide a nidus for bacterial growth. Hence they are not suitable for open-contaminated wounds, which harbour an increased risk of infection.
    - **Synthetic or natural**: to describe the source material.

Table 9.5 Characteristics of the most commonly used suture materials

Suture material	Absorbable or non-absorbable	Braided or non-braided	Tissue reactivity	Primary indications
Prolene	Non-absorbable	Non-braided	None	Skin sutures
PDS Polydioxanone	Absorbable	Non-braided	+	Intradermal sutures
Dexon Polyglycolic	Absorbable	Braided	++	Intradermal sutures Sutures in subcutaneous tissue
Nylon	Non-absorbable	Non-braided	+	Skin sutures
Silk	Non-absorbable	Braided	+++	Clean skin wounds

Inspection

- **Inspect and evaluate the wound/laceration**: look around the margins for any skin changes, depth of the wound itself, ?compromise of nerves/vessels/tendons. Continue only if suturing should be undertaken.
- **Consider**: type of suture material required, type of stitch to close the wound, need for local anaesthetic, need for tetanus prophylaxis, type of dressing to be applied post procedure.

Equipment

- **Personal protective equipment**: gloves, apron, consider face shield.
- **Suture pack contents**: needle holder, toothed forceps, scissors, gauze, plastic container for cleaning fluid.
- **Local anaesthetic**: lidocaine, syringe, one 18 or 20G and one 25 to 30G needle.
- **Wound-cleaning agents**: sterile normal saline and antiseptic fluid (e.g. 2% chlorhexidine solution).
- **Sterile drapes, sutures with needles**.

Explanation and consent

- **Introduce yourself and obtain consent from patient**: state purpose of the procedure and the possible use of LA.
- **Explain procedure to patient**: inform them that there may be some discomfort on LA injection. The LA should eliminate most of the pain but not all sensation, and pressure and tugging may still be felt. Position patient comfortably.
- **Enquire about medical history (in view of LA)**: allergies, past reactions in patient and family, relevant systemic illness, such as heart disease, liver disease, peripheral vascular disease, or seizure disorder.
- **State main benefits and potential risks**.

Procedure

Wound closure to realign tissue planes and appose edges together, providing support, eliminating dead space and promoting healing by primary intention.

- **Wash hands**.
- **Clean and prepare the skin**: Antiseptic solution such as 2% chlorhexidine solution.

- **Wound preparation**: Cleaning wounds prior to suturing reduces risk of wound infection significantly. Methods of wound preparation include:
  ○ **Saline wash**: the wound is irrigated with sterile normal saline to reduce wound contamination by the bacterial flora found on skin.
  ○ **Scrubbing**: If above is inadequate and contaminants remain, then direct, careful scrubbing of the wound may aid the removal of debris.
  ○ **Debridement**: may be required to remove contaminants which are adherent to tissue especially if they are not removed following irrigation.
  ○ Check sufficient LA given and anaesthesia established.

Simple interrupted suture method: needle and suture material are advanced through the epidermis into the subcutaneous tissue from one side, then enter the subcutaneous tissue on the opposite side, and come out the epidermis above before tying a knot to finish it off. It is good practice to start from the side of the wound farthest from you. This ensures that you are sewing toward yourself and is beneficial from a biomechanical standpoint. The needle is inserted 2–7 mm from the wound edge according to the depth and size of the wound.

- **Distal wound edge is gently everted with the toothed forcep**:
- **Suture needle is picked up by the needle holder**: approximately three-quarters of the way from its sharp edge.
- **Needle pierces skin at an angle of 90°**: 5–10 mm from the wound edge. Aim similar depth of suture across the wound itself.
- **For small wounds**: gently rotate the wrist to advance the suture needle through the epidermis and dermis and exit at the opposite site of the wound edge (in one go). Aim to exit at the same distance from the wound as the entrance to the wound with the needle. Then continue at A below.
- **For larger/deeper wounds**: gently rotating the wrist controlling the needle-holder will advance the needle through skin until it is seen within the wound. The bite size should be adequate to hold the stitch within the wound. Forceps will be needed to pull the needle through the tissues.
  ○ **Release the needle holder's grip of the needle**: reach into the wound and grasp the needle with the needle holder and pull it free so that there is enough suture material to enter the opposite side of the wound (same depth as previous entry into wound)
  ○ **Using the forceps evert the other wound edge and advance the needle through the opposite edge of the wound**: exit perpendicular to skin. Continue at A below.
- **A – Release the needle holder's grip of the needle**: grasp the portion of the needle protruding from the skin with the needle holder.
- **Pull the needle through the skin**: until you have approximately 3–5 cm of suture strand ('free end') protruding from the initial bite site (site farthest away from you).
- **Release the needle from the needle holder**: and wrap the suture around the needle holder two times.
- **Pull the 'free end' through this to make a knot**: a couple more knots, each in a different direction, is required to secure the suture in place (try keeping the knots of all sutures placed on one side of the wound margin). Cut with scissors 5 mm from knot.
- **Suture placement**: sutures placed on the face should be approximately 2–3 mm from the skin edge and 3–5 mm apart. Sutures placed elsewhere on the body should be approximately 3–7 mm and 5–10 mm apart.
- **Post suturing**: cleanse the suture site with antiseptic agent (e.g. chlorhexidine 2%) and apply dressing.
- **Dispose of waste and all sharps safely**.

Box 9.1 Other common stitches (Figure 9.14)

- **The interrupted suture**: is the commonest and most versatile of suturing techniques. An alternative to the interrupted stitch is the continuous or running suture which is less time consuming.

- **Continuous suture**: involves placing an initial 'interrupted suture' which is, however, not cut; successive sutures are then placed along the length of the wound without tying or cutting the suture material after each pass. It is a faster method and knotting occurs at the start and finish of the procedure.

- **Mattress suture**: a variation of the simple interrupted suture (two kinds are described, the vertical and horizontal). It consists of two simple interrupted stitch placed in continuity. One is placed very wide and deep into the wound edge and a second more superficial interrupted stitch is then placed closer to the wound edge and in the opposite direction (see image). Further variations exist.

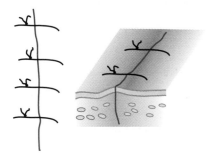

Interrupted

Placement: Each suture is individually placed and tied. The finished closure appears better if all sutures are knotted on one side of the wound margin

Indication: Technique of choice if wound is contaminated or at risk of infection

Disadvantage: Lengthier procedure as each suture must be individually tied

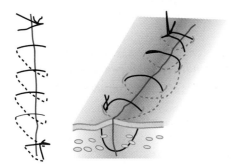

Continuous

Placement: The sutures are continuous through the length without tying each individual suture

Indication: Technique of choice when rapid closure of a wound is required, especially to stop bleeding

Disadvantage: If one suture comes out the entire suture is disrupted.

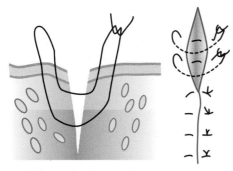

Interrupted mattress suture

Placement: suture involves placing an initial suture deeper and wider from the wound margin and re-entering the skin more superficially and closer to the wound to place the second suture before knotting.

Best eversion of wound edges

Indication: Skin-to-skin eversion is best achieved with this technique

Disadvantage: Lengthy and technically more challenging

Figure 9.14 Basic suturing techniques.

Post-procedure care

- Explain to patient and carers what you have done and how the procedure was conducted. State problems if any. Inform patient to check for signs of complications in the next 24 hours.

- Administer antibiotic and or tetanus prophylaxis if indicated.

- Postoperative care should aim at minimizing pain, adequate analgesia should be prescribed.
- Removal of suturing:
  ○ Sutures must be removed in a timely fashion to avoid complications such as cross-scarring across the wound.
  ○ Facial sutures are removed between 3 and 4 days; most other body sutures will need to be removed between 7 and 10 days.
  ○ Removal of sutures involves cutting the sutures with appropriate scissors below the knot and as close to skin as possible and pulling the suture through with forceps. Conclude by counting the number of sutures removed and ensuring it matches with the number of sutures placed.

Professionalism: working with colleagues

Inform key colleagues: nurses, doctors, carers. and family.

Write clear notes, e.g.:

'Suturing of skin cut to left forearm (3 cm). Informed consent given and recorded on form.

- **Indication**: Cut to skin following accident using sharp knife while doing DIY .
- **Procedure**: 1% lidocaine 5 mL. Standard procedure. 4 stitches using 4/0 non-absorbent material after cleaning wound. No complications and patient comfortable.
- **Post procedure**: Patient will return in 5 days for removal of sutures. Advise on infection, opening of wound given. If problems to return to A&E or see GP.

'Staff nurse informed re procedure, discharge and follow-up.'

Patient safety tips

✔ **Warn patient about possible wound infection and more systemic infection as well**.

✔ **Warn of signs of tetanus**: headaches, cramping or spasms of jaw muscles (lockjaw) or back.

✔ **Optimal size needle holder**: a large needle holder will not grip onto a small needle very well and will impair suture placement. A small needle holder likewise may limit the grasp on a large needle, control will be impaired and may cause slipping during insertion.

✔ **Forceps should be chosen carefully**: to ensure optimal grip of skin while minimizing trauma to the tissue. Gentle tissue handling is paramount.

✔ **Accurate suture placement with optimum tension**: for best apposition of wound edges and best chances of healing adequately.

✔ Local anaesthesia with adrenaline should not be used in sites where there is an end-artery circulation. This includes: fingers, toes, penis, pinna.

Student name:	Medical school:	Year:

Surgical suturing

This skin wound simulation is typical of an injury that is commonly encountered in an accident and emergency department. The patient is a 56-year-old keen DIY enthusiast who has, yet again, cut himself with a box knife. He is known to have diabetes and on insulin. His other hobbies include growing his own vegetables on his field.

Please demonstrate how you would suture this wound using interrupted stitches. Use at least 4 stitches. You will also be asked some questions related to suturing.

		Self	Peer	Peer /tutor	Tutor
What are the clinical indications for suturing?	• To join tissues together (wounds, operative incisions)	☐	☐	☐	☐
	• To tie off vessels such as arteries and ducts	☐	☐	☐	☐
	• To join tubular structures together (blood vessels or bowel anastomoses)	☐	☐	☐	☐
	• To close defects/holes and reinforce tissues	☐	☐	☐	☐
	•	☐	☐	☐	☐
Relative contraindications	• Inflammation, infection, puncture wounds or animal bites	☐	☐	☐	☐
	• Consider alternatives to suturing: stapling, adhesives, adhesive tapes	☐	☐	☐	☐
	•	☐	☐	☐	☐
What factors must be considered before suturing?	• **Time lapse** (<12 hours, may not be possible), **size of a wound, ? tetanus prophylaxis needed, depth of wound, tendon/nerve involvement, persistent bleeding**	☐	☐	☐	☐
	•	☐	☐	☐	☐
Anatomical and physiological principles	• What are three layers of the skin and their function?	☐	☐	☐	☐
	• What are the four stages of wound healing? Discuss briefly.	☐	☐	☐	☐
	• What local factors can affect wound healing?	☐	☐	☐	☐
	• What systemic factors can affect wound healing?	☐	☐	☐	☐
	•	☐	☐	☐	☐
Suturing equipment	• Identify which of these is a curved cutting needle: discuss its use	☐	☐	☐	☐
	• Identify which of these is a curved tapered needle: discuss its use	☐	☐	☐	☐
	• Suture material: briefly discuss size, absorbable/non-absorbable, braided/non-braided, synthetic/natural	☐	☐	☐	☐
	•	☐	☐	☐	☐
Inspection	• **Inspect and evaluate the wound/laceration:** margins, depth, extent of tissue damage	☐	☐	☐	☐
	• **Consider:** Type of suture material, type of stitch, ? need for LA, tetanus prophylaxis	☐	☐	☐	☐
	•	☐	☐	☐	☐
Equipment	• **Personal protective equipment:** gloves, apron, consider face shield	☐	☐	☐	☐
	• **Suture pack contents:** needle holder, forceps, scissors, gauze	☐	☐	☐	☐
	• **Local anaesthetic:** 1% lidocaine 5 or 10 mL, syringe, needles	☐	☐	☐	☐
	• **Wound-cleaning agents:** sterile normal saline and antiseptic fluid	☐	☐	☐	☐
	• **Sterile drapes, sutures with needles**	☐	☐	☐	☐
	•	☐	☐	☐	☐
Explanation and consent	• Introduce yourself, gain consent from patient, explain procedure to patient	☐	☐	☐	☐
	• **Enquire about medical history (in view of LA):** allergies, past reactions in patient	☐	☐	☐	☐
	• State main benefits and potential risks	☐	☐	☐	☐
	•	☐	☐	☐	☐
Procedure	• Wash hands	☐	☐	☐	☐
	• **Clean and prepare the skin:** antiseptic solution such as 2% chlorhexidine solution	☐	☐	☐	☐
	• **Wound preparation:** consider cleaning wound with saline, scrubbing or debridement	☐	☐	☐	☐
	•	☐	☐	☐	☐
Sequence	• Distal wound edge is gently everted with the toothed forcep	☐	☐	☐	☐
	• Suture needle is picked up by the needle holder: three-quarter way from its sharp edge	☐	☐	☐	☐
	• Needle pierces skin at an angle of 90° 5–10 mm from the wound edge	☐	☐	☐	☐
	• **For small wounds:** gently rotate the wrist to advance the suture needle through the epidermis and dermis and exit at the opposite site of the wound edge (in one go)	☐	☐	☐	☐
	• **For larger/deeper wounds:** controlling the needle-holder advance needle through skin until it is in eye-view within the wound.				
	• Release the needle holder's grip of the needle and grasp needle in wound	☐	☐	☐	☐
	• Using forceps evert the other wound edge and advance the needle through the opposite edge of the wound: exit perpendicular to skin.	☐	☐	☐	☐

	• **Continue – release the needle holder's grip of the needle**: grasp the portion of the needle protruding from the skin with the needle holder.	☐	☐	☐	☐
	• **Pull the needle through the skin:** until you have approximately 3–5 cm of suture strand ('free end') protruding from the initial bite site (site farthest away from you).	☐	☐	☐	☐
	• **Release the needle from the needle holder:** and wrap the suture around the needle holder two times.	☐	☐	☐	☐
	• **Pull the 'free end' through this to make a knot:** a couple more knots to secure the suture in place (keep knots of all sutures placed on one side of the wound margin).	☐	☐	☐	☐
	• **Suture placement:** face, approximately 2-3 mm from the skin edge and 3-5 mm apart. Elsewhere on the body should be approximately 3-7 mm and 5-10 mm apart	☐	☐	☐	☐
	• **Post suturing:** cleanse the suture site with antiseptic agent (e.g. chlorhexidine 2%) and apply dressing	☐	☐	☐	☐
	• Dispose of waste and all sharps safely	☐	☐	☐	☐
	•	☐	☐	☐	☐
Post-procedure care: please can you now remove the sutures	• Explain to patient and carers what was done. State problems if any. Inform patient to check for signs of complications in the next 24 hours	☐	☐	☐	☐
	• Administer antibiotic and or tetanus prophylaxis if indicated	☐	☐	☐	☐
	• Postoperative care should aim at minimizing pain,	☐	☐	☐	☐
	• Removal of suturing: plan made for timely removal: facial sutures removed between 4-5 days; others 7-10 days.	☐	☐	☐	☐
	• Cut below the knot, as close to skin as possible and pulling the suture through with forceps. Count number of sutures removed and ensure matches that inserted	☐	☐	☐	☐
	•	☐	☐	☐	☐
Professionalism: working with colleagues	• Inform key colleagues: nurses, doctors, carers, and family	☐	☐	☐	☐
	• Write clear notes:	☐	☐	☐	☐
	•	☐	☐	☐	☐
Patient safety tips	• **Warn patient about possible wound infection and more systemic infection as well.**	☐	☐	☐	☐
	• **Warn of tetanus:** headaches, cramping or spasms of jaw muscles (lockjaw) or back	☐	☐	☐	☐
	• **Forceps should be chosen carefully:** to minimize trauma to the tissue	☐	☐	☐	☐
	• **Accurate suture placement with optimum tension:** for best apposition of wound edge	☐	☐	☐	☐
	• Do not use LA with adrenaline in end-artery sites.	☐	☐	☐	☐
	•	☐	☐	☐	☐

			U B S E	U B S E	U B S E	U B S E
Self-assessed as at least borderline:	Signature:	Date:				
Peer-assessed as ready for tutor assessment:	Signature:	Date:				
Tutor-assessed as satisfactory:	Signature:	Date:				

Notes

9.9 Nasogastric tube insertion

Background

A nasogastric (NG) tube is a long plastic tube that is designed to be passed into the stomach through the nose. It can be used either to drain the contents of the stomach or to facilitate maintenance of nutritional intake. The procedure is usually undertaken by nursing staff and junior doctors. The latter particularly if the tube has fallen out or is difficult to place. The UK's National Patient Safety Agency has highlighted the fact that 11 deaths and one case of serious harm due to misplaced nasogastric feeding tubes over a 2-year period.

Clinical indications

To facilitate drainage of stomach contents:

- **Treatment of severe nausea and vomiting**: relief of upper abdominal distension and pain.
- **Clinical emergencies**: conditions which require drainage of the contents of the stomach in order to prevent distension of the stomach, or aspiration of gastric contents into the upper respiratory system and especially the lungs. This is to prevent aspiration pneumonia/pneumonitis. For this purpose a wider bore tube is used, and the end of the tube needs to be connected to a drainage bag or to suction.
  - Intestinal obstruction
  - Upper gastrointestinal bleed
  - Acute pancreatitis
  - Postoperative ileus
  - Gastric outflow obstruction
  - Gastric volvulus (beware that gaseous content will need frequent removal from the drainage bag in some cases).

To facilitate maintenance of nutritional intake:

- **Patients who have an unsafe swallow reflex**: e.g. due to motor neurone disease or post stroke.
- **Patients unable to maintain sufficient nutritional intake**: with a functioning gastrointestinal tact.
- **Patient unable to swallow**: This would apply in intensive care unit (ITU) patients, for example. A standard NG tube can be inserted for the purpose of feeding or administering medications enterally in patients who are unable to swallow. If more than a few days are needed, then consideration should be given to a fine-bore tube that is introduced using an inner hard stylus which is removed following insertion when position has been checked.

Anatomical and physiological principles

Anatomically a conduit is created between the external environment, via the upper respiratory tract (nasal) through the oesophagus and into the stomach (Figure 9.15).

Nasopharynx: extends superiorly with the inferior, middle, and superior nasal concha encountered medially. Laterally, there are the sinuses and eustachian tubes. Inferiorly, the soft palate is present where discomfort during this procedure is usually encountered.

Oropharynx: this begins just below the soft palate and extends inferiorly to the glottis and epiglottis and then to the oesophageal opening. It is inferior to the glottis that the nasogastric tube can 'ride' into the mouth and present as a coiled tube. Pushing the NG tube against inflamed tonsils can be traumatic for the patient.

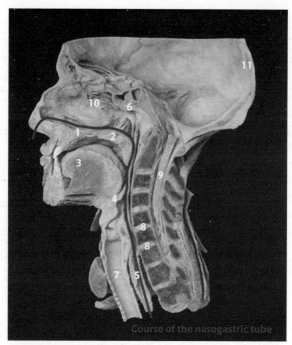

Anatomy of the head and neck in relation to nasogastric tube insertion

Sagittal section of the head with the brain removed showing:
1 hard palate
2 soft palate
3 tongue
4 epiglottis
5 oesophagus
6 cribriform plate
7 trachea
8 intervertebral discs of cervical vertebrae
9 spinal cord
10 inferior nasal concha
11 occiput

Course of the nasogastric tube

Figure 9.15 Anatomy of the head and neck.

Laryngopharynx: inferior to the epiglottis and above the vocal cords is yet another opportunity for the NG tube to be misdirected, this time into the trachea through to the vocal cords and towards the thyroid cartilage. This would manifest as an intense 'gagging'. It is the swallowing manoeuvre that closes the epiglottis over the glottis to prevent this happening.

Oesophagus: has proximal striated muscle which will be activated by the swallowing reflex and help move the NG tube into the lower oesophagus, which is characterized by smooth muscle with its involuntary peristalsis movement. After traversing the distal oesophagus smooth muscle sphincter the NG tube reaches the stomach.

Contraindications

Absolute

- Severe facial trauma
- Disruption to the cribriform plate, which may allow intracranial insertion of the tube.
- Unstable cervical spine injury to C4 or above.

Caution advised

- Base of skull fracture, this may also allow intracranial placement of tube (signs include rhinorrhoea, raccoon eye bruising, Battle's sign).
- Coagulopathy; either intrinsic to patient or iatrogenic (e.g. warfarin treatment).
- Recent surgery to the stomach, oesophagus, nose, or mouth.
- Any potential obstacles to insertion including the presence of nasopharyngeal tumours or oesophageal stricture.
- Oesophageal varices.

Equipment

- Personal protective equipment: apron, gloves, protective eyewear in some cases.

Ear Clinical Picture Suite

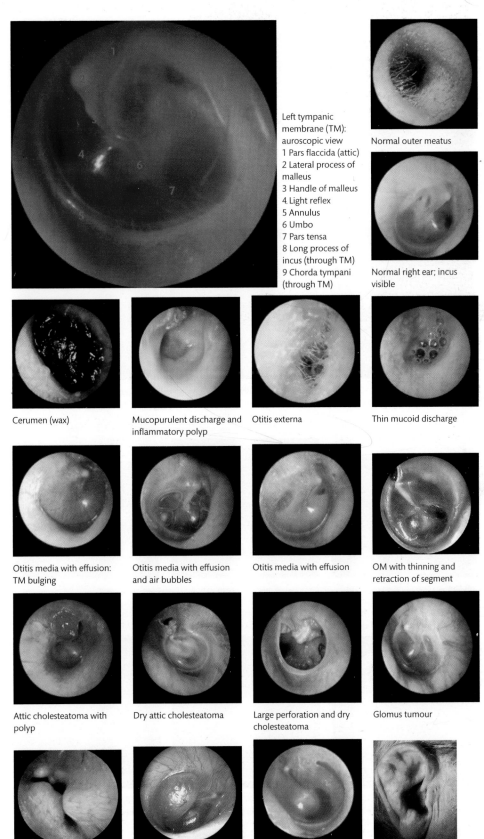

Left tympanic membrane (TM): auroscopic view
1 Pars flaccida (attic)
2 Lateral process of malleus
3 Handle of malleus
4 Light reflex
5 Annulus
6 Umbo
7 Pars tensa
8 Long process of incus (through TM)
9 Chorda tympani (through TM)

Normal outer meatus

Normal right ear; incus visible

Cerumen (wax)

Mucopurulent discharge and inflammatory polyp

Otitis externa

Thin mucoid discharge

Otitis media with effusion: TM bulging

Otitis media with effusion and air bubbles

Otitis media with effusion

OM with thinning and retraction of segment

Attic cholesteatoma with polyp

Dry attic cholesteatoma

Large perforation and dry cholesteatoma

Glomus tumour

Meatal osteomata

Bullous (viral) myringitis

Barotrauma with small haematoma

Cauliflower ear: Resolved haematoma

Ophthalmology Clinical Picture Suite I

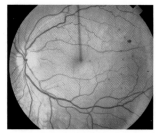

Diabetic Retinopathy (DR):
If the visual acuity is 6/12 or worse this is maculopathy. Otherwise background diabetic retinopathy
Lesions: microaneurysm (MA), dot haemorrhage

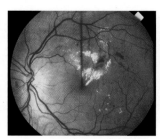

Diabetic Maculopathy:
Hard exudates within the macular area. Lesions: hard exudates, circinate hard exudates, MA, haemorrhages

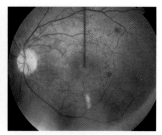

Pre-proliferative DR:
Lesions: intra-retinal micro-vascular abnormalities (IRMA), cotton wool spots, haemorrhages

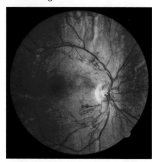

Proliferative DR
Lesions: new vessels on the disc (NVD), haemorrhages

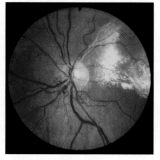

Proliferative DR with hypertensive changes.
Lesions: new vessels on the disc, hard exudates, A-V nipping, haemorrhages

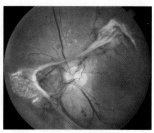

Advanced Proliferative DR:
Lesions: new vessels on the disc and elsewhere, pre-retinal fibrosis, exudates haemorrhages

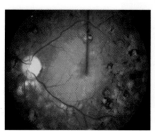

Pan Retinal Laser Photocoagulation
Macular spared, NVD have regressed and no longer seen. Lesions: laser scars, retinal pigment epithelium and fibrosis.

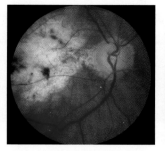

Age-related macular degeneration (ARMD) and glaucoma
Lesions: dry macular degeneration, pale optic disc with glaucomatous cupping

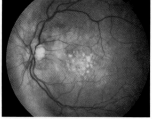

Macular Drusen
Precursor to ARMD in many cases. Can just be normal variant
Lesions: drusen

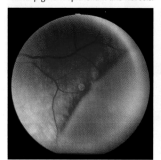

Retinal Detachment
Due to trauma in this case can be DR. Lesions: margin between normal and detached retina

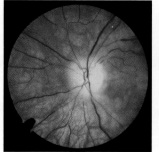

Optic Atrophy
Pale disc. Incidental findings: blurring of the disc margin due to myelinated nerve fibres, choroidal vessels

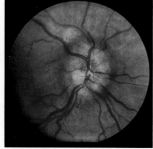

Papilloedema:
The optic disc is swollen and raised. Lesions: papilloedema, congested retinal veins, blurred disc margin.

Ophthalmology Clinical Picture Suite II

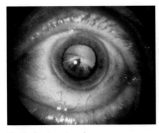

Cortical cataract and corneal arcus:
The red reflex is abnormal due to cataract most apparent "4-8pm"
Lesions: cataract, corneal arcus

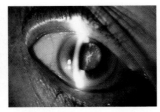

Central cataract formation seen with slit lamp
This can be due to steroid use or more commonly due to aging alone.

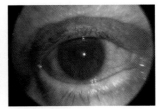

Thrombotic Glaucoma due to Diabetes:
The pupil is irregular, cornea suffused, abnormal mesh of vessels in the iris can be seen with difficulty (rubeosis iridis).

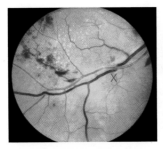

Branch Retinal Vein Occlusion:
At point X there is marked A-V nipping with thrombotic occlusion of the distal retinal vein. Lesions: haemorrhages, hard exudates

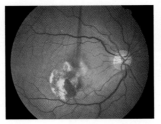

Macular degeneration with haemorrhage:
This will be associated with marked oedema Lesions: retinal scarring, haemorrhages

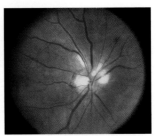

Myelinated Nerve Fibres:
This is a normal variant, enlargement of the blind spot is rarely clinically apparent. Lesion: myelinated nerve fibres

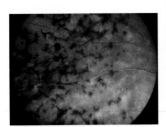

Retinitis Pigmentosa
Results in poor rod function with night blindness and tunnel vision. Lesions: spiculated peripheral lesions

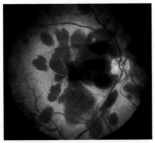

Severe Retinal Haemorrhage in Hyperviscosity Syndrome
Often due to myeloma and bleeding diatheses. Lesions: haemorrhages

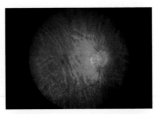

Tigroid retina with myopic crescent
The tiger skin appearance is a normal but striking variant. In myopia the elongated eyeball stretches the globe
Lesions: tigroid retina, myopic crescent

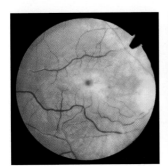

Central Retinal Artery Occlusion
This results in a pale retina and optic disc, the choroidal artery supply is still present and is seen as the "cherry red spot" (also seen in lipid storage disorders)

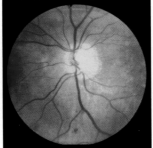

Cholesterol Embolus
Also known as a Hollenhorst Plaque, causes retinal TIA (amaurosis fugax). Embolus can originate from carotid artery, aortic valve or arch.

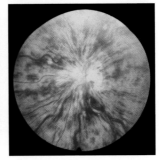

Central Retinal Vein Occusion
Retinal artery is patent and allows blood into the retinal but there is no outflow. Lesions: papilloedema, haemorrhages,

Endocrinology Clinical Picture Suite

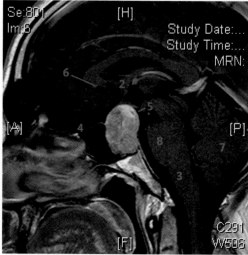

Anatomical labels:
1 Pituitary oedema
2 Pituitary stalk
3 Medulla oblongata
4 Sphenoidal sinus
5 Optic chiasm
6 Hypothalamus
7 Cerebellum
8 Pons

Clinical findings due to pituitary mass effect:
Bitemporal hemi-anopia
Diplopia
Reduced or absent corneal reflex
CSF rhinorrhoea
headaches

MRI Pituitary in patient with macro-adenoma prolactinoma

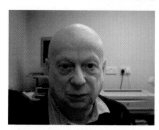

Alopecia universalis with hypothyroidism

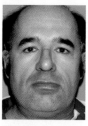

Acromegaly

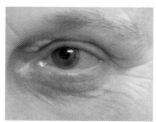

Xanthelasmata and corneal arcus

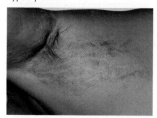

Axillary striae in Cushing's disease

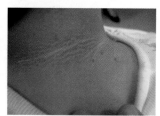

Acanthosis nigricans in PCOS

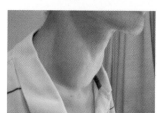

Large goitre in Graves' disease

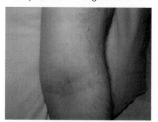

Eruptive xanthoma in familial hyperlipidaemia

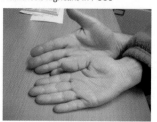

Carotinaemia due to hypothyroidism

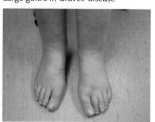

Pre-tibial myxoedema in Graves' Disease

Dermatology Picture Suite

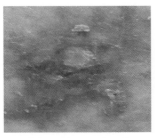

Bowen's disease (intra-epidermal carcinoma in-situ)

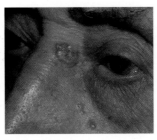

Basal cell carcinoma, in a common location.

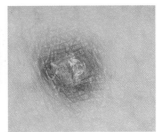

Histiocytoma

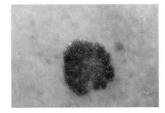

Malignant melanoma (superficial spreading type).

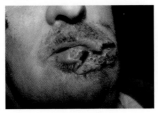

Squamous cell carcinoma

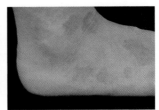

Granuloma annulare. Non-scaly erythematous rings.

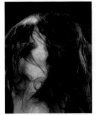

Alopecia areata.

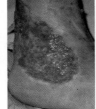

Venous leg ulceration.

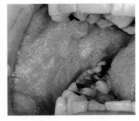

Lesions of lichen planus on the buccal mucosa.

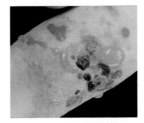

Bullous pemphigoid. Bullae (blisters) of various ages on the elbow, arising on an erythematous background.

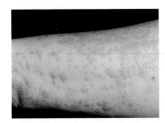

Lichen planus. Pink polygonal papules, becoming confluent in places, and demonstrating white lines on the surface (Wickham's striae).

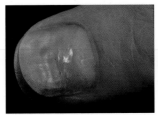

Psoriatic onycholysis.

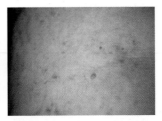

Dermatitis herpetiformis. Excoriated vesicles.

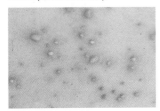

Chicken pox. Vesicles and pustules.

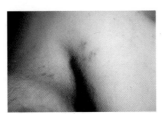

Chicken pox. Vesicles and pustules.

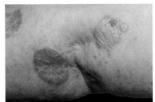

Psoriasis. Scaly, well marginated erythematous plaques on the elbow.

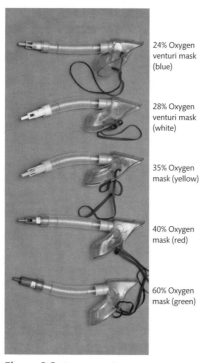

24% Oxygen
venturi mask
(blue)

28% Oxygen
venturi mask
(white)

35% Oxygen
mask (yellow)

40% Oxygen
mask (red)

60% Oxygen
mask (green)

Figure 9.2 Oxygen masks.

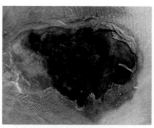

Necrotic (black coloured): debride remove eschar. Needs specialist care by either surgical team or a tissue viability nurse.

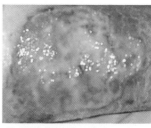

Sloughy (yellow coloured): remove slough, provide clean base for granulation tissue to develop.

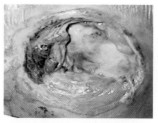

Infected (green coloured): manage infection and odour. Debride

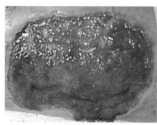

Granulation (red coloured): promote granulation. Provide base for epithelializing.

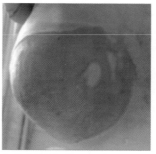

Epithelial (pink): allow wound maturation to continue.

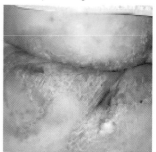

Excoriation/maceration: prevent progression to ulceration.

Figure 9.17 Wound classification and management.

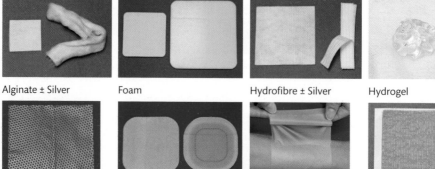

Alginate ± Silver

Foam

Hydrofibre ± Silver

Hydrogel

Non-adherent ± Silver

Hydrocolloid

Transparent non-adhesive dressing

Iodine impregnated

Figure 9.18 Examples of wound dressings.

- Kidney bowl, 50 mL purple enteral syringe, lubricating jelly or water, glass of water, pH paper, plaster or tape to secure, drainage bag or bag of enteral feed.
- Nasogastric tube: wide bore is for the removal of gastric contents, Narrow bore is for feeding purposes. Estimate the length of the tube required by the length from the bridge of the nose to the tragus of ear to the bottom of the xiphisternum. Usually 60 cm in adults.

Preparation

- If using a large bore tube, it is helpful to place the tube in the fridge for 30 minutes before use. This will make the tube rigid and easier to insert.
- Measure length of tube insertion necessary by measuring line from bridge of nose to tragus of ear then on down to xiphisternum.
- Sit patient upright and check patency of nostrils.
- It may also be helpful to ask the patient to blow their nose before starting.

Explanation and consent

Introduce yourself and gain consent from patient. Main points to emphasize are:
- State purpose of the tube. Use simple diagram or drawing.
- State specific reason in this patient and how long the tube is likely to remain *in situ*.
- State main steps. Show tube to patient.
- Explain procedure to patient including need to swallow and possible discomfort/gag as tube passes through oropharynx.
- State main risks and an idea of the prevalence.

Procedure

This is the insertion of the tube from the external nasal passage to the stomach. The tube is inserted backwards through the nostril and is passed horizontally beneath the inferior nasal concha into the nasopharynx. It then passes downwards through the oropharynx, and as the patient swallows the epiglottis closes closing off the entrance to the trachea and directing the tube into the oesophagus.

- Give the cup of water to patient and ensure that there is a vomit bowl to hand.
- Pass lubricated tube into nostril, aim horizontally backwards towards occiput, advance tube gently.
- Ask patient to take a sip of water and swallow when tube is felt at back of throat. Advance tube gently during swallow. Inspect oropharynx to ensure tube not coiled but passing straight down.
- Encourage patient to keep sipping and swallowing if this is uncomfortable.
- Stop passing tube when desired length of tube has been passed (from above estimate, usually at least 60 cm).

Post-procedure management

- Post procedure, explain to patient and carers what you have done and how the procedure was conducted (state problems if any).
- Aspirate fluid from tube. Confirm pH of less than 5.5 using pH paper. The colour change seen with litmus paper is not thought to be sensitive enough to distinguish between the acid pH of gastric contents and other fluids. For this reason, only pH paper is used.

- Secure NG tube to patient's nose/face using specially shaped adhesive dressing or use simple tape for skin. The tube position should be checked visually and functionally daily, especially to ensure that the position is correct. Check against record of length of tube inserted.
- Connect wide-bore NG tube to drainage bag and secure bag below the level of the patient's stomach to aid drainage. In some cases suction can be useful.
- Request plain chest film if needed according to local policy. Correct placement is confirmed by seeing that the radio-opaque tip of the NG tube is below the level of both diaphragms on a plain posteroanterior chest X-ray. X-Rays are used second line to pH paper testing.
- If the procedure fails, get senior help. Consider placement using mild sedation and endo-scopic placement.
- Always check position every time by checking pH and length before administering anything via NG tube.

Professionalism: working with colleagues

Inform key colleagues: nurses, dietitian, speech, and language therapist, other doctors, carers and family. Dietician may need to write up a feeding regimen and rota.

Write clear notes, e.g.:

- 'Insertion of naso-gastric tube
- Indication: Feeding post recent stroke. Assessed by speech and language therapist and NG tube advised.
- Procedure: Inserted on first passage after using standard procedure. No complications and patient comfortable. Record length of tube inserted.
- Post-procedure: Chest X-ray and pH paper test indicate that NG tube is in the correct position.

'Staff nurse informed and feeding plan written.'

Complications

- Traumatic discomfort for patient, affecting future care.
- Epistaxis, sinusitis, nasal trauma.
- Tracheal intubation: failure to recognize misplacement may lead to intrapulmonary place-ment of drugs, feeds, and other fluids.
- Tube coiling in nasopharynx, oropharynx, or laryngopharynx instead of passing downwards.
- Local trauma including ulceration over nose and face due to overzealous securing of NG tube.
- Rare: intracranial intubation through cribriform plate and intracranial placement, submucosal dissection in nasopharynx, serious bleeding, vocal cord paralysis, oesophageal perforation.
- Refeeding syndrome.

Refeeding syndrome

Refeeding syndrome is a phenomenon which can occur following enteral or parenteral feeding. During prolonged periods of starvation, there is utilization of fat and protein stores to produce energy. This leads to a loss of intracellular electrolytes and in particular a loss of phosphate. The sudden re-instigation of food leads to an increase in insulin which drives phosphate and potassium into cells, leading to electrolyte imbalance and particularly, hypophosphataemia and hypokalaemia.

Clinical consequences of the refeeding syndrome include massive oedema, cardiac failure, respiratory failure, hypotension, rhabdomyolysis, seizure, coma, and death. Patients who are known to have been without nutrition or present with a significant amount of unintentional weight loss should always prompt consideration of a risk for refeeding syndrome. There is a set of clinical indicators which can be used to identify patients at high risk. These are listed in the table below.

All patients at risk of re-feeding syndrome should have plasma levels of potassium, magnesium and phosphate checked. Any abnormal values must then be corrected prior to the administration of nutritional support. It is also advisable to measure serum calcium, urea and creatinine. Patients should then be fed according to the hospital protocol, initially at a reduced rate. Nutritional intake is gradually increased where further clinical and biochemical monitoring of the patient suggests there are no refeeding problems. Biochemical monitoring is indicated for at least 4 days.

Table 9.6 Patients at high risk of the refeeding syndrome

One of	Two of
● Body mass index (BMI) <16	● BMI <18.5
● Unintentional weight loss greater than 15% in past 3–6 months	● Unintentional weight loss greater than 10% in past 3–6 months.
● Little or no nutritional intake for 10 days	● Little or no nutritional intake for 5 days
● Low levels of potassium, magnesium or phosphate prior to feeding	● History of alcohol abuse or drugs including insulin, diuretics, chemotherapy, and antacids

NICE guidance (2006), *Nutrition Support in Adults.*

Patient safety tips

✔ **Anatomical course**: consider the anatomy of the route that the tube has to take. Check the back of the oropharynx after initial swallowing to ensure correct direction of tube. If no fluid is aspirated advance the tube 5 cm further and try again. Slow continuous sipping and swallowing can make the procedure more comfortable for the patient.

✔ **Always be suspicious that the tube is in the trachea**: until you have proven otherwise. A chest X-ray may be needed to confirm placement.

✔ **Measuring the pH of aspirate using pH indicator strips, not litmus paper**.

✔ **A chest X-ray is recommended to check placement**: but should not be used routinely. Local policies are recommended for particular groups of patients, e.g. intensive care units and neonates.

✔ **Fully radio-opaque NG tubes**: with markings will enable accurate measurement, identification and documentation of the position of the NG tube.

✔ **Do not use the 'whoosh' test**: previously 50 mL or so of air was injected and the epigastrium auscultated. A 'whoosh' was supposed to indicate correct placement. This was often not the case. This practice must cease immediately.

✔ **Do not interpret absence of respiratory distress as an indicator of correct positioning**.

✔ Review NG tube at least daily for position and whether it is still needed, if feeding via the NG tube, check position before every administration. Refer to the length of NG tube inserted.

Student name:	Medical school:	Year:

Nasogastric tube

How would you carry out nasogastric tube insertion on this mannikin/patient?
I will ask for answers based around some clinical headings and ask you to carry out the procedure.

		Self	Peer	Peer /tutor	Tutor
Background and clinical indications	• Understands indications: drain stomach	☐	☐	☐	☐
	• contents, prevent aspiration of gastric contents,	☐	☐	☐	☐
	• enteral feeding, drug therapy	☐	☐	☐	☐
Anatomical and physiological principles	• Nasopharynx: main structures, structures causing discomfort to patients	☐	☐	☐	☐
	• Oropharynx: main structures, complications	☐	☐	☐	☐
	• Laryngopharynx: main structures, complications, effect on patient	☐	☐	☐	☐
	• Oesophagus: muscle structure	☐	☐	☐	☐
Contraindications	• Base of skull fracture	☐	☐	☐	☐
	• Nasopharynx, oropharynx, laryngopharynx trauma or surgery	☐	☐	☐	☐
	• Coagulopathy: common examples, how tested	☐	☐	☐	☐
	• Nasopharyngeal tumours, oesophageal varices	☐	☐	☐	☐
Procedure	• Handwash with water and soap and alcohol gel; this is a clean technique, not aseptic	☐	☐	☐	☐
	• Personal protective clothing as appropriate	☐	☐	☐	☐
	• Introduction and identifies patient	☐	☐	☐	☐
	• Consent: informed of reason for NG tube and risks	☐	☐	☐	☐
	• Clear explanation: e.g. 'I am going to insert this tube via your nose down into your stomach. We will use this to feed you and stop you feeling sick'	☐	☐	☐	☐
	• Equipment selection: apron, non-sterile clean gloves, NG tube (adult sizes: aspiration 12–16), or small feeding tube. Kidney bowl and NG drainage bag, Lubricating jelly, glass of water, 50 mL enteral syringe and pH testing strips	☐	☐	☐	☐
	• Measures approximate length of tube, taking proximal end of tube from xiphisternum to bridge of nose, earlobe to xiphisternum	☐	☐	☐	☐
	• Sits patient upright with chin slightly forward and in line with the sternum, asks patient to blow nose	☐	☐	☐	☐
	• Explains to patient that they will need to swallow when specified to help the tube go down	☐	☐	☐	☐
	• Lubricates tube with water and inserts into a patent nostril. NG tube is gently advanced towards the occiput. Patient asked to swallow when they feel tube at the back of throat	☐	☐	☐	☐
	• The tube is advanced during the swallow, sipping water at this stage may help with this manoeuvre	☐	☐	☐	☐
	• To assess position, aspirates a few mL of gastric content and checks with pH testing strip or check chest X-ray	☐	☐	☐	☐
	• Attaches drainage bag or enteral feed. Ensures tube is secure	☐	☐	☐	☐
	• Good communication demonstrated throughout the procedure and allows patient to ask questions	☐	☐	☐	☐
Post-procedure management	• Documents procedure into clinical notes, including pH and length inserted	☐	☐	☐	☐
	• Tube length checks on daily basis, pH regularly, check pH each time tube is used	☐	☐	☐	☐
Professionalism: working with colleagues	• Communicates sensitively, thanks the patient, addresses any questions or concerns, washes hands	☐	☐	☐	☐
	• Completes all documentation legibly and unambiguously	☐	☐	☐	☐
	• Communicates appropriately with nursing staff	☐	☐	☐	☐
Complications	• Traumatic for patients, tracheal intubation, epistaxis	☐	☐	☐	☐
	• Misplacement of NG tube and intra-pulmonary placement of fluids, medication	☐	☐	☐	☐
	• Local trauma due to poor securing of tube onto nose/face	☐	☐	☐	☐
	• Rare: intracranial intubation, vocal cord paralysis, submucosal dissection, bleeding, oesophageal perforation	☐	☐	☐	☐
Patient safety tips	• Considers anatomical route that the NG tube has to take and watch out for misplacement	☐	☐	☐	☐
	• Checks position of tube before each use	☐	☐	☐	☐
	• Reviews need for NG tube daily	☐	☐	☐	☐
Global assessment	• Would you be happy for this student to be supervised to insert a nasogastric tube into a real patient?	Yes/No/Unsure			

		U B S E	U B S E	U B S E	U B S E
Self-assessed as at least borderline:	Signature:	Date:			
Peer-assessed as ready for tutor assessment:	Signature:	Date:			
Tutor-assessed as satisfactory:	Signature:	Date:			

Notes

285

9.10
Wound care and
diabetic foot ulcer
management

9.10 Wound care and diabetic foot ulcer management

Background

Leg ulcers affect around 2% of the population in the developed countries. In patients with diabetes mellitus, this is a significant cause of morbidity and mortality. Prevention is of paramount importance. This can be achieved by patient education and self-management, with regular comprehensive foot and leg examination of patients with diabetes. A patient with a septic diabetic leg ulcer admitted as an acute medical admission should rarely be seen. The admission can be prevented in the vast majority of cases by early aggressive treatment of any lower limb ulcers or infection.

Meticulous attention to preventing pressure sores and wound care, similarly, can reduce progression to more advanced wound lesions, sepsis, and even death.

This section will focus on diabetic lower limb ulcers and provide a brief overview of the principles of wound management.

Diabetic ulcers

Diagnosis: history of diabetes mellitus with neuropathy and/or peripheral vascular disease with presence of a leg ulcer. The ulcer can be painless because of the neuropathy. In the absence of severe neuropathy, ischaemic ulcers can be very painful.

Predisposing factors: Important predisposing factors for development of diabetic foot ulcers are smoking, peripheral vascular disease, neuropathy, poor glycaemic control, foot deformity and previous foot ulceration. A neuropathic joint (Charcot foot) is at particularly high risk of ulceration with poor potential heal completely.

Risk classification

Developed by the International Working Group on the Diabetic Foot for predicting risk of development of foot ulcers in patients with diabetes:

- **Group 0**: No evidence of neuropathy
- **Group 1**: Neuropathy present but no evidence of foot deformity or peripheral vascular disease (PVD)
- **Group 2**: Neuropathy with evidence of deformity or peripheral vascular disease
- **Group 3**: History of foot ulceration or lower extremity amputation.

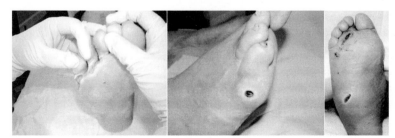

A macerated foot with multiple interdigital ulcers: earlier advice on prevention may have stopped this from occurring

A small, clean, innocuous-looking foot ulcer: must be treated aggressively to prevent progression to amputation

Charcot foot: note distortion of the arch and that an ulcer has developed at site of increased pressure

Figure 9.16 Images in diabetes foot disease.

Complications

Early aggressive management is essential. Osteomyelitis, amputation and death from sepsis are common complications of non-aggressively treated diabetic foot ulcers. The psychological and social complications, in a surviving patient, will be life-changing, for the worse.

Management

Phase 1 Initial management

History and examination

- History: duration of ulcer, whether painful or not.
- Previous treatment if any, smoking history in pack years, known macrovascular or microvascular complications of diabetes, trauma.
- Examination: assess for wound infection: erythema, warmth, pain, swelling, tenderness, pus discharge, systemic infection (fever, tachycardia, tachypnoea), assess for neuropathy with 10 g monofilament, feel foot and leg pulses for PVD ischaemia or gangrene.

Investigations

Wound swab for cultures, FBC, U&Es, CRP, HbA1c, lipid profile, B_{12}/folate, blood cultures if pyrexial, X-ray ulcer region (foot usually), Doppler studies if leg pulses absent, ankle–brachial blood pressures for ABPI (ankle-brachial pressure index). ABPI <0.8 indicates significant PVD.

Antimicrobial treatment

Antibiotic therapy is indicated for infected ulcers only or if there is cellulitis. Empirical antibiotic until wound swabs results are known. Antibiotics active against *Streptococcus* and anaerobes commonly used (such as amoxicillin, flucloxacillin, and metronidazole). Non-infected ulcers require local care or debridement.

Wound dressing

After local care and debridement, if granulating tissue is seen, simple dressings will usually suffice. The basic principles are to keep the ulcer clean and prevent it drying out. A non-adherent silicone jelly dressing would be adequate in most cases. This should be changed every 48–72 hours and the wound inspected and cleaned. Whenever possible, a tissue viability specialist nurse should be consulted for more expert advice.

Phase 2 Ongoing management

Maintain good glycaemic control

This affords the best circumstances for the wound to heal and systemic infection becomes less likely. If patient is systemically unwell and unable to take orally, consider insulin sliding scale. In many cases a long-acting background insulin with rapid-acting insulin at mealtimes will give similar excellent control (aim: glucose levels 4–7 mmol/L pre-meals and fasting).

Review antibiotic therapy

Use wound swab results to use most appropriate antibiotics. Consider route ? IV or will oral suffice? Antibiotics with a high degrees of tissue penetration such as rifampicin or clindamycin are often used after expert microbiological advice.

Investigations

Especially for ischaemic ulcers: Doppler studies, magnetic resonance angiography (MRA), then revascularization surgery or amputation. Magnetic resonance imaging (MRI) of the limb if osteomyelitis suspected.

Wound dressing

As above, a tissue viability specialist nurse should be involved at this stage for expert advice and review. Larval therapy, vacuum-assisted wound closure or hyperbaric oxygen therapy may also be considered to help accelerate healing of the ulcer.

Phase 3 Long-term management: alphabet strategy format

Advice

Ensure that the patient has been strongly advised to give up smoking, if current smoker. Offer help in terms of referral to smoking cessation services, information leaflets and telephone helplines. Also use simple behavioural change methods to help patient to change behaviour. Advice should also be given on physical activity, weight reduction if needed, and diet.

Blood pressure

Aim for blood pressure of 130/85 mmHg or less as the patient has complications and is likely to have PVD or existing other complications of diabetes.

Cholesterol control

Statin will be indicated in most patients with diabetes over the age of 40 years and others at high risk. Absolutely ensure excellent contraception in women of reproductive potential because of the risk of fetal malformation (or do not use statin). The usual aim is a total cholesterol ≤5 mmol/L (low-density lipoprotein [LDL]:high-density lipoprotein [HDL] ≤3). If there is cardiovascular disease (CVD), the total cholesterol target is ≤4 mmol/L (LDL:HDL ≤2).

Diabetes control

Aim for good glycaemic control (usually HbA1c ≤7.5%), This value must be individualized to the patient. In many patients a normal HbA1c will be the aim in other higher values will be safer.

Eye examination

Yearly with appropriate follow-up for ophthalmic opinion and laser therapy if indicated.

Feet examination

Annual comprehensive feet examination with close inspection, pulses (dorsalis pedis, posterior tibial), neuropathy testing (usually with a 10 g monofilament). Inspect for skin breaks, ulcers, fungal infection. A full assessment, if problems are detected would include testing vibration sense, proprioception, and temperature. Doppler studies and/or ABPI if absent pulses and consider referral to vascular surgeon for full assessment. Footcare and hygiene advice must be given: regular chiropody or podiatry to remove callus, no barefoot walking, comfortable shoes with no foot pressure areas, seek attention for any superficial ulcers, cellulitis, or fungal infections promptly.

Guardian drugs

Appropriate use of CVD and renal protective drugs such as aspirin, angiotensin-converting enzyme (ACE) inhibitors and statin (note: ACE inhibitors and angiotensin II antagonists are teratogenic and must not be used in women of reproductive potential without effective contraception).

General wound management

Objective

To allow the wound to heal in a moist environment unless maintenance of an eschar is clinically indicated in a dry and non-infected condition. Many of the general principles for treatment of the diabetic ulcer will apply.

Principles

- **Assessment of patient**: past medical history; current and past drugs; risk factors for wounding and delayed healing, e.g. nutrition, smoking, direct pressure.
- **Wound bed assessment**: should include: type of wound and its cause, location size, condition of wound bed (e.g. necrotic, slough, granulating), presence of infection, pain, odour or foreign body and the condition of surrounding skin.

Treatment

Employ local wound care unless there are signs of systemic infection, then use antibiotics.

Wound cleansing

The primary aim is to remove foreign materials and reduce the 'bio-burden' of dead and dying tissue/exudate and bacteria. Techniques used:

- **Aseptic technique** – used in immunocompromised patients or when a wound enters a sterile body cavity.
- **Clean wound technique** – washing or showering wound when aseptic technique not indicated. Potable tap water is suitable.

Wound classification and management

See Figure 9.17.

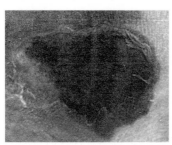

Necrotic (black coloured): debride remove eschar. Needs specialist care by either surgical team or a tissue viability nurse.

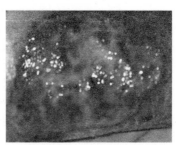

Sloughy (yellow coloured): remove slough, provide clean base for granulation tissue to develop.

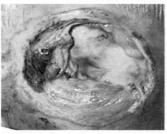

Infected (green coloured): manage infection and odour. Debride

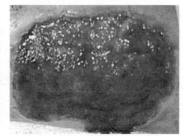

Granulation (red coloured): promote granulation. Provide base for epithilializing.

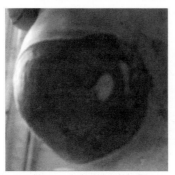

Epithelial (pink): allow wound maturation to continue.

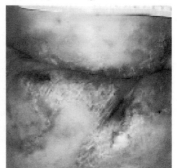

Excoriation/maceration: prevent progression to ulceration.

Figure 9.17 Wound classification and management. (See picture suite for colour version.)

Wound dressings

Choice of dressing depends on: type of wound; amount of exudate; condition of wound bed; presence or absence of infection; location of wound; patient's skin condition; characteristic of dressings available and treatment goals.

Types of wound dressing (Figure 9.18)

- **Hydrogel** (debridement of low exudate slough and necrosis). Allows dry wounds to rehydrate. Cover with film dressing to keep moist and warm to encourage autolytic debridement.
- **Alginate packing** (packing and absorption). For moderate exudate, leave in place to form a soft gel to encourage autolytic debridement of slough.
- **Hydrocolloid** (debridement of slough and necrosis). Promotes epithelial growth. Rehydrates dead tissue so encourages autolytic debridement.
- **Silicone sheet** (gentle protection/atraumatic removal). Gentle adhesion, not absorbent and allows exudate through pores to secondary absorbent dressing. Suitable for skin tears, abrasions, burns and blistering.
- **Hydrofibre** (packing and high absorption). For high levels of exudate. Allows light packing and forms a soft gel that encourages debridement of slough.
- **Povidine iodine** (antimicrobial). To prevent and treat infection. Certain contraindications may apply, e.g. hypersensitivity to iodine, renal disease, thyroid dysfunction.
- **Foam** (adhesive and non-adhesive components). Absorbs moderate amounts of exudate.
- **Transparent adhesive film**. Semipermeable allowing gas exchange. Used over blanching and non-blanching tissue to allow protection from friction and allow observation of tissues. Can also be used as a secondary dressing for a gel or alginate.

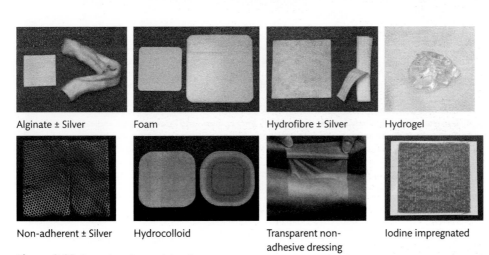

Alginate ± Silver   Foam   Hydrofibre ± Silver   Hydrogel

Non-adherent ± Silver   Hydrocolloid   Transparent non-adhesive dressing   Iodine impregnated

Figure 9.18 Examples of wound dressings.

Patient safety tips

- ✔ Most diabetes foot ulcers can be prevented by meticulous attention to all the main aspects of diabetes care, particularly patient education and self-management. Clinical expert is needed to manage all the other risk factors such as smoking and CVD risk indicators.
- ✔ Wound care poses a similar challenge. High standards of nursing, especially in relation to pressure ulcer prevention and treatment, will prevent breakdown of skin in most patients.
- ✔ Part of the general examination of a patient should be to look for pressure ulcers and skin breakdown and infection.
- ✔ Early and aggressive treatment with pressure-relieving mattresses and beds is vital.
- ✔ Early treatment with antibiotics, where indicated, will reduce the chances of the infection spreading systemically which has a very poor prognosis in the elderly.
- ✔ Seek expert opinion. In some cases maggot therapy or vacuum suction may be needed.

Student name:	Medical school:	Year:

Wound care and diabetic foot ulcer management

Your knowledge of wound care and diabetes foot ulcer management will be assessed.
You will also be asked to identify and discuss the use of some common dressings used locally.

		Self	Peer	Peer /tutor	Tutor
Diabetic ulcers	**How is a diabetes ulcer diagnosed?** History of diabetes with neuropathy ± PVD with presence of an ulcer	☐	☐	☐	☐
	What the predisposing factors for a diabetes ulcer? Smoking, PVD, neuropathy, poor glycaemic control, foot deformity, previous foot ulceration, Charcot joint	☐	☐	☐	☐
What is the risk classification for predicting risk of development of foot ulcers?	**Group 0:** No evidence of neuropathy	☐	☐	☐	☐
	Group 1: Neuropathy present but no evidence of foot deformity or PVD	☐	☐	☐	☐
	Group 2: Neuropathy with evidence of deformity or peripheral vascular disease	☐	☐	☐	☐
	Group 3: History of foot ulceration or lower extremity amputation	☐	☐	☐	☐
Phase 1 initial management	**What aspects of the history and examination should be considered?** duration of ulcer, ? painful, smoking history, macrovascular or microvascular complications, trauma, ? infection: erythema, warmth, pain, swelling, pus, systemic infection, neuropathy, pulses, gangrene	☐	☐	☐	☐
	What investigations should be considered? Swabs, FBC, U&Es, CRP, HbA1c, lipid profile, B_{12}/folate, blood cultures, X-ray, Doppler studies, ABPI	☐	☐	☐	☐
	Active against *Streptococcus*, *Staphylococcus*, and anaerobes such as amoxicillin, flucloxacillin, and metronidazole. Debridement.	☐	☐	☐	☐
	If granulating tissue is seen, simple dressings, keep ulcer clean and prevent it drying out. Consider non-adherent, silicone dressing	☐	☐	☐	☐
Phase 2 Ongoing management What are the main aspects of treatment?	Maintain good glycaemic control, review antibiotic therapy, consider further investigations, tissue viability nurse involvement	☐	☐	☐	☐
Phase 3 Long-term management What are the key aspects, use the Alphabet Strategy Format	**Advice:** smoking cessation advice, behavioural change methods, physical activity, weight, diet	☐	☐	☐	☐
	Blood pressure: Aim for 130/85 mmHg, discuss main agents that could be used				
	Cholesterol control: Statins, cholesterol ≤5 mmol/L (LDL:HDL ≤3). If CVD the total cholesterol target is ≤4 mmol/L (LDL:HDL ≤2)	☐	☐	☐	☐
		☐	☐	☐	☐
	Diabetes control: Good control (usually HbA1c ≤7.5%), individualized to the patient				
	Eye examination: Yearly, follow-up for ophthalmic opinion, and laser therapy if indicated	☐	☐	☐	☐
	Feet examination: annual with close inspection, pulses, neuropathy testing, skin breaks, ulcers, fungal infection, Doppler studies and/or ABPI if absent pulses and consider vascular referral	☐	☐	☐	☐
		☐	☐	☐	☐
	Guardian drugs: appropriate use of CVD and renal protective drugs such as aspirin, ACE inhibitors and statins (need to consider contraception in woman)	☐	☐	☐	☐
What is the objective of wound management?	To allow the wound to heal in a moist environment	☐	☐	☐	☐
What are the main principles in wound care?	Assessment of patient (past medical history; current and past drugs; risk factors) and wound bed assessment (type, cause, size, etc.)	☐	☐	☐	☐
How can wounds be cleaned?	**Aseptic technique** – in immunocompromised patients or when a wound spreads to a sterile body cavity	☐	☐	☐	☐
	Clean wound technique – washing or showering wound when aseptic technique not indicated. Potable tap water is suitable	☐	☐	☐	☐
What determines the choice of a wound dressing?	Type of wound; exudate; condition of wound bed; infection; location, patient's skin condition; characteristic of dressings, treatment goals	☐	☐	☐	☐
Please show and discuss some of these dressings	Simple gauze, amorphous hydrogels, hydrogel dressing, hydrocolloid dressing, alginate dressings, composite dressing, transparent film	☐	☐	☐	☐
What the main patient safety aspects in relation to wounds and ulcers?	Most diabetes foot ulcers can be prevented: by patient self-management and clinical care	☐	☐	☐	☐
	High standards of nursing prevents breakdown of skin in most patients	☐	☐	☐	☐
	Part of the general examination: look for pressure sores, skin breakdown/infection	☐	☐	☐	☐
	Early and aggressive treatment with pressure relieving mattresses and beds is vital	☐	☐	☐	☐
	Early treatment with antibiotics, where indicated, reduces systemic infection	☐	☐	☐	☐

		Self	Peer	Peer/tutor	Tutor
Self-assessed as at least borderline:	Signature:	Date:	U B S E	U B S E	U B S E	U B S E
Peer-assessed as ready for tutor assessment:	Signature:	Date:	U B S E	U B S E	U B S E	U B S E
Tutor-assessed as satisfactory:	Signature:	Date:	U B S E	U B S E	U B S E	U B S E

Notes

9.11 Blood glucose monitoring

Background

Blood glucose monitoring involves obtaining a small capillary blood sample from the finger which is then tested using a blood glucose monitor to ascertain the amount of glucose in the bloodstream at that time. Although there are several dozen blood glucose monitors available commercially, most use a signal generated by the reaction of glucose in the sample with glucose oxidase or hexokinase. Modern devices can measure glucose within 5 seconds with a variance of only ±5% in comparison to the biochemistry laboratory gold standard.

Other glucose sensors employing the transdermal, microdialysis, or open tissue micro-perfusion technique are currently under clinical development with a few recently released for clinical use. These glucose sensors referred are referred to as being non-invasive, but in reality they are minimally invasive and not truly non-invasive. They measure glucose concentration in the interstitial fluid of the skin or the subcutaneous tissue. Non-invasive optical glucose sensors exist and measure the characteristics of reflected light that are changed as the result of interacting with glucose. However, sufficient accuracy and precision remains a major issue precluding current widespread use.

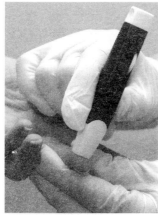
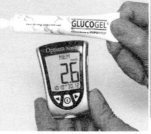
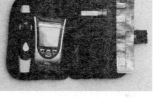
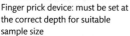

Finger prick device: must be set at the correct depth for suitable sample size

Modern meters only take a few seconds and can store several days' results as well

The full monitoring kit for patient use or ward use: testing strips, lancet device, monitor

Figure 9.19 Images in glucose monitoring.

Clinical indications

Patients with diabetes: the test is primarily used in the care and treatment of patients with both type 1 and type 2 diabetes mellitus. Almost all patients on insulin will check their glucose levels on a regular basis. This includes all patients with type 1 diabetes and those with type 2 diabetes on insulin. Many patients with type 2 diabetes and not on insulin will also monitoring glucose levels regularly to improve or maintain glycaemia and check for hypo- and hyperglycaemia. The testing regimen will differ depending on glycaemia control, insulin use, whether using glucose levels to change insulin doses, and many other factors. Meticulous control of glucose level is particularly important in gestational diabetes mellitus and regular, daily glocose monitoring is recommended, pre-meals and 1 hour after meals.

Emergency care: however, it is also a useful test to perform in any seriously ill patient and should be used as part of the A–E assessment. It is part of the 'E' or exposure. It can also be recalled as ABCDEFG: **A**irways, **B**reathing, **C**irculation, **D**on't **E**ver **F**orget **G**lucose!

Clinical principles

Type 1 diabetes

The patient needs insulin to live as the β-cells of the pancreas no longer produce insulin. There is a peak of onset in the early teens. Regular insulin injections are essential to life otherwise the patient will quickly decompensate and die from diabetic ketoacidosis. Regular and frequent monitoring of blood sugar levels allows the patient/carer and healthcare professional to tailor the insulin dose, diet, and physical activity to maintain near-normal blood glucose levels. The ideal blood glucose level is the normal physiological range, which is 4 –6 mmol/L fasting and pre-meals, or <7.9 mmol/L 2 hours after a meal. The HbA1c% value is used as measure of the average glycaemic control over the subsequent 60 days.

Type 2 diabetes

Type 2 diabetes is characterized by insulin resistance. Initially, there may be hyperinsulinaemia. With time, however, there is relative insulin deficiency and specific treatment required. Treatment is geared towards improving insulin action (metformin, 'glitazone'), augmenting insulin release from the β-cells of the pancreas (sulfonylureas), increasing glucagon-like peptide actin (gliptins and the injectable incretins) or using insulin itself in its many forms. Type 2 diabetes is a condition of middle to later life. However, in the obese and South Asian population it is frequently diagnosed in the late thirties and forties. There are now many children with type 2 diabetes in UK. Blood glucose monitoring is used to monitor 'trends' in the patient's blood glucose levels. It can also be used if the patient becomes symptomatic to confirm hypoglycaemia or hyperglycaemia.

Hypoglycaemia

Hypoglycaemia describes blood sugar levels. This can be caused by not enough food, too much medication, unplanned exercise such as housework or gardening. Alcohol and hot weather can also affect blood sugar levels.

Signs of hypoglycaemia

- **Mild**: shaking/trembling, pale and sweaty, irritable, hunger, tingling of mouth and fingers.
- **Moderate**: palpitations, tachycardia, confusion, irrational or uncontrolled behaviour, headache, and visual disturbance.
- **Severe**: loss of consciousness, seizure, coma.

Treatment

- Check for signs and symptoms, rest blood glucose levels.
- Give a quick-acting sugar, followed by a long-acting carbohydrate, e.g.:
  - ○ Three to four glucose tablets and a sandwich
  - ○ A small glass of Lucozade/fruit juice, and two plain biscuits
  - ○ Two teaspoons of sugar in a cup of tea and the next meal.
- Glucose gel can be inserted into the pouch of the mouth and massaged into the cheek. To do this the patient ideally must be cooperative and compliant.
- If the patient is unconscious, ABC is a priority, airway should be maintained and the patient put in the recovery position. The patient should then be given 75–100 mL of 20% glucose over 10–15 minutes or 150–200 mL of 10% glucose over 10–15 minutes. Repeat as necessary into large vein. Put up 10% dextrose infusion. Also consider IM glucagon.

Hyperglycaemia

Hyperglycaemia describes high blood sugar levels, usually above 13 mmol/L. This can be caused by too much food, not enough medication, lack of exercise, and especially any new illness such as infection or acute coronary syndrome. The patient may start to show ketones in their blood stream or urine if the blood sugar levels are elevated.

Signs of hyperglycaemia:

- Polydipsia, polyuria, tiredness, vomiting, abdominal pain, weight loss.

Treatment

- Check for signs and symptoms and test blood glucose levels
- Check urine for ketones and treat for diabetic ketoacidosis or hyperosmolar hyperglycaemic state.

Contraindications

The one question that needs to be considered is: will the glucose reading obtained be accurate and clinically relevant? If the patient is peripherally shut down or has dirty or food residue on the fingers then the result can be highly erroneous. In these cases only a blood sample will suffice.

Equipment

- Gloves, apron, tray for all the necessary equipment.
- Glucose monitoring device in good working order, not stained with blood!
- Lancet to obtain finger-prick blood sample.
- Ensure monitor is quality controlled and calibrated.
- Check expiry dates on the glucose monitoring strips.

Explanation and consent

- Clearly explain what you going to do and why.
- State the main steps involved.
- Obtain verbal consent.
- Position patient comfortably, arm hanging below level of the heart will serve to engorge the finger circulation.

Procedure

Obtaining a blood glucose sample from the patient/subject.

- **Wash hands, don gloves**:
- **Place test strip**: into the blood glucose monitor.
- **Load lancet device**: set for correct depth of penetration of skin.
- **Identify suitable site for pricking the skin**: the side of a finger is generally used. Other sites can also be used such as the heel in a baby. Ensure site is clean – there is no need to clean the site unless visibly unclean. Wash patient's hand if contaminated with food or drink. Note that the thumb and index are more sensitive than other fingers. The finger-print area is the most sensitive.
- **Warn the patient that they will feel a sharp scratch**.
- **Fire lancet and obtain a drop of blood. Place blood drop onto the test strip**. Offer tissue to patient to hold onto site of puncture. Ask patient to hold hand higher if bleeding.
- **Blood glucose monitor then tests the blood** and gives a reading of the blood glucose level on the screen. This can take between 5 and 30 seconds.
- **Record glucose level immediately**.
- **Dispose of sharps and other disposable equipment safety**.
- **Act on any abnormal values**.

Working with colleagues

● Inform nursing staff if needed. The monitoring regimen may need to be adjusted for example. Advise on time of next test.

Patient safety tips

✔ **Not checking glucose levels**: so frequently in clinical practice glucose testing is forgotten in an emergency. This can result in rapid decompensation and death. This is both in the case of hypoglycaemia or hyperglycaemia.

✔ **Not acting aggressively when hypoglycaemia or hyperglycaemia is diagnosed**: The glucose level is often corrected by appropriate management which is then not followed up resulting the same problem arising again. A clear plan of management must be outlined for hypoglycaemia and hyperglycaemia.

✔ Adjustment to the patient's treatment may be needed to prevent future hypo-or hyperglycaemia.

Student name:	Medical school:	Year:

Blood glucose monitoring

Please can you monitor this patient's/manikin's blood glucose level and interpret the result?

		Self	Peer	Peer /tutor	Tutor
Washes hands	● Handwash with soap and water using the Ayliffe technique	☐	☐	☐	☐
	●	☐	☐	☐	☐
Understands indications and anatomy	● The student is able to name three situations where blood glucose monitoring is required	☐	☐	☐	☐
	● Asks the patient for the preferred site for the fingerprick test. (Does **not** use thumb or index finger)	☐	☐	☐	☐
	●	☐	☐	☐	☐
Obtains informed consent	● Introduction and ensures they have the correct patient by checking both verbally and against wrist band	☐	☐	☐	☐
	● Gains informed consent	☐	☐	☐	☐
	●	☐	☐	☐	☐
Explanation to patient, often including complications	● Gives a clear explanation, e.g.: 'I need to prick your finger to check your blood sugar levels. You will feel a sharp scratch from the needle. I will then test a drop of your blood'	☐	☐	☐	☐
	●	☐	☐	☐	☐
Communication skills	● Assessment throughout the procedure, allows patient to ask questions	☐	☐	☐	☐
	●	☐	☐	☐	☐
Appropriate preparation	● Selects equipment	☐	☐	☐	☐
	● Checks machine has been quality controlled tested for that day	☐	☐	☐	☐
	● Checks expiry date on test strips	☐	☐	☐	☐
	● Cleans patient's hands with soap and water. Does *not* use alcohol wipe	☐	☐	☐	☐
	●	☐	☐	☐	☐
Technical ability especially with any special equipment and sharps	● Washes hands using the Ayliffe technique	☐	☐	☐	☐
	● Dons apron and gloves	☐	☐	☐	☐
	● Ensures patient's hands are warm and clean	☐	☐	☐	☐
	● Asks patient preferred fingerprick site	☐	☐	☐	☐
	● Prepares blood glucose monitor, inserts test strip and checks calibration	☐	☐	☐	☐
	● Rests patients arm on a firm surface	☐	☐	☐	☐
	● Performs fingerprick using a disposable lancet	☐	☐	☐	☐
	● Does not use finger pads, does not use index finger or thumb	☐	☐	☐	☐
	● Immediately disposes lancet into the sharps bin	☐	☐	☐	☐
	● Puts blood onto test strip, states would not squeeze finger	☐	☐	☐	☐
	● Offers patient a tissue for finger	☐	☐	☐	☐
	● Reads results	☐	☐	☐	☐
	● Disposes of all contaminated equipment appropriately	☐	☐	☐	☐
	● Washes hands using the Ayliffe technique	☐	☐	☐	☐
	●	☐	☐	☐	☐
Aseptic technique	● Appropriate cleansing of the site. Does not use alcohol wipe	☐	☐	☐	☐
	● Understands need for disposal of sharps and other waste materials	☐	☐	☐	☐
	●	☐	☐	☐	☐
Seeks help as appropriate	● Discusses implications of test results. Is able to recognize hypo and hyperglycaemia and can give appropriate advice	☐	☐	☐	☐
	●	☐	☐	☐	☐
Post-procedure management	● Documents in patient's notes results of test	☐	☐	☐	☐
	● Offers appropriate advice according to blood results obtained	☐	☐	☐	☐
	●	☐	☐	☐	☐
Professionalism	● Communicate to patient re: procedure and need for test	☐	☐	☐	☐
	● Allows patient opportunity to ask questions	☐	☐	☐	☐
	● Thanks patient	☐	☐	☐	☐
	● Considers change in medication for patient	☐	☐	☐	☐
	●	☐	☐	☐	☐
Overall ability to perform procedure	● Assess globally, would you be happy for this student to be supervised monitoring blood glucose levels on a real patient?	☐	☐	☐	☐
	●	☐	☐	☐	☐

				Self	Peer	Peer /tutor	Tutor
Self-assessed as at least borderline:	Signature:	Date:		U B S E	U B S E	U B S E	U B S E
Peer-assessed as ready for tutor assessment:	Signature:	Date:		U B S E	U B S E	U B S E	U B S E
Tutor-assessed as satisfactory:	Signature:	Date:		U B S E	U B S E	U B S E	U B S E

Notes

Suite 3 Emergency skills

Unit 10 Emergency life support skills

10.1 Approach to the acutely ill patient

Background

The ability to recognize serious illness, and to effectively treat it, is an essential skill for most clinicians and especially newly qualified doctors. The primary assessment often adopts an ABCDE approach which immediately allows the clinician to resuscitate and provide early management in a logical way that maximizes patient safety. After the patient has been stabilized, a more detailed secondary examination of the patient and their clinical notes should be done to make an accurate diagnosis. The immediate aim is to make the patient safe for ongoing care, with early appropriate intervention and calling for help.

The ABCDE approach

A rapid assessment is made by evaluating the patient with the key point of moving from one stage to the other only after correcting life-threatening events at that particular stage.

Initial approach

- **Ask the patient 'How are you?'**. A normal verbal response means that the patient has an intact airway, is breathing, and his brain is adequately perfused. If patient can speak only a few words or phrases/sentences then there is likelihood of severe respiratory distress.
- **Get help**: pulse oximetry, blood pressure measurement, electrocardiographic (ECG) monitor
- **If there is no response or reduced response**: this indicates serious illness and you should fully assess in seconds.
- **Use ABCDE approach**: Airway, Breathing, Circulation, Disability, Exposure.

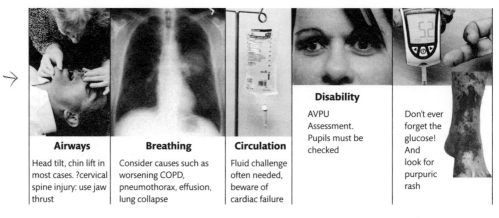

| **Airways** | **Breathing** | **Circulation** | **Disability** | |
| Head tilt, chin lift in most cases. ?cervical spine injury: use jaw thrust | Consider causes such as worsening COPD, pneumothorax, effusion, lung collapse | Fluid challenge often needed, beware of cardiac failure | AVPU Assessment. Pupils must be checked | Don't ever forget the glucose! And look for purpuric rash |

Figure 10.1 Images in ABCDE assessment. Exposure component requires a thorough inspection (examination of the whole body).

Airway in ABCDE approach

Look

- Obstruction: blood, vomit, secretions, tongue, foreign body, dentures, neck constriction (collar, rope etc)
- Symmetrical movement of both sides of chest ? chest deformity
- ? paradoxical see-saw abdomen/chest movement (normally chest/abdomen move outwards in expiration and vice versa, in complete or near-complete airway obstruction chest/abdomen moves in on inspiration and outwards on expiration
- ? use of accessory muscles of respiration (sternocleidomastoid and muscles of the neck, back and shoulder girdle).
- Sweating and central cyanosis.

Feel

- Presence of air movement at the mouth by placing your face or hand immediately in front of the patient's mouth. Caution advised in viral illnesses, chemical inhalation.
- Position of the trachea in the suprasternal notch as deviation to one side may be due to tension pneumothorax, lung fibrosis or pleural fluid.
- Surgical emphysema or crepitus (assume that this is pneumothorax until proved otherwise).
- Percuss the chest as hyper-resonance indicates pneumothorax, dull percussion note may be due to pleural fluid.

Listen at mouth and nose

- In complete upper airway obstruction, there are no breath sounds at the mouth or nose.
- In partial airway obstruction, air entry is diminished and often noisy.
- **Snoring**: occurs when there is partial obstruction of the pharynx by the tongue.
- **Crowing**: occurs when there is laryngeal spasm.
- **Inspiratory stridor**: occurs when there is obstruction at or above the level of the larynx.
- **Expiratory wheeze** when there is airways collapse during expiration.
- **Rattling sounds** occur when there are secretions in the airways.

Emergency care

An intact airway is essential to life! An obstructed airway is a medical emergency.

- Call for expert help immediately.
- Clear obstruction: suction to help clear blood, vomit, secretions, tongue, foreign body. Retrieve dentures if obstructing otherwise leave in.
- Clear airway: simple methods of airway clearance usually suffice, e.g. head tilt and chin lift or jaw thrust if cervical injury suspected. Airway suction and insertion of an oropharyngeal (Guedel) or nasopharyngeal airway will suffice.
- Surgical cricothyroidotomy: rarely is indicated, by a trained individual.
- Oxygen at high concentration: use a facemask with an oxygen reservoir. Ensure that the oxygen flow rate is sufficient (usually 10–15 L/min) to prevent collapse of the oxygen reservoir during inspiration. This system will deliver approximately 85% oxygen.
- Support breathing if absent or inadequate using bag-valve-mask, 10–12 breaths per minute.

Check that the oxygen saturation is improving and move on rapidly to assess breathing.

Breathing in ABCDE approach

Respiratory rate

The normal respiratory rate is between 12 and 20 breaths per minute. Tachypnoea is a valuable sign of early crisis so must be recorded accurately.

Now that the airway is secure, there is time to think about the breathing – seconds only! Compare right and left expansion, depth of breathing, tracheal position, ? paradoxical breathing

- **Tension pneumothorax**: tracheal away from side of pneumothorax, hypo-resonant, suitable history or injury.
- **Effusion**: dullness to percussion, trachea away from effected side.
- **Collapse**: dullness to percussion, trachea towards the side of collapse.

Emergency care

Pulse oximetry on high-flow oxygen:

If pneumothorax diagnosed then consider treatment with wide-bore venous cannula in second intercostal space midclavicular line. Expert help will be needed in most cases.

Consider arterial blood gases

If any of the following three, consider urgent expert assessment for non-invasive ventilation or endotracheal (ET) intubation and ventilation:

1 Saturations less than 90% on high-flow oxygen
2 Respiratory acidosis: pH <7.3, $PaCO_2$ >6.0 kPa
3 Failure of oxygenation: $PaCO_2$ <8.0 kPa.

Further details are given in Section 11.3.

Circulation in ABCDE approach

Circulation assessment

- **Blood pressure** (absolute value and any change from recent more stable state).
- **Pulse**: tachycardia >100, bradycardia <60.
- **Capillary return**: ? cool, cyanosed, mottled skin centrally and peripherally suggesting poor perfusion. Capillary refill time (less than 2–3 seconds).
- **Peripheral temperature and peripheral pulses**.
- **Major pulses**: assessment of both radials/brachials/carotids pulses and aorta.
- **Urine output** in the last 4 hours.

Notes

- **A thready pulse suggests a poor cardiac output. A bounding pulse may indicate sepsis.** Pulse rate >120 is abnormal.
- Measure the capillary refill time (CRT). Apply cutaneous pressure for 5 seconds on a fingertip held at heart level. Count the time in seconds that it takes for capillary refill (colour to return to the compressed area) once the pressure has been released. Usually, CRT is less than 2 seconds. Remember that CRT may be affected by the environmental temperature.

Normal blood pressure:

- Systolic 90–140 mmHg
- Diastolic 60–90 mmHg
- Normal pulse is less than the systolic.

Tachycardia + hypotension = SHOCK.

Shock is a multifactorial syndrome resulting in inadequate tissue perfusion and tissue oxygenation.

Emergency care

- **Fluid challenge**: most patients will respond initially. In all cases, insert one or more large (14–16G) intravenous cannulae. Use short, wide-bore cannulae, as they have the highest flow rate.

- **Take bloods** from the cannula for routine investigations; full blood count (FBC), urea and electrolytes (U&Es), coagulation, blood culture and blood grouping and ? cross-matching.

- **Attach the fluid and give a rapid fluid challenge** (over 5–10 minutes). Ideally warmed but do not wait:

  ○ 500 mL of crystalloid solution, if the patient has a systolic blood pressure>100 mmHg

  ○ 1000 mL of crystalloid solution, if the patient has a systolic blood pressure<100 mmHg

  ○ 250 mL of crystalloid solution, if pre-existing cardiac failure.

- **Reassess and document pulse rate and blood pressure** regularly (every 5 minutes), watching for signs of improvement (decrease in pulse rate, increase in blood pressure, increase in level of consciousness).

- **Urinary catheter**: Urine output 0.5–1.0 mL/kg/hour. Keep an accurate input/output fluid balance record.

- **Cardiac failure**: closer monitoring; listen to the chest for crepitations after each bolus, consider a central venous pressure (CVP) line and if possible an arterial line. If cardiac failure (dyspnoea, increased heart rate, raised jugular venous pressure [JVP], pulmonary crepitations), fluid infusion rate should be reduced or stopped.

- No signs of improvement, repeat fluid challenge. Consider:

  ○ Massive or ongoing blood loss

  ○ Septic shock

  ○ Cardiogenic shock.

Seek expert help as alternative means of improving tissue perfusion will be required:

- Inotropes to increase myocardial contractility (e.g. dobutamine)

- Vasodilators to reduce after load

- Nitrates or diuretics to reduce the preload to the left ventricle.

Consider arterial blood gases? metabolic acidosis: acidosis (pH <7.35) with raised lactate in circulation collapse with base excess greater than 2 and lactate greater than 2 mmol/L.

Disability in ABCDE approach

Assessment

Disability assessment is basically a global assessment from a neurological standpoint with the usual addition of a glucose assessment at the bedside and lab value:

AVPU score: record best response

- Alert

- Responsive to Voice

- Responsive to Pain

- Unresponsive.

Glasgow Coma Scale (Figure 10.2)

Glasgow Coma Scale		Best response
Eye opening	1: None, eyes closed	
	2: To pain, on limbs or trunk	
	3: To voice	
	4: Spontaneous with blinking	
Motor response	1: None	
	2: Extensor	
	3: Abnormal flexor response	
	4: Withdrawal	
	5: Localizing to pain	
	6: Obeys commands	
Verbal response	1: No vocalization	
	2: Incomprehensible vocalization	
	3: Inappropriate correct words	
	4: Confused speech	
	5: Orientated speech	
Record best response	Score record as Ex My Vz	

Figure 10.2 Glasgow Coma Scale (GCS). Highest GCS score is 15 and the lowest 3. Patients in a coma have a GCS score of 8 or less; they have no eye-opening (1), have no recognizable speech (2), and do not obey commands (5).

Pupils

Look at the pupils and check their size and reactivity to light:

- **Small, pinpoint pupils and reactive**: opioids, pontine haemorrhage
- **Mid-sized, unreactive**: midbrain lesion
- **Widely dilated, unreactive**: severe brain ischaemia, hypoglycaemia, brainstem lesion, postictal, tricyclic antidepressant drug overdose, recent intravenous administration of adrenaline
- **Unilateral dilatation, unreactive**: intracerebral haemorrhage/haematoma, cerebral infarction with oedema.

Emergency care

Treat the underlying cause:

Hypoglycaemia (glucose less than 3.5 mmol/L): correct with

- 25–50 mL of 50% glucose
- Consider glucagon 1 mg intramuscularly

Most hypoglycaemic attacks outside of a critical emergency can be managed by oral intake of glucose as a drink or sweet snack followed by a mixed carbohydrate (CHO) snack.

Hyperglycaemia due to diabetic ketoacidosis or hyperosmolar hyperglycaemic state should be considered: often missed.

Drug chart: check for reversible drug-induced causes of depressed consciousness.

Drug appropriate antagonist, where available, e.g.:

- Naloxone for opioids.
- Flumazenil for benzodiazepines.

Exposure in ABCDE approach

Urgent observations

- blood pressure, pulse, respiratory rate, temperature, oxygen saturations (modified early warning score [MEWS])
- Urine output: 'output' from body: bleeding, discharge, secretion.

History

Full history is essential from healthcare professionals, clinical notes and family. Drug chart must be reviewed together with charts on IV fluid infusion or blood transfusion. Usually a quick physical examination will need to be undertaken to diagnose or exclude the main causes of acute illness.

Examination

Full general and systems examination:

- ABCDE and pupils as above but specifically look for signs of meningitis: purpuric rash, neck stiffness
- Look at wounds and all drains and any intervention sites, e.g. venous cannulae, urinary catheter, CVP line, central line, arterial line, etc.

Emergency care

Treat the underlying cause.

Investigations

- **Standard blood tests**: U&Es, glucose, FBC, liver function tests, calcium
- **Other blood tests**: consider coagulation screen especially if bleed, ? blood culture and ? blood grouping and ? cross-matching ? thyroid function ? plasma osmolality ? lactate level.
- **ECG and cardiac monitoring**.
- **Arterial blood gases**: needed in many cases
- **Other investigations will be dictated by the differential diagnosis that you are considering**: Chest X-ray, cranial computed tomography (CT), toxicology screen, lumbar puncture (LP) commonly needed.

Other general aspects of care

- **Urine output**: Oliguria is usually defined as less than 0.5 mL/kg per hour.
- ? Urinary catheter blocked, irrigate or replace.
- Review medication list and medical history to elicit potential factors causing acute renal failure (ARF): stop any agents that could contribute. (e.g. diclofenac/gentamicin).
- Consider the i:Think xyz approach to differential diagnoses in an acutely ill patient.

Box 10.1 The i:Think xyz approach to diagnosing acute illness.

i	**In the head:**
	Stroke: cerebral, brainstem
	Cerebral bleed especially subarachnoid
	Meningitis, encephalitis
	Epileptic seizure
	Alcohol or illicit drugs
	Poisoning: carbon monoxide, overdose, e.g. paracetamol, tricyclics, opioids
T	**Thorax:**
	Respiratory tract infection
	Pneumothorax
	Pulmonary embolus
H	**Heart and vascular:**
	Acute coronary syndrome
	Cardiac failure
	Deep vein thrombosis or pulmonary embolism
	Severe hypotension or severe hypertension with encephalopathy
	Arterial insufficiency or occlusion:
I	**Infections, inflammation, injury:**
	Infections: sepsis (e.g. urinary tract infection, cellulitis, cholecystitis), malaria
	Abscess
	Meningitis
	Trauma: fracture, tissue injury, burns, hypothermia, heat stroke
	Anaphylaxis or allergic reaction
N	**Na, K, glucose, Ca, cortisol, thyroid**
	Acidosis or alkalosis
	Hypoglycaemia or hyper
	Hypokalaemia or hyper
	Hyponatraemia or hyper (metabolic encephalopathy)
	Addison's
	Hypocalcaemia or hyper
	Thyrotoxic crisis
K	**Kidney and abdomen:**
	Acute abdomen
	Acute renal failure
	Acute liver failure
	Bleed: gastrointestinal tract, aortic aneurysm
XYZ	**Other causes not covered above**

Patient safety tips

✔ **No short cuts**: There are no short cuts in assessing an ill patient. The above assessment needs to be carried out diligently with senior support called for as needed.

✔ **Review patient's notes**: as clue to diagnosis and management especially expressions of patient's wishes, do-not-attempt resuscitation (DNAR) orders, organ donation.

✔ **Focus on specific important systems**: for example the abdomen post laparotomy.

✔ **Medication**: check that medication prescribed has actually been administered.

✔ **Review results**: review results of laboratory tests. X-ray for aspiration pneumonia, international normalized ratio (INR) in patients on warfarin.

✔ **Drain and catheters**: look at these for information and complications, for example bleeding from an urinary catheter.

✔ **Seek appropriate help early**: for example from senior colleague, emergency assessment team. Assess need for high dependency care, intensive care unit early as possible.

Assessment of the acutely ill patient: ABCDE approach

A 29-year-old woman has been brought in by ambulance having fallen off a ladder whilst decorating her house. Her partner gives a history of seeing the patient painting the ceiling and 20 minutes or so later hearing a crashing sound of a ladder falling over. The patient is brought into Accident and Emergency on a stretcher by the ambulance crew.

This assessment will be based around a discussion on the assessment of the acutely ill patient with reference to above scenario.

		Self	Peer	Peer/tutor	Tutor
What is your initial approach to the patient?	• **Ask the patient** 'How are you?', **Get help**: oximetry, blood pressure, ECG	☐	☐	☐	☐
	• **If there is no response or reduced response**: fully assess in seconds	☐	☐	☐	☐
	•	☐	☐	☐	☐
What do the letters in the ABCDE Approach stand for?		☐	☐	☐	☐
What are the main aspects of airway assessment and management?	• **Look**: (? obstruction, ? chest deformity, ? paradoxical see-saw, ?cyanosis)	☐	☐	☐	☐
	• **Feel**: (? presence of air movement, ? trachea position, ? surgical emphysema or crepitus)	☐	☐	☐	☐
	• **Listen at mouth and nose**: (no sounds complete obstruction, snoring, crowing, stridor or wheeze, rattling sounds	☐	☐	☐	
	• **Clear airway**: head tilt and chin lift or jaw thrust if cervical injury suspected, airway suction and insertion of an oropharyngeal (Guedel) or nasopharyngeal airway	☐	☐	☐	☐
	• **Clear obstruction**: suction to clear blood, vomit, secretions, tongue, foreign body	☐	☐	☐	☐
	• **Oxygen at high concentration**: use a face mask with an oxygen reservoir	☐	☐	☐	☐
	•	☐	☐	☐	☐
What are the main aspects of breathing assessment and management?	• **Respiratory rate**: normal 12 to 20 breaths per minute	☐	☐	☐	☐
	• **Compare expansion right and left, depth of breathing, tracheal position**: ? tension pneumothorax (tracheal away from side of pneumothorax), ? effusion (dullness to percussion), ?collapse (dullness to percussion, trachea towards the side of collapse)	☐	☐	☐	☐
	• **Pulse oximetry** on high-flow oxygen	☐	☐	☐	☐
	• If pneumothorax diagnosed: consider treatment with wide-bore venous cannula in second intercostal space midclavicular line. Seek expert help in most cases	☐	☐	☐	☐
	• **Consider arterial blood gases**	☐	☐	☐	☐
	• **Urgent expert assessment for non-invasive ventilation or ET intubation if any of**: saturations less than 90% on high-flow oxygen or respiratory acidosis: pH <7.3, $PaCO_2$ >6.0 kPa or Failure of oxygenation: PaO_2 <8.0 kPa	☐	☐	☐	☐
	•	☐	☐	☐	☐
What are the main aspects of circulation assessment and management?	• **Blood pressure, pulse, capillary return, peripheral temperature and pulses, major pulses, urine output**. Remember: **tachycardia + hypotension=SHOCK**.	☐	☐	☐	☐
	• **IV access and fluid challenge**: wide-bore cannulae, as they have the highest flow rate.	☐	☐	☐	☐
	• **Bloods**: FBC, U&Es, coagulation, blood culture and blood grouping, ? cross-matching	☐	☐	☐	☐
	• **Reassess and document pulse rate and blood pressure** regularly (every 5 minutes), watching for signs of improvement	☐	☐	☐	☐
	• **Urinary catheter**: Very helpful. Output 50–100 mL/hr suggests adequate perfusion	☐	☐	☐	☐
	• **Cardiac failure**: closer monitoring, listen to chest for crepitations after each fluid bolus. Seek expert help: ? inotropes, vasodilators, nitrates or diuretics	☐	☐	☐	☐
	• **Consider arterial blood gases**	☐	☐	☐	☐
	•	☐	☐	☐	☐
What are the main aspects of 'disability' assessment and management?	• **Disability assessment** is a global assess from a neurological standpoint with the usual addition of a glucose assessment at the bedside and lab value	☐	☐	☐	☐
	• **AVPU score: record best response** (?Alert, ?responsive to Voice, ?responsive to Pain, ?Unresponsive	☐	☐	☐	☐
	• **Glasgow Coma Scale and pupil responses**	☐	☐	☐	☐
	• **Glucose level**	☐	☐	☐	☐
	• **Treat the underlying cause**: Hypoglycaemia (glucose less than 3.5 mmol/L): correct with 25–50 mL of 50% glucose, consider glucagon 1 mg intramuscularly. Hyperglycaemia (?DKA); drug chart (?reversible causes); drug-appropriate antagonist (naloxone for opioids, flumazenil for benzodiazepines)	☐	☐	☐	☐
	•	☐	☐	☐	☐

What are the main aspects of 'exposure' assessment?	• **Urgent observations**: blood pressure, pulse, respiratory rate, temperature, oxygen saturations (MEWS), urine output, 'output' from body: bleeding, discharge, secretion	☐	☐	☐	☐
	• **Clinical history**: Full history is essential from all sources. Drug chart, intravenous fluid infusion, blood transfusion charts must be reviewed.	☐	☐	☐	☐
	• **Clinical examination**: full general and systems examination. Look for signs of meningitis: purpuric rash, neck stiffness Look at wounds and all drains and any intervention sites, e.g. venous cannulae, urinary catheter, CVP line, central line, arterial line	☐	☐	☐	☐
	•	☐	☐	☐	☐
What will be the main conditions that need to be considered in the clinical vignette?		☐	☐	☐	☐
What are the other main causes of acute illness? Use the i: Think xyz mnemonic	• in the head, Thorax, Heart and vascular, Infection/inflammation/injury, Na etc, Kidney and Abdomen, xyz.	☐	☐	☐	☐
	•	☐	☐	☐	☐
What are the aspects of patient safety in relation to assessment using the ABCDE approach?	• **No shortcuts**: review patient's notes, focus on specific important systems, medication review	☐	☐	☐	☐
	• **Review results**: laboratory tests, X-ray	☐	☐	☐	☐
	• **Drain and catheters**: look for information and complications: e.g. bleeding from urinary catheter	☐	☐	☐	☐
	• **Seek appropriate help early:** ? emergency assessment team, ? high dependency care, intensive care unit early as possible.	☐	☐	☐	☐
	•	☐	☐	☐	☐

			U B S E	U B S E	U B S E	U B S E
Self-assessed as at least borderline:	Signature:	Date:				
Peer-assessed as ready for tutor assessment:	Signature:	Date:				
Tutor-assessed as satisfactory:	Signature:	Date:				

Notes

10.2 Adult basic life support

Background

Adult basic life support is a sequence of interventions that is used in the out of hospital environment for victims in cardiac arrest. The sequence is based around the assumption that a single rescuer, usually without resuscitation equipment, will perform the rescue. By providing basic life support (BLS) the rescuer is aiming to ensure that the victim receives adequate perfusion and ventilation until emergency services arrive at the scene. The emergency service will then assume responsibility and transfer the victim to hospital. Bystander cardiorespiratory resuscitation (CPR) will slow down the rate of deterioration of the brain, heart, and other key organs and increase the victim's chances of survival.

Basic life support

Safety

Safety for the rescuer, bystanders, and victim should be considered as being of paramount importance. If possible the victim should be assessed and resuscitated where found.

Procedure

The sequence follows the BLS algorithm recommended by the Resuscitation Council (UK), which is based on the latest International Consensus on CPR and Emergency Cardiovascular Care Science with Treatment Recommendations (CoSTR). Always use the latest recommendations and consult the full document.

- **Diagnosis**: A diagnosis of cardiac arrest is assumed if the victim is unresponsive and not breathing normally. Non-healthcare professionals are not expected to check for pulses. If the victim is not in cardiac arrest, consider moving into recovery position and seek help if needed.

- **Confirm cardiac arrest**: on suspecting cardiac arrest gently shake the victim's shoulders and ask 'Are you alright?'.

- **Shout for help**: the rescuer should summon assistance by shouting for help, but should not leave the victim. As soon as possible following the diagnosis of cardiac arrest, a 999 call should be made to alert the emergency services and appropriate assistance should be summoned.

- **Position victim onto back**: it is easier to assess and treat if positioned lying on their back.

- **Head tilt, chin lift to open airway**: place one hand on the forehead and tilting the head back, while at the same time with the other hand using the fingertips to lift the chin.

- **Look, listen, and feel for normal breathing**: keep the airway open; the rescuer should check for normal breathing using look (for chest movement), listen (at mouth for breath sounds), feel (for air movement on rescuer's cheek approach). Assess for no more than 10 seconds. If doubts about breathing status, assume abnormal. Non-healthcare professionals are not expected to check for pulses.

- **If not breathing, start chest compressions**: as below. Start with initial 30 compressions.

- **Two rescue breaths**: if attempted should be given over 1 second each. However, it is recognized that some rescuers may choose not to perform mouth-to-mouth resuscitation.

- **If chest compressions alone**: if the rescuer is unwilling to perform rescue breaths then at least 100 compressions per minute should be given (100–120 maximum per minute). Compression only CPR is better than doing nothing, especially during the first few minutes following an arrest. Some studies indicate that outcome from chest compressions alone may be as effective as standard

- **When help arrives**: the additional rescuer is taught to place the heel of the hand in the centre of the chest when performing cardiac compressions. Definitive rescue services will take over on arrival. As a clinician you may continue to be useful to the rescue.

- **Definitive end to the rescue**: help arrives, victim resuscitated or the rescuer is unable to carry on (usually through exhaustion).

Chest compressions (Figure 10.3)

Kneel at the side of the victim. Place heel of one hand in the centre of the chest and place heel of other hand over the top of the first. Interlock fingers. Downward pressure should be applied through the heel of the hands and then the pressure should be released. The compression and recoil completes each individual compression cycle. If there are enough rescuers present the provider of chest compressions should change every 2 minutes with minimum of delay.

- **Depth**: 5–6 cm and then complete recoil.
- **Rate**: 100–120 compressions per minute. Compression and recoil should be equal length of time.
- **Ratio**: 30 compressions to 2 ventilation breaths

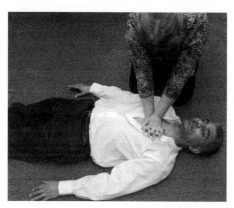

Figure 10.3 Chest compressions.

Rescue breaths (ventilation breaths) (Figure 10.4)

Open the victim's airway using a chin lift and head tilt manoeuvre (or jaw thrust if cervical spine injury).

- **Position**: one hand to pinch the victim's soft nose area immediately below the bridge of the nose (use index and thumb). The other hand maintains the chin lift.
- **Seal around mouth**: While allowing the mouth to stay open the rescuer uses his/her mouth to seal the victim's mouth.
- **Blow steadily into the victims' mouth for 1 second**: the rescuer should see chest movement. Following each breath the rescuer should remove his mouth and take a normal breath. Two rescue breaths are required between each cycle of 30 chest compressions.

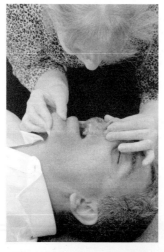

Figure 10.4 Rescue breaths.

Recovery position (Figure 10.5)

- Remove spectacles.
- Kneel beside the victim, straighten legs.
- Place near arm at right angles to body – palm up.
- Bring far arm across chest and hold hand onto victim's near cheek.
- With your other hand, lift victim's far knee up, keep foot on surface (ground, bed etc). Pull on the far leg to roll the victim towards you onto the side.
- Adjust the far (now upper) leg such that the hip and knee are bend at right angles.
- Tilt head back to ensure airway stays open. Adjust hand under the cheek to main head in tilt position.
- Check breathing regularly, and turn onto opposite side every 30 minutes.

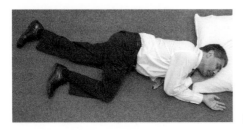

Figure 10.5 Recovery position.

Patient and rescuer safety tips

- ✔ **Summary – 'DRS ABC'**:
  - ○ Danger   Check for danger around victim
  - ○ Response   Check for victim response
  - ○ Shout   Shout for help from bystanders
  - ○ Airway   Open the victims' airway
  - ○ Breathing Check for normal breathing
  - ○ CPR   Start CPR as soon as possible.
- ✔ **Chest compressions position**: Rescuers should be taught and be given a demonstration of the fact that the ideal position for chest compressions is the middle of the lower half of the sternum. In reality, hands should be placed in the 'middle of the chest' without delay. Chest compression should not take place directly over ribs.
- ✔ **Rescue breaths not working**: check victim's mouth and remove any visible obstruction such as dentures, food, blood clot. Recheck that head tilt, chin lift is optimized to straighten the airway. Do not waste time if rescue breaths are difficult, do 2 and move straight onto the next 30 compressions.
- ✔ **Infections**: to the rescuer is theoretically possible and has been reported for tuberculosis, herpes simplex and severe acute respiratory distress syndrome. Human immunodeficiency virus (HIV) has not been reported. Filter devices especially designed for mouth to mouth resuscitation will reduce bacterial transmission.
- ✔ **Jaw thrust use**: requires expertise and only the head tilt, chin lift method is recommendation for teaching lay people.
- ✔ **Agonal gasps**: these are often confused with useful breathing. Rescuers should be taught that these occur in around 40% of cases of cardiac arrest. CPR should be started immediately.
- ✔ **Mouth to nose ventilation**: should be considered as an effective alternative to mouth to mouth ventilation. Especially useful in mouth injuries or CPR in water. Mouth to tracheostomy ventilation is possible in exceptional circumstances where the patient has an existing tracheostomy.
- ✔ **Bag mask ventilation**: useful but requires additional skills.

Student name:	Medical school:	Year:

Adult basic life support

You arrive at the GP surgery and in the car park observe a person collapsed by their car.
Please assume the mannikin is the patient and commence adult BLS.

		Self	Peer	Peer /tutor	Tutor
Ensures safety/universal precautions	• Use of standard precautions, consider latex free gloves if available	☐	☐	☐	☐
	• Awareness of environmental/clinical hazards	☐	☐	☐	☐
	•	☐	☐	☐	☐
Understands indications/ patient assessment	• Checks safe to approach	☐	☐	☐	☐
	• Checks for response	☐	☐	☐	☐
	• Call for help/emergency buzzer	☐	☐	☐	☐
	• ABC approach for unresponsive patient	☐	☐	☐	☐
	• Confirms cardiac arrest	☐	☐	☐	☐
	•	☐	☐	☐	☐
Communication skills	• Ask helper to call 999 for ambulance and gather emergency resuscitation equipment available	☐	☐	☐	☐
	•	☐	☐	☐	☐
Knowledge of i-hospital resuscitation algorithm	• Follows adult basic life support algorithm	☐	☐	☐	☐
	• Commences effective CPR	☐	☐	☐	☐
	• Attaches automated external defibrillator (AED) when equipment becomes available.	☐	☐	☐	☐
Technical ability	• Follows voice prompts on AED (VF)	☐	☐	☐	☐
	• Safe defibrillation (if VF/VT)	☐	☐	☐	☐
	• Recommences effective CPR	☐	☐	☐	☐
	• Depth: 5–6 cm, then complete recoil	☐	☐	☐	☐
	• Rate: 100–120 compressions per minute	☐	☐	☐	☐
	• Ratio: 30 compressions to 2 ventilation breaths	☐	☐	☐	☐
	•	☐	☐	☐	☐
Seeks help as appropriate	• Aware of need for advanced life support when the ambulance crew arrive.	☐	☐	☐	☐
	•	☐	☐	☐	☐
Communication	• Handover to ambulance crew	☐	☐	☐	☐
	• Utilizes initial helper appropriately	☐	☐	☐	☐
	•	☐	☐	☐	☐
Professionalism	• Acts as team leader until ambulance crew arrive	☐	☐	☐	☐
	• Remains at the scene and takes the role of a team member	☐	☐	☐	☐
	• Acts in a professional manner	☐	☐	☐	☐
	•	☐	☐	☐	☐
Documentation	• Awareness of information handover for ambulance crew	☐	☐	☐	☐
	• Completes patient documentation where appropriate	☐	☐	☐	☐
	• Completes surgery incident form if appropriate	☐	☐	☐	☐
	•	☐	☐	☐	☐

			Self	Peer	Peer/tutor	Tutor
Self-assessed as at least borderline:	Signature:	Date:	U B S E	U B S E	U B S E	U B S E
Peer-assessed as ready for tutor assessment:	Signature:	Date:	U B S E	U B S E	U B S E	U B S E
Tutor-assessed as satisfactory:	Signature:	Date:	U B S E	U B S E	U B S E	U B S E

Notes

311

10.3
Adult in-hospital
resuscitation including
do-not-attempt
resuscitation orders

10.3 Adult in-hospital resuscitation including do-not-attempt resuscitation orders

Background

The in-hospital resuscitation algorithm developed by the Resuscitation Council (UK) is aimed at providing a resuscitation sequence more suited to healthcare professionals attending in-hospital cardiac arrest events or collapse generally. The guidelines are based on joint statement Cardio-pulmonary resuscitation – standards for clinical practice and training from the Royal College of Anaesthetists, Royal College of Physicians, Intensive Care Society and Resuscitation Council (UK). These guidelines will also apply to other clinical settings. For all in-hospital cardiac arrests it is expected that:

- Cardiorespiratory arrest is recognized immediately
- Help is summoned using a standard hospital-wide number emergency number, often 2222
- CPR is started immediately using airway adjuncts (e.g. pocket mask)
- Defibrillation, if indicated, attempted immediately, and certainly within 3 minutes of confirmed cardiac arrest.

Chain of survival

All the basic sequence of skills from the adult BLS are needed with important provisions for extra equipment and additional clinical skills. These guidelines will apply to any suitable cardiac arrest or collapsed patient.

For the patient suffering a cardiac arrest or collapse within a hospital environment the following would be expected to addition to stipulations above:

- **Standardized, resuscitation equipment, including defibrillators and drugs**: must be available in all clinical areas and be immediately accessible
- **All clinical staff should be trained on in-hospital resuscitation** to a level appropriate to their role and experience
- **Seamless transition between the in-hospital resuscitation algorithm and the advanced life support (ALS) algorithm**: when the cardiac arrest team arrives
- **Post-resuscitation care**: within an appropriate high dependency area.

These expectations largely focus on the 'chain of survival' (Figure 10.6).

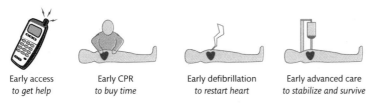

Early access | Early CPR | Early defibrillation | Early advanced care
to get help | *to buy time* | *to restart heart* | *to stabilize and survive*

Figure 10.6 Chain of survival.

Sequence after ensuring personal safety

- **Shout for help and confirm cardiac arrest or collapse**: Gently shake the patient's shoulders and ask 'Are you alright?'.
- **Involve additional team members**: as per availability. If cardiac arrest is confirmed call cardiac arrest team.

- **If patient responds**: Urgent medical assessment using the ABCDE approach, give O_2 100%, attach ECG monitoring leads, IV cannula for venous access.
- **If there is no patient response**:
  ○ Turn patient onto their back
  ○ Open airway: head tilt, chin lift
  ○ Remove mouth contents if obstruction breathing: use suction or forceps, leave well fitting dentures in-situ
  ○ If cervical injury risk: jaw thrust or more specialized manoeuvres such as manual in-line stabilization and chin lift. If life-threatening obstruction prioritize airway patency over cervical spine injury.
- **Look, listen, and feel for normal breathing**: keep the airway open; the rescuer should check for normal breathing using look (for chest movement), listen (at mouth for breath sounds), feel (for air movement on rescuer's cheek approach). Assess for no more than 10 seconds. If doubts about breathing status, assume abnormal.
- **Consider carotid pulse assessment**: no more than 10 seconds. Perform at same time as breathing check or immediately after. If there is a pulse, treat as above for responding patient.
- **If there is no pulse**:
  ○ One person should do CPR, other (s) call cardiac arrest team and get resuscitation trolley with monitor and defibrillator. More help needed urgently
  ○ 30 chest compressions to 2 rescue breath using an adjunct airway. Compression at a rate of 100–120 per minute.
  ○ Adjunct airways include: pocket mask, Guedal airway with pocket mask, laryngeal mask airway (LMA), or bag and mask. Endo-tracheal intubation should only be decided upon and inserted by an experienced clinician
  ○ Defibrillator: once this arrives the pads should be placed on the patient's chest without interrupting chest compression. Brief pauses will be required to assess rhythm. If indicated, perform defibrillation without delay.
- If there is no breathing but a pulse is present (respiratory arrest), maintain airway as above and seek expert opinion and management of definitive airway.
- Many patients will have both cardiac and respiratory arrest and will need activation of the ALS pathway. The eventual sequence will depend on a full assessment of the patient's clinical state and co-morbidities and expressed wishes. Expert advice should be sought and obtained at all times needed.
- **In a witnessed and monitored arrest**: it may be possible to mechanically defibrillate the heart. The ventricular fibrillation (VF)/ventricular tachycardia (VT) arrest should be confirmed and a trained healthcare practitioner should deliver the precordial thump with the patient lying flat. CPR is then started if there is no pulse.

Do-not-attempt resuscitation orders

In many circumstances in hospitals, patients may be deemed not to be candidates for further resuscitation in the event of cardio-pulmonary resuscitation being needed. It must be stressed to all healthcare professionals, involved family members and particularly the patient, that a DNAR order *does not* mean the end of other appropriate treatment and care. It is specifically CPR that will not be attempted. All decisions should be carefully considered with senior clinical input and involvement of the patients and carers/family where and if possible.

There are several reasons why a DNAR request is needed:

- **Advance decision by the patient**: this will need verification by the patient themselves or in writing or in some exceptional cases relayed to the clinical team by family members.
- **Futility of CPR in certain patients**: For example, in a frail patient with metastatic disease and cardiac failure it is highly unlikely that CPR will be successful. The attempt at CPR may

be painful and very distressing for the patient. The clinical team may therefore decide that a DNAR order is appropriate. Extending life by a few days through active CPR and intensive treatment thereafter should weighed up against a more natural planned demise with effective palliative care.

- **Quality of life for the patient**: This criterion is one that is most difficult to use in clinical practice. It is almost impossible for one human to decide that the quality of life of another human is so poor as to need a DNAR order. Nevertheless this reason for why CPR would be inappropriate does overlap with the futility argument above.

Key principles and considerations

- **Easily recognizable DNAR form**: such as the red-bordered one advised by the Resuscitation Council UK for adults (and a separate one for children) should be used (this is reproduced adjacent). The council's guidance has been used to prepare this section of the book).

- **Attention to demographic details**: the potential for harm is immense if patient identity is not secure. Use black pen. Date and sign appropriately. Remember that the order is permanent unless reversed or a review date specified. Local policies must be followed.

- **Review date of DNAR order**: in many cases it will entirely appropriate to review the DNAR order. This must be clearly stated on the form.

- **Cancellation of the DNAR order**: if this is done then 'the form should be crossed through with two diagonal lines in black ball-point ink and 'CANCELLED' written clearly between them, signed and dated by the healthcare professional cancelling the order.'

- **Capacity decisions**: If there is any doubt in relation to capacity then a thorough assessment should be carried out with legal and professional advice.

- **The DNAR decision should be discussed with the patient if possible**: it will not always be appropriate or possible and the kind decision to allow the patient a natural demise to death with excellent palliation may be all that is possible. The reason why discussion was not possible or appropriate must be recorded. This discussion may cause great distress in some patients.

- **Summary of discussion with the patient's relative or friends**: if the patient does not have capacity or otherwise unable to have a full discussion then the relatives and friends must be consulted and may have important information on the patient's wishes. Life-sustaining treatment may be refused by the patient's welfare attorney on behalf of the patient. Be aware that the patient's confidentiality must be respected and not be breached. Write clear records as to the discussion and people (and role) present.

- **Involve multi-disciplinary team and senior clinician input at all times**: The latter will need to fully endorse the DNAR order and sign to do so. All parts of the form must be filled in accurately and legibly.

Student name:	Medical school:	Year:

In-hospital resuscitation and DNAR orders

You are asked to see a collapsed patient. Initially, there is no clear history available apart from the fact that the patient has just returned from endoscopy.

		Self	Peer	Peer /tutor	Tutor
Ensures safety/universal precautions	● Use of universal precautions, consider latex-free gloves	☐	☐	☐	☐
	● Awareness of clinical hazards	☐	☐	☐	☐
	●	☐	☐	☐	☐
Understands indications/ patient assessment	● Checks safe to approach	☐	☐	☐	☐
	● Checks for response	☐	☐	☐	☐
	● Call for help/emergency buzzer	☐	☐	☐	☐
	● ABC approach for unresponsive patient	☐	☐	☐	☐
	● Confirms cardiac arrest	☐	☐	☐	☐
	●	☐	☐	☐	☐
Communication skills	● Asks helper to call 2222 for cardiac arrest team and gathers emergency equipment/trolley	☐	☐	☐	☐
	●	☐	☐	☐	☐
Knowledge of in-hospital resuscitation algorithm	● Follows in-hospital resuscitation algorithm: head tilt, chin lift	☐	☐	☐	☐
	● Commences effective CPR	☐	☐	☐	☐
	● Uses pocket mask effectively	☐	☐	☐	☐
Technical ability	● Attaches and monitors defibrillator when equipment arrives	☐	☐	☐	☐
	● Follows voice prompts on AED (shockable rhythm)	☐	☐	☐	☐
	● Safe defibrillation (if VF/VT)	☐	☐	☐	☐
	● Recommences effective CPR	☐	☐	☐	☐
	● Depth: 5–6 cm, then complete recoil	☐	☐	☐	☐
	● Rate: 100–120 compressions per minute	☐	☐	☐	☐
	● Ratio: 30 compressions to 2 ventilation breaths	☐	☐	☐	☐
	●	☐	☐	☐	☐
Seeks help as appropriate	● Aware of need for ALS when the resuscitation team arrives.	☐	☐	☐	☐
	●	☐	☐	☐	☐
Communication	● Handover to resuscitation team	☐	☐	☐	☐
	● Utilizes initial helper appropriately	☐	☐	☐	☐
	●	☐	☐	☐	☐
Professionalism	● Acts as team leader until resuscitation team arrive	☐	☐	☐	☐
	● Remains at the scene and takes the role of a team member	☐	☐	☐	☐
	● Acts in a professional manner	☐	☐	☐	☐
	● Considers a DNAR if needed	☐	☐	☐	☐
	● Discusses all sections of the DNAR with understanding	☐	☐	☐	☐
	●	☐	☐	☐	☐
Documentation	● Awareness of resuscitation form	☐	☐	☐	☐
	● Completes documentation where appropriate	☐	☐	☐	☐
	●	☐	☐	☐	☐

Self-assessed as at least borderline:	Signature:	Date:	U B S E	U B S E	U B S E	U B S E
Peer-assessed as ready for tutor assessment:	Signature:	Date:	U B S E	U B S E	U B S E	U B S E
Tutor-assessed as satisfactory:	Signature:	Date:	U B S E	U B S E	U B S E	U B S E

Notes

10.4 Adult advanced life support

Background

The ALS algorithm from the Resuscitation Council (UK) is aimed at healthcare professionals trained in ALS techniques and offers a standardized approach to cardiac arrest management. Cardiac arrest teams trained in ALS have the advantage of being able to prepare for each stage of the resuscitation without having distracting discussions on management. Individual team members will understand each role required so ensuring urgent, efficient, and excellent treatment. The ALS course from the Resuscitation Council (UK) teaches and assesses competence in all the key clinical skills required to deliver ALS. This course is a vital part of the training of most doctors, coronary care staff, intensive care unit (ITU) staff, all resuscitation officers, and many other clinicians.

The commencement of ALS should follow seamlessly on from the CPR already having been commenced by initial rescuers or responders using the BLS or in-hospital resuscitation algorithms. All the main aspects of treatment are encapsulated in the ALS algorithm, which should be used extensively (see appendices). The initial sequence of events will be the same as for in-hospital resuscitation.

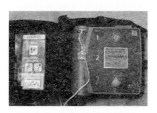

Automated Electrical Defibrillator devices are commonly found in community settings such as schools, factories and community gatherings. Generally safe to use as clear instructions are given audibly and on the screen in most devices

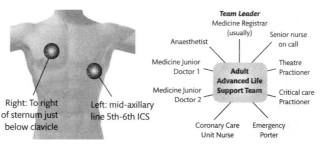

Right: To right of sternum just below clavicle   **Left:** mid-axillary line 5th-6th ICS

Accurate Debrillator pad position is essential to efficacy of defibrillation and ECG monitoring.
Right: right of sternum, infra-clavicular
Left: V6 ECG position

Team decision making: post cardiac arrest many different specialist teams are involved to make the most appropriate decision for the patient: ?diagnosis, ?ITU, ?continue care

Figure 10.7 Images in advanced life support.

Notes on treatment

General

- **Cardiac monitoring**: As soon as this is set up, patients in cardiac arrest will be categorized for treatment depending on the cardiac rhythm identified:
  - **Shockable rhythms**: VF or pulseless VT. Both require immediate defibrillation (Figure 10.7).
  - **Non-shockable rhythms**: asystole or pulseless electrical activity (PEA).
- **All patients require**:
  - Chest compressions
  - Airway management and ventilation
  - Intravenous access: adrenaline
  - Treatment of identified reversible causes.

Treatments most likely to improve survival are early defibrillation and effective uninterrupted CPR. In adults the most common initial rhythm is VF, if a defibrillator is immediately available, the treatment is defibrillation followed by 2 minutes of CPR. If there is a delay in obtaining a defibrillator and the cardiac arrest was a witnessed and monitored event then a precordial thump could be considered.

Defibrillation

- **VF or pulseless VT**: Single shock of 150–200 J using a biphasic defibrillator. Immediately resume CPR for 2 minutes (30 compression to 2 breaths). Check rhythm – if no change second shock at 150–360 J. Repeat cycle as needed and expert advice available.
- **To ensure safe and effective defibrillation**: a number of measures must be considered:
  - ○ **Position of defibrillation (and ECG monitoring pads)**: The right sternal pad is placed right of the sternum below the clavicle. The left apical pad is placed vertically in the mid-axillary line, at the V6 ECG electrode position. The alternative anteroposterior placement can also be used.
  - ○ **Chest hair**: may need to be removed prior to positioning of the self-adhesive pads, however if a razor or clippers are not immediately available then defibrillation should not be delayed.
  - ○ **Ensure safe defibrillation within an oxygen enriched atmosphere**: use self-adhesive defibrillation pads, remove the oxygen mask or nasal cannulae at least 1 m from the patient's chest. However, the bag-valve-mask device can be left connected to the LMA or ET tube (and patient) where a leak of oxygen is not suspected.
  - ○ **Healthcare team and other attendees at the cardiac arrest must stand clear of the bed during defibrillation**.

Chest compressions

Cycles of CPR: run for 2 minutes at a time during cardiac arrest treatment. Prior to the commencement of each new cycle, the cardiac rhythm will be reassessed and if appropriate, pulses checked. There is an emphasis on good quality compressions for each of the cycles so a new provider for compressions is required every 2 minutes to prevent fatigue. The team involved in resuscitation should ensure quick and coordinated changes of provider for compressions and that there is minimal delay between compressions and defibrillation and the recommencement of compressions. Once the airway has been secured with an advanced airway device there is no need for the 30:2 ratio to be followed, compressions will be delivered uninterrupted. Cardiac compressions should be at a rate of 100–120 per minute, with a 5–6 cm depth of compression.

Airway management and ventilation

Ensure adequate oxygenation and ventilation of the lungs: it is essential that the airway is patent and appropriate adjuncts are used. Basic airway opening manoeuvres and adjuncts have been described in previous sections. However, during ALS the airway would be more usually be secured using a LMA device or an endo-tracheal tube. These more advanced airway devices allow the patient to receive uninterrupted chest compressions to allow better perfusion and ventilation will be delivered at a rate of 10 breaths per minute using high-flow oxygen.

Intravenous access

- **Secure effective intravenous access**: a key priority in any deteriorating patient. Occasionally access may need to be achieved during the resuscitation attempt, it is usually easier and safer to perform peripheral venous cannulation than central venous cannulation. Drugs that are injected peripherally should be flushed with 20 mL of normal saline for injection.
- **Consider intraosseous access**: if venous access is very difficult. The intraosseous route will allow samples of bone marrow to be taken for the analysis of blood gases, electrolytes, and haemoglobin concentration. Clearly, this can only be done by an experienced clinician.

Drugs

- **Adrenaline**: Although there is clear evidence to support the use of adrenaline, it is recommended for use in the ALS guidance and algorithm due to its α-adrenergic actions causing vasoconstriction; this in turn acts on increasing myocardial and cerebral perfusion pressure during cardiac arrest. Adrenaline should be used at 3–5 minute intervals during CPR and the dose is 1 mg intravenously.

- **Atropine**: is no longer recommended for routine use in asystole or PEA. It can be used in bradycardia with haemodynamic instability.
- **Amiodarone**: if VF/VT persists after 3 defibrillation shocks, give 300 mg of amiodarone as an IV bolus. A further dose of 150 mg may be given for refractory VF/VT followed by an infusion of amiodarone 900 mg over 24 hours. Lidocaine can used only if amiodarone if not available.

Therapeutic hypothermia

Unconscious adult patients with spontaneous circulation may benefit from cooling to 32–34 °C. Expert advice needed.

Reversible causes

Specific treatments are available for some of the potential causes or aggravating factors of cardiac arrest. These causes and factors need to be systematically explored during the resuscitation attempt. To aid the advanced life support team in considering all relevant causes it is suggested that these are divided into the 4Hs and 4Ts (Table 10.1).

Table 10.1 Reversible causes of cardiac arrest

4 H	4T
Hypoxia	**Tension pneumothorax**
Hypothermia	**Tamponade**
Hypovolaemia	**Toxins**
Hyperkalaemia: hypokalaemia, hypoglycaemia, hypocalcaemia, acidaemia, and other metabolic disorders.	**Thrombosis:** pulmonary embolism or coronary thrombosis

Post-resuscitation care

Once there has been return of spontaneous circulation, high-quality post-resuscitation care is required if the patient is to make a full recovery. The A–E approach to assessing the deteriorating patient should also be used in the initial post-resuscitation phase of the recovery. Once stable the patient should be transferred to the most suitable high-dependency area, usually if the patient is breathing spontaneously this will be coronary care unit (CCU), alternatively if the patient remains ventilated it will be ITU.

Student name:	Medical school:	Year:

Adult advanced life support

You are asked to see a 60-year-old patient who was complaining of severe chest pain. The patient collapsed and cardiac arrest appears likely. You are first on the scene.

		Self	Peer	Peer /tutor	Tutor
Ensures safety/universal precautions	• Use of universal precautions (consider latex free gloves)	☐	☐	☐	☐
	• Awareness of clinical hazards	☐	☐	☐	☐
	•	☐	☐	☐	☐
Understands indications/patient assessment	• Checks safe to approach	☐	☐	☐	☐
	• Checks for response	☐	☐	☐	☐
	• Call for help/emergency buzzer	☐	☐	☐	☐
	• ABC approach for unresponsive patient	☐	☐	☐	☐
	• Confirms cardiac arrest	☐	☐	☐	☐
	•	☐	☐	☐	☐
Communication skills	• Asks helper to call 2222 for cardiac arrest team and gathers emergency equipment/trolley	☐	☐	☐	☐
	•	☐	☐	☐	☐
Knowledge of advanced life support algorithm	• Follows ALS algorithm	☐	☐	☐	☐
	• Commences effective CPR	☐	☐	☐	☐
	• Attaches defibrillator when equipment arrives	☐	☐	☐	☐
Technical ability with any special equipment	• Recognizes rhythm (shockable)	☐	☐	☐	☐
	• Safe defibrillation pathway	☐	☐	☐	☐
	•	☐	☐	☐	☐
Aware of changes in rhythm	• Recognizes rhythm (non-shockable)	☐	☐	☐	☐
	• Follows non-shockable pathway	☐	☐	☐	☐
	• Considers reversible causes and necessary interventions	☐	☐	☐	☐
	• State 4 Hs and 4 Ts of reversible causes	☐	☐	☐	☐
	•	☐	☐	☐	☐
Knowledge of drugs	• Is able to indicate when adrenaline, amiodarone, atropine should be given	☐	☐	☐	☐
	•	☐	☐	☐	☐
Post-procedure management/post-resuscitation care	• Recognizes return of spontaneous circulation	☐	☐	☐	☐
	• Follows A–E approach during post-resuscitation period	☐	☐	☐	☐
	•	☐	☐	☐	☐
Seeks help as appropriate	• Referral to appropriate team	☐	☐	☐	☐
	• Transfer arrangements to CCU/ITU/HD/theatre, etc., where appropriate	☐	☐	☐	☐
	• Thanks team	☐	☐	☐	☐
	•	☐	☐	☐	☐
Communication	• Handover to receiving team	☐	☐	☐	☐
	• Completes resuscitation audit form	☐	☐	☐	☐
	• Completes clinical notes	☐	☐	☐	☐
	•	☐	☐	☐	☐
Professionalism	• Acts as team leader until senior help available	☐	☐	☐	☐
	• Acts in a professional manner	☐	☐	☐	☐
	• Does not leave until handover and documentation complete	☐	☐	☐	☐
	•	☐	☐	☐	☐
Ethics of acute care	• Knowledge of cardiac arrest audit	☐	☐	☐	☐
	• Knowledge of DNAR guidelines and paperwork	☐	☐	☐	☐
	•	☐	☐	☐	☐

			Self	Peer	Peer/tutor	Tutor
Self-assessed as at least borderline:	Signature:	Date:	U B S E	U B S E	U B S E	U B S E
Peer-assessed as ready for tutor assessment:	Signature:	Date:	U B S E	U B S E	U B S E	U B S E
Tutor-assessed as satisfactory:	Signature:	Date:	U B S E	U B S E	U B S E	U B S E

Notes

10.5 Paediatric basic life support

Background

Cardiopulmonary arrest in children is usually due to hypoxia which has resulted from underlying illness or injury. Commonly bradycardia which deteriorates into asystole or pulseless electrical activity will result in a poor outcome.

Knowledge of paediatric basic life resuscitation is the minimum requirement for all clinical staff involved in the treatment of infants and children, anyone performing more complex skills should be taught and practise the principles of ALS.

Safety for the rescuer, bystanders, and victim should be considered as being of paramount importance. If possible the victim should be assessed and resuscitated where found.

Age definitions for resuscitation

If the rescuer assesses the victim as a child then the paediatric guidelines should be used.

- Infant: under 1 year of age
- Child: between 1 year old and puberty
- Adult: beyond puberty.

Procedure

It is important for rescuers to follow the recommended basic life support algorithm, but all will follow the sequence as below.

- S Safety
- S Stimulate
- S Shout for assistance
- A Airway
- B Breathing
- C Circulation
- R Reassess

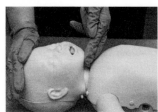
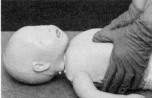
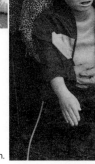

Especially in paediatric basic life support (BLS), practice must take place until a very high degree of proficiency is attained. Manikins are excellent, especially as they are available in different age groups.

Two hands clearly cannot be used as in adult CPR. In a small baby, two fingers, placed correctly and with adequate force, will be enough to deliver effective CPR. Alternatively, two thumbs can be used as shown here.

Other manoeuvres to complete the panoply of skills needed in paediatric BLS include Heimlich's manoeuvre for choking. This is best taught and practised on a manikin.

Figure 10.8 Images in paediatric basic life support.

Safety

Potential hazards will differ depending on the environment within which the emergency has occurred. The safety aspect of the sequence relates to both the rescuer and the child. The child should only be moved if they are in physical danger.

It should be recommended that all clinical staff will adopt universal precautions when dealing with a cardiac arrest due to infection risks from bodily fluids, these may include the use of gloves, aprons, goggles, or pocket masks for ventilation depending on the clinical situation and what is available.

In the clinical environment care should be taken that any access device involving needles or sharps will be disposed of at the point of use to prevent needle stick injuries, as the child may have been deteriorating for some time prior to the arrest, and may have been subject to many procedures.

Stimulate

If the child appears to be unconscious then attempts should be made to elicit a response by the use of gentle but firm verbal and tactile stimulation. If the child responds then the rescuer should follow the principles of an ABCDE assessment, if there is no response then the rescuer should continue with basic life support.

Shout

Accessing further help and support will be dependent on where the emergency has occurred and what help is initially available.

If alone in a healthcare setting verbally shouting for help or activating the emergency buzzer will alert colleagues that you require assistance; this second person can then be instructed to activate the relevant emergency service or team and to bring clinical emergency equipment to the child. In-hospital paediatric emergencies will require a 2222 call for the paediatric emergency team; out of hospital this would be a 999 or 112 phone call to request an ambulance.

Airway

The tongue is the commonest cause of airway obstruction in the unconscious child; this can usually be dealt with by using a simple airway opening manoeuvre. There are two recommended manoeuvres: the chin lift and head tilt, and the jaw thrust. Infants require the head to be placed in a neutral position and for the child a 'sniffing' position will be more appropriate.

Occasionally vomit or other substance may be the cause of further airway obstruction; suction would be required in this instance. Foreign bodies may be removed by the use of a single finger sweep if the rescuer can clearly see the obstruction and feels confident they can remove it. Finger sweeps are rarely performed on children under the age of 1 year.

Breathing

Whilst maintaining an open airway the rescuer can check the child for signs of spontaneous breathing. This check is performed for up to 10 seconds by using a three-step approach, look, listen, and feel.

- Look for chest and abdominal movement.
- Listen for breath sounds.
- Feel for air movement over the nose and mouth.

If the child is not breathing effectively then five rescue breaths should be delivered to provide oxygen to the lungs. Each breath should be delivered slowly, lasting 1–1.5 seconds duration; this will help minimize gastric distension. Chest movement will indicate successful ventilation. Mouth-to-mouth or mouth to pocket mask can be used to deliver these breaths if a bag-valve-mask device is not available. The rescuer's mouth should cover the nose and mouth of an infant.

Circulation

Following delivery of 5 rescue breaths an assessment of the circulation will be performed. If the rescuer has not received training in how to palpate for pulses, it would be appropriate to check for other signs of life; healthcare professionals, however, will also palpate for a pulse. In infants this is done by palpating a brachial pulse, in children a carotid or femoral pulse check can be performed. The assessment for circulation is performed for no longer than 10 seconds.

If an adequate pulse is felt (>60 beats/min) then breathing should be reassessed and supported. If the pulse is inadequate or below 60 beats/minute and no signs of life have been detected then chest compressions should be commenced to attempt to continue to perfuse vital organs until spontaneous circulation is achieved.

The recommended ratio for chest compressions to ventilation in infants and children is 15:2. It may be more appropriate, however, for lone rescuers or non-healthcare professionals to use the adult ratio of 30:2. Effective chest compressions are more likely to be achieved when the child is lying on a firm, flat surface and they are being delivered at a rate of 100–120 per minute. The rescuer should aim to compress the chest over the lower half of the sternum, in the midline by one third of its resting depth.

In infants the two finger or two thumb technique will be used; in the child, however, the heel of the hand will be necessary, by use of either the one- or two-handed technique.

Reassess

BLS should continue until the emergency help arrives at the scene to take over and move the resuscitation onto an ALS pathway.

BLS can be discontinued if the child shows signs of life, a reassessment of ABC will be made and supportive action taken to stabilize the child.

In certain circumstances if a second rescuer or emergency support is not immediately available, it may be necessary due to rescuer exhaustion to discontinue the resuscitation attempt.

Student name:	Medical school:	Year:

Paediatric basic life support

A mother shouts her child is not breathing; you are the only healthcare professional on the scene.

		Self	Peer	Peer /tutor	Tutor
Awareness of paediatric BLS sequence	● Uses specific order of sequence in BLS; ● safety, stimulate, shout, airway, breathing, circulation, reassess. ●	☐ ☐ ☐	☐ ☐ ☐	☐ ☐ ☐	☐ ☐ ☐
Safety: ensures safety/universal precautions	● Use of standard precautions; consider latex free gloves, aprons ● Awareness of clinical hazards ● Safe approach ●	☐ ☐ ☐ ☐	☐ ☐ ☐ ☐	☐ ☐ ☐ ☐	☐ ☐ ☐ ☐
Stimulate: establishes responsiveness of the child	● Checks for response by both tactile and verbal stimulation, for example, stabilize the child's head, tug their hair and call their name ●	☐ ☐	☐ ☐	☐ ☐	☐ ☐
Shout: demonstrates effective communication skills	● If there is no response call for help/emergency buzzer ● Commence BLS following the algorithm ● Ask for help when it arrives to telephone 999 or 2222 depending on location for emergency team or local numbers ●	☐ ☐ ☐ ☐	☐ ☐ ☐ ☐	☐ ☐ ☐ ☐	☐ ☐ ☐ ☐
Airway: ensures patent airway	● Perform appropriate airway opening manoeuvre; chin lift, head tilt, or jaw thrust ● Assess airway for obstructions; use suction if appropriate ●	☐ ☐ ☐	☐ ☐ ☐	☐ ☐ ☐	☐ ☐ ☐
Breathing: assesses breathing and ensures effective ventilation	● Assess spontaneous breathing using a look, listen, and feel approach ● If the child is not breathing, immediately deliver five rescue breaths ●	☐ ☐ ☐	☐ ☐ ☐	☐ ☐ ☐	☐ ☐ ☐
Circulation: assesses circulation and ensures effective external compressions	● Assess circulation relevant to age; brachial pulse palpation for child under 1, carotid pulse palpation for child over 1 year ● If no palpable pulse present or inadequate pulse (<60 beats/min) commence chest compressions using correct ratio, rate and depth at an appropriate landmark ● Uses 100–120 compressions per minute ● Ratio is 15 compressions to 2 rescue breaths ●	☐ ☐ ☐ ☐ ☐	☐ ☐ ☐ ☐ ☐	☐ ☐ ☐ ☐ ☐	☐ ☐ ☐ ☐ ☐
Reassesses	● After 1 minute the rescuer should reassess the child's ABC, if no signs of life then BLS should be immediately resumed ●	☐ ☐	☐ ☐	☐ ☐	☐ ☐
Seeks help as appropriate	● On arrival of emergency team and equipment the advanced paediatric life support algorithm will commence ● Rescuer acts as team member ●	☐ ☐ ☐	☐ ☐ ☐	☐ ☐ ☐	☐ ☐ ☐
Communication	● Handover to receiving team ●	☐ ☐	☐ ☐	☐ ☐	☐ ☐
Professionalism	● Acts as lead rescuer until senior help available ● Acts in a professional manner ● Does not leave until handover and documentation complete ●	☐ ☐ ☐ ☐	☐ ☐ ☐ ☐	☐ ☐ ☐ ☐	☐ ☐ ☐ ☐

			U B S E	U B S E	U B S E	U B S E
Self-assessed as at least borderline:	Signature:	Date:	U B S E	U B S E	U B S E	U B S E
Peer-assessed as ready for tutor assessment:	Signature:	Date:	U B S E	U B S E	U B S E	U B S E
Tutor-assessed as satisfactory:	Signature:	Date:	U B S E	U B S E	U B S E	U B S E

Notes

10.6 Paediatric advanced life support

Background

The transition between BLS and ALS should be seamless and CPR should be ongoing. As soon as resuscitation monitoring equipment is available the priority is to decide which treatment pathway to follow by identifying whether the rhythm is shockable or non-shockable. When following either treatment pathway CPR is delivered in 2-minute cycles. To prevent rescuer fatigue and ensure effective CPR it is recommended that the provider of cardiac compressions is changed every 2 minutes during the resuscitation attempt.

Calculations

It is necessary to ensure that the treatment delivered is appropriate for the age and weight ranges of the child; therefore calculations will need to be made to ascertain the weight of the child. Common calculations are as follows;

- **Weight in kg** $(age + 4) \times 2$
- **Energy** 4 J/kg
- **Endotracheal tube size** $(age/4) + 4$
- **Fluids** 20 mL/kg of 0.9% saline
- **Adrenaline** 10 µg/kg of 1:10 000 solution (0.1 mL/kg of 1:10 000 solution)
- **Glucose** usually 200 mg/kg of 10% glucose (2 mL/kg of 10% glucose)

Shockable rhythms

VF occurs in around 25% of cardiorespiratory arrests in children, and pulseless VT is rare. If a shockable rhythm is present then a successful outcome will depend on rapid defibrillation. VF or pulseless VT requires defibrillation at 4 J/kg, followed by 2 minutes of CPR. Adrenaline doses of 10 µg/kg are delivered prior to the third shock and thereafter every 3–5 minutes.

Procedure for VF/VT

Once arrest has been confirmed and CPR commenced the defibrillator should be prepared.

- Place the defibrillator self-adhesive pads on the child's chest.
- Confirm shockable rhythm
- Select energy level at 4 J/kg.
- Remove free flowing oxygen, instruct team to stand clear.
- Charge pads and check safety and final rhythm check.
- Deliver the shock.
- Immediately resume CPR for 2 minutes.
- If VF/VT is still present then prepare for 2nd shock and deliver.
- Continue CPR for further 2 minutes.
- If VF/VT still present administer adrenaline followed by a saline flush.
- Deliver 3rd shock and give amiodarone 5 mg/kg, repeat dose after 5th shock (if needed).
- Recommence CPR. Give adrenaline dose, as above, every 3–5 minutes.

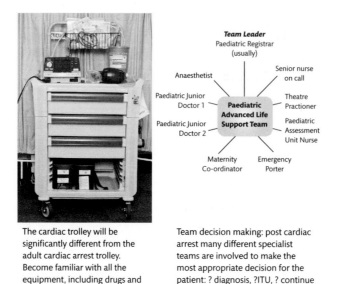

The cardiac trolley will be significantly different from the adult cardiac arrest trolley. Become familiar with all the equipment, including drugs and their dosages.

Team decision making: post cardiac arrest many different specialist teams are involved to make the most appropriate decision for the patient: ? diagnosis, ?ITU, ? continue care

Figure 10.9 Images in paediatric advanced life support.

Non-shockable rhythms

PEA or asystole are the commonest rhythms found in arrest in children. These rhythms require ongoing effective CPR. All cardiac arrest rhythms require investigation of any underlying reversible causes; however, this is particularly important with PEA. The first dose of adrenaline at 10 µg/kg is delivered as soon as intravenous access is available then repeated every 3–5 minutes.

Procedure for asystole and PEA

Once arrest has been confirmed and CPR commenced the defibrillator should be prepared.

- Place the defibrillator self-adhesive pads on the child's chest.
- Confirm non-shockable rhythm.
- Establish circulatory access if not already present.
- Administer adrenaline followed by a saline flush.
- After 2 minutes of CPR check rhythm and if electrical activity seen, check pulse.
- If no output or signs of life detected resume CPR.
- After 2 minutes of CPR check rhythm and if electrical activity seen, check pulse.
- If no output or signs of life detected administer adrenaline and resume CPR.
- Relevant history should be ascertained and reversible causes considered and treated.

Airway management and ventilation

Prior to the arrival of expert help the airway may be secured by the use of an oropharyngeal or nasopharyngeal airway and ventilation provided by the use of a bag-valve-mask device with high-flow oxygen. As soon as expert help is available the airway can be secured by tracheal intubation, ventilation can then be delivered at a rate of 12–20 breaths per minute and compressions can be performed continuously.

Circulation

Circulatory access during the cardiorespiratory arrest is vital for taking blood samples and for the administration of drugs and fluids. Any venous access devices already *in situ* will require a flush of normal saline to ensure the device is patent prior to the administration of drugs or fluids.

If there is no venous access and peripheral cannulation is difficult to obtain or will delay treatment then insertion of an intraosseous cannula is indicated, bone marrow can be aspirated for sampling and then fluids and drugs may be administered.

History and reversible causes

Obtaining relevant history and underlying medical conditions or predisposing events to the cardiorespiratory arrest can be useful in helping to identify reversible causes. Any causes identified that have specific treatments must be dealt with during the resuscitation attempt.

The mnemonic of 4Hs and 4Ts can be used to recall the most likely reversible causes (see Table 10.1).

Student name:	Medical school:	Year:

Advanced paediatric life support

You are present when a 6-year-old child with suspected sepsis becomes unresponsive.

		Self	Peer	Peer /tutor	Tutor
Ensures safety/universal precautions	• Use of standard precautions; consider latex-free gloves, aprons	☐	☐	☐	☐
	• Awareness of clinical hazards	☐	☐	☐	☐
	•	☐	☐	☐	☐
Knowledge of calculations	• Is able to calculate; weight, energy, ET tube, fluids, adrenaline, glucose	☐	☐	☐	☐
	•	☐	☐	☐	☐
Understands indications/ patient assessment	• Safe approach	☐	☐	☐	☐
	• Checks for response, if no response	☐	☐	☐	☐
	• Call for help/emergency buzzer	☐	☐	☐	☐
	• Commence BLS following paediatric BLS algorithm	☐	☐	☐	☐
	• Confirms cardiac arrest	☐	☐	☐	☐
	•	☐	☐	☐	☐
Communication skills	• Asks helper to call 2222 for paediatric emergency team and gathers emergency equipment/ trolley (or local number)	☐	☐	☐	☐
	•	☐	☐	☐	☐
Knowledge of advanced paediatric life support algorithm **Technical ability with any special equipment**	• Follows advanced paediatric life support algorithm	☐	☐	☐	☐
	• Continues effective CPR	☐	☐	☐	☐
	• Attaches defibrillator/monitor when equipment arrives	☐	☐	☐	☐
	•	☐	☐	☐	☐
Recognizes rhythm	• Recognizes rhythm (PEA)	☐	☐	☐	☐
	• Follows non-shockable pathway	☐	☐	☐	☐
	•	☐	☐	☐	☐
Considers further steps during CPR	• Considers reversible causes and necessary interventions	☐	☐	☐	☐
	• Establishes secure airway	☐	☐	☐	☐
	• Establishes IV access and sends relevant bloods	☐	☐	☐	☐
	•	☐	☐	☐	☐
Knowledge of drugs	• Is able to indicate when adrenaline should be given	☐	☐	☐	☐
	•	☐	☐	☐	☐
Post-procedure management/post-resuscitation care	• Recognizes return of spontaneous circulation	☐	☐	☐	☐
	• Follows A–E approach during post-resuscitation period	☐	☐	☐	☐
	•	☐	☐	☐	☐
Seeks help as appropriate	• Referral to appropriate team	☐	☐	☐	☐
	• Transfer arrangements to paediatric ITU/HD/theatre, etc where appropriate	☐	☐	☐	☐
	• Thanks team	☐	☐	☐	☐
	•	☐	☐	☐	☐
Communication	• Handover to receiving team	☐	☐	☐	☐
	• Completes resuscitation audit form	☐	☐	☐	☐
	• Completes clinical record	☐	☐	☐	☐
	•	☐	☐	☐	☐
Professionalism	• Acts as team leader until senior help available	☐	☐	☐	☐
	• Acts in a professional manner	☐	☐	☐	☐
	• Does not leave until handover and documentation complete	☐	☐	☐	☐
	•	☐	☐	☐	☐
Ethics of acute care	• Knowledge of cardiac arrest audit	☐	☐	☐	☐
	• Knowledge of DNAR guidelines and paperwork	☐	☐	☐	☐
	•	☐	☐	☐	☐

			U B S E	U B S E	U B S E	U B S E
Self-assessed as at least borderline:	Signature:	Date:	U B S E	U B S E	U B S E	U B S E
Peer-assessed as ready for tutor assessment:	Signature:	Date:	U B S E	U B S E	U B S E	U B S E
Tutor-assessed as satisfactory:	Signature:	Date:	U B S E	U B S E	U B S E	U B S E

Notes

10.7 Anaphylaxis

Background

Anaphylaxis is an acute reaction that can involve several systems. It is potentially life-threatening and extremely unpleasant for the victim. It is a type I hypersensitivity reaction, which means that it is an allergic response to the re-exposure to a previously identified or known allergen such as peanuts or due to an immediate hypersensitivity to a new allergen. Some reports from the USA state that 1500 deaths per year may be due to anaphylaxis. There is some evidence from UK that attendances to the Accident and emergency department due to anaphylaxis may be increasing. A dramatic representation of anaphylaxis was by Will Smith in the film *Hitch*, the reaction to seafood is very accurately portrayed!

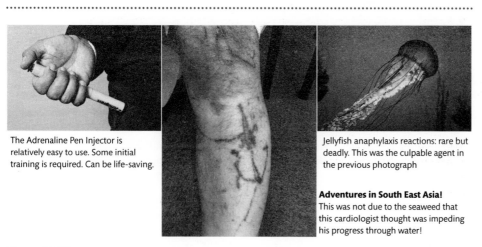

The Adrenaline Pen Injector is relatively easy to use. Some initial training is required. Can be life-saving.

Jellyfish anaphylaxis reactions: rare but deadly. This was the culpable agent in the previous photograph

Adventures in South East Asia!
This was not due to the seaweed that this cardiologist thought was impeding his progress through water!

Figure 10.10 Images in anaphylaxis. Right © Cristian Lazzari/iStockphoto.

Pathophysiological principles

Anaphylaxis occurs after degranulation of mast cells or basophils mediated by immunoglobulin E activated by the allergen. This is not the only mechanism, however, and the reaction can also be due to non-allergic non-immunological triggered events. The clinical definition and the treatment protocol is the same.

Definition

Anaphylaxis is an IgE immune-mediated or non-allergic non-immunological event that leads to certain clinical symptoms and signs (see Table 10.2). Three criteria need to be fulfilled in most definitions:

- **Acute onset of an illness (minutes to hours) with skin and/or mucosal involvement**: generalized hives, pruritus or flushing, swollen lips or tongue or uvula. There may be respiratory compromise (dyspnoea, wheeze, bronchospasm, stridor, or reduced peak expiratory flow rate, hypoxaemia), or hypotension or syncope or collapse.

- **Two or more classical reactions after exposure**: involvement of the skin or mucosal tissues ± respiratory compromise ± hypotension or syncope or collapse ± persistent abdominal symptoms (cramp, abdominal pain, vomiting).

- **Reduced blood pressure after exposure**: to a known allergen for that patient, this can be minutes or longer. Defined as systolic blood pressure <90 mmHg or 30% decrease from that person's baseline.

Differential diagnosis

- Bronchial asthma
- Cardiogenic pulmonary oedema
- Foreign body inhalation
- Irritant chemical exposure
- Facial swelling or angioedema: bacterial/viral usually cause fever and pain.
- C1 esterase deficiency
- Carcinoid syndrome
- Systemic mastocytosis
- Alcohol induced flushing
- Shock.
- Tension pneumothorax

Table 10.2 Grades of anaphylaxis

Grade	Definition
Mild (skin and subcutaneous tissues only) Mild can be sub-classified depending on those with and without angioedema)	Generalized erythema, urticaria, periorbital oedema or angioedema)
Moderate (features suggesting cardiovascular / respiratory/gastrointestinal involvement)	Dyspnoea, stridor, wheeze, nausea, vomiting, dizziness (presyncope), diaphoresis, chest or throat tightness, or abdominal pain.
Severe (hypoxia, hypotension or neurological compromise)	Cyanosis or O_2 saturations <92% at any stage Hypotension (systolic blood pressure (BP) <90 mmHg in adults) confusion, collapse, loss of consciousness or incontinence

Treatment

- **Systematic assessment of ABCDE.**
- **Stop any potential causative agent**: and call for help.
- **Give adrenaline**: 0.001 mg/kg intramuscularly into lateral thigh to a maximum of 0.5 mg (0.5 mL). May be repeated every 5–15 minutes.
- **Give high-flow oxygen**: by facemask with reservoir bag and 15 L/min oxygen in all patients aiming for oxygen saturation >92%.
- **Airway care**: Elevate the head and body torso, if signs of worsening stridor/tachypnoea and wheeze.
- **Call for anaesthetic help**: cyanosis and wheeze indicate impending respiratory arrest.
- **Place patient supine**: preferably with legs elevated to increase venous return.
- **Intravenous access**: insert 14G or 16G cannula and give crystalloid bolus 10–20 mL/kg (0.9% saline).

Failure to respond

- **Call for anaesthetist**.
- **Intravenous adrenaline indications**:
  - Rapid cardiovascular collapse with shock
  - Imminent airways obstruction
  - Critical bronchospasm.

- **Start adrenaline infusion**: 1 mL (1 mg) of 1:1000 adrenaline in 100 mL of normal saline at 30–90 mL/h (5–15 µg/min) titrated to response continuing up to 60 minutes after the resolution of anaphylaxis, then weaning over 30 minutes and stopping watching closely for recurrence. Nebulized adrenaline (5 mg which is undiluted 1:1000 adrenaline) can be given while parenteral adrenaline is being prepared.
- **Consider assisted ventilation and ET intubation**.
- **Other drugs**: can be considered once patient is cardiorespiratory stable. These are less evidence based than above. They are indicated for relief of skin symptoms such as urticaria, mild angioedema, and pruritus.
  - ○ Intramuscular 10–20 mg of chlorphenamine or very slow intravenously
  - ○ Intravenous ranitidine 50 mg three times daily change to oral when patient can tolerate.
  - ○ Prednisone 1 mg/kg up to a maximum of 50 mg orally or hydrocortisone 1.5–3 mg/kg intravenously.
  - ○ Consider glucagon (1–5 mg intravenously): in patients taking β-blockers who are resistant to the action of adrenaline.

Continuing treatment: drugs

- Chlorphenamine oral supply for 2–3 days
- Oral prednisolone : 50 mg once daily
- Consider cetirizine 10 mg once daily
- Ranitidine 150 mg twice daily.

Patient safety tips

- ✔ **Referral to allergist/immunologist**: provide a detailed letter with nature and circumstances and treatment of the anaphylactic reaction.
- ✔ **Consider providing an adrenaline injection pen**: responsibility for use of an adrenaline pen injection and an action plan should be discussed. Indications include:
  - ○ Anaphylaxis after known allergen exposure outside of a medical setting.
  - ○ Known food allergy (e.g. nuts, peanuts, fish, shellfish)
  - ○ Reaction was severe and/or the cause unknown including idiopathic anaphylaxis.
- ✔ **Patient to identify themselves at risk**: this can be done using a suitable clinical alert bracelet or necklace or card.

Student name:	Medical school:	Year:

Anaphylaxis

A 51-year-old cardiologist physician is admitted to the hospital where you are doing an elective, in South East Asia. He is breathless and has the rash that is shown in Figure 10.10.

This assessment will be based around this clinical vignette and the management of anaphylaxis generally.

		Self	Peer	Peer /tutor	Tutor
What is anaphylaxis?	• Anaphylaxis is an acute reaction that can involve several systems. It is potentially life-threatening.	☐	☐	☐	☐
	• Type I hypersensitivity reaction	☐	☐	☐	☐
	•	☐	☐	☐	☐
What three criteria need to be met for the diagnosis of anaphylaxis?	• **Acute onset of an illness (minutes to hours) with skin and/or mucosal involvement**	☐	☐	☐	☐
	• **Two or more classical reactions after exposure**: involvement of the skin or mucosal tissues ± respiratory compromise ± hypotension or syncope or collapse ± persistent abdominal symptoms	☐	☐	☐	☐
	• **Reduced blood pressure after exposure**: to a known allergen for that patient, this can be minutes or longer. Defined as systolic blood pressure <90 mmHg or 30% decrease from that person's baseline	☐	☐	☐	☐
	•	☐	☐	☐	☐
What are the differential diagnosis to consider when anaphylaxis is suspected?	• Bronchial asthma, cardiogenic pulmonary oedema, foreign body inhalation, irritant chemical exposure, facial swelling or angioedema, C1 esterase deficiency, carcinoid syndrome, systemic mastocytosis, alcohol induced flushing, shock, tension pneumothorax	☐	☐	☐	☐
	•	☐	☐	☐	☐
What are the main aspects of treatment?	• **Stop any potential causative agent**: and call for help	☐	☐	☐	☐
	• **Give adrenaline**: repeated every 5–15 minutes	☐	☐	☐	☐
	• **Give high-flow oxygen**: by reservoir face mask aiming for O_2 saturation >92%	☐	☐	☐	☐
	• **Airway care**: elevate the head and body torso, if signs of worsening stridor/tachypnoea and wheeze	☐	☐	☐	☐
	• **Call for anaesthetic help**: cyanosis and wheeze indicate impending respiratory arrest				
	• **Place patient supine**: preferably with legs elevated to increase venous return	☐	☐	☐	☐
	• **IV access**: insert 14G or 16G cannula and give crystalloid bolus 10–20 mL/kg (0.9% saline)	☐	☐	☐	☐
	•	☐	☐	☐	☐
What if there is failure to respond to the early measure?	• **Call for anaesthetist**	☐	☐	☐	☐
	• **Start adrenaline infusion 1 mL (1 mg)**	☐	☐	☐	☐
	• **Consider assisted ventilation and ET intubation**.	☐	☐	☐	☐
	• **Other drugs**:	☐	☐	☐	☐
	• IM 10–20 mg of chlorphenamine or very slow IV	☐	☐	☐	☐
	• IV ranitidine 50 mg three times daily change to oral when patient can tolerate	☐	☐	☐	☐
	• Prednisone 1 mg/kg up to a maximum of 50 mg orally or hydrocortisone 1.5–3 mg/kg IV.	☐	☐	☐	☐
	• Consider glucagon (1 to 5 mg IV): in patients taking β-blockers	☐	☐	☐	☐
	•	☐	☐	☐	☐
What are the key patient safety tips	• **Referral to allergist/immunologist**: detailed letter, treatment of the anaphylactic reaction	☐	☐	☐	☐
	• **Consider providing an adrenaline injection pen**: education and action plan should be discussed	☐	☐	☐	☐
	• **Patient to identify themselves at risk**: using a suitable clinical alert bracelet or necklace or card	☐	☐	☐	☐
	•	☐	☐	☐	☐
What are the indications for an adrenaline pen to be considered for issue to a patient?	• Anaphylaxis after known allergen exposure outside of a medical setting.	☐	☐	☐	☐
	• Known food allergy (e.g. nuts, peanuts, fish, shellfish)	☐	☐	☐	☐
	• Reaction was severe and/or the cause unknown including idiopathic anaphylaxis	☐	☐	☐	☐
	•	☐	☐	☐	☐

			Self	Peer	Peer /tutor	Tutor
Self-assessed as at least borderline:	Signature:	Date:	U B S E	U B S E	U B S E	U B S E
Peer-assessed as ready for tutor assessment:	Signature:	Date:	U B S E	U B S E	U B S E	U B S E
Tutor-assessed as satisfactory:	Signature:	Date:	U B S E	U B S E	U B S E	U B S E

Notes

10.8 Basic airway management

Background

Maintenance of a patent airway is essential to prevent a patient's condition deteriorating and leading to hypoxia. Unless airway obstruction can be relieved to enable adequate ventilation within a few minutes, brain injury will result and lead to cardiac arrest. Prompt assessment and treatment is essential. This can be achieved by the use of simple manoeuvres and/or the use of airway adjuncts.

Causes of airway obstruction

Obstruction of the airway may be partial or complete. It can occur at any level from the nose and the mouth down to the bronchi. Studies of the human in the unconscious state have shown that the site of airway obstruction is often at the soft palate and epiglottis but can also be attributed to the posterior displacement of the tongue caused by decreased muscle tone.

Obstruction may also be caused by vomit or blood, as a result of regurgitation of gastric contents or trauma, or by foreign bodies, pharyngeal swelling, laryngospasm, or bronchospasm. It must be assumed that anyone who has a decreased conscious level, regardless of the cause, is at risk of airway obstruction.

Recognition of airway obstruction: the look, listen, and feel approach

The look, listen and feel approach is a method of assessing a patient's breathing and airway patency. It is essential to check that interventions have been effective and this approach is a useful tool.

- **Look for**: foreign bodies (e.g. dentures, food), use of accessory muscles in particular seesaw pattern of respiration. There may also be intercostal and subcostal recession and a tracheal tug.
- **Listen for**: normal breathing should be quiet, completely obstructed breathing will be silent, gurgling sounds (fluid), stridor, wheezes, snoring sounds may be present as in partial obstruction, air entry is diminished and usually noisy.
- **Feel for**: breaths from nose/mouth.

Wherever possible, give high concentration oxygen while attempting to relieve airway obstruction. As airway patency is restored, oxygen saturation will rise more rapidly if the inspired oxygen concentration is high.

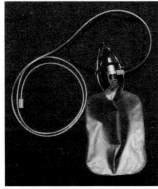

High Concentration Oxygen must be given immediately. A basic mask can be used with a reservoir bag which will allow 90-100% O$_2$ to be delivered

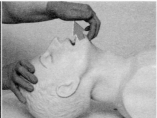

Head tilt, chin lift is the standard manoeuvre to open up the airways. This allows the oropharyngeal, laryngopharyngeal and trachea are all straightened out to improve airway patency

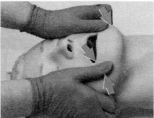

Jaw thrust manoeuvre
If cervical spine injury is suspected, the jaw thrust manoeuvre will allow opening of the airway without movement of the cervical spine

Figure 10.11 Images in basic airway management

Airway opening manoeuvres

These are designed to lift the tongue away from the posterior pharyngeal wall. After each manoeuvre, check for success using the look, listen, and feel approach. If a clear airway cannot be achieved, look for other causes of airway obstruction. Remove broken or displaced dentures but leave well fitting dentures in place as they help maintain the contours of the mouth.

- **Head tilt, chin lift**: involves placing one hand on the forehead and gently tilting the head back while placing the fingertips of the other hand under the point of the patient's chin and lifting upwards to stretch the anterior neck structures. **This manoeuvre is contraindicated in patients with suspected cervical spine injury**. If spinal injury is suspected, if the patient has fallen or been struck on the head for example, maintain the head, neck, and chest in the neutral position and establish a clear upper airway by using the jaw thrust manoeuvre.

- **Jaw thrust**: involves placing the index and other fingers behind the angle of the mandible and applying a steady upwards and forward pressure to lift the mandible. The thumbs should be used to open the mouth by downward displacement of the chin.

If any of the above manoeuvres are implemented the patient must always be assessed to ensure the intervention has been effective.

- **Suction**: involves the removal of blood/vomit or other liquids to clear the airway. This can be achieved by the use of a suction device and suction catheters. Suctioning should be performed at the inner sides of the mouth and used to remove only what can be visualized. Gagging can be stimulated if the catheter is passed across the soft palate and care should be taken to prevent damage to soft tissue when using hard plastic suction catheters. After suction is used the patient must be reassessed to ensure the intervention has been effective. Occasionally forceps or a gloved hand will be needed to remove obstructions such as food, debris, or dentures out of the mouth.

- **Nasopharyngeal tube**: this is a soft plastic tube with a bevel at one end (to aid insertion) and a flange at the other (to prevent displacement into the nose). It is tolerated in a conscious patient and can be used to:

  ○ Remove secretions from the back of the pharynx

  ○ Ensure adequate oxygenation in patients with clenched jaws/ maxillofacial injuries

  ○ **Insertion**: size 6 and 7 mm tubes are suitable for adults, though measuring from the tragus on the ear to the external nares will estimate the appropriate length of the tube. It is inserted by introducing a lubricated tube, bevel end first, vertically along the floor of the nose (Figure 10.12) . The right nostril is used first (usually larger). Insertion should stop immediately if any obstruction is met.

- **Oropharyngeal airways**: commonly known as a Guedel airway, is a curved plastic tube with a reinforced bite plate at one end. It comes in several sizes and is designed to fit from the incisors over the tongue to the pharyngeal wall; it is used for unconscious patients to help maintain the airway.

  ○ **The airway size**: is estimated by measuring the tube against the **vertical** distance from the angle of the mandible to the level of the incisors.

  ○ **Insertion**: insert the oropharyngeal airway 'upside down' into a clear airway as far as the junction of the hard and soft palate. It is then rotated through 180° and advanced till it lies against the pharynx. Re-assess to ensure that the intervention has been effective.

The oropharyngeal airway cannot be used on conscious patients.

If an oropharyngeal airway is used the patient must be re-assessed to ensure the intervention has been effective.

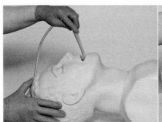
Suction using a soft plastic catheter

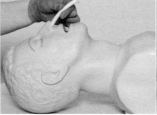
Nasopharyngeal airway being inserted

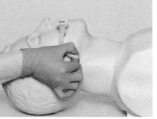
Measuring up for a oropharyngeal airway

Figure 10.12 Basic airway adjuncts.

Patient safety tips

✔ **Always give high-flow oxygen**: while sorting out inserting any basic airway adjunct.

✔ **Nasopharyngeal tubes are contraindicated in patients with suspected base of skull fractures due to the theoretical possibility of entering the brain**. If a nasopharyngeal tube is used the patient must be reassessed to ensure the intervention has been effective.

Student name:	Medical school:	Year:

Basic airway management

A patient with a compromised airway has been admitted to the emergency department, please show how you will manage his airway.

		Self	Peer	Peer /tutor	Tutor
Washes hands Uses appropriate PPE	• Handwash using the Ayliffe technique • Puts on gloves and apron •	☐ ☐ ☐	☐ ☐ ☐	☐ ☐ ☐	☐ ☐ ☐
Understands indications and anatomy	• Explains why it is important to maintain a patent airway • Explains the anatomy of the airway •	☐ ☐ ☐	☐ ☐ ☐	☐ ☐ ☐	☐ ☐ ☐
Consent issues Explanation to patient, often including complications	• Explains procedures correctly for a semiconscious patient • Explains the ethical issues concerning consent in an unconscious patient •	☐ ☐ ☐	☐ ☐ ☐	☐ ☐ ☐	☐ ☐ ☐
Communication skills	• Communicates effectively and politely with colleagues •	☐ ☐	☐ ☐	☐ ☐	☐ ☐
Appropriate preparation	• Ensures all airway equipment is ready for use • Demonstrates what checks need to be undertaken prior to using airway equipment •	☐ ☐ ☐	☐ ☐ ☐	☐ ☐ ☐	☐ ☐ ☐
Technical ability especially with any special equipment and sharps	**Initial airway assessment** • Demonstrates how to use the look, listen, and feel technique to assess the airway. • Airway opening manoeuvres • Explains when chin lift, head tilt should be used • Demonstrates chin lift and head tilt correctly • Explains when jaw thrust should be used • Demonstrates jaw thrust correctly • Assesses airway and ventilation following the intervention **Suction** • Explains when suctioning is indicated • Demonstrates the correct method for suctioning • Assesses airway and ventilation following the intervention **Oropharyngeal airway** • Discusses the indications and contraindications • Demonstrates the correct sizing technique • Demonstrates the correct insertion technique • Assesses airway and ventilation following the intervention. **Nasopharyngeal airway** • Discusses the indications and contraindications • Demonstrates the correct sizing technique • Demonstrates the correct insertion technique • Assesses airway and ventilation following the intervention •	☐ (×24)	☐ (×24)	☐ (×24)	☐ (×24)
Seeks help as appropriate	• Calls for help when required • Discusses when expert help should be sought •	☐ ☐ ☐	☐ ☐ ☐	☐ ☐ ☐	☐ ☐ ☐
Post-procedure management	• Escalates interventions as appropriate • Correctly disposes of used equipment safely •	☐ ☐ ☐	☐ ☐ ☐	☐ ☐ ☐	☐ ☐ ☐
Professionalism	• Demonstrates appropriate professional behaviour •	☐ ☐	☐ ☐	☐ ☐	☐ ☐
Overall ability to perform procedure	• Assess globally, would you be happy for this student to be supervised using appropriate interventions to manage the airway in a real patient? •	☐ ☐	☐ ☐	☐ ☐	☐ ☐

		Self	Peer	Peer /tutor	Tutor
Self-assessed as at least borderline:	Signature:	Date:	U B S E	U B S E	U B S E	U B S E
Peer-assessed as ready for tutor assessment:	Signature:	Date:	U B S E	U B S E	U B S E	U B S E
Tutor-assessed as satisfactory:	Signature:	Date:	U B S E	U B S E	U B S E	U B S E

Notes

10.9 Laryngeal mask airway insertion

Background

An LMA is a plastic tube with an anatomically shaped air-filled silicone end. It is designed to be inserted into the oropharynx where it provides a patent airway. A gel LMA airway device is a plastic tube with an anatomically shaped silicone end, it has a ventilation channel and a channel for gastric drainage.

Clinical indications

To facilitate the maintenance of a patent airway:

- For elective anaesthesia with a spontaneously breathing or ventilated patient
- For emergency maintenance of the airway during a cardiac arrest
- For emergency maintenance of the airway in the unconscious patient when ventilation with bag-valve-mask and other airway adjuncts is difficult.

Anatomical and physiological principles

In the unconscious patient airway patency can be compromised. This is often due to the tongue falling posteriorly, particularly due to relaxation of other airway muscles. In order to maintain ventilation (either spontaneously or with controlled intermittent positive pressure ventilation) a patent airway is required.

Contraindications

The laryngeal mask airway is only supraglottic and does not fully protect the airway from aspiration of stomach contents and therefore should not be used in an unfasted patient for elective procedures.

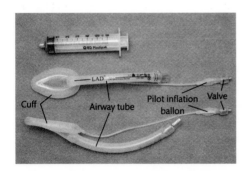

LMA (Laryngeal mask airway) with component parts labelled

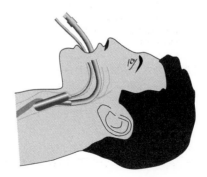

LMA *in situ*: this clearly shows the tight seal over the entrance to the trachea while occluding the oesophageal opening

Figure 10.13 Images in laryngeal mask insertion.

Explanation and consent

An LMA or gel LMA will be inserted during an emergency into an unconscious patient's airway. There must a clear indication and complications should be considered. It is unnecessary to explain the procedure to the patient. However, where possible, carers and/or relatives should be informed.

Equipment and preparation

A suitably sized LMA is required. The weight range is indicated on the LMA. Also needed is a 20 mL or 50 mL syringe and a means of ventilating the patient, e.g. a bag-valve-mask. The upper side (without the hole) of the LMA is lubricated with a suitable aqueous jelly. If a standard LMA is to be used the cuff should be checked by inflating with the correct volume of air (as indicated on the LMA). The cuff should be fully deflated before insertion.

Procedure

The patient will be unconscious and in respiratory or cardiac arrest.

- **Pre-oxygenation**: by ventilating with the bag-valve-mask and 100% oxygen, if possible.
- **LMA insertion**: stand at the head of the patient. The LMA should be held so that the curvature matches that of the hard palate. Hold the tube of the LMA placing index finger in the angle between the tube and the silicone end. It should be inserted into the mouth and advanced into the posterior pharynx, following the curve of the hard palate, until resistance is felt. It may aid insertion to get an assistant to administer a jaw thrust manoeuvre. If insertion is difficult the LMA can be turned through 90° to get around the tongue.
- **Cuff inflation**: Once the LMA is in position the balloon should be inflated with the correct volume of air. The bag-valve should be attached and ventilation attempted. Attempts at LMA insertion should not continue for more than 30 seconds before ventilating with bag-valve-mask prior to the next attempt.

Post-procedure management

The LMA is usually an intermediate measure prior to the insertion of a definitive airway (e.g. endotracheal tube) by a specifically trained person. The patient should continue to be ventilated and should be monitored at all times. If the patient regains consciousness and is breathing effectively the LMA should be removed.

Professionalism

It is essential that the person inserting the LMA communicates effectively with other team members to reflect what they are doing. They should remain with the patient at all times following the insertion of the LMA until appropriate further care has been administered.

Complications

- Aspiration of stomach contents
- Inability to ventilate
- Bleeding
- Sore throat

Patient safety tips

- **LMA for early ventilation only**: The LMA should only be used for maintenance of the airway in the unconscious patient with respiratory or cardiac arrest until a definitive assessment is made, usually by a trained anaesthetist.
- **Balloon inflation**: under-inflation results in a less than optimal seal for ventilation and over-inflation will have the same effect. Read the volume of air to be inserted carefully and inflate accordingly.
- **Evidence or suspicion of aspiration**: definitive assessment and, usually, an ET tube is required.

Student name:	Medical school:	Year:

Laryngeal mask airway insertion

This assessment is based around insertion of the LMA airways and questions in relation to this procedure.

		Self	Peer	Peer /tutor	Tutor
What are the clinical indications for an LMA?	• To facilitate the maintenance of a patent airway:	☐	☐	☐	☐
	• For elective anaesthesia with a spontaneously breathing or ventilated patient	☐	☐	☐	☐
	• For emergency maintenance of the airway during a cardiac arrest	☐	☐	☐	☐
	• For emergency maintenance of the airway in the unconscious patient when ventilation with bag-valve-mask and other airway adjuncts is difficult	☐	☐	☐	☐
	•	☐	☐	☐	☐
What are the main contraindications?	• The LMA does not fully protect the airway from aspiration of stomach contents and therefore should not be used in an unfasted patient for elective situation	☐	☐	☐	☐
	•	☐	☐	☐	☐
Please insert the LMA as you would in real time		☐	☐	☐	☐
Please go through the procedure again explaining each step	• **Explanation and consent**	☐	☐	☐	☐
	• **Equipment and preparation**: suitable sized LMA is required. Note weight range on the LMA. 20 mL or 50 mL syringe, bag-valve-mask needed. LMA is lubricated with aqueous jelly. Check balloon	☐	☐	☐	☐
	• **Procedure**:	☐	☐	☐	☐
	• **Pre-oxygenation**: ventilating with bag-valve-mask and 100% oxygen	☐	☐	☐	☐
	• **LMA insertion**: Hold LMA placing index finger in the angle between the tube and the silicon end. Insert into mouth and advance into posterior pharynx. Consider assistant to administer a jaw thrust manoeuvre	☐	☐	☐	☐
	• **Balloon inflation**: inflate with correct volume of air. Attach bag-valve and attempt ventilation. Continue for no more than 30 seconds before ventilating with bag-valve-mask prior to the next attempt.	☐	☐	☐	☐
	• **Post-procedure management**: Seek help for definitive airway (e.g. ET tube).	☐	☐	☐	☐
	• **Professionalism**: Communicate with team, remain with the patient at all times following the insertion of the LMA until appropriate further care has been administered.	☐	☐	☐	☐
	•	☐	☐	☐	☐
What are the main complications in relation to LMA insertion?	• Aspiration of stomach contents, inability to ventilate, bleeding, sore throat	☐	☐	☐	☐
	•	☐	☐	☐	☐
What are the key patient safety tips in relation to LMA insertion?	• **LMA for early ventilation only**: until definitive assessment by a trained anaesthetist	☐	☐	☐	☐
	• **Balloon inflation**: under-inflation and over-inflation must be avoided	☐	☐	☐	☐
	• **Evidence or suspicion of aspiration**: definitive assessment and, usually, ET tube.	☐	☐	☐	☐
	•	☐	☐	☐	☐

			U B S E	U B S E	U B S E	U B S E
Self-assessed as at least borderline:	Signature:	Date:	U B S E	U B S E	U B S E	U B S E
Peer-assessed as ready for tutor assessment:	Signature:	Date:	U B S E	U B S E	U B S E	U B S E
Tutor-assessed as satisfactory:	Signature:	Date:	U B S E	U B S E	U B S E	U B S E

Notes

10.10 Cardiac arrest

Background

Cardiac arrest is the most serious medical emergency that clinicians encounter. It can occur suddenly without warning or may be the inexorable outcome of a prolonged illness. Apart from a few specific situations the mortality from both in- and out-of-hospital cardiac arrest remains high. Significant improvements in the management of this condition have stemmed from widely followed guidelines from a number of national and international agencies. These guidelines have standardized the initial care for all patients undergoing cardiorespiratory arrest. Instruction in these guidelines has been formalized with the development of specific courses, e.g. Advanced Life Support, Paediatric Advanced Life Support, Advanced Trauma Life Support, which are widely taught. The reader is directed to literature produced by such bodies for the exact details of management. The Resuscitation Council UK is the body that sets national guidelines in the UK.

Diagnosis

Cardiac arrest is defined as a sustained severe failure of either the circulatory or respiratory system. In a severely compromised state, cardiorespiratory function may be detected, e.g. shallow breathing, but the functional output may be inadequate for the normal functioning of the body necessitating intervention. For diagnosis the patient must be unresponsive (a sign of severe brain dysfunction) and have been for at least a period of 10 seconds

- Absent central pulse, e.g. carotid
- Absent or inadequate breathing.

Causes

These are manyfold but essentially the final common pathway is either a failure of the circulation or a failure of oxygenation/ventilation. Respiratory failure will inevitably lead to circulatory failure. See also Figure 10.14.

Cardiac/vascular

- Myocardial infarction, cardiac rupture, cardiac tamponade
- Cardiac arrhythmia: ischaemia, electrolyte/acid–base imbalance or structural disease
- Massive pulmonary embolism
- Massive haemorrhage
- Natural/accidental severe damage to a critical organ, e.g. ruptured aorta
- Severe intravascular volume depletion
- Septic/anaphylactic shock

Airway/respiratory

- Occluded upper airway, e.g. foreign body, angioedema etc.
- Overwhelming lung pathology, e.g. pulmonary oedema, severe pneumonia, pulmonary haemorrhage
- Tension pneumothorax

Central nervous system

- Intracranial pathology, e.g. bleed impairing normal brainstem function (controlling respiration and cardiac function)

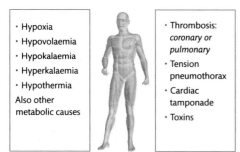

- Hypoxia
- Hypovolaemia
- Hypokalaemia
- Hyperkalaemia
- Hypothermia

Also other metabolic causes

- Thrombosis: *coronary or pulmonary*
- Tension pneumothorax
- Cardiac tamponade
- Toxins

Figure 10.14 Reversible causes of cardiac arrest.

- Drug/toxin/metabolic-induced CNS depression.
- Organ failure, e.g. liver, kidney causing progressive CNS dysfunction.

Management

See the Resuscitation Council (UK) 2010 Advanced life support guidelines for specific details on management (http://www.resus.org.uk/pages/guide.htm). A general outline is given below. The goals are to make a prompt diagnosis and summon help, begin BLS, initiate appropriate ALS, in particular defibrillation where necessary and appropriate post-arrest care. The ABCDE approach should be used initially and as soon as cardiac arrest is confirmed treatment commenced.

Phase 1 initial management

After confirmation of cardiorespiratory arrest, help should be called and BLS should be initiated as soon as possible.

- When appropriate staff and equipment are available ALS can be started.
- The two main types of arrest are:
  ○ Shockable rhythms, i.e. VF or pulseless VT
  ○ Non-shockable, i.e. asystole or PEA, formerly known as electromechanical dissociation (EMD).
- It is important to make this distinction as soon as possible because prompt defibrillation of shockable rhythms improves patient outcomes significantly.
- Where available, the patient's history and recent investigations and treatments should be reviewed by a member of the arrest team.
- For both types of arrest the clinician should always be on the look out for potentially reversible causes of cardiac arrest. Where suspected immediate treatment should be initiated:
  ○ Hypoxia, hypovolaemia, hypo/hyperkalaemia/metabolic, hypothermia
  ○ Thrombosis (coronary or pulmonary), tension pneumothorax, tamponade, toxins.
- Investigations – in general an immediate arterial/venous sample should be drawn and taken to a multifunctional blood gas machine, which will give additional data such as haemoglobin, sodium, potassium, urea, glucose, lactate, etc. A full set of bloods should be sent to the laboratory as well but the results will generally not be back within 30 minutes. Additionally, if trained personnel are immediately available some other bedside tests may help, e.g. echocardiogram to diagnose tamponade, abdominal ultrasound for aortic aneurysm, etc.
  ○ The following will be required post arrest: FBC, U&Es, bicarbonate, glucose, LFT, bone, CRP, clotting, magnesium, lactate; repeat ABG; cardiac enzymes, e.g. creatine kinase (CK) MB, troponin etc. if a cardiac event is suspected; 12-lead electrocardiogram (ECG); chest X-ray; additional specialized investigations may be needed where appropriate, e.g. CT pulmonary angiogram, CT brain etc.

Phase 2 management

- If resuscitation has been successful (ROSC – return of spontaneous circulation) the patient may still be in a critical condition with one or more modalities of organ support *in situ*, e.g. intubation and ventilation.
- A repeat ABCDE survey should be undertaken. Important to recheck the capillary glucose at this point.
- There is a high chance that the patient will arrest again so adequate monitoring and clinical vigilance should be employed.
- Difficult clinical decisions have to be made at this point as to further care. Firstly, it should be decided whether to pursue further resuscitation in the event of another cardiac arrest. Patient wishes, pre-morbid condition, the potential reversibility of any underlying pathologies and potential quality of life after recovery should all be considered when making this decision.
- If the cause of the arrest has been identified, definitive treatment for this condition should be undertaken where possible, e.g. percutaneous coronary intervention (PCI) for myocardial infarction.
- If the patient remains critically unwell and requires intensive monitoring or organ support, they will need to be transferred to an intensive therapy unit (ITU) unless it is felt that this would be not in the patient's best interests.

Ongoing management

- If a reversible/treatable cause has been found appropriate treatment should continue.
- Further interventions which may improve outcome in post-arrest patients include:
  - Tight blood glucose control
  - Therapeutic hypothermia.
- Even after successful resuscitation, it may be necessary to consider whether further resuscitation attempts should be made. In some patients, a 'DNAR' (do not attempt resuscitation) order may be needed.

Other aspects of treatment

- In patients who do not want CPR or whose clinical situation would make CPR unlikely to succeed, early decisions on resuscitation including the use of DNAR orders should be considered by senior members of the clinical team.

Patient safety tips

- ✔ **Prevention**: In retrospect many patients who arrest have been shown to be deteriorating over some time, the use of patient scoring scales, e.g. MEWS and timely intervention may help prevent some arrests.
- ✔ **Cardiac arrest team**: When making decision during the cardiac arrest the right balance between quick directed commands and team involvement should be attained. There must be no delays in aspects such as CPR and defibrillation. Decisions, such as the one to consider stopping CPR, should be discussed with all present with an expression by the lead such as 'I think we should discontinue CPR in this patient. This is because we have tried unsuccessfully for 24 minutes. The patients was brought into hospital with fixed dilated pupils after severe chest pain and collapse. What do you all think?'. The lead can then ask all team members individually for their opinion, gain a consensus and make a final decision, often after senior opinion if needed. This is to ensure that all aspects in relation to the cardiac arrest, particularly reversible factors have all been considered.

Student name: Medical school: Year:

Cardiac arrest

This assessment will be based around asking you questions in relation to cardiac arrest and demonstrating how to lead a cardiac arrest using this manikin and the team that you have available. You are the lead for the cardiac arrest team. You arrive first on the scene. The team arrive 45 seconds later.

The patient is a 73-year-old man who has been brought into hospital and collapsed. He is known to have oesophageal varices and was recently started on spironolactone.

		Self	Peer	Peer/tutor	Tutor
How is the diagnosis confirmed?	● Absent central pulse, e.g. carotid	☐	☐	☐	☐
	● Absent or inadequate breathing	☐	☐	☐	☐
What are the main causes of cardiac arrest	● Myocardial infarction, cardiac rupture, cardiac tamponade	☐	☐	☐	☐
	● Cardiac arrhythmia due to ischaemia, electrolyte/acid–base imbalance	☐	☐	☐	☐
	● Massive pulmonary embolism, massive haemorrhage	☐	☐	☐	☐
	● Natural/accidental severe damage to a critical organ, e.g. ruptured aorta	☐	☐	☐	☐
	● Severe intravascular volume depletion, e.g. septic/anaphylactic shock	☐	☐	☐	☐
	● Occluded upper airway, e.g. foreign body, angioedema, etc.	☐	☐	☐	☐
	● Overwhelming lung pathology, e.g. pulmonary oedema, severe pneumonia, pulmonary haemorrhage, tension pneumothorax	☐	☐	☐	☐
	● Massive intracranial pathology, e.g. bleed impairing normal brainstem function	☐	☐	☐	☐
	● Drug/toxin/metabolic-induced CNS depression.	☐	☐	☐	☐
	● Organ failure e.g. liver, kidney causing progressive CNS dysfunction.	☐	☐	☐	☐
What are the main aspects of phase 1 initial management (first 30 minutes)?	● Confirm arrest. Call for help	☐	☐	☐	☐
	● Initiate BLS including opening airway, chest compression and respirations	☐	☐	☐	☐
	● When equipment and personnel available start ALS	☐	☐	☐	☐
	● Distinguish between shockable and non-shockable rhythms and initiate appropriate treatment	☐	☐	☐	☐
	● Look for reversible causes (4 Hs and 4 Ts)	☐	☐	☐	☐
	● Review patient details and recent clinical details, e.g. bloods etc.	☐	☐	☐	☐
	● Take immediate blood gas and for analysis. Send venous bloods	☐	☐	☐	☐
	● Understanding of when resuscitation efforts should be discontinued	☐	☐	☐	☐
	● Post-arrest tests; FBC, U&E, glucose, LFT, bone, CRP, bone, magnesium, troponin (later), clotting	☐	☐	☐	☐
	● Repeat ABG, 12-lead ECG, chest X-ray	☐	☐	☐	☐
What are the main aspects of phase 2 management (30 minutes to 1 hour)?	● Appropriate full reassessment post cardiac resuscitation including full ABCDE survey	☐	☐	☐	☐
	● Aware that patient may re-arrest	☐	☐	☐	☐
	● If possible ensure definitive plan for underlying condition is present	☐	☐	☐	☐
	● Additional advanced tests may be needed, e.g. CTPA.	☐	☐	☐	☐
	● Awareness of need for intensive monitoring in appropriate setting, e.g. CCU, ITU, etc.	☐	☐	☐	☐
	● Understanding of when DNAR order and palliation may be appropriate	☐	☐	☐	☐
What are the main aspects of phase 3 (ongoing management)?	● Tight control of blood glucose	☐	☐	☐	☐
	● Therapeutic hypothermia may be beneficial to a subgroup of patients	☐	☐	☐	☐
Other aspects of treatment?	● Role of DNAR orders in patients at risk of having a cardiac arrest, ethical aspects	☐	☐	☐	☐
What are the main complications?	● Despite adequate treatment mortality and morbidity is high	☐	☐	☐	☐
	● Patients may develop complications during CPR including rib fractures, burns from defibrillation (rare)	☐	☐	☐	☐
What are the key patient safety tips?	● Prevention – in retrospect many patients who arrest have been deteriorating over some time, use MEWS and timely intervention to prevent some arrests	☐	☐	☐	☐
	● Cardiac arrest team: check key decisions with other team members	☐	☐	☐	☐
Clinical note writing and handover	● Adequate documentation in notes including cardiac arrest audit forms	☐	☐	☐	☐

Self-assessed as at least borderline:	Signature:	Date:	U B S E	U B S E	U B S E	U B S E
Peer-assessed as ready for tutor assessment:	Signature:	Date:	U B S E	U B S E	U B S E	U B S E
Tutor-assessed as satisfactory:	Signature:	Date:	U B S E	U B S E	U B S E	U B S E

Notes

DO NOT ATTEMPT CARDIOPULMONARY RESUSCITATION

Adults aged 16 years and over

DNAR adult (June 2010)

George Eliot Hospital **NHS**

NHS Trust

Name _____

Address _____

Date of birth _____

NHS or hospital number _____

Date of DNAR order:

/ /

DO NOT PHOTOCOPY

In the event of cardiac or respiratory arrest no attempts at cardiopulmonary resuscitation (CPR) will be made. All other appropriate treatment and care will be provided.

1 Does the patient have capacity to make and communicate decisions about CPR? If "YES" go to box 2 — YES / NO

If "NO", are you aware of a valid advance decision refusing CPR which is relevant to the current condition?" If "YES" go to box 6 — YES / NO

If "NO", has the patient appointed a Welfare Attorney to make decisions on their behalf? If "YES" they must be consulted. — YES / NO

All other decisions must be made in the patient's best interests and comply with current law. Go to box 2

2 Summary of the main clinical problems and reasons why CPR would be inappropriate, unsuccessful or not in the patient's best interests:

3 Summary of communication with patient (or Welfare Attorney). If this decision has not been discussed with the patient or Welfare Attorney state the reason why:

4 Summary of communication with patient's relatives or friends:

5 Names of members of multidisciplinary team contributing to this decision:

6 Healthcare professional completing this DNAR order:

Name _____ **Position** _____

Signature _____ **Date** _____ **Time** _____

7 Review and endorsement by Consultant:

Signature _____ **Name** _____ **Date** _____

Review dates (if appropriate)

Signature _____ **Name** _____ **Date** _____

Signature _____ **Name** _____ **Date** _____

Top copy in patient notes, Carbonated copy to Resuscitation Officer, GETEC.

Unit 11 General clinical emergencies

11.1 Sepsis

Background

Sepsis and septic shock are life-threatening medical emergencies. Despite clinical advances in treatment, mortality is high (50%) and morbidity even higher. A source of infection is always the trigger for a recognized sequence of events which progress to septicaemia. The mechanism responsible for the progression of an infective process to sepsis and septic shock is unclear. However, risk factors that predispose to infection and septicaemia have been identified. In sepsis, microorganisms provoke an intense inflammatory response leading to severe derangement of normal physiological function in tissues and organs. The net effect is hypoperfusion, which leads to organ dysfunction initially and progressively to end-organ failure. The main targets in the management of sepsis and septic shock are:

1 To intervene fast, accurately and efficiently in the process of sepsis in order to prevent reversible cellular dysfunction becoming irreversible

2 To reverse the hypoperfusion and restore homeostasis and organ function.

The treatment is focused on ensuring adequate delivery of oxygen to tissues and end organs. Oxygen delivery is regulated by four elements: amount of haemoglobin, haemoglobin saturation, cardiac output, and peripheral perfusion. The UK Surviving Sepsis Campaign has produced guidelines on rapid and effective recognition of sepsis and septic shock, and appropriate interventions based on the best-available evidence. These interventions involve measures to restore the four key elements that regulate oxygen delivery to the organs to their normal limits in an organized and efficient framework.

The 'sepsis six' are 6 key topics that must be completed urgently as soon as is currently diagnosed:

1 Give high flow O_2: via non-rebreathable bag.

2 Take blood cultures.

3 Give IV antibiotics considering presumed source of infection.

4 IV fluid resuscitation: Hartmann's or local policy.

5 Measure haemoglobin and lactate.

6 Monitor hourly urine output: urinary catheter usually needed.

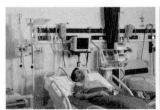
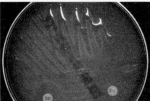
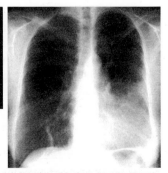

History, examination, investigations: essential parts of early management

Ensure appropriate microbiological specimens are taken prior to antibiotic therapy in most cases

Early recourse to intensive care if rapid improvement not forthcoming

Figure 11.1 Images in sepsis.

Clinical definitions in sepsis

Sepsis is defined as the presence of two or more markers for systemic inflammatory response syndrome (SIRS) plus confirmed or suspected infection.

Systemic inflammatory response syndrome

- Temperature >38 °C or <36 °C,
- Heart rate >90/min
- Respiratory rate >20/min
- White cell count (WCC) >12 × 10^9/L or <4 × 10^9/L
- Acutely altered mental state
- Glucose >8.3 mmol/L (in absence of known diabetes mellitus).

Severe sepsis

Severe sepsis is the addition of organ dysfunction or hypoperfusion, or hypotension. Defined by one or more single organ dysfunction or single hypoperfusion criteria.

- Organ dysfunction
  - Respiratory: New or increased O_2 requirement to maintain O_2 saturation >90%
  - Renal: Urine output <0.5 mL/kg/hr for 2 hours
  - Hepatic: Bilirubin >34 µmol/L
  - Coagulation: Platelets <100 × 10^9/L, INR >1.5 or aPTT >60 s
- Tissue hypoperfusion
  - BP: Systolic <90 mmHg or mean arterial pressure < 65 mmHg
  - BP: Reduced by >40 mmHg from patients normal systolic
  - Lactate >2 mmol/L

Septic shock

Septic shock is the persistence of severe sepsis and hypotension despite adequate fluid resuscitation. Signs include hypotension, mottled skin, delayed capillary refill and oliguria.

Causes and possible source of infection

Most common causative agents are bacteria but viruses, parasites, and fungi have the potential to cause sepsis in specific conditions. Risk factors for sepsis include: immunosuppression, diabetes especially if poorly controlled, chemotherapy, radiation, steroid treatment, acquired immune deficiency syndrome (AIDS), splenectomy. Common conditions predisposing to sepsis include: pneumonia, urinary tract infection, cellulitis, severe burns or injuries, peritonitis, appendicitis, meningitis, and post operatively, central and peripheral line infections.

Management

For most sections in this unit we have divided management into: phase 1 initial management (first hour), phase 2 management (2–6 hours), phase 3 ongoing management. This section deviates a little from this plan to accord with the guidelines of the UK Surviving Sepsis campaign. The guidelines propose two 'management bundles' for the initial resuscitation (first 6 hours) and further management (first 24 hours) of sepsis based on the best available evidence. The elements of each bundle are therapies/interventions that achieve better outcomes when implemented together rather than when implemented individually. The UK Surviving Sepsis management bundles are described after a summary of initial management actions (phase 1 initial management).

Phase 1 initial management (first hour)

- **ABCDE assessment and management**: high-flow oxygen, irrespective of medical history. Resuscitate with intravenous (IV) fluids. Exclude or treat hypoglycaemia.

- **Large-bore intravenous cannula**: send bloods for investigation (full blood count [FBC], urea and electrolytes [U&Es], clotting profile, lactate, random glucose, venous bicarbonate). Continue IV fluids.

- **Arterial blood gases**: to establish degree of metabolic acidosis and evaluate partial oxygen and carbon dioxide pressures.

- **Cultures**: blood, midstream urine (MSU) or catheter specimen of urine (CSU), injury sites, pressure sores, ulcers, cerebrospinal fluid (CSF) (if indicated), central lines, peripheral lines. Preferably before antibiotic administration.

- **IV antibiotics**: to be initiated as soon as possible and should be guided by clinical assessment and suspicion of likely source of infection and according to hospital antibiotic guidelines.

- **Urinary catheterization**: for urine output hourly monitoring.

- **Imaging**: chest radiograph (CXR) and abdominal X-ray (AXR) if indicated, ultrasound scan abdomen or computed tomography (CT) abdomen in case of intra-abdominal abscess suspicion, CT brain if brain abscess is suspected.

- **Venous thromboembolism (VTE) assessment**: TED stockings (after ruling out peripheral vascular disease) and anti-deep vein thrombosis (DVT) prophylaxis (usually low-molecular-weight heparin [LMWH]).

- **Observations**: hourly or more frequent observations to be recorded, medical early warning score (MEWS) calculated, general intake and output chart.

- **Consider abscess**: in cases of abscess (intra-abdominal or intracranial) or presence of source of infection that might need debridement urgent surgical review must be sought.

- **Intensive care unit (ICU) team**: should be contacted after the early steps of management.

UK surviving sepsis campaign management bundle A: resuscitation (management within 6 hours)

The resuscitation bundle is a combination of evidence-based goals that must be completed within 6 hours for patients with severe sepsis, septic shock, and/or lactate >4 mmol/L (36 mg/dL). Begin resuscitation immediately in patients with hypotension or elevated serum lactate >4 mmol/L; do not delay pending ICU admission.

Resuscitation goals

- **Central venous pressure** (CVP) 8–12 mm Hg

- **Mean arterial pressure** ≥70 mm Hg (MAP = diastolic blood pressure [BP] + (33% of systolic-diastolic BP)

- **Urine output** ≥0.5 mL/kg/h

- **Central venous (superior vena cava) oxygen saturation** ≥70%, or mixed venous ≥65%

Bundle element 1: measure lactate

- Hyperlactatemia is typically present in severe sepsis or septic shock and may be secondary to anaerobic metabolism due to hypoperfusion. Lactate level is used to identify tissue hypoperfusion in patients who are not yet hypotensive but are at risk for septic shock.

- Elevated serum lactate does not always reflect global hypoperfusion but can be a result of cellular metabolic failure.

Rx: fluid resuscitation and treatment of underlying cause, antibiotics, oxygen.

Bundle element 2: obtain blood cultures prior to antibiotic administration

Indications: Fever, chills, hypothermia, leucocytosis, left shift of neutrophils, neutropenia, and the development of otherwise unexplained organ dysfunction, e.g. renal failure or signs of haemodynamic compromise.

- 30–50% of severe sepsis or shock patients have positive blood cultures. Specific antibiotic treatment is best, therefore, two or more blood cultures are recommended. In suspected vascular access device-related infection, obtain blood cultures through the suspected device and a peripheral site simultaneously. If the vascular access device culture is positive earlier than a peripheral site culture, the former is strongly implicated as the source of infection. **Rx: broad-spectrum antibiotics urgently, ideally within 1 hour of admission**.

- Treat empirically while awaiting culture and sensitivities. Early administration of appropriate antibiotics reduces mortality in patients with Gram-positive and Gram-negative sepsis. Duration of therapy is typically 7–10 days, guided by clinical response.

Bundle element 3: treat hypotension and/or elevated lactate with fluids

Rx: Fluid therapy:

- Fluid resuscitation should be commenced as early as possible in the course of septic shock (even before intensive care unit admission).
- Initially 20 mL/kg IV of crystalloid, bolus fluid if hypoperfusion or actual cases of serum lactate >4 mmol/L (36 g/dL). A colloid is an acceptable alternative to crystalloid.
- Rate of fluid administration: depends on clinical urgency (after 500–1000 mL every 30 minutes) but should be reduced if cardiac filling pressures increases without concurrent haemodynamic improvement. In septic shock 5 litres of IV fluid may be needed initially.

Fluid challenge versus fluid overload

- *Fluid challenge* is used to describe the initial volume expansion period in which the response of the patient to IV fluid is carefully evaluated. During this process, large amounts of fluids may be administered over a short period of time under close monitoring to evaluate the patient's response.
- Safety margins: observe for evidence of pulmonary and systemic oedema during fluid resuscitation. During the first 24 hours, input is typically much greater than output, and input/output ratio is of no utility to judge fluid resuscitation needs during this time.

Bundle element 4: vasopressors for ongoing hypotension

- **Administer vasopressors**: for hypotension not responding to initial fluid resuscitation to maintain mean arterial pressure (MAP) >65 mmHg. Adequate fluid resuscitation is a prerequisite for the successful and appropriate use of vasopressors in patients with septic shock.
- **Noradrenaline**: through a central catheter, is the first-choice vasopressor agent to correct hypotension in septic shock. Adrenaline or phenylephrine should not be used as first-line vasopressors as part of the treatment of septic shock. Inotropic support with dobutamine may be needed.
- **Volume resuscitation**: is a prerequisite, otherwise vasopressor use may worsen already inadequate organ perfusion.

Bundle element 5: in septic shock and/or lactate >4 mmol/L maintain adequate CVP and central venous oxygen saturation (ScvO$_2$)

A. Achieve a CVP of >8 mmHg

- **CVP catheter** and deliver repeated fluid challenges until the target CVP value is achieved.
- **Packed red cell transfusion**: for hypovolaemia with haematocrit <30%. Oxygen delivery to ischaemic tissues will increase and CVP >8 mmHg will be maintained for longer periods than with fluids alone.
- *Blood transfusion*: when haemoglobin decreases, transfuse to obtain target haemoglobin of at least >10 g/dL in adults. A higher haemoglobin level may be required in special circumstances (e.g. myocardial ischaemia, severe hypoxaemia, acute haemorrhage, cyanotic heart disease, or lactic acidosis).
- **Platelet transfusion**: when:
  ○ Platelet counts are ≤5 × 10^9/L regardless of bleeding.
  ○ Platelet counts are 5–30 × 10^9/L and there is significant bleeding risk.

○ Higher platelet counts ≥50 × 10^9/L are typically required for surgery or invasive procedures.

B. Achieve $ScvO_2$ >70% or mixed venous oxygen saturation (SvO_2) >65%

By combination of fluid resuscitation, fluid challenge, blood transfusion, inotropes, and mechanical ventilation.

UK Surviving Sepsis campaign bundle B

Sepsis management bundle to be completed within 24 hours in severe sepsis, septic shock, and/or lactate >4 mmol/L (36 mg/dL).

Bundle element 1: Low-dose steroids for septic shock in accordance with local policy

- **IV corticosteroids**: hydrocortisone 200–300 mg/day, for 7 days in three or four divided doses or by continuous infusion is suggested for adult septic shock patients if blood pressure (BP) is poorly responsive to fluid resuscitation and vasopressor therapy. Evidence suggests decreased mortality and earlier shock reversal. Do not use corticosteroids to treat sepsis in the absence of shock unless the patient's endocrine or corticosteroid history warrants it.

Bundle element 2: Recombinant human activated protein C (rhAPC) in accordance with local policy

- **rhAPC**: is recommended for sepsis-induced organ dysfunction associated with a clinical assessment of high risk of death, most of whom will have APACHE II ≥25 (see below) or multiple organ failure (if there are no contraindications).

Bundle element 3: maintain adequate glycaemic control

- **Glucose control**: use IV insulin to control hyperglycaemia in patients with severe sepsis following stabilization in ICU. Aim to keep blood glucose <8.3 mmol/L using a validated protocol for insulin dose adjustment.
- **Provide a glucose calorie source and monitor blood glucose values**: every 1–2 hours (4 hours when stable) in patients receiving IV insulin.
- **Beware of biochemical and clinical hypoglycaemia**: interpret low glucose levels obtained with point of care testing with caution, as these techniques may overestimate arterial blood or plasma glucose values.
- **Effective glucose control in the ICU** has been shown to decrease morbidity and mortality but optimal target range for blood glucose in critically ill patients remains unclear. Intensive insulin therapy halved the prevalence of: bloodstream infections, acute renal failure dialysis or haemofiltration, critical illness polyneuropathy, transfusion requirements.

Bundle element 4: inspiratory plateau pressures maintained <30 cm H_2O for mechanically ventilated patients for acute lung injury or Adult Respiratory Distress Syndrome

Inspiratory plateau pressure of <30 cm H_2O: results in a 9% decrease of all-cause mortality in patients ventilated with tidal volumes of 6 mL/kg of estimated lean body weight (as opposed to 12 mL/kg).

Other aspects of sepsis care

- **Renal replacement**: intermittent haemodialysis and continuous veno-venous haemofiltration (CVVH) are considered equivalent. CVVH offers easier management in haemodynamically unstable patients
- **Bicarbonate therapy**: do not use bicarbonate therapy for the purpose of improving haemodynamics or reducing vasopressor requirements when treating hypoperfusion-induced lactic acidaemia with pH ≥7.15. Bicarbonate is only used in more very severely acidotic haemodynamically unstable patients.
- **VTE prophylaxis**: LMWH is usually used, unless contraindicated. Mechanical prophylactic devices, such as compression stockings or an intermittent compression device are used, when heparin is contraindicated. A combination of pharmacological and mechanical therapy

is used for patients who are at very high risk for deep vein thrombosis (DVT) or pulmonary embolism.

● Stress ulcer prophylaxis: using H_2 blocker or proton pump inhibitor should be considered in all ICU patients. Benefits of prevention of upper gastrointestinal bleed must be weighed against the potential for development of ventilator-acquired pneumonia. The incidence of the latter is increased by H_2 blocker or proton pump inhibitors.

APACHE II physiological scoring systems

The reason for briefly introducing the APACHE II scoring system is that it acts as summary or 'algebra' of the main physiological and pathological states that influence morbidity and mortality in virtually any clinical setting. There are many other scoring systems. Clinicians should therefore always be aware of these 'risk factors' for a poor clinical outcome and make all attempts to address them effectively where possible.

● A general measure of disease severity based on: current physiological measurements, age, previous health condition.

● Scores range from 0 to 71: allocated in similar fashion to the MEWS score.

● Increasing score associated with an increasing risk of hospital death.

APACHE II score = (acute physiology score) + (age points) + (chronic health points)

Acute physiology score parameters

(Maximum four points each depending on degree of abnormality, high or low):

1 Temp (C)
2 MAP (mmHg)
3 Heart rate (bpm)
4 Respiratory rate (per minute)
5 Oxygen delivery (mL/min)
6 PO_2 (mmHg)
7 Arterial pH
8 Serum sodium (mmol/L)
9 Serum potassium (mmol/L)
10 Creatinine (μmol/L)
11 Haematocrit (ratio or %)
12 White cell count (10^3/mL).
13 Glasgow Coma Scale (GCS) points: 15 minus the GCS Score = maximum 12 points (see Table 11.8 below).

Age points

Age: 44 (0 points), 45–54 (2 points), 55–64 (3 points), 65–74 (5 points), >75 (6 points)

Chronic health points

History of severe organ insufficiency or immunocompromised state points:

● Non-operative patients or emergency postoperative patients = 5
● Elective postoperative patients = 2.

Organ insufficiency or immunocompromised state must have preceded the current admission.

- **Immunocompromised if**: receiving therapy reducing host defences (immunosuppression, chemotherapy, radiation therapy, long-term steroid use, high-dose steroid therapy) or has a disease interfering with immune function such as malignant lymphoma or leukaemia.
- **Hepatic insufficiency if**: biopsy proven cirrhosis or portal hypertension or episodes of upper gastrointestinal bleeding due to portal hypertension or prior episodes of hepatic failure, coma or encephalopathy.
- **Cardiovascular insufficiency if**: New York Heart Association (NYHA) class IV cardiac failure (Table 11.1).
- **Respiratory insufficiency if**: severe exercise restriction due to chronic restrictive or obstructive or vascular disease or documented chronic hypoxia or hypercapnia or secondary polycythaemia or severe pulmonary hypertension or respirator dependency.
- **Renal insufficiency if**: on chronic dialysis.

Table 11.1 New York Heart Association (NYHA) functional classification for cardiac failure

Class I	No limitation of physical activity Ordinary physical activity does not cause undue fatigue, palpitation, or dyspnoea
Class II	Slight limitation of physical activity. Comfortable at rest, but ordinary physical activity results in fatigue, palpitation, or dyspnoea
Class III	Marked limitation of physical activity. Comfortable at rest, but less than ordinary activity results in fatigue, palpitation, or dyspnoea
Class IV	Unable to carry on any physical activity without discomfort Symptoms at rest. If any physical activity is undertaken, discomfort is increased

APACHE II score: maximum 71

(acute physiology score: max 60) + (age points: max 6) + (chronic health points: max 5)

Risk of death: Range from 4% with score of 0 to 4 through to 85% with score of >34.

Patient safety tips

✔ **Meticulous attention**: to history, examination, results of investigations.

✔ **Use MEWS**: or similar system to track improvement or deterioration in patient.

✔ **Close observation**: keep patient close to nursing station.

✔ **Seek help early**: early recourse for help from critical care team or ICU team.

Sepsis

A 79-year-old woman has been brought in from home with a BP of 84/58 mmHg. She is confused and incoherent and coughing up green, blood stained sputum. The peripheries are cold to touch despite the hot warm summer day. Her initial observations are:

- Temperature 38.7 °C
- Heart rate 104/min
- Resp. rate 24
- WCC 19.3×10^9/L,
- Neutrophils 13.7×10^9/L

This Assessment will be based around a discussion on the management of sepsis with reference to the above scenario.

		Self	Peer	Peer /tutor	Tutor
What are the aims of management of sepsis?	To intervene to prevent reversible cellular dysfunction to become irreversible	☐	☐	☐	☐
	To reverse the hypoperfusion and restore homeostasis and organ function. This is especially in relation to oxygen delivery to the tissues, cardiac output, and peripheral perfusion	☐	☐	☐	☐
	What are the 'sepsis six' tasks: give high flow O_2, take blood cultures, give IV antibiotics, give IV fluid resuscitation, measure Hb and lactate, monitor hourly urine output	☐	☐	☐	☐
		☐	☐	☐	☐
What are the four main definitions in sepsis?	**SIRS**: Temperature >38 °C or <36 °C, heart rate >90/min, respiratory rate >20/min, WCC >12/<4, altered mental state, glucose >8.3 in absence of diabetes	☐	☐	☐	☐
	Sepsis: at least two markers for SIRS plus confirmed or suspected infection	☐	☐	☐	☐
	Severe sepsis: Sepsis plus organ dysfunction or hypoperfusion, or hypotension (oliguria, confusion, lactate >4 mmol/L, poor peripheral perfusion	☐	☐	☐	☐
	Septic shock: severe sepsis and hypotension despite adequate fluid resuscitation	☐	☐	☐	☐
		☐	☐	☐	☐
What category does the patient in the above vignette fit into?	Phase 1: initial management (first hour): Please outline what this is in relation to the above case:				
	ABCDE assessment and management: high-flow oxygen, IV fluids, check glucose, and treat	☐	☐	☐	☐
	Large-bore IV cannula: send bloods for investigation	☐	☐	☐	☐
	Arterial blood gases: ? metabolic acidosis, evaluate pO_2, pCO_2	☐	☐	☐	☐
	Cultures: blood, sputum. Ideally, before antibiotic administration	☐	☐	☐	☐
	IV antibiotics: as soon as possible, consider streptococcal or atypical pneumonia.	☐	☐	☐	☐
	Urinary catheterization: for urine output hourly monitoring	☐	☐	☐	☐
	Imaging: CXR.	☐	☐	☐	☐
	VTE assessment: DVT prophylaxis (usually LMWH), ? TED stockings if no peripheral vascular disease	☐	☐	☐	☐
	Observations: hourly or more frequent MEWS scores, intake and output chart	☐	☐	☐	☐
	Consider ICU team: should be contacted after the early steps of management	☐	☐	☐	☐
	UK Surviving Sepsis Campaign management bundle a: resuscitation (within 6 hours)	☐	☐	☐	☐
		☐	☐	☐	☐
What are the resuscitation goals?	CVP 8–12 mm Hg, MAP ≥70 mm Hg, urine output ≥0.5 ml/kg/hr, central venous (superior vena cava) oxygen saturation ≥70%, or mixed venous ≥65%	☐	☐	☐	☐
		☐	☐	☐	☐
What is the MAP in the patient in the clinical vignette? How is it calculated? **What the main 'bundle elements' in management bundle A and how are they treated?**	**Bundle element 1: measure lactate. Rx**: fluid resuscitation and treatment of underlying cause, antibiotics, oxygen	☐	☐	☐	☐
	Bundle element 2: obtain blood cultures and urgent antibiotic administration 30–50% positive blood cultures. Specific antibiotic treatment is best	☐	☐	☐	☐
	Bundle element 3: treat hypotension and/or elevated lactate with fluids. Rx: fluid therapy: initially 20 mL/kg IV of crystalloid or colloid	☐	☐	☐	☐
	Bundle element 4: vasopressors for ongoing hypotension: To maintain MAP >70 mmHg. Adequate fluid resuscitation is needed prior to noradrenaline or dopamine	☐	☐	☐	☐
	Bundle element 5: maintain adequate CVP and $ScvO_2$: Repeated fluid challenges until target CVP achieved. ? blood transfusion, inotropes and mechanical ventilation	☐	☐	☐	☐
		☐	☐	☐	☐

What the main 'bundle elements' in management bundle B and how are they treated?	• **Bundle element 1: steroids for septic shock in accordance with local policy**. Hydrocortisone if BP is poorly responsive to fluid resuscitation and vasopressor therapy	☐	☐	☐	☐
	• **Bundle element 2: rhAPC in accordance local policy**. For organ dysfunction associated with high risk of death	☐	☐	☐	☐
	• **Bundle element 3: maintain adequate glycaemic control**. Use IV insulin to control hyperglycaemia. Aim to keep blood glucose <8.3 mmol/L. Monitor every 1–2 hours	☐	☐	☐	☐
	• **Bundle element 4: Inspiratory plateau pressures maintained <30 cm H$_2$O for mechanically ventilated patients**	☐	☐	☐	☐
	•	☐	☐	☐	☐
What are the key patient safety tips in relation to managing sepsis?	• **Meticulous attention**: to history, examination, results of investigations	☐	☐	☐	☐
	• **Use MEWS**: or similar system to track improvement or deterioration in patient	☐	☐	☐	☐
	• **Close observation**: keep patient close to nursing station	☐	☐	☐	☐
	• **Seek help early**: early recourse for help from critical care team or ICU team.	☐	☐	☐	☐
	•	☐	☐	☐	☐

			U B S E	U B S E	U B S E	U B S E
Self-assessed as at least borderline:	Signature:	Date:				
Peer-assessed as ready for tutor assessment:	Signature:	Date:	U B S E	U B S E	U B S E	U B S E
Tutor-assessed as satisfactory:	Signature:	Date:	U B S E	U B S E	U B S E	U B S E

Notes

11.2 Acute abdomen

Background

'Acute abdomen' (Figure 11.2) is widely used to describe a clinical condition of rapid onset or rapidly worsening abdominal pain in patients, severe enough to warrant emergency admission to the hospital. Initial assessment of such patients is of pivotal importance as many of them are likely to have underlying life-threatening conditions that would need immediate surgical interventions after initial resuscitation. Other patients need intensive monitoring and may be considered for surgery if the condition worsens or fails to improve. An acute abdomen can also result from abdominal trauma. Epigastric pain implicates foregut structures. Peri-umbilical pain suggests mid-gut and supra-pubic pain implies hindgut structures are affected.

1 Stomach: peptic ulcer disease
2 Heart: ACS
3 Liver: hepatitis, cardiac failure, cholangitis
4 Gallbladder: Cholecystitis, biliary colic
5 Omentum: inflammation (local sepsis)
6 Appendix: appendicitis ± perforation
7 Bladder & ureters: cystitis, obstruction, stones
8 Lungs: basal pneumonia
9 Oesophagus: reflux, rupture
10 Aorta: rupture of aneurysm, dissection
11 Renal: sepsis, stones
12 Pancreas: acute pancreatitis
13 Small bowel: infarction
14 Sigmoid colon: diverticulitis, perforation
15 Ectopic pregnancy, testicular torsion, hernial obstruction

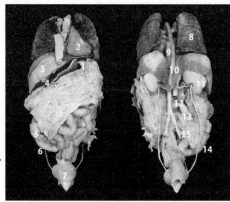

Figure 11.2 Acute abdomen: common diagnoses.

Main anatomical sites and causes of an acute abdomen

Causes arising from retroperitoneum and thorax

- Pancreas: acute and necrotizing pancreatitis
- Aorta: aortic aneurysm, dissection of aorta
- Kidneys, ureter: calculi, pyelonephritis, pyonephrosis
- Heart: inferior myocardial infarction
- Lungs: basal pneumonia, especially in elderly

Systemic and other causes

- 'Internal medicine causes': diabetic ketoacidosis (DKA), mesenteric adenitis (*Yersinia pseudotuberculosis* infection), porphyria, familial Mediterranean fever (autosomal recessive condition), sickle cell disease
- Non-specific acute abdominal pain: irritable bowel syndrome, constipation

Causes arising from upper abdomen

- Liver: any condition stretching Glisson's capsule, e.g. hepatitis, congestive cardiac failure (CCF), liver metastases

- Biliary system: acute cholecystitis, biliary colic, and cholangitis
- Oesophagus: gastro-oesophageal reflux disease (GORD)
- Spontaneous rupture or the oesophagus (Boerhaave's syndrome)
- Stomach and duodenum: peptic ulcer perforation or bleed, acute gastritis, gastric volvulus, hiatus hernia, gastric cancer (rare)
- Spleen: injury, torsion (rare), infarction

Causes arising from lower abdomen and pelvis

- Small bowel: obstruction, perforation, ischaemia, Meckel's diverticulitis, Crohn's disease
- Large bowel: colitis (ulcerative colitis, Crohn's colitis, pseudo-membranous colitis), diverticulitis, ischemia, perforation, pelvic abscess, volvulus
- Appendix: acute appendicitis, perforation
- Omentum: torsion and ischaemia
- Reproductive organs: mid-cycle pain (Mittelschmerz), torsion of ovarian cyst, ectopic pregnancy, pelvic inflammatory disease, fibroids in uterus, testicular torsion
- Hernias: Strangulated inguinal or femoral hernias

Diagnosis of acute abdomen

History

A full clinical is needed, a few points specific to the acute abdomen will be emphasized.

The history of pain may be elaborated under following subheadings (SQITAS):

- **Site**: The site of pain correlates well but not perfectly with the anatomical location of specific organs. This should only be used as a guide to the final diagnosis. Pain is referred from the gallbladder or diaphragm to shoulder tips and renal colic is referred from 'loin (renal angle) to groin'. Pain from retroperitoneal organ is often referred to the back. Pain in appendicitis is generalized and is shifted and localized to right iliac fossa with progression of disease.
- **Quality**: Pain from abdominal aortic aneurysm (AAA) rupture or dissection is described as 'stabbing', 'piercing', or 'tearing' in nature, and severe in intensity.
- **Intensity**: nature and severity (scale of 0–10), where 0 is no pain at all and 10 the worst pain you have ever had.
- **Timing**: when did it start, is it constant, does it come and go, how long does it last, is it getting worse?
- **Aggravating and relieving factors**: Spicy food tends to aggravate pain from GORD and fatty food makes cholecystitis worse. If inflamed organ or omentum is present, movement in general can make pain worse. Pain from a duodenal ulcer can be improved by food or antacids.
- **Symptoms-associated**:
  - ○ Weight and appetite: significant loss of weight and appetite may indicate underlying malignancy or chronic illness such as inflammatory bowel disease
  - ○ Collapse or loss of consciousness: in AAA rupture and dissection of aorta, massive gastrointestinal bleed
  - ○ Temperature: infections such as cholangitis, cholecystitis, urinary tract infections
  - ○ Nausea and vomiting: intestinal obstruction, pancreatitis, ? haematemesis
  - ○ Diarrhoea: associated with colitis and constipation associated with intestinal obstruction

○ Urinary symptoms: blood in urine in renal calculi, tumour or urinary tract infection (UTI). Urinary retention in bladder outflow obstruction

○ Abdominal distension: and associated vomiting in intestinal obstruction

○ Jaundice: in obstructed biliary system, cholangitis

○ Melaena or any change in bowel habit.

Past medical history and medications

- Medical: peptic ulcer disease, inflammatory bowel disease, diabetes, porphyria, ischaemic heart disease, jaundice.

- Surgical: previous operations which may result in adhesions and intestinal obstruction.

- Gynaecological: pregnancy, contraceptives, menstrual cycles.

- Investigations: endoscopy or scans and what did they reveal, for example patients on surveillance for aortic aneurysm have yearly scans.

- Medications: patients on anticoagulants such as aspirin, warfarin, and clopidogrel are at risk of bleeding if operated on. β-blockers may mask signs of hypovolaemic shock.

- Allergies: especially to antibiotics such as penicillin.

- Social history: occupation, alcohol, smoking.

Examination

General survey

- Hands: clubbing, koilonychia and leuconychia in nails, evidence of rheumatoid arthritis in fingers (often co-exists with inflammatory bowel disease), palmar erythema, Dupuytren's contracture.

- Pulse: rate, rhythm, and volume. Atrial fibrillation (irregularly irregular pulse can be responsible for embolism and mesenteric ischemia), Low volume pulse and cold periphery in hypovolaemic shock.

- Blood pressure: Low BP is associated with advanced stage of shock.

- Face: Jaundice in sclera and pallor on conjunctivae.

- Neck: For lymph nodes and jugular venous pulse.

- Oedema: on the ankles and sacrum.

Systemic examination

Ideally started from foot end of bed, with the head end as flat as possible. Does the patient look ill? Is he/she lying still or rolling about, watching TV calmly and walking to the toilet, or unable to move and very stressed? Practise these observations, they are crucial.

- Inspection: For scars (previous operations), hernias, prominent veins (example 'caput medusa' in portal hypertension due to end-stage liver disease), distension due to intestinal obstruction, etc.

- Palpation: superficial and deep palpation of all abdominal areas (nine areas: epigastrium, right and left hypochondrium, right and left lumbar, right and left iliac, umbilical, and hypogastrium; see Unit 2, Figure 2.1). Tenderness in respective areas is due to specific abdominal conditions. Generalized abdominal tenderness is often elicited in extensive peritonitis (example faecal peritonitis from large intestinal perforation). ? Guarding. Rebound tenderness is too painful for patients, do percussion tenderness instead.

- Percussion: dull note is elicited over solid or fluid filled cavity; underlying hollow viscus gives a resonant note. Severe tenderness on percussion is due to peritonitis.

- Auscultation: bowel sounds are normally present. Acute intra-abdominal sepsis can result in paralytic ileus with no bowel sounds (auscultation should be continued for at least 1 minute before reaching this conclusion). Intestinal obstruction results in 'hurried' bowel sounds.

Hugely distended bowel loops give a 'high pitched cavernous' sound. Bruits are heard over narrowed arteries (often renal).

- Hernial orifices and external genitalia: inguinal, femoral, and abdominal wall hernias are excluded. Testicular palpation in males to rule out torsion.
- Rectal examination: initial anal inspection then digital examination to exclude rectal mass or blood, 'ballooned rectum' in intestinal obstruction, Proctoscopy and rigid sigmoidoscopy to exclude haemorrhoids or rectal neoplasm.

Investigations

- Venepuncture investigations: FBC with differential, U&Es, creatinine kinase (CK), liver function tests (LFTs), amylase, inflammatory markers (C-reactive protein [CRP]).
- Arterial blood gases (ABGs): may be used to diagnose acidosis or alkalosis and detect levels of partial pressure of oxygen and carbon dioxide.
- Culture and sensitivity: blood cultures to rule out septicaemia.
- Chest X-ray: Erect chest X-ray with 'gas under diaphragm' signifies intestinal perforation. Gas (bowel loop) in the chest can be found in hiatus hernia.
- Abdominal X-ray: this helps to rule out intestinal obstruction. Small bowel is characterized by 'step ladder' pattern (valvulae conniventes across the whole width of the dilated bowel) in contrast to large bowel (haustral folds, only extend up to one-third of the width of large bowel).
- KUB X-ray (kidneys, ureters, bladder): to rule out radio-opaque calculi in renal tract.
- Endoscopy: upper gastrointestinal up to the second part of duodenum, rigid and flexible sigmoidoscopy and colonoscopy to detect causes of gastrointestinal bleed and neoplasms. Endoscopic retrograde cholangiopancreatography (ERCP) is used to extract calculi from bile duct with or without stent placement and to relieve obstruction of common bile duct.
- Contrast radiography: barium contrast meal or enema (generally water soluble in acute cases) to find the site of obstruction, rate of emptying or filling defects (neoplastic lesions).
- IVU: IV urography to rule out obstruction in renal tract.
- Other contrast radiography: contrast through fistula tract gives an indication of its extent.
- Ultrasound scan: ultrasound waves used to investigate intra-abdominal hollow viscus and related pathology.
- CT scan or magnetic resonance imaging (MRI): for diagnosis and anatomical delineation of problem. This is now a common investigation in most ill patients but must not be allowed to delay the management or surgery required if this is obvious.
- Radiology-guided biopsy and drainage: unknown mass or collection found on abdominal imaging (ultrasound scan and CT scan).
- Radionuclide scans: rarely used, but can define sites of bleeding or infection.

Management of acute abdomen

Phase 1 initial management (first hour)

- ABCDE assessment and management: 'nil by mouth' until senior review of diagnosis.
- Large-bore IV cannula: send bloods for investigation, group and save, start IV fluids, if patient is dehydrated or colloids if hypotensive.
- Urine: for dipstick and pregnancy test (in females).
- Analgesia: morphine 10 mg, IV, or intramuscular. This is very important and can help the accuracy of clinical examination. Only avoid if the patient is in shock.
- Electrocardiogram (ECG) and imaging: erect chest X-ray and abdominal X-ray.
- Nasogastric tube: consider if patient is vomiting, with antiemetic (e.g. metoclopramide 10 mg IV).

- Urinary catheter: monitor urine output hourly,
- VTE assessment: TED stockings (after ruling out peripheral vascular disease) and anti-DVT prophylaxis (usually LMWH).
- Observations: hourly or more frequent observations to be recorded, MEWS score calculated, general intake, and output chart.
- Antibiotics: if indicated give as soon as possible.

Phase 2 management (2–6 hours)

- Observations, blood and imaging results, consider antibiotics if indicated and not given already. Re-examination of the patient is probably the most useful investigation for most patients, especially when appendicitis is under consideration.
- If pancreatitis is suspected: ABG and assess patient using Glasgow pancreatitis score (see Box 11.1). If score is more than 3, ask for urgent ICU review.
- If renal colic is suspected: ask for CT scan KUB or IVU (following local guidelines). Monitor patient for complications of obstructive uropathy (e.g. pyonephrosis). Continue hydration and analgesia.
- If surgery is imminent (e.g. bowel perforation, uncontrolled gastrointestinal bleed), cross match for at least 2–4 units of blood. If aortic aneurysm is suspected, urgent referral to vascular on-call.
- If ECG suspicious: ask for urgent medical advice.
- If cause for acute abdomen is unknown: further imaging (CT scan, ultrasound scan) may be needed.

Phase 3 Further management after 6 hours

Most patients respond to conservative approach. Those who fail to respond are treated by definitive management, which may be as follows:

- Laparotomy: This remains the mainstay treatment for acute abdomen where all other modalities have failed to improve the patient's condition. Generally employed approaches are:
  - Midline laparotomy.
  - Right subcostal (Kocher's incision, generally used for open cholecystectomy).
  - Right Iliac fossa incision (Lanz's incision over or McBurney's point for acute appendicitis).
- Laparoscopy: The use of diagnostic laparoscopy in acute abdomen is increasing. Its use as a diagnostic tool has decreased rates of negative laparotomies. Laparoscopic procedures in experienced hand are found to have lower postoperative recovery time as compared with open procedures. It is used:
  - To diagnose abdominal and pelvic pathologies (example non-specific lower abdominal pain in young women, where it is used to view the appendix, uterus, ovaries and fallopian tubes).
  - For therapeutic procedures such as cholecystectomy, appendicectomy, closure of duodenal ulcer perforation.
  - Drainage: It is used to drain abdominal or pelvic collections and take specimens for culture and/or biopsy (e.g. localized pelvic abscess).

Box 11.1 Glasgow prognostic score for pancreatitis
Score 1 for each factor

- Age >55 years
- WBC $>15 \times 10^9$/L
- Urea >16 mmol/L
- Glucose >10 mmol/L
- PO_2 <8 kPa
- Albumin <32 g/L
- Calcium <2.0 mmol/L
- Lactate dehydrogenase (LDH) >600 units/L
- Aspartate aminotransferase (AST) /alanine aminotransferase (ALT) >200 units/L

A useful mnemonic to recall the Glasgow prognostic score for pancreatitis is PANCREAS: PO_2, Age, Neutrophils, Calcium, Renal function (urea), Enzymes (AST/ALT, LDH), Albumin, Sugar (glucose).

Complications

Acute abdominal problems not treated quickly or correctly can have disastrous complications. Some conditions such as advanced colitis are resistant to most modalities of treatment and often have complications even after the best possible management. Following complications often arise as a consequence of an acute abdomen.

- Generalized peritonitis resulting into sepsis
- Shock (sepsis, hypovolaemic)
- Wound (postoperative) dehiscence
- Enterocutaneous fistula
- Prolonged ICU/hospital stay
- Intestinal failure resulting into malnutrition
- Death.

Patient safety tips

- ✔ Review diagnosis: if the diagnosis is unclear, revisit the history and clinical examination and reconsider all the main diagnoses considered in this section.
- ✔ Review all results: as in all emergency situations the blood, radiology, ECG and all other investigation results must be known as soon as possible and acted on urgently.
- ✔ Seek senior review and consider involvement of other specialists: for example urologists, gynaecologists, ICU team, vascular surgeons, medical team.
- ✔ **Use prophylactic antibiotics for surgery as per local guidelines**: check for allergies.

Acute abdomen

Mr John Raffles (45-year-old white Caucasian man), presents to A&E with a 1-day history of continuous acute abdominal pain and discomfort which has been associated with light-headedness and nausea. He is extremely distressed and anxious to know the cause.

This assessment will be based around a discussion on the management of acute abdomen with reference to above scenario.

		Self	Peer	Peer /tutor	Tutor
What is the definition of an acute abdomen?	• 'Acute abdomen' is used to describe a clinical condition of rapid onset or rapidly worsening abdominal pain, severe enough to warrant emergency admission to hospital. Initial assessment is of pivotal importance as may indicate an underlying life-threatening condition requiring immediate surgical intervention	☐	☐	☐	☐
What aspects of the history are important?	**Details about the pain:**				
	• Site: epigastric implicates foregut structures; umbilical pain implicates mid-gut and supra-pubic hindgut. Is the pain localized? Generalized? Site of pain may correlate with anatomical location of specific organ	☐	☐	☐	☐
	• Referring: pain from gallbladder/diaphragm referred to shoulder tip, renal colic referred from 'loin to groin', retroperitoneal organs referred 'to the back'	☐	☐	☐	☐
	• Shifting: pain in appendicitis may be generalize around the umbilicus then shifting and localized to the right iliac fossa with disease progression	☐	☐	☐	☐
	• Duration.	☐	☐	☐	☐
	• Nature and severity (0–10 scale): pain from AAA rupture or dissection is described as stabbing, piercing or tearing and is severe in intensity. Colic tend to be described as pain in waves on top of a background pain	☐	☐	☐	☐
	• Aggravating factors: spicy food and GORD, fatty food and cholecystitis	☐	☐	☐	☐
	• Relieving factors: upper abdominal pain from inferior myocardial infarction may be relieved by glyceryl trinitrate (GTN) spray	☐	☐	☐	☐
	• Weight loss and appetite: recent significant weight loss and appetite may suggest underlying malignancy or chronic illness such as inflammatory bowel disease	☐	☐	☐	☐
What are the associated symptoms and key aspects of examination?	• Collapse/loss consciousness and AAA rupture/dissection aorta	☐	☐	☐	☐
	• Pyrexia may suggest infection e.g. cholangitis, cholecystitis, UTIs	☐	☐	☐	☐
	• Nausea + vomiting (intestinal obstruction, pancreatitis)	☐	☐	☐	☐
	• Urinary: blood in urine in renal calculi; urinary retention in bladder outflow obstruction	☐	☐	☐	☐
	• Abdominal distension and vomiting: intestinal obstruction	☐	☐	☐	☐
	• Jaundice: obstructed biliary system, cholangitis	☐	☐	☐	☐
	• Menstrual history (possibility of ectopic pregnancy?)	☐	☐	☐	☐
	• Previous abdominal surgery?	☐	☐	☐	☐
	• General examination: signs of shock (low volume pulse, low BP)?	☐	☐	☐	☐
	• Abdominal examination: caput medusa? Abdominal distension? Tenderness? Percussion note? Guarding? Bowel sounds present? (no bowel sounds: paralytic ileus due to sepsis, hurried bowel sounds: intestinal obstruction).	☐	☐	☐	☐
	• Testicular palpation to rule out torsion, hernial orifices to exclude hernia.	☐	☐	☐	☐
	• PR examination: for intestinal obstruction.	☐	☐	☐	☐
What are the main causes of acute abdomen?	**Causes arising from chest:**				
	• Heart: inferior myocardial infarction, lungs: basal pneumonia (especially elderly)	☐	☐	☐	☐
	Causes arising from upper abdomen:				
	• Liver: hepatitis, CCF, Liver metastases, etc. (stretching of Glisson's capsule)	☐	☐	☐	☐
	• Biliary system: acute cholecystitis, biliary colic, cholangitis.	☐	☐	☐	☐
	• Oesophagus: GORD, spontaneous rupture (Boerhaave's syndrome).	☐	☐	☐	☐
	• Stomach and duodenum: peptic ulcer perforation/bleed, acute gastritis, gastric volvulus, hiatus hernia, gastric cancer (rare).	☐	☐	☐	☐
	• Spleen: injury, torsion (rare), Infarction.	☐	☐	☐	☐
	Causes arising from lower abdomen and pelvis:				
	• Small bowel: obstruction, perforation, ischaemia, Meckel's diverticulitis, Crohn's disease.	☐	☐	☐	☐
	• Large bowel: colitis (ulcerative colitis, Crohn's colitis, pseudo-membranous colitis) diverticulitis, ischaemia, perforation, pelvic abscess	☐	☐	☐	☐
	• Appendix: acute appendicitis, perforation	☐	☐	☐	☐
	• Omentum: torsion and ischaemia	☐	☐	☐	☐
	• Reproductive organs: mid-cycle pain (Mittelschmerz), torsion of ovarian cyst, ectopic pregnancy, pelvic inflammatory disease, fibroids in uterus, testicular torsion	☐	☐	☐	☐
	• Strangulated hernias	☐	☐	☐	☐

	Causes arising from retroperitoneum:				
	● Pancreas: acute and necrotizing pancreatitis	☐	☐	☐	☐
	● Aorta: aortic aneurysm, dissection of aorta	☐	☐	☐	☐
	● Kidneys, ureter: calculi, pyelonephritis, pyonephrosis	☐	☐	☐	☐
	Other causes:				
	● DKA, mesenteric adenitis, non-specific abdominal pain, porphyria, familial Mediterranean fever, sickle cell disease	☐	☐	☐	☐
Phase 1 (initial management: first hour)	● Clinically: history, examination focus on respiratory rate, temperature, BP, pulse, oxygen saturations, Glasgow Coma Score, MEWS	☐	☐	☐	☐
	● Investigations: ECG, erect chest X-ray and abdominal X-ray, urine dipstick, pregnancy test if female, bloods (FBC, U&Es, CK, LFTs, CRP and blood group.	☐	☐	☐	☐
	● Oxygen via mask and non-rebreathing bag (100%) if saturations <92%.	☐	☐	☐	☐
	● Analgesia: morphine 10 mg IV or intramuscularly (IM).	☐	☐	☐	☐
	● Start IV fluids (if dehydrated) or colloids (if hypotensive)	☐	☐	☐	☐
	● Nasogastric (NG) tube with metoclopramide 10 mg IV if patient is vomiting	☐	☐	☐	☐
	● More intensive monitoring: catheter (hourly input/output chart)	☐	☐	☐	☐
	● Nil by mouth and hourly observations/MEWS	☐	☐	☐	☐
Phase 2 management (2-6 hours)	● Continue to monitor patient and give analgesia and fluids as above	☐	☐	☐	☐
	● Start antibiotics if indicated from test results	☐	☐	☐	☐
	● Suspected pancreatitis: ABG and assess GCS (score >2 urgent ICU review)	☐	☐	☐	☐
	● Suspected renal colic: CT KUB or IVU. Monitor for complications (obstruction). Continue fluids and analgesia	☐	☐	☐	☐
	● If surgery indicated, cross-match for 2–4 units blood	☐	☐	☐	☐
	● Suspected AA: urgent referral to on-call vascular	☐	☐	☐	☐
	● Suspicious ECG: urgent medical advice	☐	☐	☐	☐
	● Unknown cause: further imaging (CT, ultrasound)	☐	☐	☐	☐
Phase 3 (ongoing management)	● Most respond to conservative approach	☐	☐	☐	☐
	Definitive management:				
	● Laparotomy (where all other possibilities failed to improve patient)	☐	☐	☐	☐
	● Laparoscopy (reduce need for laparotomy) to diagnose pathologies: to view appendix, uterus, ovaries, fallopian tubes, etc.	☐	☐	☐	☐
	● Laparoscopy for cholecystectomy, appendectomy, closure duodenal ulcer, perforation, etc.	☐	☐	☐	☐
	● Drainage of localized abscess or abdominal/pelvic collections – send sample for culture and biopsy.	☐	☐	☐	☐
Other aspects of treatment	● High-risk patients (continued vomiting) should have an NG tube and metoclopramide 10 mg IV to avoid aspiration	☐	☐	☐	☐
	● Catheter to ensure fluid balance	☐	☐	☐	☐
	● Look for infection and treat vigorously	☐	☐	☐	☐
	● TED stockings and low dose heparin prophylaxis should be considered – (usually enoxaparin 40mg subcutaneously once daily).	☐	☐	☐	☐
Complications	● Generalized peritonitis leading to sepsis	☐	☐	☐	☐
	● Shock (septic, hypovolaemic)	☐	☐	☐	☐
	● Postoperative wound dehiscence or enterocutaneous fistula	☐	☐	☐	☐
	● Prolonged ICU/hospital stay	☐	☐	☐	☐
	● Intestinal failure resulting in malnutrition	☐	☐	☐	☐
	● Death	☐	☐	☐	☐
Patient safety tips	● Patient monitoring: for early signs of complications, e.g. shock, sepsis	☐	☐	☐	☐
	● Fluid balance: meticulous attention to fluid balance. Too little and renal dysfunction precipitated with cardiovascular instability. Too much and cardiac failure precipitated	☐	☐	☐	☐
	● Subcutaneous heparin: to prevent VTE	☐	☐	☐	☐
Clinical note writing and handover	● Liaise with colleagues for consultations and preparation for theatre	☐	☐	☐	☐

Self-assessed as at least borderline:	Signature:	Date:	U B S E	U B S E	U B S E	U B S E
Peer-assessed as ready for tutor assessment:	Signature:	Date:	U B S E	U B S E	U B S E	U B S E
Tutor-assessed as satisfactory:	Signature:	Date:	U B S E	U B S E	U B S E	U B S E

Notes

11.3 Respiratory failure

Background

Respiratory failure indicates failure of the lungs to provide adequate ventilation between the atmosphere and the lungs and hence oxygenation of the blood (i.e. inadequate gas exchange) at a rate to meet the metabolic demands of the body. Acute respiratory failure specifically is defined as the inability to maintain gas exchange at a rate to meet the metabolic demands of the body. More precisely, respiratory failure is a clinical syndrome in which the respiratory system fails in one or both of its gas-exchanging functions; oxygenation of pulmonary arterial blood or elimination of CO_2 from it. Respiratory failure can result from both pulmonary and extra-pulmonary conditions.

Ventilation requires a healthy cardiovascular, respiratory, neurological, and musculoskeletal system, and therefore there are many potential causes of ventilatory and therefore respiratory failure.

Pathophysiologically, there are two types of respiratory failure:

● **Type 1**: PaO_2 <8.0 kPa
● **Type 2**: Hypercapnic, $PaCO_2$ >6.5 kPa

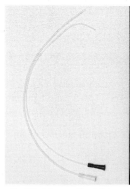 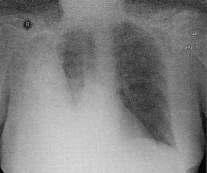 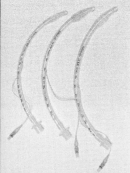

Occasionally a suction tube can lead to dramatic relief of breathing difficulties due to retained secretions.

A chest x-ray (CXR) can reveal treatable causes of acute respiratory distress such as pleural effusion, pneumothorax, or chest infection.

Early recourse to intensive care and possible endotracheal intubation if rapid improvement not forthcoming.

Figure 11.3 Images in respiratory failure.

In many cases, hypoxaemic and hypercapnic respiratory failure co-exist. Disorders that initially cause hypoxaemia may be complicated by hypercapnia due to respiratory pump failure (e.g. failure of respiratory muscle and or respiratory drive). Conversely hypercapnic respiratory pump failure may be complicated by hypoxaemia due to pulmonary parenchymal disease (e.g. pneumonia or atelectasis) or vascular disorders (e.g. pulmonary embolism). This defining level of PaO_2 has been rather arbitrarily defined based on a critical point on the oxygen–haemoglobin dissociation curve. Below this critical point, the curve becomes much steeper and a small fall in PaO_2 is associated with a large decrease in blood oxygen content and subsequent oxygen supply to the tissues.

Clinically: Respiratory failure may present in three different ways:

● **Acute respiratory failure:** develops in minutes to hours and leads to life threatening derangement in blood gases and acid-base balance

● **Chronic respiratory failure:** develops over several days and may be more indolent

● **Acute on chronic respiratory failure:** acute deterioration of chronic respiratory failure

Acute hypercapnic respiratory failure is associated with an elevated $PaCO_2$ (>6.5 kPa) with accompanying acidosis (pH <7.35) and normal bicarbonate. In chronic hypercapnic respiratory failure, pH is within the normal range but the bicarbonate level (which acts as a buffer) is elevated due to renal compensation. Acute or chronic respiratory failure is associated with an elevated bicarbonate level and acidosis (pH <7.35). In these patients, bicarbonate and $PaCO_2$ is significantly higher than seen in patients with acute hypercapnic respiratory failure.

Diagnosis

Since there are numerous causes of respiratory failure, the patient may have a wide range of symptoms, however, all patients will invariably present with a change in their normal breathing pattern. The patient may commonly present with:

- **Symptoms**: shortness of breath, cough, increased sputum production, haemoptysis, chest pain or tightness, wheeze, stridor
- **Signs**: cyanosis, tachycardia, tachypnoea, hypotension, reduced respiratory rate (? opioid overdose, check pupil size), unable to speak in full sentences, agitation, impaired consciousness, coma, papilloedema
  - **Use of accessory muscles of respiration** – including intercostal muscles, neck muscles, and abdominal wall muscles
  - **Paradoxical respiration** – all or part of a lung is deflated during inspiration and inflated during expiration, such as in flail chest or paralysis of the diaphragm. This can result in abdominal paradox, which is inward displacement of the abdomen during inspiration because of a weakened or paralysed diaphragm
  - **Respiratory alternans** – cyclical alteration between predominantly rib cage and abdominal breathing
  - **Kussmaul's breathing** – deep rapid breathing as seen in metabolic acidosis as a compensatory mechanism
  - **Cheyne–Stokes breathing** – breathing with rhythmic waxing and waning of depth of breaths and regularly recurring apnoeic periods

Awareness should also be made of patients at risk of respiratory failure presenting with altered breathing who do not have obvious chest pathology, e.g. stroke, drug intoxication, head injury, chest wall deformity, metabolic acidosis.

Causes of respiratory failure

Type 1 (acute hypoxaemic) respiratory failure: occurs due to V/Q mismatch, impaired diffusion, R to L shunt or alveolar hypoventilation.

- *Parenchymal disease (V/Q mismatch)*:
  - Pulmonary embolism
  - Asthma
  - Pneumothorax
  - Pulmonary oedema, e.g. left heart
  - Arrhythmia
  - Acute lung injury/ARDS
- *Interstitial lung disease*:
  - Acute respiratory distress syndrome (ARDS)
  - Pneumonia
  - Emphysema, interstitial lung disease
- *Others*:
  - A-V malformation, high altitude, opiate overdose

Type 2 (ventilatory) respiratory failure: due to imbalance between respiratory drive and respiratory effort or capacity.

- *Reduced breathing effort (drive failure):*
  - ○ Fatigue, drug intoxication
  - ○ Neurological disease, head injury, stroke. Encephalitis (high load)
- *Inability to overcome increased resistance to breathing*
  - ○ COPD
  - ○ Obesity, hypoventilation
  - ○ Foreign body, tumour
  - ○ Kyphoscoliosis
- Respiratory muscle abnormalities (neurotransmitter abnormalities)
  - ○ Spinal cord (above C3), myasthenia gravis, neuromuscular blocking agents (e.g. aminogly-cosides), hypokalaemia.
  - ○ Motor neurone disease, musculuar dystrophies, Guillain-Barré syndrome.

There can often be a combination of these factors.

Management of acute respiratory failure

The triage decision is a critical initial step in management to determine the appropriate setting for care: standard in-patient emergency bed, High Dependency Unit (HDU) or Intensive Care Unit (ICU). Factors determining this decision include acuteness of onset of respiratory failure, degree of hypoxia, hypercapnia, acidosis, presence of co-morbidities.

Phase 1 initial management (first hour)

- **ABCDE assessment**
- **Secure airway**
  - ○ **Clear any upper airway obstruction**: suction, is tracheostomy required? Use simple airway measures such as oropharyngeal, nasopharyngeal or laryngeal mask airway (LMA) if required, assess breathing, assess circulation and achieve IV access, call anaesthetic team and initiate form of mechanical ventilation if clinically indicated.
  - ○ **Consider tension pneumothorax**: immediate insertion of a large-bore cannula into second intercostal space, midclavicular line. Always ask the question ? pneumothorax, especially in previous history, trachea deviated, asymmetrical ventilation, cardiac arrest, pulseless electrical activity (PEA)
- **Correction of hypoxemia**: Once the airway is secured, hypoxaemia, the most life threatening aspect of acute respiratory failure should be corrected. The goal is to assure adequate oxygen delivery to the tissues. In a critically ill patient high flow oxygen should be administered short term via a non-rebreathing mask. In more stable patients, adequate oxygen delivery may be achieved by nasal prongs or face mask at 40% or 60% oxygen. In patients who are at risk of hypercapnic respiratory failure (e.g. COPD, neuromuscular weakness) controlled oxygen should be administered by use of a Venturi-mask. If acceptable level of oxygenation, as judged by arterial blood gas analysis cannot be achieved, or if supplemental O_2 causes hypercapnia to worsen significantly, either non-invasive ventilation or endotracheal intubation and mechanical ventilation are required.
- **Correction of hypercapnia**: The urgency of correction of hypercapnia depends on its magnitude and its effect on the patient. Controlled oxygen therapy is used for those who are at risk of hypercapnia. Treatment of underlying conditions such as an opiod overdose, or use of noninvasive or mechanical ventilation may be needed.
- **If known asthma/COPD**: if reduced air entry, use salbutamol nebulizers (back-to-back if required), consider steroids and further adjuncts such as ipratropium nebulizer, IV magnesium (for asthma).

Phase 2 management (2–6 hours)

Sign and symptoms of underlying disease process may now become clearer. These may be localized to pulmonary conditions (e.g. pneumonia, COPD or pulmonary oedema) or may be more remote and systemic (e.g. sepsis, pancreatitis or a fracture of a long bone leading to ARDS).

Repeated assessment by bedside methods and/or invasive techniques is critical in monitoring patients with respiratory failure. Simple observation of respiratory rate, use of accessory muscles, paradoxical breathing, oxygen saturation monitoring by pulse oximetry or arterial blood gas analysis will help detect worsening respiratory failure. In mechanically ventilated patients, indwelling arterial or central venous catheters or measurement of lung compliance and airway pressure are needed.

- **Continue oxygen and consider serial ABG measurements**.
- **Review CXR**: does patient require IV antibiotics, IV furosemide?, pleurocentesis, chest drain,
- **Consider steroids again**.
- **Reassess need for ICU support and mechanical ventilation** –
  - ○ **Variable/bi-level positive airway pressure (BiPAP)**: provides two levels of pressure, inspiratory positive airway pressure and an expiratory positive airway pressure
  - ○ **Continuous positive airway pressure (CPAP)**: initially and primarily used for treatment of chronic sleep apnoea, but also used in intensive care units. Provides continuous positive airway pressure at a level determined by the physician and which can be changed quickly and easily. Additionally useful in reducing pulmonary oedema
  - ○ Positive end-expiratory pressure
  - ○ **Mechanical ventilation**: pressure support ventilation, intermittent mandatory ventilation, extracorporeal membrane oxygenation (ECMO)

Phase 3 ongoing management

- Repeat general and cardiorespiratory examination
- Repeat ABG if required
- Treat underlying cause of acute respiratory failure
- Refer for ventilation in ICU if indicated
- Further investigations: these may include pulmonary function testing, sleep studies, bronchoscopy, imaging or specialized tests such as muscle enzymes, EMG or muscle biopsy.

Box 11.2 Summary of the British Thoracic Society (BTS) guidelines for emergency oxygen therapy in acute ill adult patients

- *Oxygen should be used for treatment of hypoxaemia*, not merely the symptom of breathlessness.
- *Oxygen should be prescribed* according to a target saturation range and there should be close monitoring of these saturations to remain within this range
- *Aim for normal or near-normal saturations*: for all acutely ill patients apart from those at risk of hypercapnic respiratory failure or those treated palliatively
- *High concentration oxygen should be administered*: immediately for all critically ill patients and documented in the patient notes
- *Oxygen saturation should be checked by pulse oximetry*: and supplemented if clinically indicated by ABGs, the inspired oxygen concentration should also be recorded. Pulse oximetry must be available in all locations where oxygen therapy is used
- *All critically ill patients should be monitored*: using a recognized physiological tracking system such as MEWS
- *Oxygen should be prescribed to achieve the target saturation*: 94–98% for most acutely ill patients or 88–92% for those at risk of hypercapnic respiratory failure. The target saturation should be written on the drug chart
- *Oxygen should be administered by trained staff*: using appropriate devices and flow rates in order to achieve target saturation range
- *Oxygen should be signed for on the drug chart on each ward round*
- Oxygen should be reduced in stable patients with satisfactory oxygen saturation, and crossed off the drug chart once discontinued

Complications

- Pulmonary: PE, pneumothorax, ARDS, pulmonary fibrosis
- Related to use of mechanical ventilation: ventilator associated pneumonia, tracheal stenosis if prolonged intubation or tracheostomy
- Gastrointestinal: stress ulceration, paralytic ileus
- Cardiovascular: hypotension, arrhythmias, MI, pulmonary hypertension
- Renal: acute renal failure, fluid retention
- Others: severe sepsis, nutritional compromise, psychological sequelae
- ARDS has a survival of 60% only and at 50% of the survivors will be left with neuro-cognitive dysfunction or reduced respiratory function.

Patient safety tips

- ✔ **High flow oxygen initially to all critically ill patients**: However, giving high flow oxygen to a patient with an acute exacerbation of COPD may reduce their respiratory drive by removing their hypoxic stimulus for ventilation. Hypoxia causes mortality and in an acute setting a trial of high-flow oxygen is recommended until an airway and patient's breathing are stabilized. Blood gases are crucial to determining % oxygen and ventilation needed in a given patient.
- ✔ **Risk of chest drain insertion**: bleeding, infection, pneumothorax, re-expansion pulmonary oedema, injury to adjacent organs. Therefore employ a clinician experienced in chest drain insertion.
- ✔ **Fluid mismanagement**: Pulmonary oedema or acute renal failure. Therefore fully assess with full history and examination, vital signs, urine output, U&Es, CVP if needed.
- ✔ **Risk of endotracheal intubation**: oedema, bleeding, tracheal and oesophageal perforation, pneumothorax (collapsed lung), aspiration. Therefore employ anaesthetic assistance.

Respiratory failure

A 49-year-old man has been brought in by ambulance having collapsed while out walking in the local hills. He had forgotten to pack his inhalers and is known to have asthma for the last 17 years. He is distressed and obviously wheezy. His ABGs are shown:

pH	PaO_2	$PaCO_2$	HCO_3^-	Temperature 37.1 °C
7.45–7.35	10.5–13.5 kPa	4.7–6.0 kPa	22–28 mmol/L	Heart rate 124/minute
pH	PaO_2	$PaCO_2$	HCO_3^-	Respiratory rate 26
7.54	23.5	3.8	24.1	

This assessment will be based around a discussion on the management of respiratory failure with reference to the above scenario.

		Self	Peer	Peer /tutor	Tutor
What are the types of respiratory failure? And how are they defined?	● **Type 1** (hypoxia, PaO_2 <8): failure of oxygenation	☐	☐	☐	☐
	● **Type 2** (hypoxia and hypoxemia, $PaCO_2$ > p > 6.5): failure of alveolar ventilation.	☐	☐	☐	☐
	● **Acute**	☐	☐	☐	☐
	● **Chronic**	☐	☐	☐	☐
	● **Please name some common causes of type 1 and type 2 respiratory failure stated in this chapter**	☐	☐	☐	☐
	●	☐	☐	☐	☐
What other symptoms could the above patient have?	● Shortness of breath, cough, haemoptysis, chest pain or tightness, wheeze, stridor	☐	☐	☐	☐
	●	☐	☐	☐	☐
What signs could the above patient have?	● Cyanosis, tachycardia, tachypnoea, hypotension, reduced respiratory rate, unable to speak in full sentences, agitation	☐	☐	☐	☐
	●	☐	☐	☐	☐
What are the main aspects of phase 1 initial management (first hour) in this patient?	● **ABCDE assessment**	☐	☐	☐	☐
	● **Secure airway**: **clear any upper airway obstruction**: ? suction, IV access, ? airway needed.	☐	☐	☐	☐
	● **Consider tension pneumothorax**: immediate insertion of a large-bore cannula into second intercostal space, midclavicular line. ? trachea deviated, asymmetrical ventilation	☐	☐	☐	☐
	● **Administer oxygen**: high-flow O_2 through a non-rebreathe mask.	☐	☐	☐	☐
	● **Assess breathing and assess globally**: respiratory rate, O_2 saturations, heart rate, blood pressure, cyanosis	☐	☐	☐	☐
	● **Re-assess history**: collateral history from family/carers, GP, previous clinical records	☐	☐	☐	☐
	● **Investigations**: ABG, FBC, U&Es, glucose, CXR, ECG	☐	☐	☐	☐
	● **Reduce O_2 administration to 2-4 L**: if patient is retaining CO_2 on ABG	☐	☐	☐	☐
	● **As known asthma**: salbutamol nebulizers, steroids and further adjuncts such as ipratropium nebulizer, IV magnesium	☐	☐	☐	☐
	●	☐	☐	☐	☐
What are the main aspects of phase 2 management (2–6 hours)?	● Continue oxygen and consider serial ABG measurements	☐	☐	☐	☐
	● **Review CXR**: does patient require IV antibiotics, exclude pneumothorax.	☐	☐	☐	☐
	● Consider steroids again.	☐	☐	☐	☐
	● Re-assess need for ICU support and mechanical ventilation	☐	☐	☐	☐
	●	☐	☐	☐	☐
What are the main aspects of phase 3 (ongoing management)?	● Repeat general and cardiorespiratory examination	☐	☐	☐	☐
	● Repeat ABG if required	☐	☐	☐	☐
	● Change to inhalers and oral treatments as soon as able to do so	☐	☐	☐	☐
	● In some patients specialized investigations: bronchoscopy, imaging, EMG, etc.	☐	☐	☐	☐
	●				
What are the key patient safety tips in relation to this case?	● 100% oxygen initially, caution if hypercapnic	☐	☐	☐	☐
	● Consider tension pneumothorax	☐	☐	☐	☐
	● Discuss with colleagues to optimize care and consider. Ventilation early if patient is deteriorating	☐	☐	☐	☐
	● Exclude infection, if infection consider antibiotics	☐	☐	☐	☐

Self-assessed as at least borderline:	Signature:	Date:	U B / S E	U B / S E	U B / S E	U B / S E
Peer-assessed as ready for tutor assessment:	Signature:	Date:	U B / S E	U B / S E	U B / S E	U B / S E
Tutor-assessed as satisfactory:	Signature:	Date:	U B / S E	U B / S E	U B / S E	U B / S E

Notes

11.4 Cardiac chest pain

Background

Chest pain is common medical emergency associated with significant morbidity and mortality. In this section we will focus on cardiac chest pain. Cardiac chest pain is due to cholesterol-rich plaque on coronary artery walls narrowing the artery lumen, compromising blood supply to myocardium and causes pain on exertion. Coronary artery spasm can also cause the same symptoms (Prinzmetal's angina). An unstable plaque may rupture and expose the underlying atheroma leading to clot (thrombus) formation. Cardiac chest pain is divided into acute coronary syndrome (ACS) and stable angina.

There are three main pathological and clinical presentations of acute coronary syndromes (ACS):

- **Unstable angina**: myocardial ischaemia without myocardial necrosis.
- **Non-ST elevation myocardial infarction** (**NSTEMI**): this is myocardial ischaemia without ST elevation changes on the ECG but with biochemical evidence of myocardial necrosis. This is usually not a transmural infarct.
- **ST elevation myocardial infarction** (**STEMI**): this is myocardial ischaemia with ST elevation changes on the ECG and with biochemical evidence of myocardial necrosis.

Cardiac pain is central, retrosternal chest pain, discomfort, heaviness or tightness and/or other areas, e.g. arms, shoulders, back or jaw lasting longer than 15 minutes. This may or may not be associated with nausea, vomiting, shortness of breathing, sweating, or combination of these with or without haemodynamic instability. These features may be atypical in many cases.

Stable angina or angina pectoris is a specific type of cardiac chest pain which has the following features:

- Cardiac pain as above.
- Precipitated by physical exertion
- Relieved by rest or GTN within about 5 minutes

Presence of all of above factors is called typical angina, presence of two factors is called atypical angina and presence of one or none of any above-mentioned features is defined as non-anginal chest pain.

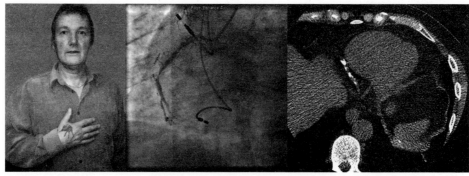

Levine's sign: holding a clenched fist held over the chest to describe and locate ischaemic chest pain

Coronary angiograms accurately define location of new MI or existing narrowing of coronary arteries for PCI

Calcification in the coronary vessels on CT scan: increasingly used in screening for coronary disease

Figure 11.4 Images in cardiac chest pain.

There is a long list of differential diagnoses to consider when a patient with chest pain presents. Clearly, ACS has to be excluded and requires urgent treatment. Other important conditions to consider are:

- **Cardiovascular**: dissecting aortic aneurysm, pericarditis, arrhythmias, hypertrophic cardiomyopathy, aortic stenosis, takotsubo stress cardiomyopathy, myocarditis
- **Respiratory**: pulmonary embolism, pneumothorax, asthma, infection, tumour, lymphadenopathy
- **Gastrointestinal**: reflux oesophagitis, gastritis, hiatus hernia, dysphagia
- **Chest**: shingles, costochondritis (Tietze's), trauma (e.g. broken rib), musculoskeletal pain.

Factors intensifying cardiac chest pain

- Reduced oxygen supply, e.g. anaemia, coronary spasm
- Increased oxygen demand, e.g. increased heart rate, left ventricular hypertrophy (LVH)
- Large mass of ischaemic myocardium
- Proximally located lesion.

Myocardial infarction

Myocardial infarction is defined by detection of rise in cardiac biomarkers including troponin at least one value above 99th percentile with at least one of following;

- ECG changes (new ST changes or new left bundle branch block [LBBB])
- Imaging evidence of new loss of myocardium
- Chest pain within last 12 hours.

Coronary artery disease

Coronary artery disease (CAD) is diagnosed on invasive coronary angiography if there is >70% stenosis of one of the major epicardial artery segment or narrowing of more than 50% of the left main stem coronary artery.

Diagnosis

This is based on history, risk factors, physical examination, ECG and cardiac enzymes. Classical symptoms include central retrosternal chest pain, heaviness, discomfort or tightness with or without radiation to left arm and/or jaw. However, the following features help in making a diagnosis of cardiac chest pain.

- Ongoing chest pain or chest pain within last 12 hours.
- Risk factors, e.g. previous known history of ischaemic heart disease (IHD), hypertension (HTN), diabetes mellitus (DM), smoker, male sex, family history of CAD, dyslipidaemia.
- Resting ECG: may show STEMI, ST depression, T wave inversion, non-specific changes or can be completely normal. Arrhythmias can result in ischaemic pain, e.g. AF, heart block.
- Cardiac enzymes including troponin on arrival and 12 hours after chest pain.
- Haemodynamic status of patient.
- Signs of any complication, e.g. pulmonary oedema or cardiogenic shock.
- Chest X-ray: may be normal, primarily done to rule out complications, e.g. pulmonary oedema.
- Think of other serious causes, e.g. aortic dissection, pulmonary embolism.

ECG changes

- **STEMI**: Presenting with cardiac sounding chest pain as described above along with ST elevation of 1 mm in two contiguous limb leads or 2 mm in two contiguous chest leads (V leads), or new-onset LBBB. Cardiac enzymes and troponin levels are raised after onset of the STEMI. Highly sensitive troponin assays can detect myocardial necrosis within 1–2 hours of onset of necrosis.
- **NSTEMI**: Presenting with cardiac sounding chest pain as described above. ECG may be abnormal ranging from ST depression to non-specific ST changes or T wave inversion, or

can be completely normal. Cardiac enzymes and troponin levels are raised after onset of the STEMI.

- **Unstable angina**: presenting with cardiac sounding chest pain as described above on minimal exertion or at rest. ECG may be abnormal, ranging from ST depression to non-specific ST changes or T waves inversion, or can be completely normal. Cardiac enzymes including troponin levels are not raised.

- **Stable angina**: presenting with cardiac sounding chest pain as described above on exertion. ECG may be abnormal, ranging from ST depression to non-specific ST changes or T waves inversion, or can be completely normal. Cardiac enzymes including troponin levels are not raised.

Management strategies for ACS and stable angina are different and will be considered separately.

Acute coronary syndrome

Phase 1 initial management (first hour) (Table 11.2)

- **Clinically**: history, examination focus on cardiorespiratory system, BP, pulse, oxygen saturation, and MEWS.
- **Investigations**: FBC, U&Es, cholesterol, blood glucose, and cardiac enzymes/troponin initially; if normal repeat 8–12 hours after onset of ACS event.
- **Initial steps**:
  - IV access, pain relief with IV morphine, antiemetic with IV metoclopramide or other preferred agent, GTN spray or sublingual GTN tablet
  - Supplemental O_2: if O_2 saturation is less that 94%. In patients not at risk of hypercapnic respiratory failure aim for saturations between 94% and 98%, in patients at risk of hypercapnic respiratory failure aim for saturations above 92% until ABGs are available
  - Load with anti-platelet agents
  - Chest X-ray
  - Intensive monitoring for heart rate, rhythm, BP, respiratory rate, oxygen saturations, pain relief and repeated 12-lead ECGs if necessary

Table 11.2 Phase 1 management of acute coronary syndromes

STEMI	NSTEMI	Unstable angina
Take initial steps	Take initial steps	Take initial steps
Load with aspirin 300 mg stat	Load with aspirin 300 mg stat	Load with aspirin 300 mg stat
Load with clopidogrel 600 mg stat	Load with clopidogrel 300 mg stat	Load with clopidogrel
Transfer urgently to cardiac catheterization lab for revascularization in the form of primary percutaneous coronary intervention (PPCI) or consider thrombolysis if no facility for PPCI available	Anticoagulant, e.g. LMWH. Consider once daily if glomerular filtration rate (GFR) <30. IIb/IIIa blockers, e.g. tirofiban, in high-risk patients. This will be determined from local protocols such as TIMI scores	300 mg stat LMWH twice daily. Consider once daily if GFR <30

Phase 2 management (2–6 hours)

- **Elevated glucose level**: any patient with blood glucose of >11.0 mmol/L, irrespective of their diabetes status, should be considered for an insulin regimen.
- **Troponin**: 8–12 hours after presumed acute cardiac event in all patients diagnosed with ACS.
- **Urgent U&E results**: Correct any electrolyte imbalance, especially hypokalaemia which can lead to life-threatening arrhythmias
- **Monitor fluid input and output**: watch out for hypotension and renal failure

- **Serial ECGs**: If diagnosis of ACS in doubt, take serial ECGs and also consider other serious causes, e.g. aortic dissection and pulmonary embolism.
- **Dynamic ECG changes**: this often indicates incipient coronary narrowing and obstruction or spasm or plaque rupture. Seek expert help.

Phase 3 management

- **Inpatient angiogram**: All intermediate- or high-risk NSTEMI patients should be offered inpatient angiograms within 96 hours unless contraindicated.
- **Consider further testing**: exercise tolerance test (ETT), stress echocardiogram, stress cardiac MRI or invasive testing, e.g. coronary angiogram to diagnose coronary artery disease.
- **Cardiac rehabilitation**: at earliest point.
- **Patient education**: extremely important, especially as many risk factors are amenable to patient and healthcare professional intervention such as smoking, low levels of physical activity, and increased weight or waist circumference. Booklets and leaflets alone do not suffice, basic behavioural change techniques have greater success in achieving lower rates of smoking and concordance with treatment.
- **Control risk factors**: smoking, glycaemic control, hypertension, lipid profile.
- **Follow up trans-thoracic echocardiograph**: usually 4–6 weeks after the ACS event.
- **Cardiologist follow-up**: in outpatient clinic in usually 4–12 weeks.
- **All ACS patients should be considered for the following evidence-based treatment to reduce future cardiovascular disease (CVD) events and readmission**:
  - ○ Lifelong aspirin 75 mg once daily unless contraindicated
  - ○ Clopidogrel for 12 months except unstable angina
  - ○ Clopidogrel for 12 months after coronary artery stent insertion
  - ○ Lifelong statins unless contraindicated usual total cholesterol target is ≤4 mmol/L, intermediate density lipoprotein (IDL) cholesterol ≤2 mmol/L
  - ○ β-blockers unless contraindicated, aim a heart rate of <70.
  - ○ Lifelong angiotensin-converting enzyme (ACE) inhibitor/angiotensin receptor blocker (ARB) unless contraindicated
  - ○ Eplerenone in all patients with left ventricular ejection fraction (LVEF) less than 40% after acute myocardial infarction or spironolactone in patients with severe heart failure (HF) with LVEF less than 35%
  - ○ Formal testing for diabetes in all patients with ACS. At least 25% will be expected to have **undiagnosed** diabetes at the time of ACS.

Other aspects of treatment

- Watch for pain and provide adequate pain relief.
- Anxiolytics may help some patients.
- Monitor fluid balance of ACS patients closely. This group of patients are prone to develop pulmonary oedema secondary to cardiac failure.
- Monitor electrolytes and replace if necessary. Patients with electrolyte imbalance are at risk of cardiac arrhythmias.
- Monitor functions of other vital function, as ACS patients with multi-organ disease are prone to develop multi-organ failure if not treated properly.
- Seek expert help in patients developing ACS post operatively and/or in ICU.
- Treatment of ACS is not straightforward in patients with active bleeding and/or at risk of bleeding, e.g. upper gastrointestinal bleeding, intracranial bleeding. Involve experts of related specialities early.

Complications of ACS

Cardiovascular mortality remains the most important cause of death in Europe in terms of number of people affected. ACS, if not optimally treated, is associated with a high rate of mortality and morbidity. Patients should be monitored for any complications and treated appropriately. Following complications are common:

- **Bradycardia**: withhold rate-limiting agents. Temporary or permanent pacemaker may be indicated
- **Tachycardia**: ventricular tachycardia, supraventricular tachycardia, atrial fibrillation/flutter: rate limiting agents, and/or electrical cardioversion may be necessary
- **Ventricular fibrillation**: immediate direct current defibrillation shock is needed to treat this immediately life-threatening arrhythmia
- **Conduction abnormalities**: heart blocks of varying degrees and bundle branch blocks: temporary or permanent pacemaker may be indicated
- **Pericarditis**: treat with non-steroidal anti-inflammatory drugs (NSAIDs). Heparin is contraindicated in presence of this condition.
- **Pulmonary oedema or cardiogenic shock**: transfer patient to intensive care or specialized coronary care unit. Inotropes will be indicated in many cases. Patient will need to be monitored very closely.
- **Papillary muscle rupture leading to acute mitral regurgitation**: urgent cardiothoracic surgical input is required to treat this condition.
- **Ventricular septal defect**: urgent cardiothoracic surgical input is required to treat this condition.
- **Ventricular aneurysm**: may cause arrhythmias, e.g. ventricular tachycardia or false ST elevation. Seek expert help.
- **Heart failure**: treat as per protocol.

Stable angina

Diagnosis of stable angina is made clinically. In patients presenting with cardiac sounding chest pain the diagnosis of stable angina is likely and they should be started on anti-anginal medication. Risk factors need to be controlled and/or treated. The following factors make the diagnosis of stable angina likely:

- Increasing age
- Male sex
- Known ischaemic heart disease, e.g. myocardial infarction, revascularization
- Cardiac risk factors e.g. smoking, HTN, hyperlipidaemia, diabetes mellitus, family history of CAD (before age of 55 years) or other form of cardiovascular disease.

All stable angina patients should be on:

- Lifelong aspirin unless contraindicated
- Lifelong statins unless contraindicated
- Lifelong β-blockers unless contraindicated, aim a heart rate of <60
- Lifelong ACE inhibitor/ARB unless contraindicated
- Nitrates can be used for symptom control.
- Treat modifiable risk factors, e.g. diabetes mellitus, HTN, hypercholesterolaemia, advice against smoking, advice regarding regular exercise.

However, if diagnosis of stable angina is difficult to make then the following strategy should be adopted as per the National Institute for Health and Clinical Excellence (NICE) guidelines;

- Estimated likelihood of CAD 61–90%, invasive coronary artery imaging should be performed if coronary revascularization is being considered, provided it is clinically indicated and acceptable to patient.
- Estimated likelihood of 30–60%, functional imaging, e.g. myocardial perfusion scanning, Stress echocardiogram or stress cardiac MRI is the first line of diagnostic investigation.
- Estimated likelihood of 10–30%, CT coronary angiogram is recommended for calcium scoring.

Stable angina is treated in community or as an outpatient. However, if patients become more symptomatic and get chest pain on minimal exertion and/or on rest then follow ACS protocol for unstable angina.

Patient safety tips

✔ **Watch out for atypical manifestations of ACS**: not all patients with ACS present with central chest pain as predominant feature. Patient can present with chest discomfort, chest tightness, chest heaviness, referred pain as presentation and shortness of breathing. Silent myocardial infarction can occur in patients with diabetes mellitus and other neuropathies.

✔ **Consider the differential diagnoses of ACS symptoms and signs**: many of these require urgent treatment, e.g. pulmonary embolism, aortic dissection, pneumothorax.

✔ **Normal ECG does not mean no ACS**: do not exclude the diagnosis of ACS in patients who have a normal 12-lead resting ECG but do have symptoms or a strong likelihood of ACS from the current or past history.

✔ **Ethnic and gender differences do not really help in emergency care**: do not assess symptoms of an ACS differently in ethnic groups, there are no major differences in symptoms of an ACS among different ethnic groups, similarly, do not assess symptoms of an ACS differently in men and women

✔ **Exercise ECG**: do not use just exercise ECG testing to diagnose or exclude stable angina for people without known CAD.

✔ **GTN spray**: Do not use people's response to GTN to make a diagnosis of CAD. A beneficial response is neither sensitive or specific enough to accurately diagnose significant angina.

✔ Do not use biochemical markers such as natriuretic peptide and high sensitivity CRP to diagnose an ACS.

✔ Correct timing of samples for troponin. Some highly sensitive assays will detect very low levels only a few hours after the onset of myocardial necrosis.

Cardiac chest pain

Magan Tagores is a 56-year-old man with type 2 diabetes mellitus has an episode of severe chest pain in the morning at 7.30 am. He catches a bus to see his GP. After history and examination by the GP, an ECG shows evidence of STEMI. An ambulance is called and he is immediately admitted to the local coronary care unit. He usually takes metformin 500 mg tds only. His ECG is shown below.

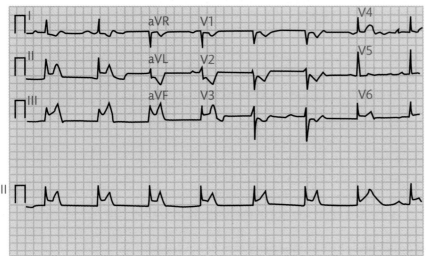

This assessment will be based around a discussion on the management of cardiac chest pain with reference to above scenario.

		Self	Peer	Peer /tutor	Tutor
What are the three main pathological and clinical presentations of ACS?	● **Unstable angina**: myocardial ischaemia without myocardial necrosis	☐	☐	☐	☐
	● **NSTEMI**: myocardial ischaemia and necrosis, without ST elevation	☐	☐	☐	☐
	● **STEMI**: myocardial ischaemia and necrosis with ST elevation changes	☐	☐	☐	☐
	●	☐	☐	☐	☐
What are the classic clinical features of angina pectoris?	● Cardiac chest pain, triggered by physical exertion or stress	☐	☐	☐	☐
	● Relieved by rest or GTN within about 5 minutes	☐	☐	☐	☐
	●	☐	☐	☐	☐
What the main differential diagnoses to consider when dealing with suspected cardiac chest pain?	● **Cardiovascular**: aneurysm, pericarditis, arrhythmias, hypertrophic obstructive cardiomyopathy (HOCM), aortic stenosis, takotsubo stress cardiomyopathy	☐	☐	☐	☐
	● **Respiratory**: pulmonary embolism, pneumothorax, asthma, infection, tumour, lymphadenopathy	☐	☐	☐	☐
	● **Gastrointestinal**: reflux oesophagitis, gastritis, hiatus hernia, dysphagia	☐	☐	☐	☐
	● **Chest**: shingles, costochondritis (Tietze's), trauma (e.g. broken rib), musculo-skeletal pain	☐	☐	☐	☐
	●	☐	☐	☐	☐
How is a myocardial infarction defined?	Detection of rise in cardiac biomarkers including troponin at least one value above 99th percentile with at least one of following;				
	● ECG changes (new ST changes or new LBBB)	☐	☐	☐	☐
	● Imaging evidence of new loss of myocardium	☐	☐	☐	☐
	● Chest pain within last 12 hours	☐	☐	☐	☐
	●	☐	☐	☐	☐
What kind of ACS does the above patient have? How and why was the presentation atypical? ACS: What are the key aspects of phase 1 initial management (first hour)?	● **Clinically**: history, examination, BP, pulse, oxygen saturations and MEWS	☐	☐	☐	☐
	● **Investigations**: FBC, U&Es, lipids, glucose and cardiac enzymes/troponin	☐	☐	☐	☐
	● **Initial steps**: IV access and morphine, IV antiemetic, GTN spray or sublingual tablet	☐	☐	☐	☐
	○ Supplemental O_2: if O_2 saturation is less than 94%.				
	○ Load with antiplatelet agents and CXR				
	○ Intensive monitoring, pain relief and repeated 12-lead ECGs if necessary (see Table 11.2)				
	●	☐	☐	☐	☐

What are key aspects of phase 2 management (2nd to 6th hour)?	● **Elevated glucose level**: >11.0 mmol/L, commence on insulin if necessary	☐	☐	☐	☐
	● **Troponin**: 12 hours after presumed acute cardiac event in all patients diagnosed with ACS	☐	☐	☐	☐
	● **Urgent U&Es results**: Correct imbalance, especially hypokalaemia arrhythmias	☐	☐	☐	☐
	● **Monitor fluid input and output**: watch out for hypotension and renal failure	☐	☐	☐	☐
	● **Serial ECGs**: consider other serious causes, e.g. aortic dissection and pulmonary embolism	☐	☐	☐	☐
	● **Dynamic ECG changes**: Seek expert help	☐	☐	☐	☐
	●	☐	☐	☐	☐

What are the key aspects of phase 3 management?	● **Inpatient angiogram, consider non-invasive tests**	☐	☐	☐	☐
	● **Cardiac rehabilitation and patient education**: many risk factors amenable to intervention	☐	☐	☐	☐
	● **Control risk factors**: smoking, glycaemic control, hypertension, lipid profile				
	● **Follow-up transthoracic echocardiograph**: usually 4–6 weeks after the ACS event	☐	☐	☐	☐
	● **Cardiologist follow-up**: in outpatient clinic, usually 4–12 weeks.	☐	☐	☐	☐
	● **Evidence-based treatments to reduce future CVD event and readmission (unless contraindicated)**:	☐	☐	☐	☐
	○ Aspirin 75 mg od lifelong, clopidogrel for 12 months except unstable angina				
	○ Clopidogrel for 12 months after coronary artery stent insertion				
	○ Lifelong statins: usual total cholesterol target is ≤4 mmol/L, LDL-cholesterol ≤2 mmol/L				
	○ Lifelong β-blockers, aim a heart rate of <70.				
	○ Lifelong ACEI/ ARB unless contraindicated.				
	○ Eplerenone in all patients with LVEF <40% after acute MI or spironolactone in patients with severe HF with LVEF <35%.				
	○ Formal testing for diabetes in all patients with ACS. At least 25% will be expected to have **undiagnosed** diabetes at the time of ACS				
	●	☐	☐	☐	☐

What are the main complications of ACS and how are they treated?	● Bradycardia, tachycardia, ventricular fibrillation, conduction abnormalities, pericarditis, pulmonary oedema or cardiogenic shock, papillary muscle rupture leading to acute mitral regurgitation, VSD, ventricular aneurysm, HF	☐	☐	☐	☐
	●	☐	☐	☐	☐

What are the main patient safety tips in relation to managing ACS?	● Watch out for atypical manifestations of ACS	☐	☐	☐	☐
	● Consider the differential diagnoses of ACS symptoms and signs	☐	☐	☐	☐
	● Normal ECG does not mean no ACS	☐	☐	☐	☐
	● **GTN spray**: the response is neither sensitive or specific to diagnose angina	☐	☐	☐	☐
	●	☐	☐	☐	☐

Self-assessed as at least borderline:	Signature:	Date:	U B / S E	U B / S E	U B / S E	U B / S E
Peer-assessed as ready for tutor assessment:	Signature:	Date:	U B / S E	U B / S E	U B / S E	U B / S E
Tutor-assessed as satisfactory:	Signature:	Date:	U B / S E	U B / S E	U B / S E	U B / S E

Notes

11.5 Acute heart failure

Background

Heart failure is a common clinical emergency with considerable mortality and morbidity. Acute cardiogenic pulmonary oedema (ACPOE) is one of the more dramatic presentation forms of acute heart failure (AHF). It is characterized by the development of dyspnoea, generally associated with the rapid accumulation of fluid within the alveolar and interstitial spaces of the lung as a result of acutely elevated cardiac filling pressures. In-hospital mortality from HF is about 5%, and is higher for ACPOE (12%). Six-month mortality rates of AHF in clinical trials have ranged from 14% to 26%.

Definitions

HF is a clinical syndrome in which patients have the following features:

- **Symptoms typical of HF**: breathlessness at rest or on exertion, fatigue, tiredness, ankle swelling.

- **Signs typical of HF**: tachycardia, raised jugular venous pressure (JVP), tachypnoea, pulmonary rales, pleural effusion, peripheral oedema, hepatomegaly.

- **Evidence of a structural or function abnormality of the heart at rest**: third heart sound, murmurs, cardiomegaly, ECG or ECHO abnormality, raised brain natriuretic peptide (BNP).

AHF can be defined as a rapid onset or change in the symptoms and signs of HF requiring urgent therapy. The clinical presentation of AHF is a spectrum of conditions dominated by pulmonary congestion in some patients, to a picture of reduced cardiac output and hypoperfusion in others. Patients generally present in one of six categories:

- **Worsening or decompensated chronic HF**: progressive deterioration of a patient with chronic HF on treatment, with evidence of systemic and pulmonary congestion

- **Pulmonary oedema**: severe respiratory distress, tachypnoea, and orthopnoea. Hypoxaemia with arterial O_2 saturations <90% on air. Widespread pulmonary rales

- **Hypertensive HF**: HF decompensation accompanied by high BP. Sympathetic system activation with tachycardia and vasoconstriction. Left ventricular systolic function is usually preserved with rapid response to treatment with low hospital mortality

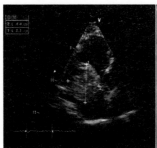 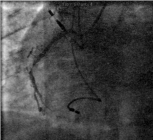

Echocardiography: essential element in diagnosis and to exclude valvular abnormalities, detect areas of previous damage, and exclude pericardial effusion.

LV architecture using an ECHO 3-D reconstruction – can detect areas of hypokinesis in cardiac failure

Figure 11.5 Images in acute heart failure.

- **Cardiogenic shock**: HF with tissue hypoperfusion after correction of preload and rhythm disturbance. Typically: systolic <90 mmHg and absent or low urine output (<0.5 mL/kg/h). Rapid onset organ hypoperfusion and pulmonary congestion
- **Isolated right HF**: Raised JVP, peripheral oedema, ascites, hepatomegaly, low cardiac output without pulmonary congestion
- **Acute coronary syndrome (ACS) and HF**: Clinical and laboratory evidence of ACS.

Causes and precipitants of acute heart failure

- **Coronary artery disease**: ACS, mechanical complications of acute myocardial infarction, right ventricular infarction.
- **Valvular heart disease**: valve stenosis, valve regurgitation, endocarditis, aortic dissection.
- **Myopathies**: postpartum cardiomyopathy, acute myocarditis.
- **Hypertension and arrhythmias**.
- **Circulatory failure**: septicaemia, thyrotoxicosis, anaemia, arteriovenous (AV) shunts, cardiac tamponade, pulmonary embolism.
- **Decompensation of pre-existing chronic HF**: lack of concordance to treatment, volume overload, infections (especially respiratory), cerebrovascular insult, surgery, renal dysfunction, asthma/COPD, drug abuse, alcohol abuse.

Diagnosis

The diagnosis of AHF is based on presenting symptoms and clinical signs and objective evidence, especially echocardiography. Table 11.3 illustrates the common clinical manifestations.

Table 11.3 Common clinical manifestations of heart failure (HF)

Dominant clinical feature	Symptoms	Signs
Peripheral oedema/ congestion	Breathlessness, fatigue, anorexia	Peripheral oedema, raised JVP, pulmonary rales, hepatomegaly, ascites
Pulmonary oedema	Severe breathlessness at rest	Widespread rales over lungs, effusion Tachycardia, tachypnoea
Cardiogenic shock	Confusion, weakness Cool peripheries	Poor peripheral perfusion, SBP <90 mmHg Anuria or oliguria
Hypertensive HF	Breathlessness	Raised JVP, congestion Left ventricular hypertrophy, preserved ejection fraction
Right HF	Breathlessness Fatigue	Evidence of right ventricular dysfunction, raised JVP, peripheral oedema, hepatomegaly, ascites

Having compiled a differential diagnosis from the history and physical examination, refinement of the diagnosis is achieved by ECG, chest X-ray, echocardiography, and laboratory investigations with specific biomarkers.

- **Chest X-ray**: perform as soon as possible to confirm diagnosis and exclude pulmonary causes of breathlessness (pneumonia, lung cancer, pneumothorax).
- **CXR findings**: cardiothoracic ratio often >50%, perihilar confluent alveolar shadowing ('bat's wing' shadow), upper lobe blood diversion, Kerley B lines (short horizontal lines perpendicular to pleural surface at base of lungs due to oedema of interlobular septa), Kerley A lines (lines extending from periphery to hila, caused by oedematous distention of anastomotic channels

between peripheral and central lymphatics), Kerley C lines (reticular opacities at lung base, representing Kerley's B lines en face).

- **ECG**: to confirm heart rhythm (atrial fibrillation common precipitant or accompanying rhythm. Look for conduction defects, chamber hypertrophy, or myocardial ischaemia

- **ABG analysis**: On all patients in respiratory distress. Enables assessment of oxygenation (pO_2), respiratory function (pCO_2), and acid-base balance (pH) to be determined. Pulse oximetry does not provide information on pCO_2 or acid–base status. Pulse oximetry unreliable in low-output or vasoconstricted shocked states.

- **Echocardiography**: Essential for evaluating functional and structural changes underlying or associated with AHF to direct subsequent treatment/management. A full evaluation should give information on regional and global left and right systolic function, diastolic dysfunction, valvular structure and function, pericardial disease, left ventricular filling pressures, pulmonary artery pressures, and abnormal atrial or ventricular septal defects.

- **Laboratory tests**: FBC, electrolytes and renal function, glucose, albumin and hepatic enzymes, international normalized ratio (INR), troponin (small rise may be seen in AHF without ACS).

- **Natriuretic peptides**: B-type natriuretic peptides (BNP and NT-proBNP) are useful markers in the diagnosis of HF and management of patients with established chronic HF. However, there is no general consensus regarding reference values in AHF.

Management

The aims of the initial management of AHF are haemodynamic stabilization, support of oxygenation and ventilation, and relief of symptoms.

Phase 1 initial management (first hour)

- **Clinical history – key features**:
  - Symptoms (breathlessness, orthopnoea, paroxysmal nocturnal dyspnoea, fatigue, angina, palpitations, syncope)
  - Cardiovascular events (CAD, myocardial infarction, intervention including thrombolysis and percutaneous coronary intervention [PCI], coronary artery bypass graft [CABG] and other surgery, stroke, peripheral vascular disease, valvular disease).
  - Risk profile (smoking, alcohol, hypertension, hyperlipidaemia, diabetes, family history), Response to current and previous therapy.

- **Clinical examination**: focus on cardiorespiratory system, BP, pulse, oxygen saturations, and MEWS. Clinical features:
  - Breathless and sitting upright, accessory muscle use
  - Pale, sweaty, cool to touch reflecting sympathetic nervous system activation
  - Cough productive of blood stained/pink frothy sputum (relatively uncommon)
  - Central or peripheral cyanosis with reduced oxygen saturations
  - Leg oedema (may not be present)
  - Jugular venous distension, though often hard to estimate
  - Resting tachycardia, ?atrial fibrillation with rapid ventricular response
  - Displaced left ventricular apex if left ventricular dilatation is present
  - Chest auscultation should reveal bilateral fine basal crepitations that do not clear on coughing. High-pitched expiratory wheezes (rhonchi) may be heard
  - S3 gallop is suggestive of diagnosis. Murmurs of aortic or mitral valve disease are useful diagnostic pointers.

- **Investigations**: CXR, ECG, FBC, laboratory tests. ABG if in respiratory distress and hypoxic (<94%). Thyroid-stimulating hormone (TSH) if atrial fibrillation.

- **Treatment**: initiated based on strong clinical suspicion and before all the confirmatory tests are back. General expert consensus opinion is represented below.
  - ○ **Supplemental high-flow oxygen**: in hypoxaemic patients to achieve an arterial oxygen saturation ≥95% (>90% in COPD, care required in those with serious obstructive lung disease to avoid hypercapnia).
  - ○ **Consider morphine**: (2.5–5.0 mg IV) if patient presents with restlessness, dyspnoea, anxiety, or chest pain (relieves dyspnoea and, as vasodilator, other symptoms of AHF, antiemetic therapy may be required, monitor respiration rate). Caution with hypotension, atrioventricular (AV) block, bradycardia, or CO_2 retention.
  - ○ **Loop diuretics**: if symptoms secondary to congestion and volume overload. Dosing, individualized and depends on patient status and renal function (higher doses in renal failure). Diuretic-naïve patients, 40 mg of IV furosemide bolus. If on chronic loop diuretics, use IV equivalent of their maintenance dose. A continuous infusion can be considered after an initial bolus. Patients should be assessed frequently to follow urine output; a urinary catheter may be needed.
  - ○ **Vasodilators**: nitrates, nitroprusside, and nesiritide are useful in AHF patients with systolic BP >110 mmHg (caution between 90 and 110 mmHg) without serious obstructive valvular disease. **Nitrate use**: particularly in patients with ACS, Initial starting dose of IV GTN is 10–20 μg/minute increasing in increments of 5–10 μg/minute every 3–5 minutes as needed. Frequent BP measurements to avoid large falls in systolic BP especially in renal failure. Headache is a frequent side-effect. Tachyphylaxis (tolerance) is common necessitating dose increase.
  - ○ **IV digoxin**: in atrial fibrillation with rapid ventricular response to control heart rate to <100. IV amiodarone is an alternative agent. Consider synchronized DC cardioversion if haemodynamically unstable.
  - ○ **Inotropic agents**: in patients with low output states, in the presence of hypoperfusion and congestion despite the use of vasodilators and/or diuretics. Therapy usually for those with dilated, hypokinetic ventricles. Infusion of inotropes is associated with an increase incidence of both atrial and ventricular arrhythmias. **Dobutamine** – start at 2–3 μg/kg/min infusion without loading dose, increasing according to symptoms, diuretic response, and clinical status up to 20 μg/kg/min. Other agents, expert advice only: dopamine, milrinone, enoximone, levosimendan, and noradrenaline
  - ○ **Monitor**: BP, pulse, respiratory rate, ECG monitor, continuous pulse oximetry, urine output (? urinary catheter), consider arterial line if haemodynamically unstable or need for frequent ABG analysis. Consider central venous line for delivery of drugs/fluid, and monitoring of CVP.

Phase 2 management (2–6 hours)

- **Consider non-invasion positive-pressure ventilation (NIPPV)**: if unable to correct hypoxaemia.
- **Consider ventilation**: if patient exhaustion, hypoxaemia despite high-flow O_2 (<8 kPa), hypercapnia (>8 kPa), acidosis (pH <7.2), and failure to respond to NIPPV.
- **Treat underlying aetiology and precipitating factors**.
- **VTE prophylaxis**: LMWH.

Phase 3 management (after 6 hours)

- **Serial ECGs/enzymes/troponin**: to exclude ACS.
- **Continued loop diuretic**: with adjustments according to fluid balance, daily weights, and volume status. Combination of thiazide and loop diuretics may be useful in volume-overloaded patients with diuretic resistance. Metolazone is often used in this context with furosemide.

- **Monitor renal function and electrolytes**: adverse effects of diuretic therapy include hypokalaemia, hyponatraemia, hyperuricaemia, and hypovolaemia.
- **Aldosterone antagonists**: can also be used in combination with loop diuretics, particularly in patients with hypokalaemia.
- **ECHO**: arrange transthoracic echocardiogram. Initiate on-going therapy based on results.
- **Discharge medication may include**: ACE inhibitor (e.g. ramipril, lisinopril, perindopril) or angiotensin II blocker (candesartan), β-blockers (e.g. bisprolol, carvedilol), spironolactone (if patient remains in NYHA Class III or IV), statin, other diuretics, nitrates.
- New York Heart Association Function Classification of Heart Failure
  - ○ Class I: No limitation of physical activity. Ordinary activity does not cause undue fatigue, palpitations or shortness of breath (SOB).
  - ○ Class II (mild): Slight limitation of physical activity. Comfortable at rest but ordinary physical activity results in fatigue, palpitations or SOB.
  - ○ Class III (moderate): Marked limitation of physical activity. Comfortable at rest. Minimal activity causes fatigue, palpitations or SOB.
  - ○ Class IV (severe): Unable to carry out any physical activity without discomfort. Cardiac failure symptoms at risk.
- **Digitoxin in AF**.
- **Patient education** on aspects of HF management particularly rehabilitation, concordance with therapy and risk factor management.

Patient safety tips

- ✔ **Daily weights**: aiming for a loss of 0.5–1.0 kg per day. Too brisk a diuresis (>1 kg weight loss) increases risk of renal failure, and hypokalaemia.
- ✔ **Strict fluid balance**: ensure patient is not drinking excessively or overloaded with IV fluids and therapies.
- ✔ **COPD is not a contraindication for β_1-selective β-blockers**: such as bisoprolol and metoprolol.
- ✔ **Screen for diabetes mellitus**: so often remains undiagnosed or sub-optimally treated in patient with HF both acute and chronic.
- ✔ β-blockers are contraindicated in the acute phase but should be administered as soon as the patient is stable.

Student name: **Medical school:**   **Year:**

Cardiac failure

Mr Spiegelman is a 76-year-old gentleman who has presented to the emergency department with acute shortness of breath. His past medical history includes two previous myocardial infarctions and well-controlled diabetes. On inspection he is pale and wheezing with cool and clammy skin. On examination he tachypnoeic with a weak and thready pulse at a rate of 102 beats/min. On auscultation he has bilateral bi-basal crepitations; a third heart sound is audible alongside a pansystolic murmur.

This assessment will be based around a discussion on the management of cardiac chest pain with reference to above scenario.

		Self	Peer	Peer /tutor	Tutor
Diagnosis	• *Chest X-ray* – exclude pulmonary causes of breathlessness, cardiothoracic ratio estimation, alveolar oedema shadowing.	☐	☐	☐	☐
	• *ECG* – confirm heart rhythm, estimate hypertrophy or myocardial ischaemia	☐	☐	☐	☐
	• *ABG* – estimation of oxygenation (pO_2), respiratory function (pCO_2) and acid–base balance	☐	☐	☐	☐
	• *Echocardiography* – evaluation structure and function of the heart, including wall and valvular movement, to direct subsequent management	☐	☐	☐	☐
	• *Biochemistry* – FBC, electrolytes and renal function, glucose levels, LFTs and INR, cardiac biomarkers (troponin)	☐	☐	☐	☐
	• *Natriuretic* peptides – B-type natriuretic peptides useful marker in chronic HF	☐	☐	☐	☐
	•	☐	☐	☐	☐
Causes of cardiac failure	• *CAD* – ACS, complication of acute myocardial infarction	☐	☐	☐	☐
	• *Valvular heart disease* – valve stenosis and regurgitation	☐	☐	☐	☐
	• *Hypertension*	☐	☐	☐	☐
	• *Arrhythmias*	☐	☐	☐	☐
	• *High output circulatory failure* – septicaemia, thyrotoxicosis, anaemia	☐	☐	☐	☐
	• *Decompensation of chronic HF* – poor compliance, volume overload, infections, surgery, obstructive lung disease, drug/alcohol abuse	☐	☐	☐	☐
	• *Myopathies*	☐	☐	☐	☐
	•	☐	☐	☐	☐
Phase 1 initial management (first hour)	• *Clinically* – history, examination focus on haemodynamic status (BP, pulse, oxygen saturation), GCS, MEWS	☐	☐	☐	☐
	• *Investigations* – CXR, ECG, FBC, repeat ABGs if in respiratory distress and hypoxic (<94%), TSH if in atrial fibrillation.	☐	☐	☐	☐
	• *Airway* – high-flow oxygen (pO2 ≥95%), beware the patient with COPD	☐	☐	☐	☐
	• *Circulation* – two wide-bore venous cannulae, consider central line	☐	☐	☐	☐
	• *Loop diuretics IV* – monitor renal function and assess urine output	☐	☐	☐	☐
	• *Opiates IV* – relieves dyspnoea/restlessness/chest pain, may require the use of an antiemetic	☐	☐	☐	☐
	• *Venous vasodilators* – useful when systolic BP >110 mmHg in absence of serious valvular obstruction, slowly titrate in small increments and measure BP often	☐	☐	☐	☐
	• *Inotropic agents* – consider in low output states or hypoperfusion.	☐	☐	☐	☐
	• *Digoxin* – whether atrial fibrillation is present or not.	☐	☐	☐	☐
	•	☐	☐	☐	☐
Phase 2 management (2–6 hours)	• *Airway* – consider non-invasive positive pressure ventilation if unable to correct hypoxaemia.	☐	☐	☐	☐
	• *Airway* – consider mechanical ventilation if hypoxaemia or patient exhausted	☐	☐	☐	☐
	• *Secondary assessment* – look for and treat underlying cause	☐	☐	☐	☐
	• *Thromboprophylaxis* – give LMWH	☐	☐	☐	☐
	•	☐	☐	☐	☐
Phase 3 on-going management	• *ECGs* – serial ECGs/troponin T or I to exclude acute coronary syndrome	☐	☐	☐	☐
	• *Echocardiogram* – prognostic transthoracic echocardiogram	☐	☐	☐	☐
	• *Diuretics* – continued loop diuretic with adjustments according to fluid balance, daily weights, and volume status	☐	☐	☐	☐
	• *Monitor renal function* – beware dangerous electrolyte imbalances	☐	☐	☐	☐
	• *Volume overload* – a combination of thiazide and loop diuretics may be useful in volume-overloaded patients with diuretic resistance	☐	☐	☐	☐
	• *Aldosterone antagonists* – can be used in combination with loop diuretics, particularly in patients with hypokalaemia	☐	☐	☐	☐
	• *Initiate long-term therapy* – based on results of echocardiogram, based on an ACE inhibitor/ ARB with the potential addition of a β-blocker, digoxin, a diuretic and spironolactone.	☐	☐	☐	☐
	• *Patient education* – aspects of heart failure management and lifestyle alteration	☐	☐	☐	☐
	•	☐	☐	☐	☐

Other aspects of treatment	• *Pulse oximetry* – unreliable in low-output or vasoconstricted shocked states	☐	☐	☐	☐
	• High-risk patients should have an NG tube to avoid aspiration.	☐	☐	☐	☐
	• *Catheterize* – ensure accurate measurement of fluid balance	☐	☐	☐	☐
	• *Daily weights* – aiming for a loss of 0.5–1.0 kg per day	☐	☐	☐	☐
	•	☐	☐	☐	☐
Complications	• *ARF* – low blood pressure and fluid restriction can lead to acute renal failure with oliguria and electrolyte disturbance	☐	☐	☐	☐
	• *Cardiac arrest* – due to arrhythmia or electrolyte disturbance	☐	☐	☐	☐
	• *CHF* – increasingly frequent admissions for decompensation leading to increasing disability.	☐	☐	☐	☐
	• Progression of any underlying condition independently	☐	☐	☐	☐
	• What is the NYHF Function Classification of Heart Failure	☐	☐	☐	☐
	•	☐	☐	☐	☐
Patient safety tips	• *Thromboprophylaxis* – usually subcutaneous low-molecular weight heparin	☐	☐	☐	☐
	• *β-blockers* – COPD itself not a contraindication for beta$_1$ selective agents such as bisoprolol and metoprolol	☐	☐	☐	☐
	• Screen for diabetes and other cardiovascular risk factors	☐	☐	☐	☐
	•	☐	☐	☐	☐
Clinical note writing and handover	• Clear recording of clinical status and a regular review of electrolytes	☐	☐	☐	☐
	•	☐	☐	☐	☐

Self-assessed as at least borderline:	Signature:	Date:	U B S E	U B S E	U B S E	U B S E
Peer-assessed as ready for tutor assessment:	Signature:	Date:	U B S E	U B S E	U B S E	U B S E
Tutor-assessed as satisfactory:	Signature:	Date:	U B S E	U B S E	U B S E	U B S E

Notes

11.6 Acute liver failure

Background

Acute hepatic failure occurs when there is damage to the liver to the extent that the hepatocytes can no longer regenerate. This tends to manifest clinically as hepatic encephalopathy and jaundice. Urgent investigation is required as there is often only a small window of opportunity to reverse some treatable causes. Classification is determined by the length of time between onset of jaundice to development of encephalopathy:

- **Hyperacute**: 7 days
- **Acute**: 8–28 days
- **Subacute**: 5–12 weeks.

Diagnosis

Classically patients will present with symptoms of jaundice and encephalopathy. It is important to classify the onset and severity of the encephalopathy as below

- **History**: non-specific symptoms (anorexia, lethargy, pruritis, confusion, dark urine, pale stools, bruising, colicky pain if gallstones, recent blood transfusion, recent infectious disease, IV drugs, sexually transmitted disease, recent travel, certain foods, e.g. shellfish).
- **Examination**: impaired mental state which can guide the severity. Look for signs of liver dysfunction such as palmar erythema, asterixis (liver flap), jaundice, ascites, hepatomegaly and splenomegaly, scratch marks, leuconychia.
- **Investigations**: INR will be raised (>2.0 indicates severe dysfunction). LFTs may shows marked elevation of transaminases, alkaline phosphate (ALP) can be normal or slightly high. Bilirubin will often be elevated. Renal failure and other abnormalities such as hyponatraemia and hypoglycaemia are common. Most patients will need an ultrasound of the liver/pancreas and or CT scan of the abdomen.

Causes of acute liver failure

Acute liver failure is caused by a number of diverse aetiologies:

- **Toxins**: alcohol, overdose (paracetamol), medication (e.g. co-amoxiclav, rifampicin, statins, methotrexate), illicit drugs (Ecstasy and cocaine)

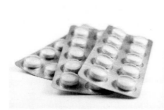 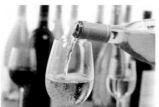 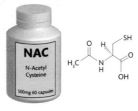

Paracetamol overdose: still the commonest cause of acute liver failure. Limiting paracetamol to only 16 tablets per pack has significantly reduced rate of overdoses

Alcohol in all manifestations: commonest cause of long-term liver disease in Europe. Advise on safe limits to alcohol use at every opportunity for health promotion

N-Acetyl Cysteine: given intravenously for significant paracetamol overdose. It acts by repleting intracellular glutathione in the hepatocytes.

Figure 11.6 Images in acute liver failure.

- **Infections**: sepsis, viral hepatitis (A, B, E), adenovirus, Epstein–Barr virus (EBV), cytomegalo-virus (CMV)
- **Neoplastic**: hepatocellular carcinoma or metastatic carcinoma
- **Metabolic**: Wilson's disease, α-1 antitrypsin deficiency, haemochromatosis
- **Pregnancy-related**: acute fatty liver of pregnancy, intrahepatic cholestasis of pregnancy, HELLP syndrome (Haemolytic anaemia, Elevated Liver enzymes and Low Platelets)
- **Vascular**: ischaemia, veno-occlusive disease, Budd–Chiari syndrome
- **Others**: autoimmune liver disease, idiopathic (15% of cases).

Management

Phase 1 Initial management (first hour)

Management is dependent on the severity of the patient's condition and the complications that may arise subsequently. The primary marker should be the grade of encephalopathy (Box 11.3). There is a high risk of cerebral oedema and multiorgan failure at grades 3 and 4. Urgent correction of any aggravating factors should be initiated.

- **Clinically**: history, examination, focus on GCS (see Table 11.8 below).
- **Investigations**: bloods: coagulation (INR, partial thromboplastin time of kaolin [PTTK]), glucose, potassium, FBC, group and save (G&S), U&Es, LFTs, amylase and paracetamol levels (4 hours after ingestion of overdose). Urine dip (culture), blood culture (even in absence of pyrexia), CXR. Consider ascitic tap for biochemistry and microbiology culture and sensitivity.
- **Consider**: ABG, hepatitis screen (A, B, E, CMV), immunology screen (antinuclear antibody (ANA), anti-smooth muscle antibody, chronic active hepatitis, primary biliary cirrhosis).
- **Monitoring**: hourly: blood glucose, urine output, vital signs and neurological observations. Consider transfer to an ICU/high-dependency unit (HDU) setting.
- **Interventions**:
  - Fluid resuscitation (avoid normal saline – secondary hyperaldosteronism)
  - Treat reversible factors that may complicate encephalopathy (hypoglycaemia, hypo-kalaemia, and hypoxia, infection, bleeding)
  - Avoid: sedatives (can mask signs of hepatic encephalopathy, and even cause it)
  - *N*-acetyl cysteine – established role in paracetamol toxicity, developing role in other forms of acute liver failure
  - Lactulose at earliest stage of encephalopathy
  - Prophylactic antibiotics, including anti-fungals in some cases.

Box 11.3 Grades of hepatic encephalopathy

- **Grade 0**: Normal mental status. Minimal disturbance of memory, concentration, cognition, and coordination
- **Grade 1**: Mild confusion, euphoria/depression, poor attention, impaired cognition, irritability, sleep disturbances (inverted sleep pattern)
- **Grade 2**: Drowsiness, lethargy, gross cognitive impairment, personality changes, inappropriate behaviour, intermittent disorientation
- **Grade 3**: Marked confusion, worsening drowsiness but rousable, inability to perform cognitive tasks, disorientation in time and place, amnesia, incomprehensible speech
- **Grade 4**: Coma with or without response to pain

Phase 2 management (2–6 hours)

- **Continued fluids**: 10% dextrose at 100 mL/h with 400 mmol KCL. Care must be taken to prevent fluid overload.
- **Continued treatment of hypoglycaemia, hypokalaemia, and hypoxia**.

- **Further investigations**: paracetamol levels (4 hours after overdose), ultrasound scan liver/pancreas.
- **Continued monitoring**: twice daily: U&Es, LFTs, FBC, CK, albumin, and coagulation.

Phase 3 ongoing management

- **Fluids as above and continued monitoring**.
- **Consider steroids**: according to local protocols (often based on Glasgow Alcoholic Hepatitis Score; see Figure 11.7). Usually prednisolone 40 mg daily for 28 days.
- **Further investigations**: reconsider hepatitis serology, serum copper and caeruloplasmin, 24-hour copper (in presence of appropriate clinical picture), ferritin
- **Seek specialist advice**: local according to expertise or liver unit.
- **If continued liver impairment consider transfer to a specialist liver unit**.
- **At discharge**: advice on lifestyle and self-management. Advise on alcohol cessation or safer limits to alcohol use (usually 14 units/week for females, 21 units/week for males).

	1 point	2 points	3 points
Age	<50	≥50	
White Cell Count (10^9/l)	<15	≥15	
Urea (mmol/l)	<5	≥5	
Prothrombin Time Ratio/INR	<1.5	1.5-2.0	>2.0
Bilirubin (µmol/l)	<125	125-250	>250

Score 9 or more: identifies patients who may benefit from corticosteroids

Figure 11.7 Glasgow Alcoholic Hepatitis Score.

Other aspects of treatment

Management of developing complications:

- **Cardiovascular**: patients may need inotropes (adrenaline and noradrenaline) for maintenance of mean arterial pressure.
- **Infection**: these patients are at increased risk of infection and potentially sepsis which can complicate hepatic encephalopathy. Meticulous catheter and cannula care (use of local care bundles), Blood, urine and ascites cultures before antibiotic therapy starts, consider use of prophylactic antibiotics and nystatin (patients often lack common clinical signs of sepsis).
- **Hepatic coagulopathy**: consider – parenteral vitamin K, fresh frozen plasma (only used in patients who are bleeding or waiting invasive procedures), ranitidine (reduces bleeding complications).
- **Cerebral oedema**: patient positioned at 30° to the horizontal, hyperventilation, and consider the use of steroids.
- **Diet**: usually high protein, low salt, with general nutritional support.
- **Consider**:
  - **Artificial liver support** – improves survival in patients waiting for transplant

○ **Liver transplantation** – improves survival rates considerably from 10% to nearly 75%. A liver transplant is contraindicated if there is metastatic disease, continued high alcohol intake, sepsis or a recent variceal haemorrhage.

Complications

● Prognosis depends on the underlying pathology behind the liver failure (Figure 11.8). Unfortunately death still occurs in many liver failure patients.

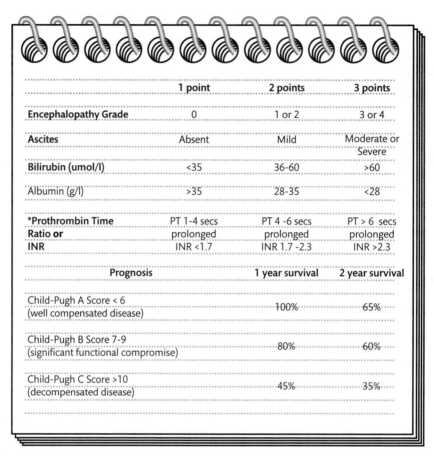

	1 point	2 points	3 points
Encephalopathy Grade	0	1 or 2	3 or 4
Ascites	Absent	Mild	Moderate or Severe
Bilirubin (umol/l)	<35	36-60	>60
Albumin (g/l)	>35	28-35	<28
*Prothrombin Time Ratio or INR	PT 1-4 secs prolonged INR <1.7	PT 4 -6 secs prolonged INR 1.7 -2.3	PT > 6 secs prolonged INR >2.3

Prognosis	1 year survival	2 year survival
Child-Pugh A Score < 6 (well compensated disease)	100%	65%
Child-Pugh B Score 7-9 (significant functional compromise)	80%	60%
Child-Pugh C Score >10 (decompensated disease)	45%	35%

Figure 11.8 Child-Pugh classification of severity of liver disease.

● The main complications that lead to death are variceal haemorrhage, sepsis, cerebral oedema, renal failure, and respiratory failure.

Patient safety tips

✔ **Assessment** – accurate history and examination to guide treatment to causative agent as aetiology of acute liver failure is diverse.

✔ **Management** – avoid normal saline and high salt diet due to possibility of hyperaldosteronism. Lactulose to reduce complications from ammonia build-up in the gut.

✔ **Careful monitoring** – look for signs of bleeding and have a high index of suspicion. May need emergency endoscopy. Monitor blood glucose and potassium regularly and correct as appropriate. Manage in the appropriate setting with regular observations. Consider HDU/ICU/specialist liver unit.

✔ **Infection** – Patients may not show signs of infection; have a high index of suspicion and take blood, urine and ascites cultures prior to starting prophylactic antibiotic regimens.

Acute liver failure

Louise Noble (43 years old; date of birth 3 July 1966; hospital number AL45612845) is brought to a local NHS walk-in centre by her husband who complains of her increasing levels of confusion. She has noticed her urine change colour recently and on examination she has yellow sclera. She has no known allergies. She weighs 71 kg.

This assessment will be based around a discussion on the management of acute liver failure with reference to above scenario.

		Self	Peer	Peer /tutor	Tutor
Background	Acute hepatic failure occurs when there is damage to the liver to the extent that the hepatocytes can no longer regenerate. Clinically there can be hepatic encephalopathy and jaundice. Classification is determined by the length of time between onset of jaundice to development of encephalopathy:				
	● Hyperacute: 7 days	☐	☐	☐	☐
	● Acute: 8–28 days	☐	☐	☐	☐
	● Subacute: 5–12 weeks	☐	☐	☐	☐
	●	☐	☐	☐	☐
Diagnosis	● Classically patients present with symptoms of jaundice and encephalopathy. It is important to classify the onset and severity	☐	☐	☐	☐
	● Examination may show an impaired mental state which can guide the severity. Look for signs of liver dysfunction such as palmar erythema, asterixis (liver flap), jaundice, ascites, hepatomegaly and splenomegaly.	☐	☐	☐	☐
	● On investigation INR will be raised (>2.0 indicates severe dysfunction). Liver function test may shows marked elevation of transaminases, ALP can be normal or slightly high. Bilirubin will often be elevated. Consider ultrasound of the liver/pancreas	☐	☐	☐	☐
	●	☐	☐	☐	☐
Causes of acute liver failure	● **Toxins**: alcohol, overdose (paracetamol), medication (e.g. co-amoxiclav, rifampicin, statins, methotrexate), illicit drugs (Ecstasy and cocaine)	☐	☐	☐	☐
	● **Infections**: viral hepatitis, adenovirus, EBV, CMV	☐	☐	☐	☐
	● **Neoplastic**: hepatocellular carcinoma or metastatic carcinoma	☐	☐	☐	☐
	● **Metabolic**: Wilson's disease, α-1 antitrypsin deficiency, haemochromatosis	☐	☐	☐	☐
	● **Pregnancy related**: Acute fatty liver of pregnancy, cholestasis, HELLP	☐	☐	☐	☐
	● **Vascular**: ischaemia, veno-occlusive disease, Budd–Chiari syndrome	☐	☐	☐	☐
	● **Others**: autoimmune liver disease, idiopathic (15% of cases)	☐	☐	☐	☐
	●	☐	☐	☐	☐
Phase 1 initial management (first hour)	● **Clinically**: history, examination, focus on GCS	☐	☐	☐	☐
	● **Investigations**: Bloods: coagulation, glucose, potassium, FBC, G&S, U&Es, LFTs, amylase and paracetamol levels (4 hours after ingestion of overdose). ABG – hypoxia	☐	☐	☐	☐
	● **Consider**: urine dip (culture), blood culture (even in absence of pyrexia), CXR	☐	☐	☐	☐
	● **Monitoring**: hourly: blood glucose, urine output, vital signs and neurological observations. Consider transfer to an ICU/HDU setting	☐	☐	☐	☐
	● **Interventions**:	☐	☐	☐	☐
	○ Fluid resuscitation (avoid normal saline – secondary hyperaldosteronism)				
	○ Treat reversible factors that may complicate encephalopathy (hypoglycaemia, hypokalaemia and hypoxia), infection, bleeding				
	○ N-acetyl cysteine – established role in paracetamol toxicity, developing role in other forms of acute liver failure				
	○ Lactulose at earliest stage of encephalopathy				
	○ Prophylactic antibiotics ? anti-fungals				
	○ Avoid: sedatives (can mask signs and even cause hepatic encephalopathy)				
	●	☐	☐	☐	☐
Phase 2 management (2–6 hours)	● Continued fluids: 10% dextrose at 100 mL/h with 400 mmol KCL. Care must be taken to prevent fluid overload	☐	☐	☐	☐
	● Continued treatment of hypoglycaemia, hypokalaemia, and hypoxia.	☐	☐	☐	☐
	● Further investigations – paracetamol levels (4 hours after overdose), ultrasound scan liver/pancreas	☐	☐	☐	☐
	● Continued monitoring – twice daily: potassium, FBC, albumin, and coagulation	☐	☐	☐	☐
	●	☐	☐	☐	☐

Phase 3 ongoing management	• Fluids as above.	☐	☐	☐	☐
	• Continued monitoring.	☐	☐	☐	☐
	• Further investigations – hepatitis serology, serum copper and caeruloplasmin, 24 hour copper (in presence of appropriate clinical picture)	☐	☐	☐	☐
	• If continued liver impairment consider transfer to a specialist liver unit	☐	☐	☐	☐
	•	☐	☐	☐	☐
Other aspects of treatment	• **Cardiovascular**: Patients may need inotropes (adrenaline and noradrenaline), for maintenance of mean arterial pressure	☐	☐	☐	☐
	• **Infection**: These patients are at increased risk of infection and potentially sepsis which can complicate hepatic encephalopathy. Meticulous catheter and cannula care (use of local care bundles), Blood, urine and ascites cultures before antibiotic therapy starts, consider use of prophylactic antibiotics and nystatin (patients often lack common clinical signs of sepsis)	☐	☐	☐	☐
	• **Hepatic coagulopathy**: Consider – parenteral vitamin K, fresh frozen plasma (only used in patients who are bleeding or waiting invasive procedures), ranitidine (reduces bleeding complications).	☐	☐	☐	☐
	• **Cerebral oedema**: Patient positioned at 30 degrees to the horizontal, hyperventilation and consider the use of steroids.	☐	☐	☐	☐
	• **Diet**: high protein, low salt, nutritious	☐	☐	☐	☐
	• **Consider**: ○ **Artificial liver support –** Improves survival in patients waiting for transplant ○ **Liver transplantation –** Improves survival rates considerably from 10% to nearly 75%. A liver transplant is contraindicated if there is metastatic disease, continued high alcohol intake, sepsis or a recent variceal haemorrhage.	☐	☐	☐	☐
	•				
Complications	• Prognosis depends on the underlying pathology behind the liver failure. Unfortunately death still occurs in many liver failure patients.	☐	☐	☐	☐
	• The main fatal complications are variceal haemorrhage, sepsis, cerebral oedema, renal failure, and respiratory failure	☐	☐	☐	☐
	•	☐	☐	☐	☐
Patient safety tips	• **Assessment –** accurate history and examination to guide treatment to causative agent as aetiology of acute liver failure is diverse	☐	☐	☐	☐
	• **Management** – avoid normal saline and high salt intake. Lactulose to reduce complications from ammonia build-up in the gut	☐	☐	☐	☐
	• **Careful monitoring** – look for signs of bleeding and have a high index of suspicion. May need emergency endoscopy. Monitor blood glucose and potassium regularly and correct as appropriate. Manage in the appropriate setting with regular observations. Consider HDU/ICU/specialist liver unit	☐	☐	☐	☐
	• **Infection** – patients may not show signs of infection, have a high index of suspicion and take blood, urine and ascites cultures prior to starting prophylactic antibiotic regimens	☐	☐	☐	☐
	•	☐	☐	☐	☐
Clinical note writing and handover	• Stress that patient's clinical state and electrolytes must be reviewed regularly	☐	☐	☐	☐
	•	☐	☐	☐	☐

			U B S E	U B S E	U B S E	U B S E
Self-assessed as at least borderline:	Signature:	Date:				
Peer-assessed as ready for tutor assessment:	Signature:	Date:	U B S E	U B S E	U B S E	U B S E
Tutor-assessed as satisfactory:	Signature:	Date:	U B S E	U B S E	U B S E	U B S E

Notes

11.7 Upper gastrointestinal bleeding

Background

Upper gastrointestinal bleeding (UGIB) is one of the most common clinical emergencies and has a significant morbidity and mortality in patients with underlying co-morbidities. Prompt initial assessment of patient and resuscitation with IV fluids and/or blood as well as urgent upper gastrointestinal endoscopy if indicated is important to limit complications.

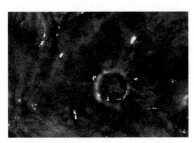

Peptic ulcer disease: common but remains significant cause of mortality in acute upper gastrointestinal bleeding

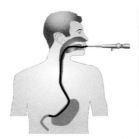

Oesophago-gastro-duodenoscopy (OGD): early recourse to this investigation for accurate intervention such as coagulation of bleeding peptic ulcer

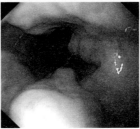

Oesophageal varices: frequent complication of portal hypertension due to cirrhosis of the liver; can be treated if actively bleeding by sclerotherapy, banding, or tamponade

Figure 11.9 Images in upper gastrointestinal bleeding. Left © CNRI/Science Photolibrary; right © Gastrolab/Science Photo Library.

Diagnosis

Haematemesis (vomiting blood or coffee-ground-like material), and/or melaena (passing of black, tarry stool) are the hallmarks to the diagnosis of UGIB. Fresh blood can also be observed from the rectum in UGIB following a massive haemorrhage due to rapid transit through the gastrointestinal tract. Good history taking is important in making the diagnosis where the bleeding has not been observed by the clinician as melaena is not always present on rectal examination (see Table 11.4).

Table 11.4 Causes of upper gastrointestinal bleeding

Cause	Frequency (%)
Peptic ulcer	40–50
Oesophagitis	28
Gastritis/erosion	26
Erosive duodenitis	15
Varices	13–14
Portal hypertensive gastropathy	7
Malignancy	4–5
Mallory–Weiss tears	5
Vascular malformations	3
Other causes, e.g. Osler–Weber–Rendu syndrome, blood dyscrasias, haemobilia, etc.	11

Management

Phase 1 Initial management (first hour)

- **Clinical history**: previous UGIB, dyspepsia, known peptic ulcers, liver disease, weight loss, drugs (NSAIDs, aspirin, corticosteroids, cyclo-oxygenase-2 [COX-2] inhibitors, bisphosphonates), and co-morbidities.

- **Clinical examination**: assess for signs of shock, evidence of chronic liver disease and other co-morbidities such as heart and renal failure. ? telangiectasia due to hereditary haemorrhagic telangiectasia (Osler–Weber–Rendu syndrome).

- **Resuscitation**: Two large-bore IV cannulae are inserted. IV fluids (colloids or crystalloids), avoid crystalloids in patients with cirrhotic ascites. Blood transfusion if haemoglobin <10 g/dL and patient in shock or active heavy bleeding, otherwise wait for FBC results.

- **Investigations**: FBC, G&S, LFTs, U&Es, coagulation screen, AXR and CXR if suspected ruptured peptic ulcer. Consider ECG if patient has history of ischaemic heart disease or HF.

- **Monitoring**: patients with significant bleeding need continuous cardiac monitoring, and those with shock might need CVP and renal function monitoring.

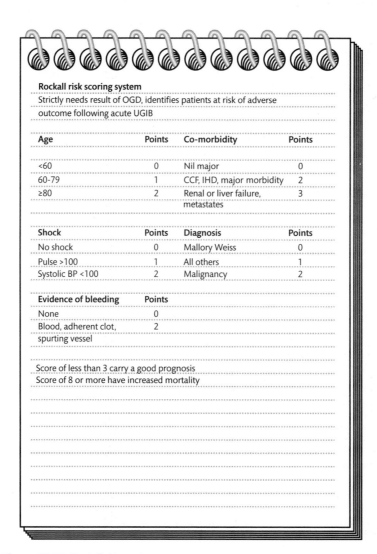

Rockall risk scoring system

Strictly needs result of OGD, identifies patients at risk of adverse outcome following acute UGIB

Age	Points	Co-morbidity	Points
<60	0	Nil major	0
60-79	1	CCF, IHD, major morbidity	2
≥80	2	Renal or liver failure, metastates	3

Shock	Points	Diagnosis	Points
No shock	0	Mallory Weiss	0
Pulse >100	1	All others	1
Systolic BP <100	2	Malignancy	2

Evidence of bleeding	Points
None	0
Blood, adherent clot, spurting vessel	2

Score of less than 3 carry a good prognosis
Score of 8 or more have increased mortality

Figure 11.10 Rockall risk scoring system.

Phase 2 management (2–6 hours)

- **Continue with fluid resuscitation**: monitor urine output and cardiac monitoring where indicated.

- **Consider oesophagogastroduodenoscopy (OGD)**: conduct Rockall score (pre-OGD; see Figure 11.10); score of 0, consider no admission or early discharge. If the score is >0, endoscopy required in most cases after resuscitation. Or use Glasgow–Blatchford Score (Figure 11.11): score greater than 3 consider OGD.

- **Start a proton pump inhibitor (PPI)**: there is only minimal evidence that pre-endoscopic PPI improves the clinical outcome. Most clinical protocols include their use at this stage. IV PPI, e.g. omeprazole 80 mg bolus followed by 8 mg/h infusion for 72 hours, in patients with high-risk ulcers on OGD, i.e. active bleeding, non-bleeding visible vessel or adherent clot.

- **IV terlipressin or similar agent**: prior to endoscopy in acute variceal bleeding; 2 mg then repeated at 4-hour intervals up to 72 hours.

- **Start antibiotics**: preferably IV ceftriaxone or oral norfloxacin, in patients with chronic liver disease presenting with acute UGIB.

- **Full (post-OGD) Rockall score**: is predictive of mortality in acute gastrointestinal bleed but less so in predicting re-bleeding.

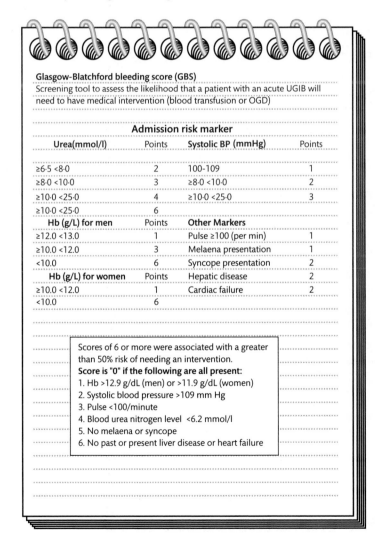

Glasgow-Blatchford bleeding score (GBS)

Screening tool to assess the likelihood that a patient with an acute UGIB will need to have medical intervention (blood transfusion or OGD)

Admission risk marker			
Urea(mmol/l)	Points	Systolic BP (mmHg)	Points
≥6·5 <8·0	2	100-109	1
≥8·0 <10·0	3	≥8·0 <10·0	2
≥10·0 <25·0	4	≥10·0 <25·0	3
≥10·0 <25·0	6		
Hb (g/L) for men	Points	**Other Markers**	
≥12.0 <13.0	1	Pulse ≥100 (per min)	1
≥10.0 <12.0	3	Melaena presentation	1
<10.0	6	Syncope presentation	2
Hb (g/L) for women	Points	Hepatic disease	2
≥10.0 <12.0	1	Cardiac failure	2
<10.0	6		

> Scores of 6 or more were associated with a greater than 50% risk of needing an intervention.
> **Score is "0" if the following are all present:**
> 1. Hb >12.9 g/dL (men) or >11.9 g/dL (women)
> 2. Systolic blood pressure >109 mm Hg
> 3. Pulse <100/minute
> 4. Blood urea nitrogen level <6.2 mmol/l
> 5. No melaena or syncope
> 6. No past or present liver disease or heart failure

Figure 11.11 Glasgow-Blatchford bleeding score (GBS).

Phase 3 ongoing management

- **Repeat OGD**: within 24 hours if patient continues to bleed or if initial OGD was suboptimal.
- **Re-bleeding**: following repeat OGD requires surgery or selective arterial embolization.
- **Review and stop implicated medications**: aspirin, NSAIDs, COX-2 inhibitors if an ulcer diagnosed on OGD.
- *Helicobacter pylori* **eradication**: therapy for a week and a further 8 weeks of antisecretory treatment if *H. pylori* positive.
- **Discontinue antacid treatment**: after successful healing of the ulcer and *H. pylori* eradication treatment in non-NSAIDs users.
- **Continue PPI**: in patients who require continued use of NSAID, aspirin, or COX-2 inhibitors.
- **Use selective serotonin reuptake inhibitors (SSRIs) with caution**: in patients with increased risk of UGIB, especially if on NSAIDs or aspirin.
- **Repeat OGD in 6–8 weeks** to confirm healing in case of gastric ulcer or suspicion of malignancy.
- **Consider referral for transjugular intrahepatic portosystemic shunt (TIPS)**: to prevent oesophageal and gastric variceal re-bleeding in patients with intolerance to or failure of endoscopic and/or pharmacological therapy.

Other aspects of treatment

- Intubation in unconscious patients.
- Monitor FBC and U&Es closely.
- Terlipressin for 72 hours in variceal bleeding after endoscopic treatment.

Complications

- **Re-bleeding**: endoscopic and pharmacological treatment reduce incidence of re-bleeding but not so with mortality. Unfortunately re-bleeding still occurs in 20% of cases within 72 hours.
- **Mortality**: rates of 7–10% do occur especially in patients >60 years old. Most deaths are due to co-morbidities.

Patient safety tips

- ✔ **Resuscitation**: assess promptly for shock, prompt resuscitation before endoscopy. Cardiac monitoring in patients with HF, ischaemic heart disease, renal failure.
- ✔ **OGD endoscopy**: Rockall or Glasgow–Blatchford Score in all patients. All patients with an initial Rockall score >0 must have an endoscopy.
- ✔ **PPI infusion**: needs to be handed over to make sure that the patient gets the continuous 72 hrs of omeprazole infusion following OGD if indicated.
- ✔ **Drugs**: stop any antithrombotic drugs, NSAIDs, aspirin, COX-2 inhibitors in patients with acute UGIB.
- ✔ **Advise patient in relation to self-management**: risk factors (alcohol) and watching out for future bleeds.

Gastrointestinal bleeding

John Raffles, a 64-year-old well-known patient, presents to the emergency department with massive haematemesis which he described as being 'bright red'. It is elicited from the history that Mr Raffles drinks a bottle of vodka per day and has been on warfarin long term. On examination he is tachycardic (112 rate), has a blood pressure of 92/64 mmHg and is pale with cool peripheries. His urea is 9.3 mmol/L with and Hb of 9.2 g/dL. He is known to have cardiac failure due to a previous anterior myocardial infarction 4 years ago.

This assessment will be based around a discussion on the management of UGIB with reference to above scenario.

		Self	Peer	Peer /tutor	Tutor
What diagnoses are likely in this patient as a cause of his UGIB? Consider at least four possible causes	•	☐	☐	☐	☐
	•	☐	☐	☐	☐
What are the key aspects of phase 1 initial management (first hour)	• **Clinical history**: **?** previous UGIB, peptic ulcer disease, drugs, co-morbidities	☐	☐	☐	☐
	• **Clinical examination**: ? signs of shock, ? liver disease, ? telangiectasia, ? heart disease	☐	☐	☐	☐
	• **Resuscitation**: two IV cannulae, IV fluids, blood treatment if Hb <10 g/dL and shock or active heavy bleeding, otherwise wait for FBC results	☐	☐	☐	☐
	• **Investigations**: FBC, G&S, LFTs, U&Es, coagulation screen, ? AXR and CXR.	☐	☐	☐	☐
	• **Monitoring**: continuous cardiac monitoring, ? CVP, renal output and function monitoring	☐	☐	☐	☐
	•	☐	☐	☐	☐
What are the key aspects of phase 2 management (2–6 hours)?	• **Continue with fluid resuscitation**: urine output and cardiac monitoring where indicated	☐	☐	☐	☐
	• **Consider OGD**: Conduct Rockall Score and Glasgow–Blatchford Score. What are these scores in this patient?	☐	☐	☐	☐
	• **Start a PPI**: e.g. omeprazole 80 mg bolus followed by infusion.	☐	☐	☐	☐
	• **IV terlipressin or similar agent**: prior to endoscopy in acute variceal bleeding	☐	☐	☐	☐
	• **Start antibiotics**: preferably IV ceftriaxone or oral norfloxacin, in chronic liver disease	☐	☐	☐	☐
	•	☐	☐	☐	☐
What are the key aspects of phase 3 ongoing management?	• **Repeat OGD**: within 24 hours if bleeding continues or if initial OGD was suboptimal	☐	☐	☐	☐
	• **Re-bleeding**: following repeat OGD requires surgery or selective arterial embolization	☐	☐	☐	☐
	• **Review and stop implicated medications**: aspirin, NSAIDs, COX-2 inhibitors	☐	☐	☐	☐
	• **H. pylori eradication**: therapy for a week and a further 8 weeks of PPI	☐	☐	☐	☐
	• **Continue PPI**: in patients who require continued use of NSAID, aspirin or COX-2 inhibitors	☐	☐	☐	☐
	• **Repeat OGD in 6–8 weeks** to confirm healing in gastric ulcer or suspicion of malignancy	☐	☐	☐	☐
	• **Consider referral for TIPS** to prevent oesophageal and gastric variceal re-bleeding in failure of endoscopic or pharmacological therapy	☐	☐	☐	☐
	•	☐	☐	☐	☐
What are the main complications of UGIB?	• **Re-bleeding**: endoscopic and pharmacological treatment reduce incidence of re-bleeding	☐	☐	☐	☐
	• **Mortality**: rates of 7–10% do occur especially in patients >60 years old	☐	☐	☐	☐
	•	☐	☐	☐	☐
What the main aspects to consider in relation to patient safety?	• **Resuscitation**: assess promptly for shock, prompt resuscitation before endoscopy	☐	☐	☐	☐
	• **OGD endoscopy**: do not delay if indicated.	☐	☐	☐	☐
	• **Advise patient in relation to self-management**: risk factors (alcohol) and watching out for future bleeds	☐	☐	☐	☐
	• **PPI infusion**: once IV phase completed start oral treatment	☐	☐	☐	☐
	• **Drugs**: stop any antithrombotic drugs, NSAIDs, aspirin, COX-2 inhibitors	☐	☐	☐	☐
	•	☐	☐	☐	☐

				Self	Peer	Peer /tutor	Tutor
Self-assessed as at least borderline:	Signature:		Date:	U B S E	U B S E	U B S E	U B S E
Peer-assessed as ready for tutor assessment:	Signature:		Date:	U B S E	U B S E	U B S E	U B S E
Tutor-assessed as satisfactory:	Signature:		Date:	U B S E	U B S E	U B S E	U B S E

Notes

11.8 Acute kidney injury

Background

Acute kidney injury (AKI; commonly known as acute renal failure) is a common medical condition which is associated with significant mortality and morbidity. Prompt diagnosis and treatment can often be rewarding and can reduce the morbidity associated with this condition. Risk factors for developing AKI include age, chronic kidney disease, heart disease, diabetes, hypertension, and history of collagen vascular diseases. The incidence of community-acquired AKI has been estimated at 384/100 000 person years (not requiring dialysis) and 24.4/100 000 person years (requiring dialysis), which has a 50% mortality.

Diagnosis

AKI refers to a sudden change in kidney function which has occurred over hours-days. The clinical presentation varies considerably due to the multitude of causes. Patients often present with the history of a condition which has caused the AKI (e.g. post operation) or may be asymptomatic, being diagnosed purely on the basis of abnormal laboratory investigations. Some non-specific symptoms can occur with uraemia per se such as nausea/vomiting, lethargy and confusion. If there is longstanding unexplained history of this, severe chronic kidney disease (CKD) should be considered. It is important to determine whether the patient's presentation is AKI, acute-on-chronic kidney injury or severe chronic kidney disease. The RIFLE criteria for AKI takes into account rises in serum creatinine as well as changes in urine output. It classes patients into 'at-risk', injury and failure. The criteria for AKI are one or more of:

● A threefold rise in serum creatinine from baseline

● A ≥75 % decrease in the patient's glomerular filtration rate (GFR)

● Serum creatinine >350 µmol/L (with an acute rise of at least 44 µmol/L)

● Urine output <0.3 mL/kg/h for at least 12 hours

● Anuria for 12 hours.

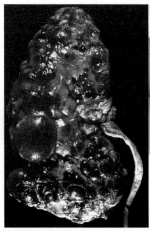
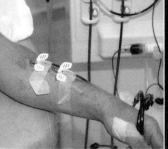
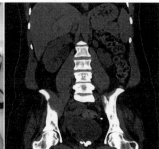

Haemodialysis: adds years to patients' lives. Certain renal disease is very amenable to prevention, especially hypertensive and diabetic renal disease – treat risk factors aggressively.

Bladder stones: a rare cause of AKI due to outflow obstruction.

Polycystic kidneys: can often present with hypertension, haematuria or CKD

Figure 11.12 Images in acute renal injury. Right © Mr Hashim Hashim and Mr Dan Wood, University College Hospital, London.

Causes

These are divided into pre-renal, renal and post-renal.

- **Pre-renal – renal hypoperfusion**:
  - ○ Hypovolaemia, e.g. bleeding, severe diarrhoea/vomiting, diuretic use, burns
  - ○ Hypotension, e.g. cardiac failure, sepsis, medication induced
  - ○ Abnormal intrarenal blood flow, e.g. ACE inhibitors, A_2 receptor blocks, NSAIDs
- **Renal causes** (**intrinsic kidney disease**):
  - ○ Renal vascular disease (arteries, arterioles or veins)
  - ○ Glomerulonephritis, e.g. lupus nephritis, Wegener's
  - ○ Tubulo/interstitial disease, e.g. drugs – NSAIDs, gentamicin, penicillins
- **Post-renal** (**obstruction of urine flow from kidneys**):
  - ○ Ureteric stone/stricture, retroperitoneal fibrosis, extrinsic tumour
  - ○ Bladder – stone/tumour, neurogenic bladder, drugs, e.g. tricyclics
  - ○ Prostate – benign prostatic hypertrophy, prostate carcinoma
  - ○ Urethra – stricture/tumour, blocked urinary catheter

Management

Phase 1 management (first hour)

- **Clinical history**: consider causes above. Take a detailed past medical history and accurate drug history (including over-the-counter and herbal remedy use). Try to find patient's baseline renal function, e.g. previous clinical record and ? GP.
- **Clinical examination**: assess ABCDE as usual. Full set of vital signs including postural blood pressure if possible. Look for potentially causative condition, in particular post renal causes, e.g. enlarged bladder, enlarged prostate, enlarged kidneys. Assess whether the patient is hypovolaemic, euvolaemic, or hypervolaemic. Assess if the patient has any indications for immediate dialysis (see below).
- **Investigations**:
  - ○ **In all patients**: urine (inspection, dipstick, microscopy, culture), random protein/creatinine (PCR) ratio, FBC, U&Es, bicarbonate, bone profile, glucose, LFTs, clotting, CRP/erythrocyte sedimentation rate (ESR). ECG (? hyperkalaemia ? ischaemic heart disease), CXR (? fluid overload, ? infection), ABGs (if acidosis suspected or respiratory failure), renal ultrasound.
  - ○ **In some patients according to clinical state and differential diagnoses**: blood culture, urate, CK, immunology screen (antineutrophilic cytoplasmic antibodies [ANCA], anti-glomerular basement membrane antibodies, ANA, anti-DsDNA Ab, C3, C4. Myeloma screen (IgG/A/M + serum electrophoresis, serum free light chains). Urine sodium and osmolality are often very useful. Prostate-specific antigen (PSA) indicated if prostatic pathology suspected.
- **Monitoring**: nurse in area appropriate to degree of illness. At least hourly observations, cardiac monitoring, urine output. Accurate fluid balance charting. Daily weight. Consider CVP monitoring.
- **Treatment**: this will vary considerably depending on the cause. The goal is to prevent further renal injury, correction of the underlying cause if possible and treat the complications of AKI. A senior doctor should review the patient at the earliest opportunity. The immediate causes of death in AKI are (the latter four are indications for urgent dialysis):
  - ○ Severe causative illness, e.g. massive haemorrhage, sepsis
  - ○ Refractory hyperkalaemia causing fatal cardiac dysrhythmia
  - ○ Refractory fluid overload causing pulmonary oedema
  - ○ Severe metabolic acidosis.
  - ○ Severe uraemic complication, e.g. pericarditis, encephalopathy etc.

- **General management**:
  - ○ The only proven treatment, apart from treating the underlying cause, is prompt administration of IV fluids (crystalloid)
  - ○ Stop any nephrotoxic agents, e.g. ACE inhibitors, A$_2$ receptor blockers, diuretics, NSAIDs, gentamicin
  - ○ Catheterize the bladder, noting residual volume
  - ○ Establish good IV access. Avoid forearm veins if likely to need long-term dialysis
  - ○ Does the patient need high level care? HDU, ICU
  - ○ If hypovolaemic, administer a fluid challenge, e.g. 500 mL 0.9% NaCl over 30 minutes and assess response. Replace volume briskly till patient is euvolaemic. The euvolaemic patient should be given a daily quota of fluid at around 300–500 mL of fluid plus the previous day's urine output and fluid losses
  - ○ If the patient is fluid overloaded discuss with senior. Treatment may include diuretics and vasodilators. A diuretic may be tried, e.g. 120 mg IV furosemide. A GTN infusion can reduce pre- and after-load while definitive treatment is undertaken. The definitive treatment of dialysis may be needed.
- **Hyperkalaemia**: common cause of cardiac arrest and death in AKI. If potassium level is raised or ECG changes of hyperkalaemia are present, immediate treatment is needed. ECG changes include: peaked T waves, prolonged PR interval, absent P waves, widening of the QRS complex. Again if refractory, dialysis will be the definitive treatment (see Table 11.5).

Table 11.5 Treatments for hyperkalaemia

Any ECG changes of hyperkalaemia	Calcium Resonium® + insulin/dextrose + calcium gluconate ± salbutamol Withdraw offending drug
K⁺ value	
5.5–6 mmol/L	Calcium Resonium®
6.0–6.4 mmol/L	Calcium Resonium® + insulin/dextrose
>6.4 mmol/L	Calcium Resonium® + insulin/dextrose + calcium gluconate ± salbutamol
Standard initial doses	
Oral Calcium Resonium®	15 g four times daily: causes constipation, unpalatable, also enema formulation
IV insulin/dextrose	50 mL of 50% glucose with 10 units soluble insulin, IV into a large vein over 20 minutes. Monitor glucose levels
IV calcium gluconate	10 mL of 10% calcium gluconate: injected slowly (with cardiac monitoring) over 5 minutes into large vein. Can repeat once if electrocardiogram (ECG) changes still present
Nebulized salbutamol	5–10 mg salbutamol, nebulized over 10–20 minutes with air or oxygen if indicated

U&Es every 1–4 hours.

If infection is suspected: take appropriate cultures, e.g. urine, blood, wound and promptly administer non-nephrotoxic, broad-spectrum antibiotics as per local guidelines.

Phase 2 management (2–6 hours)

- **Monitor the patient's response to treatment**: especially urine output.
- **Ensure definitive plan**: for treating underlying condition is present.

- **Regular assessment of fluid balance**: tailor IV fluid replacement to each patient.
- **Bicarbonate**: consider if there is a persistent metabolic acidosis (expert supervision).
- **Consider CVP measurement**: if fluid balance is difficult to assess.
- **Repeat U&Es frequently**: this will be required after hyperkalaemia treatment and 6-hourly through the day as rebounds in the serum potassium can occur.
- Ensure K$^+$ <6.0 mmol/L as soon as possible, hand patient onto next team of doctors if needed.
- **Liaise with nephrology team**: transfer of patient not always indicated. General advice on management will be invaluable.

Phase 3 ongoing management

- **Diagnosis should be clear**: if not seek help.
- **Organize an ultrasound scan of the renal tract**: looking for kidney size, evidence of obstruction, e.g. hydronephrosis, Doppler of the renal arteries may be possible.
- **Consider urology and radiology advice and management**: if an obstruction is present, one or two nephrostomies may be required.
- **Consider renal biopsy**: if an intrinsic renal cause is suspected such as glomerulonephritis.
- **Dietician consultation**: may be required as patients are often in a catabolic balance and special diets (e.g. low potassium) may be of clinical benefit.
- **Treat potential complications proactively**: patients with AKI of any aetiology (as with any critically ill patient) are at risk of developing sepsis, gastrointestinal bleeds, VTE, pressure sores, and malnutrition. Look out for these and treat aggressively.
- **Watch out for recovery phase diuresis**: Patients with post-renal failure who have relief of the obstruction and those with recovering acute tubular necrosis (ATN) can develop a massive diuresis, which may require large amounts of volume replacement.

Other aspects of treatment

- Look for infection and treat vigorously. Avoid nephrotoxic antibiotics, when possible. Under expert advice a single dose of gentamicin may be used.
- Avoid administration of nephrotoxins, e.g. NSAIDs, aminoglycosides, IV contrast.
- Many drugs, e.g. antibiotics, digoxin will need dose changes in patients with impaired renal function. Refer to the drug data sheet.

Patient safety tips

- ✔ **Hyperkalaemia**: commonest cause of avoidable cardiac arrest. Must be treated obsessively and meticulously. U&Es need to be checked frequently in the early phase of the illness as sharp rebound rises in serum potassium can occur as the effect of insulin-dextrose is temporary and Calcium Resonium® takes several hours to start working.
- ✔ **Post-renal causes**: very important not to miss a post-renal cause as it is often easily treatable and recovery of renal function can be good.
- ✔ **Fluid balance must be frequently assessed**: uncorrected hypovolaemia and hypotension can lead to acute tubular necrosis. Conversely, injudicious excess fluid replacement can lead to fluid overload and pulmonary oedema.
- ✔ **Intrinsic AKI**: in patients with suspected intrinsic AKI, early review by the nephrology team with a view to kidney biopsy should occur. Specific treatments such as steroids and immunosuppressants can then be given.
- ✔ **Watch out for AKI in hospitalized patients admitted for other reasons**: adequate clinical and laboratory monitoring can help prevent this issue.

Acute renal failure

Matthew Tantripp, aged 76, was admitted with acute urinary retention, nausea and vomiting and confusion. He is known to have a history of rheumatoid arthritis and hypertension. His medications from general practice are as follows: ramipril 10 mg once daily, naproxen 1 g once daily, omeprazole 20 mg once daily.

He has no known drug allergies. His results on admission are: urea 24.6 mmol/L, creatinine 452 µmol/L, K$^+$ 7.2 mmol/L.

This assessment will be based around a discussion on the management of acute kidney injury with reference to above scenario.

Student name: Medical school: Year:

		Assessments			
		Self	Peer	Peer/tutor	Tutor
Background	● Also known as acute kidney injury. Common, significant morbidity and mortality, which can be reduced with prompt assessment, diagnosis, and treatment	☐	☐	☐	☐
	●	☐	☐	☐	☐
Diagnosis	A sudden change in kidney function occurring over hours-days. Try to decide whether it is AKI, acute-on-chronic, or severe chronic kidney failure. Risk factors for development include advancing age, chronic kidney disease, heart disease, diabetes, hypertension and collagen vascular diseases. Non-specific symptoms include nausea and vomiting, lethargy, and confusion. The criteria for *failure* is *any* of:				
	● Threefold rise in serum creatinine from baseline	☐	☐	☐	☐
	● ≥75% decrease of GFR	☐	☐	☐	☐
	● Serum creatinine >350 µmol/L (with acute rise of ≥44 µmol/L)	☐	☐	☐	☐
	● Urine output <0.3 mL/kg/h for ≥12 hours	☐	☐	☐	☐
	● Anuria for 12 hours	☐	☐	☐	☐
	●	☐	☐	☐	☐
Causes of AKI	**Pre-renal (renal hypoperfusion):**				
	● Hypovolaemia (e.g. bleeding, severe diarrhoea/vomiting, diuretic use, burns)	☐	☐	☐	☐
	● Hypotension (e.g. cardiac failure, sepsis, medication induced)	☐	☐	☐	☐
	● Abnormal intrarenal blood flow (e.g. ACE inhibitors, NSAIDs)	☐	☐	☐	☐
	Renal (intrinsic kidney disease):				
	● Renal vascular disease (artery-arteriole-vein)	☐	☐	☐	☐
	● Glomerulonephritides (e.g. lupus nephritis, Wegner's granulomatosis), vasculitis	☐	☐	☐	☐
	● Tubulo/interstitial disease (e.g. drugs – NSAIDs, gentamicin, penicillins)	☐	☐	☐	☐
	Post-renal (obstruction of urine outflow):				
	● Ureteric – stone/stricture, retroperitoneal fibrosis	☐	☐	☐	☐
	● Bladder – stones/tumour, neurogenic bladder, drugs (e.g. tricyclics)	☐	☐	☐	☐
	● Prostate – benign prostatic hypertrophy (BPH), prostate carcinoma	☐	☐	☐	☐
	● Urethra – stricture, blocked urinary catheter	☐	☐	☐	☐
	●	☐	☐	☐	☐
Phase 1 initial management (first hour)	● **History** – take detailed past medical history and drug history, considering risk factors above. If possible, ascertain patient's baseline renal function (e.g. from old U&Es).	☐	☐	☐	☐
	● **Examination** – ABCDE. Full set of vital signs including postural BP and whether patient is hypo-, eu-, or hypervolaemic. Consider causes (e.g. enlarged bladder or prostate). Assess need for immediate dialysis	☐	☐	☐	☐
	● **Investigations** – urine dipstick and microscopy + culture ± PCR, FBC, U&Es, bicarbonate, bone profile, glucose, LFTs, clotting, CRP/ESR, CXR, ABG, renal US	☐	☐	☐	☐
	● **Consider** – blood culture, urate, CK, immunology screen	☐	☐	☐	☐
	● **Monitoring** – at least hourly observations, cardiac monitoring, urine output, fluid balance charting, daily weight. Consider CVP monitoring	☐	☐	☐	☐
	● **Treatment** – aim to correct underlying cause and treat complications.	☐	☐	☐	☐
	● In **hypovolaemia** – administer fluid challenge (e.g. 500mL 0.9% NaCl over 30 min and assess response.	☐	☐	☐	☐
	● In **fluid overload** – discuss with senior. Consider diuretics (e.g. IV furosemide 120 mg) and vasodilators (e.g. GTN infusion). Definitive treatment is dialysis.	☐	☐	☐	☐
	● In **hyperkalaemia** – indicated by ECG changes including peaked T-waves, prolonged PR interval, absent P-waves, widening QRS complex. Treat with calcium gluconate + insulin/dextrose + Calcium Resonium® ± salbutamol ± sodium bicarbonate. Dialysis is definitive treatment if refractory	☐	☐	☐	☐
	●	☐	☐	☐	☐

Phase 2 management (2–6 hours)	• Monitor response to treatment	☐	☐	☐	☐
	• Ensure definitive plan for underlying condition is present	☐	☐	☐	☐
	• Tailor IV fluid replacement and regularly assess fluid balance and urine output	☐	☐	☐	☐
	• Consider CVP line if fluid balance difficult to assess	☐	☐	☐	☐
	• If persistent metabolic acidosis, consider bicarbonate	☐	☐	☐	☐
	•	☐	☐	☐	☐
Phase 3 on-going management	• Cause of AKI should be known	☐	☐	☐	☐
	• Ultrasound renal tract – look for kidney size and hydronephrosis in obstruction	☐	☐	☐	☐
	• Consider nephrostomy if obstruction is suspected and consult with urology and radiology teams	☐	☐	☐	☐
	• Consider renal biopsy if intrinsic cause is suspected	☐	☐	☐	☐
	• Consider dietician involvement (e.g. low potassium diet maybe of clinical benefit)	☐	☐	☐	☐
	• Check for sepsis, gastrointestinal bleeds, VTE, pressure sores and malnutrition, and treat aggressively	☐	☐	☐	☐
	• Check for massive diuresis requiring volume replacement following relief of obstructive renal failure				
	•	☐	☐	☐	☐
Other aspects of treatment	• Check for infection and treat aggressively, avoiding nephrotoxic antibiotics (e.g. gentamicin)	☐	☐	☐	☐
	• Avoid nephrotoxins (e.g. NSAIDs, aminoglycosides, IV contrast)	☐	☐	☐	☐
	• Amend drug doses (e.g. digoxin, antibiotics) in patients with impaired renal function. Refer to *BNF*/data sheet	☐	☐	☐	☐
	•	☐	☐	☐	☐
Complications	• Death from severe causative illness (e.g. massive haemorrhage)	☐	☐	☐	☐
	• Cardiac dysrhythmia – fatal in refractory hyperkalaemia	☐	☐	☐	☐
	• Pulmonary oedema – in refractory fluid overload	☐	☐	☐	☐
	• Severe metabolic acidosis	☐	☐	☐	☐
	• Severe uraemic complications (e.g. pericarditis, encephalopathy)	☐	☐	☐	☐
	•	☐	☐	☐	☐
Patient safety tips	• Check for post-renal causes as they are often easily treatable and recovery of renal function is favourable	☐	☐	☐	☐
	• Regularly reassess patient	☐	☐	☐	☐
	• **Fluid balance –** frequently assess to avoid acute tubular necrosis in uncorrected hypovol-aemia/hypotension: and pulmonary oedema in excess fluid replacement/fluid overload	☐	☐	☐	☐
	• **U&Es –** frequently assess in early phase of the illness as sharp rebound rises in serum potassium can occur as the effect of insulin-dextrose is temporary and Calcium Resonium® takes several hours to start working	☐	☐	☐	☐
	• In patients with suspected intrinsic AKI, early review by the nephrology team with a view to kidney biopsy should occur	☐	☐	☐	☐
	• AKI can develop in hospitalized patients admitted for other reasons. Adequate clinical and laboratory monitoring can help prevent this issue	☐	☐	☐	☐
	•	☐	☐	☐	☐
Clinical note writing and handover	• Examiner checks for accuracy and adequacy of clinical note taking and verbal handover	☐	☐	☐	☐
	•	☐	☐	☐	☐

Self-assessed as at least borderline:	Signature:		Date:	U B S E	U B S E	U B S E	U B S E
Peer-assessed as ready for tutor assessment:	Signature:		Date:	U B S E	U B S E	U B S E	U B S E
Tutor-assessed as satisfactory:	Signature:		Date:	U B S E	U B S E	U B S E	U B S E

Notes

11.9 Deep vein thrombosis and pulmonary embolism

Background

VTE covers a range of presentations including DVT and pulmonary embolism. All patients should be assessed for risk of VTE and bleeding risk on admission to hospital. VTE prophylaxis should be initiated, if deemed appropriate according to current guidelines. A high index of suspicion should be maintained for considering the diagnosis of VTE in hospital inpatients despite use of VTE prophylaxis. This is especially in patients who deteriorate rapidly or indeed are in the throes of a cardiac arrest. It is estimated that 25 000 people in the UK die from preventable hospital-acquired VTE each year.

Definitions

- **Thrombus**: blood clot formed within a blood vessel and remaining attached to its place of origin.
- **Embolus**: an abnormal clot circulating within the blood, detached from its place of origin.
- **DVT**: a thrombus in the deep venous system typically in the calf or thigh.
- **Pulmonary embolism**: blockage of the pulmonary artery by a clot usually originating from a DVT or other foreign matter. Pulmonary embolism can arise *de novo* in the pulmonary arteries, especially in conditions such as right heart failure.

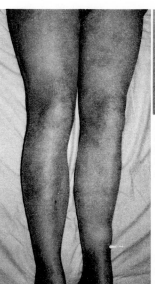

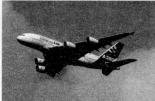

Meticulous attention to VTE assessment and prophylaxis: in all inpatients, also advise in relation to long-haul flights and other high-risk situations.

DVT: common presentation in acute medicine with effective local protocols, can be managed as an outpatient.

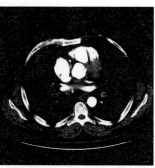

CT Pulmonary Angiography: now the gold standard for diagnosis of PE. More sensitive and specific than VQ scanning.

Figure 11.13 Images in pulmonary embolism and deep vein thrombosis. Middle © Apply Pictures

Risk factors

Pathophysiologically, Virchow's triad helps us understand the clinical risk factors for VTE. This triad is a group of three factors known to affect clot formation: rate of flow of blood, the consistency (viscosity) of blood, and qualities of the vessel wall. Causes of DVT can be classified according to Virchow's triad

- **Changes in vessel wall**: injury, inflammation or infection.

- **Increased blood coagulation or increased viscosity**: dehydration, myeloma, haematological disorders, post surgery, obstetrics patients, oral contraceptive pill, HRT.
- **Decreased blood flow**: immobility, obstetrics patients, pelvic pathology.

Main risk factors for DVT and pulmonary embolism

- **General**: smoking, prolonged travel, dehydration, oral contraceptive pill.
- **Surgery**: major abdominal, pelvic, hip replacement, knee replacement.
- **Obstetrics**: late pregnancy, post-partum, caesarean section.
- **CVD**: myocardial infarction, stroke, peripheral vascular disease (PVD).
- **Lower limb**: fracture, cellulitis, varicose veins.
- **Malignancy**: especially pancreatic, lung, gastric, haematological.
- **Reduced mobility**: prolonged bed rest, hospitalization.
- **Previous DVT or pulmonary embolism**: especially if thrombophilia such as factor V Leiden deficiency, protein S or C deficiency, antithrombin deficiency, antiphospholipid syndrome.
- **Not receiving VTE prophylaxis in hospitals**: frequently omitted still.

Diagnosis

Suspect DVT in patient presenting with:

- Localized limb swelling, warmth and tenderness
- Pyrexia or tachycardia
- May be asymptomatic.
- Well's score 1 or 2 (moderate probability), ≥3 (high probability) (Table 11.6).

Table 11.6 Well's score: Prediction of pre-test probability of deep vein thrombosis (DVT)	
Active cancer	+1
Paralysis, paresis or recent plaster immobilization of lower extremities	+1
Recently bedridden for more than 3 days or major surgery within 4 weeks	+1
Localized tenderness along the distribution of deep venous system	+1
Entire leg swollen	+1
Calf swelling by more than 3 cm when compared to asymptomatic leg	+1
Pitting oedema greater in symptomatic leg	+1
Collateral superficial veins (non-varicose)	+1
Alternative diagnosis as likely or greater than DVT	−2

Suspect pulmonary embolism in patient presenting with:

- Acute breathlessness
- Chest pain especially pleuritic chest pain or haemoptysis
- Acute collapse, especially cardiac arrest with PEA.

Details on management are given below. In the diagnosis of both DVT and pulmonary embolism, the D-dimer level should be determined in most cases. D-dimer is a specific component of the fibrin degradation products that are formed when a thrombosis is reacted on by plasmin and dissolved. A low D-dimer result should suggest alternative diagnoses such as ruptured Baker's cyst. The D-dimer test is not highly specific and can be raised in infection such as cellulitis, post surgery, and malignancy.

399

11.9
Deep vein
thrombosis
and pulmonary
embolism

Management

DVT: phase 1 initial management (first hour)

- **Clinical history**: recent immobilization, thromboprophylaxis (? discontinued), surgery in last 3 months, smoking, oral contraceptive pill use, hormone replacement therapy (HRT), malignancy, recent long haul flight, previous thrombotic episode, family history of thrombosis or miscarriage (lupus anti-coagulant syndrome). Leg swelling as above.

- **Clinical examination**: weight (needed for prescribing LMWH), limb measurement as per Well's score, calf warmth/tenderness/swelling (Pratt's sign), cardiorespiratory examination, MEWS, in particular oxygen saturation. Avoid electing Homan's sign (this is quick flexion of the foot at the ankle joint to elicit calf tenderness, this may result in dislodging a DVT, leading to pulmonary embolism).

- **Investigations**: FBC, U&E, LFTs, clotting, CRP, D-dimer, ultrasound leg veins. In the acute event a thrombophilia screen is of little or no value as factors will be low due to the clot.

- **Treatment**: LMWH: e.g. enoxaparin 1.5 mg/kg subcutaneously once daily. In pregnancy some LMWH are given twice daily. Use local DVT pathway if available and refer to the anti-coagulation service. Adjust dose in renal failure.

DVT: phase 2 management (2–6 hours)

- **Start warfarin**: if DVT confirmed by ultrasound legs.
- **If ultrasound normal**: consider performing a repeat ultrasound legs in 1 week, if strong suspicion of DVT. Continue therapeutic LMWH in the meantime.
- **Target INR**: usually 2.5, 3 if recurrent DVT on treatment at lower INR.
- **Duration of anticoagulation**: 12 weeks if reversible cause, 6 months if no cause identified. Warfarin may be used lifelong for causes such as thrombophilia or in recurrent DVTs.

Pulmonary embolism: phase 1 initial management (first hour)

- **General considerations**: presentation will depend on size, distribution and quantity of emboli. Massive pulmonary embolism is a medical emergency. Suspect in patients with sudden collapse particularly if 1–2 weeks post surgery. If clinical features suggest pulmonary embolism, the risk is particularly high if there is absence of another reasonable explanation and a major risk factor is present. If there is high suspicion of pulmonary embolism then treatment is started without waiting for a definitive diagnosis of pulmonary embolism.

- **Clinical history**: exactly the same risk factors as for DVT. Symptoms: acute dyspnoea, haemoptysis, pleuritic chest pain, haemoptysis.

- **Clinical examination**: MEWS, in particular oxygen saturation. Cardiorespiratory examination: cyanosis, right ventricular heave, raised JVP, gallop rhythm, atrial fibrillation, loud pulmonary second heart sound, pleural rub, pleural effusion, haemoptysis. ? evidence of DVT.

- **Investigations**: FBC, U&E, LFTs, clotting, CRP, D-dimer.
  - ○ **ECG**: tachycardia and right BBB (RBBB) are the commonest features but the well described right ventricular hypertrophy and right axis deviation may also be used. $S_I Q_{III} T_{III}$ is infrequently seen.
  - ○ **ABG**: Often low PaO_2, low $PaCO_2$, pH high. If normal, consider repeating after short walk.
  - ○ **CXR**: may be normal. May see decreased vascular markings, wedge shaped infarction, small pleural effusion.
  - ○ **CT pulmonary angiogram**: Very sensitive and specific for pulmonary embolism.
  - ○ **Other investigations in special circumstances**: pulmonary angiography, VQ scan, venograms, ECHO.

401

11.9
**Deep vein
thrombosis
and pulmonary
embolism**

- **Treatment**:
  - ○ Oxygen 100%, in very severe pain morphine 5–10 mg IV with antiemetic. Aim oxygen saturations 95–100%.
  - ○ Maintain systolic BP >100 mmHg with IV fluids.
  - ○ LMWH: e.g. enoxaparin 1.5 mg/kg subcutaneously once daily. In pregnancy some LMWH are given twice daily. Use local pulmonary embolism pathway if available and refer to the anti-coagulation service for warfarin treatment once diagnosis confirmed.
  - ○ Unfractionated heparin (UFH) should only be considered as a first dose bolus in massive PE or where rapid reversal of effect may be needed.
  - ○ If haemodynamically unstable or peri-arrest state or arrhythmia: consider thrombolysis with IV alteplase (rt-PA) 10 mg over 1–2 minutes then followed by 90 mg over 2 hours.
  - ○ Rarely: embolectomy and even thoracotomy.

Pulmonary embolism: phase 2 ongoing management (2–6 hours)

- **Confirm diagnosis**.
- **Warfarin**: target INR: 2.5–3.0. INR aim will be 3.5 if recurrent pulmonary embolism.
- Duration of anticoagulation: 12 weeks if reversible cause. 6 months if no cause identified. Lifelong for causes such as thrombophilia or recurrent DVTs/PEs.
- **Investigate for underlying cause**.
- **Consider venal caval filter**: if anticoagulation contraindicated or failed or leads to serious complications.

Patient safety tips

- ✔ **Meticulous attention to VTE assessment and prophylaxis**: mobilize early after surgery and consider antithrombotic stockings according to local protocols. The oral contraceptive pill or hormone replacement therapy should be stopped 4 weeks prior to planned surgery.
- ✔ **Consider preventative measures for long haul flights**: leg exercises, increased water intake, avoidance of excess alcohol and caffeine (cause dehydration), compression stockings may decrease risk.
- ✔ **Warfarin treatment is potentially hazardous**: strict attention to warfarin follow-up and monitoring of INR. Be aware that treatments such as antibiotics will change the INR – closer monitoring is required in these situations. Take care when prescribing warfarin in patients with the following: malignancy, thrombophilia, liver disease, renal failure.
- ✔ **Consider the risk/benefit of warfarin**: especially in the elderly due to high risk of falls.
- ✔ **Ensure patient education in relation to warfarin therapy and monitoring for side effects particularly bleeding**: on discharge ensure appropriate patient education about warfarin and length of warfarin therapy required. Refer patient to outpatient anti-coagulation service.

Figure 11.14 gives the VTE NICE 2010 one-page guideline for all hospital patients.

VTE Prophylaxis

Medical patients: Risk factors
- If mobility significantly reduced for ≥ 3 days or
- If expected to have ongoing reduced mobility relative to normal state plus any VTE risk factor.

Surgical patients and patients with trauma: Risk factors
- If total anaesthetic + surgical time > 90 minutes or
- If surgery involves pelvis or lower limb and total anaesthetic + surgical time > 60 mins or
- If acute surgical admission with inflammatory or intra-abdominal condition or
- If any VTE risk factor present.

VTE risk factors in general
- Active cancer or cancer treatment.
- Age > 60 years.
- Critical care admission.
- Dehydration.
- Known thrombophilias.
- Obesity (BMI > 30 kg/m2).
- Use of HRT.
- Use of oestrogen-containing contraceptive therapy
- One or more significant medical co-morbidities (for example: heart disease; metabolic, endocrine or respiratory pathologies; acute infectious diseases; inflammatory conditions).
- Personal history or first-degree relative with a history of VTE.
- Varicose veins with phlebitis.

Patients who are at risk of bleeding:
DO NOT ANTI-COAGULATE THESE PATIENTS. See full guidelines !

All patients who have **any** of the following.
- Active bleeding.
- Acquired bleeding disorders (such as acute liver failure).
- Concurrent use of anticoagulants that increase the risk of bleeding (eg warfarin with INR > 2).
- Lumbar puncture/epidural/spinal anaesthesia within the previous 4 hours or expected within the next 12 hours.
- Acute stroke.
- Thrombocytopenia (platelets < 75 x 109/l).
- Uncontrolled systolic hypertension (≥ 230/120 mmHg).
- Untreated inherited bleeding disorders (eg haemophilia or von Willebrand's disease).

How to treat

1 Encourage patients to mobilise as soon as possible.
2 Offer pharmacological VTE prophylaxis to general medical patients assessed to be at increased risk of VTE. Choose any one of:
   - fondaparinux sodium (factor Xa inhibitor)
   - low molecular weight heparin (LMWH)
   - unfractionated heparin (UFH) (for patients with renal failure)
Assess VTE risk and assess bleeding risk
3 Balance risks of VTE and bleeding.
4 Offer VTE prophylaxis if appropriate.
5 Do not offer pharmacological VTE prophylaxis if patient has any risk factor for bleeding and risk of bleeding outweighs risk of VTE.
6 Re-assess risks of VTE and bleeding within 24 hours of admission and whenever clinical situation changes.

- Start pharmacological VTE prophylaxis as soon as possible after risk assessment has been completed. Continue until the patient is no longer at increased risk of VTE.

Figure 11.14 VTE NICE 2010 one page guideline for hospital patients.

Venous thromboembolism

Mrs Henrietta Noble (32 Holmes Road, Carlton, CL2 9SV; date of birth 22 July 1936, hospital number GE13954627, Bob Jakin Ward) is allergic to penicillin. She weighs 52 kg.

She is admitted due to swelling of left leg with shortness of breath. She is known to have hypertension and osteoporosis. Four weeks ago she had surgery following a fractured neck of femur.

This assessment will be based around a discussion on the management of VTE with reference to above scenario.

		Self	Peer	Peer /tutor	Tutor
Background	Range of presentations: DVT and pulmonary embolism. VTE prophylaxis should be initiated if appropriate. Maintain high index of suspicion for hospital inpatients	☐	☐	☐	☐
	●	☐	☐	☐	☐
Diagnosis	Consider in any hospital inpatient. Especially if any risk factors present: Surgery: major abdominal/pelvic/THR/TKR	☐	☐	☐	☐
	Obstetrics: late pregnancy/post-partum/caesarean section, recent myocardial infarction/ stroke, lower limb fracture, varicose veins, malignancy, reduced mobility/prolonged bed rest, previous pulmonary embolism, personal/family history of DVT	☐	☐	☐	☐
	DVT:				
	● Localized limb swelling, warmth and tenderness	☐	☐	☐	☐
	● Pyrexia or tachycardia	☐	☐	☐	☐
	● May be asymptomatic	☐	☐	☐	☐
	Pulmonary embolism:				
	● Acute breathlessness.	☐	☐	☐	☐
	● Pleuritic chest pain or haemoptysis	☐	☐	☐	☐
	● Acute collapse	☐	☐	☐	☐
Causes of VTE	Virchow's triad:				
	● Changes in vessel wall: injury, inflammation, or infection	☐	☐	☐	☐
	● Increased blood coagulability: dehydration, myeloma, haematological disorders, post surgery, obstetrics patients, oral contraceptive pill, HRT	☐	☐	☐	☐
	● Decreased blood flow: immobility	☐	☐	☐	☐
	●	☐	☐	☐	☐
Phase 1 initial management (first hour)	DVT				
	● History: Recent hospital stay, thromboprophylaxis, surgery in last 6 months, smoker, contraceptive pill, HRT, malignancy, recent long haul flight, previous thrombotic episode, family history of thrombosis/miscarriage	☐	☐	☐	☐
	● Examination: weight: needed for prescribing enoxaparin, limb measurement as per Well's score, calf warmth/tenderness/swelling, cardiorespiratory examination, observations, in particular saturations, avoid electing Homan's sign.	☐	☐	☐	☐
	● Investigations: bloods: FBC/U&E/LFTs/clotting/CRP/D-dimers, ultrasound.	☐	☐	☐	☐
	● Consider: thrombophilia screen if no predisposing factors, family history of DVT or recurrent DVT	☐	☐	☐	☐
	Treatment: consult and fill in DVT pathway if available, LMWH: 1.5 mg/kg subcutaneously: give stat dose and then once daily, refer to anticoagulation nurse				
	Pulmonary embolism				
	● History: consider pulmonary embolism risk factors, acute dyspnoea, haemoptysis, pleuritic chest pain, haemoptysis.	☐	☐	☐	☐
	● Examination: observations: hypotension/tachycardia/pyrexia/tachypnoea, cardiovascular system: cyanosis/right ventricular heave/raised JVP/gallop rhythm/atrial fibrillation/loud P2; respiratory system: pleural rub/pleural effusion, review for signs of cause, e.g. DVT/recent surgical scar	☐	☐	☐	☐
	● Investigations: bloods: FBC/U&Es/LFTs/CRP/clotting, ECG: sinus tachycardia/RBBB/atrial fibrillation/S1 Q3 T3, ABGs: may be normal, try after exertion. Low PaO_2, low $PaCO_2$, pH high CXR: may be normal. May see decreased vascular markings, wedge shaped infarction, small pleural effusion, CTPA	☐	☐	☐	☐
	● Consider: V/Q scan, pulmonary angiography, bilateral venograms, ECHO, D-dimer test: may help exclude pulmonary embolism	☐	☐	☐	☐

		☐	☐	☐	☐
	Massive pulmonary embolism management:				
	• Oxygen 100%	☐	☐	☐	☐
	• Morphine 10 mg IV with antiemetic	☐	☐	☐	☐
	• Call for senior help	☐	☐	☐	☐
	• If haemodynamically unstable/peri-arrest: IV alteplase (rt-PA) 10 mg over 1–2 minutes then followed by 90 mg over 2 hours	☐	☐	☐	☐
	• If not alteplase then thoracotomy + embolectomy	☐	☐	☐	☐
	• Maintain BP >90 mmHg	☐	☐	☐	☐
	Non-massive pulmonary embolism management:				
	• O_2: aim for saturations 95–97%	☐	☐	☐	☐
	• LMWH: use dose appropriate to the specific agent. This will usually be calculated according to the patient's weight and renal function	☐	☐	☐	☐
	• Start warfarin 10 mg once daily	☐	☐	☐	☐
	DVT				
	• Start warfarin if DVT confirmed by ultrasound.	☐	☐	☐	☐
	• If ultrasound –ve consider performing a repeat ultrasound at 1 week if strong suspicion of DVT	☐	☐	☐	☐
	Pulmonary embolism				
	• Confirm diagnosis.	☐	☐	☐	☐
	• Target INR: 2–3. 3.5 if recurrent	☐	☐	☐	☐
	• Refer to anticoagulation service	☐	☐	☐	☐
	• Investigate for underlying cause	☐	☐	☐	☐
	• Consider venal caval filter if anticoagulation contraindicated/failed/leads to complications	☐	☐	☐	☐
	•	☐	☐	☐	☐
Phase 2 management (2–6 hours)	**DVT**				
	• Duration of anticoagulation: 6 weeks if reversible cause/6 months if no cause identified/ lifelong for causes such as thrombophilia	☐	☐	☐	☐
	• Target INR 2–3	☐	☐	☐	☐
	Pulmonary embolism				
	• Duration of anticoagulation: 6 weeks if reversible cause/6 months if no cause identified/ lifelong for causes such as thrombophilia	☐	☐	☐	☐
	•	☐	☐	☐	☐
Phase 3 ongoing management	**VTE NICE 2010 one page guideline for all hospital patients:**				
	• Assess VTE risk and assess bleeding risk	☐	☐	☐	☐
	• Balance risks of VTE and bleeding	☐	☐	☐	☐
	• Offer VTE prophylaxis if appropriate	☐	☐	☐	☐
	• Do not offer pharmacological VTE prophylaxis if patient has any risk factor for bleeding and risk of bleeding outweighs risk of VTE	☐	☐	☐	☐
	• Re-assess risks of VTE and bleeding within 24 hours of admission and whenever clinical situation changes	☐	☐	☐	☐
	•	☐	☐	☐	☐
Other aspects of treatment	• Mobilize early after surgery	☐	☐	☐	☐
	• VTE risk assessment and prophylaxis for all patients	☐	☐	☐	☐
	• Stop HRT and contraceptive pill 4 weeks pre-operatively	☐	☐	☐	☐
	• DVT and long-haul flights: preventative measures include leg exercises, increased water intake, avoidance of alcohol and caffeine. Compression stockings may decrease risk	☐	☐	☐	☐
	• Take care when prescribing warfarin in patients with the following: malignancy, thrombophilia, liver disease, renal failure	☐	☐	☐	☐
	• Consider the risk/benefit of warfarin in the elderly due to high risk of falls	☐	☐	☐	☐
	• On discharge ensure appropriate patient education about warfarin and length of warfarin therapy required	☐	☐	☐	☐
	• Refer patient to anticoagulation service	☐	☐	☐	☐
	•	☐	☐	☐	☐
What complications can arise?	•	☐	☐	☐	☐
Patient safety tips		☐	☐	☐	☐
Self-assessed as at least borderline:	Signature:	Date:	U B / S E	U B / S E	U B / S E
Peer-assessed as ready for tutor assessment:	Signature:	Date:	U B / S E	U B / S E	U B / S E
Tutor-assessed as satisfactory:	Signature:	Date:	U B / S E	U B / S E	U B / S E
Notes					

11.10 Pneumonia

Background

Pneumonia is defined as an inflammation of the lung parenchyma. It is characterized by the presence of exudate, inflammatory cells and fibrin in the alveolar air spaces with consolidation of the affected part usually caused by infection with bacteria, viruses, fungi, and parasites. It can also result from physical and chemical injury to the lung. It is a common illness with significant morbidity and mortality in all age groups especially in elderly patients who are terminally ill and with chronic diseases. Its incidence is about 1–3/1000 population. Elderly patients and those with co-morbidities such as cardiac failure, COPD, asthma, bronchiectasis, diabetes, alcohol abuse, and human immunodeficiency virus (HIV) infection are more prone to infection with bacteria and other pathogens. The British Thoracic Society guidelines (2009) have been used extensively to prepare this section.

Diagnosis

Diagnosis is based on a complex of signs and symptoms both from the respiratory tract and general health of patient. They include:

- **Systemic features**: at least one (fever >38 °C, rigors, malaise, sweating, aches and pains, confusion, diarrhoea).
- **Tachypnoea**: usually defined as a respiratory rate greater than 30/min.
- **Cough**: with purulent sputum/haemoptysis. Other features include pleuritic pain.
- **New focal chest signs on examination**: such as bronchial breathing, increased vocal fremitus/resonance, pleuritic rub, pleural effusion.
- **New radiographic shadowing**: for which there is no other explanation such as pulmonary oedema or infarction.

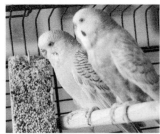 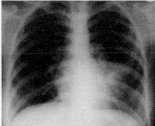 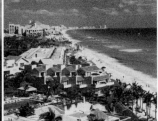

Budgerigars may harbour *Chlamydia psittaci*: detailed history critical to correct diagnosis and treatment.

Lobar pneumonia: compare with previous chest X-ray where possible. Features of pre-existing chest disease such as COPD or bronchiectasis may be evident.

Legionella pneumonia can be acquired from air-conditioning and water tanks especially from hotels. Immunocompromised patients are particularly at risk.

Figure 11.15 Images in chest infection. Left © Lee Ingram/iStockphoto; right © Corbis/Digital Stock.

In UK, the CURB-65 criteria are used to assess the severity of community-acquired pneumonia (CAP). This is useful to recognize patients at high risk of complications and death.

- **C**onfusion with Abbreviated Mental Test Score ≤8.
- **U**rea >7 mmol/L.
- **R**espiratory rate of ≥30/minute.
- **B**lood pressure of systolic <90 and/or diastolic ≤60 mmHg.
- **A**ge ≥65 years of age.

CURB-65 score should be interpreted in conjunction with clinical judgement when deciding to treat at home, hospital ward, or ICU. Mortality rates increase with increasing score. Patients with score of 0–1 are at low risk of death (<3%) and can be treated at home. Patients with score 2 are at moderate risk (about 9% mortality) and should be considered for short-stay inpatient treatment at hospital. Those who are scoring 3 and above are at high risk of death (15–40%), hence require close monitoring and should be assessed with specific consideration to be treated in critical care unit.

Other markers of severe pneumonia are:

- Involvement of one or more lobes on chest X-ray
- PaO_2 <8 kPa
- Low albumin (<35 g/L)
- WCC (<4 × 10^9/L or >20 × 10^9/L)
- Positive blood cultures
- New-onset atrial fibrillation.

Classification and causes of pneumonia

This is based on the site of the pneumonia or its aetiology. Pneumonia confined to a single lobe is called 'lobar pneumonia', and when it is diffuse affecting the lobules in association with bronchi and bronchioles is called 'bronchopneumonia'. Aetiologically pneumonia can be classified as given below.

Community-acquired pneumonia (CAP)

- *Streptococcus pneumoniae* is the most common cause of CAP worldwide. It is especially the organism most commonly implicated post splenectomy, in immunocompromised patients and those with pre-existing heart and lung diseases. It usually follows viral infection and patients may develop herpes labialis. In the UK, penicillin resistance is still less than 5%.
- *Staphylococcus aureus* causes pneumonia in the young, elderly, and IV drug abusers. It may complicate influenzal viral illness. It is also a common pathogen in hospital-acquired pneumonia (HAP).
- *Mycoplasma pneumoniae* is relatively common among residents of boarding institutions and recently has caused epidemics every 3–4 years.
- *Legionella pneumophila* causes legionnaire's disease among healthy individuals. It spreads through water tanks and air conditioning systems. Also seen in immunocompromised patients.
- *Haemophilus influenzae* causes pneumonia mainly in patients with chronic obstructive lung disease and is a frequent cause of exacerbations.
- *Chlamydia psittaci* causes psittacosis in individuals who are exposed to infected birds.
- *Viruses* – commonest is influenza A (H1N1) usually with a bacterial component. Other viruses include CMV, parainfluenza, herpes zoster.

Hospital-acquired pneumonia

The onset of HAP occurs at least 72 hours after admission. Gram-negative bacteria and anaerobes are commonly responsible for many HAPs.

- *Klebsiella pneumoniae* causes pneumonia usually in elderly patients with chronic systemic diseases.
- *Pseudomonas aeruginosa* is seen in patients with bronchiectasis, cystic fibrosis, and in patients with neutropenia following chemotherapy.
- *Moraxella catarrhalis* is seen in patients with COPD exacerbations and sometimes leading to severe pneumonia.
- Meticillin-resistant *Staphylococcus aureus* (MRSA).

Aspiration pneumonia

This is caused by aspiration of gastric contents and exogenous foreign materials into the lungs. It is commonly seen in patients with swallowing difficulties (e.g. post-stroke, Parkinson's disease, oesophageal disease, motor neurone disease) and in patients with impaired conscious levels (post-seizure, anaesthesia, alcohol binge).

- Common pathogens are anaerobes and Gram-negative bacteria.
- Any substance toxic to the lower respiratory tract (non-bacterial) causing chemical pneumonitis.

Pneumonia due to opportunistic infections

- *Pneumocystis jiroveci* is the most common infection in acquired immune deficiency syndrome (AIDS) and immunosuppressed patients.
- Others include *Mycobacterium avium-intracellulare*, *Mycobacterium tuberculosis*, *Cryptococcus* and CMV.

Management

Phase 1 initial management (first hour)

- **Clinical history**: detailed history focusing on symptoms, and their progression. This would include risk factors such as smoking, past history, co-morbidities, pets, recent travel, recent antibiotics.
- **Clinical examination**: thorough general and systemic examination with a focus on airway, breathing, and circulation. Auscultation is particularly important to allow monitoring of the pneumonia.
- **Assess severity**: clinically and CURB-65.
- **IV access and investigations**:
  - ○ **Venous bloods**: FBC, U&Es, LFTs, consider CRP, blood cultures (preferably prior to antibiotics)
  - ○ **ABGs**: correct hypoxia, maintain oxygen saturations ≥94%, correct acidosis
  - ○ **Urgent CXR**: confirm diagnosis
  - ○ **Sputum** for inspection, culture and sensitivities, Gram staining, acid-fast bacillus. *Legionella* urine antigen and acute sample for serology (*Mycoplasma pneumoniae*, *Coxiella burnetii*, *Chlamydia psittaci*, infection, etc.) in all patients with severe pneumonia
  - ○ **ECG**: ? atrial fibrillation, ? tachycardia, rule out ACS.
- **Early treatment**:
  - ○ Supplementary oxygen usually indicated
  - ○ **Fluid resuscitation**: if signs of dehydration or shock. Beware of cardiac failure
  - ○ **Start empirical antibiotics**: as indicated in Table 11.7
  - ○ **Continuous cardiac monitoring/vital signs**: MEWS (including temperature, respiratory rate, pulse, BP, GCS, oxygen saturation and inspired oxygen concentration) should be recorded at least twice a day and more frequently in moderate to severe pneumonia
  - ○ **Nebulized bronchodilators** if underlying COPD/asthma. Consider steroids.
  - ○ **VTE thromboprophylaxis**: in all hospitalized patients unless there are contraindications.

Table 11.7 Initial empirical treatment regimens for community-acquired pneumonia in adults (use local guidelines where possible)

Pneumonia severity: clinical judgement and CURB-65	Treatment site	Preferred treatment	Alternative treatment
Low severity *CURB-65: 0–1 score*	Home	Amoxicillin 500 mg three times daily orally	Doxycycline 200 mg loading dose and then 100 mg daily or clarithromycin 500 mg twice daily orally
Low severity *CURB-65: 0–1 score* Admission indicated for: unstable co-morbid illnesses	Home or hospital	Amoxicillin 500 mg three times daily Orally or IV if oral route not possible	Doxycycline 200 mg loading dose and then 100 mg daily or clarithromycin 500 mg twice daily orally
Moderate severity *CURB-65: 2 score*	hospital	Amoxicillin 0.5 gm–1 g three times daily orally plus clarithromycin 500 mg twice daily orally Benzylpenicillin 1.2 g four times daily IV or amoxicillin 500 mg three times daily IV plus clarithromycin 500 mg twice daily IV	Doxycycline 200 mg loading dose and then 100 mg daily or levofloxacin 500 mg once daily orally or Moxifloxacin 400 mg once daily orally
High severity *CURB-65: 3–5 score*	Hospital: consider critical care review	Co-amoxiclav 1.2 g three times daily IV plus clarithromycin 500 mg twice daily IV ? *Legionella* suspected (consider adding levofloxacin)	1: Benzylpenicillin 1.2 g four times daily IV plus either levofloxacin 500 mg twice daily IV or ciprofloxacin 400 mg twice daily IV *or* 2: cefuroxime 1.5 g three times daily IV or cefotaxime 1 g three times daily IV or ceftriaxone 2 g once daily IV plus clarithromycin 500 mg twice daily IV

Phase 2 management (2–6 hours)

- **Review bloods**: correct U&Es if deranged, consider severe on-going sepsis treatment.

- **Continue monitoring vital signs for early recognition of deterioration**: low BP, poor urine output, worsening confusion, hypoxia, tachypnoea. Consider ICU/HDU if worsening or progressive exhaustion.

- **Repeat ABGs**: if suspected hypercapnia or unable to correct hypoxia. Assess whether needs invasive/non-invasive ventilatory support.

- **Repeat blood cultures**: if spiking temperatures, total two sets are ideal.

- **Chest physiotherapy**: for sputum clearance in bronchiectasis patients and other patients who have difficulty clearing bronchial secretions.

- **Review patient's regular medications**: with a view of stopping them or to withhold in the acute phase (especially diuretics or NSAIDs in acute renal failure, statins if deranged LFTs), antihypertensive agents.

- **Watch for fluid overload**: especially in patients with underlying heart problems

- **Pain relief**. Use analgesics for pleuritic chest pain.

- **Consider thoracocentesis**: if present for pleural fluid, culture, pneumococcal antigen, pH, protein, LDH.

- **Consult microbiologist**: regarding antibiotic regimen if a pneumonia other than CAP is suspected.

Phase 3 ongoing management

- **Continue monitoring vital signs**: at regular intervals if patient improving. Otherwise consider ICU/HDU care.
- **Repeat ABG**: if previous hypercapnia or acidosis.
- **Continue fluids as indicated**.
- **IV antibiotics should be reviewed daily**: with a view of changing them to oral regimen as soon as there is clinical improvement with normal temperature for 24 hours.
- **Nil by mouth**: if aspiration is suspected.
- **Isolate patient**: if neutropenic or immunocompromised.
- **Repeat inflammatory markers, renal functions, and LFTs**: to check response to treatment.

Other aspects of treatment

- Check results of blood cultures/sensitivities with a view of changing to appropriate antibiotics.
- Indication for antibiotics and the duration should be clearly documented in the medical notes.
- Urinary catheter to ensure correct fluid balance in high-risk patients and with other co-morbidities.
- Patients with diabetes may need insulin therapy in the acute phase to maintain glucose level around 4–8 mmol/L.
- Repeat CXR and CRP after 3 days of treatment in patients who are not improving satisfactorily and there should be a review of presenting history, examination, prescription charts, and all results by a experienced clinician.
- Nutritional support should be provided to all patients with prolonged illness.
- Airway clearance techniques should be considered for patients who are finding it difficult to expectorate.
- Advise on lifestyle measures to reduce risk of pneumonia especially smoking cessation and optimizing physical activity.

Complications

Pneumonia is a major cause of mortality generally and hence the need for high standards of care. Specific complications include: failure of treatment (change in treatment plan and antibiotics needed), lung abscess, empyema, disseminated intravascular coagulation, renal failure, hepatic failure. Many existing co-morbidities, such as cardiac failure, can also worsen.

Patient safety tips

- ✔ **Antibiotic regimen**: Change to appropriate oral antibiotics after IV regimen. Healthcare-associated infections, especially MRSA and *Clostridium difficile*, are far less likely with careful use of antibiotics. Specific antibiotics against the microorganism thought culpable should be used in preference to broad-spectrum antibiotics. Co-amoxiclav, levofloxacin, moxifloxacin, and clindamycin in particular should be reviewed and discontinued as soon as the clinical condition and other antibiotic choice allow.
- ✔ **Review in the clinic with repeat chest X-ray in 6 weeks**: to check resolution and exclude complications such as abscess formation. Persisting pneumonia raises the suspicion of an underlying bronchial carcinoma.
- ✔ **Patients aged >65 years should receive pneumococcal vaccine**.
- ✔ **Smoke cessation advice**: should be offered to all patients with CAP who need this.
- ✔ **Community treatment**: Patients should be reviewed after 48 hours, or earlier if clinically indicated. Patients with suspected CAP should be advised to rest, drink plenty of fluids and not to smoke. Early treatment prior to expected hospital admission for more serious cases could be benzylpenicillin 1.2 g IV or amoxicillin 1 g orally.

Pneumonia

Anna Karenski, a 69-year-old woman, has been brought in by ambulance having been treated at home for a chest infection. She is known to have COPD and currently smokes 20 cigarettes a day. Her sputum has been green with tinges of blood. Her GP gave her amoxicillin 500 mg three times daily 4 days ago but there has been no improvement. She is alert and orientated but anxious and has pleuritic pain. Her key results are shown.

pH	PaO$_2$	PaCO$_2$	HCO$_3^-$	
7.45–7.35	10.5–13.5 kPa	4.7–6.0 kPa	22–28 mmol/L	• Temperature 38.1 °C
				• Heart rate 124/min
pH	PaO$_2$	PaCO$_2$	HCO$_3^-$	• Respiratory. rate 26
7.31	9.2	7.8	24.4	• WCC 18.6 × 10^9/L, urea 11.6 mmol/L
				• Chest X-ray: as per the central image in Figure 11.11
				• ECG: sinus tachycardia

This assessment will be based around a discussion on the management of pneumonia with reference to above scenario.

		Self	Peer	Peer/tutor	Tutor
How is the diagnosis of pneumonia made?	• Systemic features, tachypnoea, cough, new focal chest sign, CXR changes •	☐ ☐	☐ ☐	☐ ☐	☐ ☐
What are the criteria for severity of pneumonia using CURB-65?	• **C**onfusion, **U**rea >7 mmol/L, **R**espiratory rate of ≥30/minute, **B**P systolic <90 or diastolic ≤60, Age ≥**65** •	☐ ☐	☐ ☐	☐ ☐	☐ ☐
What are the other markers of severity that can be used?	• Involvement lobe (s) on CXR, PaO$_2$ <8 kPa, low albumin (<35 g/L), WCC (<4 × 10^9/L or >20 × 10^9/L), Positive blood cultures, new-onset atrial fibrillation •	☐ ☐	☐ ☐	☐ ☐	☐ ☐
How severely affected is the patient in the vignette above?	•	☐	☐	☐	☐
Classification and causes of pneumonia	• This is based on the site of the pneumonia or its aetiology. Pneumonia confined to a single lobe is called 'lobar pneumonia' and when it is diffuse affecting the lobules in association with bronchi and bronchioles is called 'bronchopneumonia' Pneumonia can be classified in two ways, by site and by aetiology •	☐ ☐	☐ ☐	☐ ☐	☐ ☐
What are the main micro-pathogens implicated in CAP?	• S. pneumonia, S. aureus, M. pneumonia, L. pneumophila, H. influenza, C. psittaci, viruses •	☐ ☐	☐ ☐	☐ ☐	☐ ☐
What are the main pathogens implicated in HAP?	• Anaerobes, Gram-negatives such as K. pneumoniae, P. aeruginosa, M. catarrhalis, MRSA. •	☐ ☐	☐ ☐	☐ ☐	☐ ☐
What are the main aspects of phase 1 initial management (first hour)?	• **Clinical history and examination** • **Assess severity**: clinically and CURB-65. • **IV access and Investigations**: venous bloods, ABG, CXR, sputum, ECG • **Early treatment**: resuscitation, supplementary oxygen, nebulized bronchodilators if wheezy, start empirical antibiotics, cardiac monitoring/vital signs, VTE thromboprophylaxis •	☐ ☐ ☐ ☐ ☐	☐ ☐ ☐ ☐ ☐	☐ ☐ ☐ ☐ ☐	☐ ☐ ☐ ☐ ☐
Which antibiotic could be used in the above patient?	• Discusses choice of antibiotics in accordance with local guidelines •	☐ ☐	☐ ☐	☐ ☐	☐ ☐
What are the main aspects of phase 2 management (2nd–6th hour)?	• **Review and repeat bloods** and **continued monitoring of vital signs** for early recognition of deterioration. • **Chest physiotherapy:** for sputum clearance in bronchiectasis, poor expectoration • **Review patient's regular medications**: e.g. diuretics, NSAID, statins, antihypertensives • **Watch for fluid overload, pain relief** • **Consider pleural aspiration, consult microbiologist** •	☐ ☐ ☐ ☐ ☐ ☐	☐ ☐ ☐ ☐ ☐ ☐	☐ ☐ ☐ ☐ ☐ ☐	☐ ☐ ☐ ☐ ☐ ☐

What are the main aspects of phase 3 ongoing and further management?	• **Continue monitoring vital signs and ? repeat ABG. Consider insulin treatment**	☐	☐	☐	☐
	• **IV antibiotics should be reviewed daily**	☐	☐	☐	☐
	• **Isolate patient**: if neutropenic or immunocompromised	☐	☐	☐	☐
	• **Repeat inflammatory markers, renal functions and LFTs**: to see response to treatment. Chase results.	☐	☐	☐	☐
	• Repeat CXR after 3 days of treatment if not improving satisfactorily	☐	☐	☐	☐
	• Airway clearance techniques: in those finding it difficult to expectorate	☐	☐	☐	☐
	•	☐	☐	☐	☐
What the main complications of pneumonia?	• Failure of treatment, lung abscess, empyema, disseminated intravascular coagulation, renal failure, hepatic failure	☐	☐	☐	☐
	• Non-resolution	☐	☐	☐	☐
	•	☐	☐	☐	☐
What are the key patient safety tips in relation to pneumonia?	• **Antibiotic regimen**: Change to oral antibiotics as soon as possible clinically. High risk of MRSA, *C. difficile*. Review: co-amoxiclav, levofloxacin, moxifloxacin, and clindamycin	☐	☐	☐	☐
	• **Review in the clinic with repeat chest X-ray in 6 weeks**: to check resolution and exclude complications such as abscess formation	☐	☐	☐	☐
	• **Patients aged >65 years should receive pneumococcal vaccine**	☐	☐	☐	☐
	• **Smoke cessation advice**: should be offered to all patients with CAP who need this	☐	☐	☐	☐
	• **Community treatment**: Review after 48 hours. Community treatment prior to admission: benzylpenicillin 1.2 g IV or amoxicillin 1 g orally	☐	☐	☐	☐
	•	☐	☐	☐	☐

Self-assessed as at least borderline:	Signature:	Date:	U B S E	U B S E	U B S E	U B S E
Peer-assessed as ready for tutor assessment:	Signature:	Date:	U B S E	U B S E	U B S E	U B S E
Tutor-assessed as satisfactory:	Signature:	Date:	U B S E	U B S E	U B S E	U B S E

Notes

11.11 Coma

Background

Coma is a common medical emergency which all medical personnel should be able to deal with. This condition has a myriad of causes but a relatively small number of causes account for the majority of cases seen in hospital; the remainder can present a clinical challenge. A good working knowledge of neuroanatomy and neurophysiology is essential for diagnosis. It should be stressed that dealing with immediate complications of coma often takes precedence over the exact diagnosis which can determined later after results of investigations, including further clinical or drug history, is made available. This section gives a broad outline of the management of coma only. It is important to read other related sections and other literature for full and complete guidance.

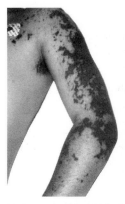

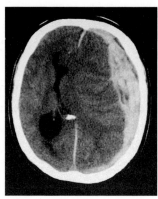

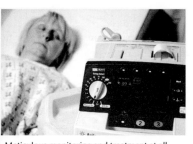

In coma management think of potentially reversible causes and exclude them: drug overdose, meningitis, meningococcal sepsis, encephalitis, hypoglycaemia, metabolic disturbances are commonly missed.

Early referral for urgent CT head is needed to exclude potentially treatable causes such as stroke, cerebral abscess, sub-dural haematoma.

Meticulous monitoring and treatment at all stages in the management of coma: consider organ donation from patients with clearly diagnosed brain stem death and otherwise preserved tissue perfusion and tissues not globally damaged.

Figure 11.16 Images in coma.

Definition

Coma is a severe depression in the level of consciousness characterized by unresponsiveness to external stimuli. The Glasgow Coma Scale (GCS) is an internationally accepted method for grading the level of consciousness. A score of less than 8 is generally accepted to be consistent with coma. A patient is allocated a score out of 15 as shown in Table 11.8.

Causes of coma

Coma with neck stiffness

- Subarachnoid haemorrhage (SAH).
- Meningitis/encephalitis.
- Intraventricular/subarachnoid extension of other intracranial haemorrhage.

Coma without neck stiffness

- *Vascular*
  - ○ Stroke, cerebral venous thrombosis, systemic shock of any cause
  - ○ Hypertensive encephalopathy, cerebral vasculitis (e.g. systemic lupus erythematosus).

Table 11.8 Glasgow Coma Scale

Eye opening	Best verbal response	Best motor response
1 No eye opening	1 No verbal response	1 No movement
2 Opening in response to pain	2 Incomprehensible sounds	2 Extension response to pain: decerebrate posturing
3 Opening in response to voice	3 Inappropriate words	3 Flexion response to pain: decorticate posturing
4 Spontaneous eye opening	4 Confusion or disorientation	4 Withdrawal response to pain
	5 Oriented, normal speech	5 Localizes pain
		6 Obeys commands

The best response from each category is added up: maximum 15, minimum 3, <8 is coma.

- *Metabolic*
  - Hypoglycaemia of any cause, hepatic encephalopathy, severe hypoxia/hypercapnia, diabetic ketoacidosis, hyperosmolar hyperglycaemic non-ketotic state, severe hypothyroidism, severe hyperthyroidism, severe hypoadrenalism
  - Severe metabolic acidosis, uraemic encephalopathy, hypo/hyperthermia
  - Severe electrolyte abnormality, e.g. hypo/hypernatraemia, hypercalcaemia
- *Drug/toxin*
  - Opiates, benzodiazepines, alcohol, barbiturates, neuroleptic malignant syndrome, carbon monoxide poisoning. Many other drugs in overdose, e.g. tricyclics, SSRI.
- *Structural*
  - Subdural haematoma, extradural haematoma, depressed skull fracture, intracranial tumour (primary/secondary), brain abscess, obstructive hydrocephalus of any cause.
- *Other*
  - Psychogenic coma.

Management

Phase 1 management: first hour

Initially a quick history and focused examination should be performed to allow stabilization. A detailed history is always important in clinical medicine, particularly so to define the cause of coma. Inevitably, this will be from carers, family, friends, and any other sources and witnesses.

- *Clinical history*
  - **How long has the patient been unwell?** Coma is a late stage of many of the underlying pathologies. Ascertain the disease progression in the patient. In non-traumatic and non-vascular causes, the patient may show a gradually declining or fluctuating consciousness level. Earlier indications include altered behaviour, disorientation, increased sleep, fever, headache.
  - **Recent trauma should be asked about**.
  - **Past medical and social history and drug history**: in particular does the patient have any risk factors for hypoglycaemia (e.g. diabetes medication), do they take drugs (e.g. heroin, amfetamines), could they have taken an overdose? Consider counting tablets remaining from supply to patient or access to patient. ? Suicide note. Detailed enquiry should be made about alcohol intake and recent foreign travel (? malaria, viral encephalitis). Consider carbon monoxide poisoning from, for example, a faulty heating/boiler system.

- *Clinical examination*
  - ○ **ABCDE assessment**: call for help.
  - ○ **Airway and observations**: patients in coma cannot protect their airway and will experience fatal aspiration or anoxia if untreated. Unless trauma to the spine is suspected, open the airway with head tilt, chin lift. Insert a nasopharyngeal or oropharyngeal airway (unless facial/skull fracture suspected). Place the patient in the recovery position and administer high-flow oxygen. Full set of vital signs including capillary glucose and oxygen saturations should be checked. Attach the patient to a cardiac monitor and continuous pulse oximetry monitoring. Obtain good IV access. The only definitive airway is a cuffed endotracheal tube and an anaesthetist should be called immediately.
  - ○ **Detailed examination**: fever may suggest an infective aetiology or may be due to stimulant drugs. Look for needle tracks, signs of chronic liver or kidney disease. Asterixis may occur in some metabolic comas. Check the breath for ketotic odour. Observe the respiration pattern and look for abnormal hiccoughing and yawning. Check for neck stiffness. Look for a petechial rash which may be present in meningococcaemia. Look for signs of a basal skull fracture (raccoon eyes, CSF rhinorrhoea or otorrhoea, blood behind ear drum). Observe the muscle tone. A detailed neurological examination should be performed including retinal examination and all major cranial nerve reflexes (pupillary, corneal, consider vestibulocochlear and caloric).
- *Investigations*
  - ○ **In all patients**: FBC, U&Es, glucose, LFTs, bone, CRP, INR, ECG, ABGs, urinalysis, chest X-ray. CT/MRI brain (unless obvious, easily reversed metabolic cause).
  - ○ **Consider**: blood culture, T_4, TSH, cortisol, paracetamol and salicylates, ethanol, serum/urine drug screen, lumbar puncture, blood film for malarial parasite, pregnancy test, arterial ammonia level, autoimmune screen, electroencephalogram (EEG).
  - ○ **Monitoring**: nurse in area appropriate to degree of illness. Any patient with persistent deep coma should be nursed in an ICU unless it is felt that admission to such a facility would be medically futile or the patient is not to undergo resuscitation. At least hourly observations, cardiac monitoring, urine output. Accurate fluid balance charting.
- *Treatment*
  - ○ This will vary considerably depending on the cause. Treatment should be coordinated between intensive care physicians, neurosurgeons, neurologists and general physicians.
  - ○ **Initial stabilization and rapid reversal of cause**: if possible (see below).
  - ○ **Optimize physiological parameters**: to prevent secondary brain injury (pO_2, pCO_2, pH, arterial BP, intravascular volume, body temperature, glucose, intracranial pressure, treatment of seizures).
  - ○ **Urgent neuroimaging**: undertake whatever is appropriate (usually CT scan ± contrast). Identify patients who require urgent neurosurgical intervention and transfer to appropriate facility as soon as possible.
  - ○ **If meningitis is suspected**: take blood cultures and administer antibiotics promptly. For suspected herpes simplex encephalitis, aciclovir should be started without delay. It should be stressed that in patients with suspected meningoencephalitis *initial* treatment should *not* be delayed while waiting for CT scanning or lumbar puncture or even blood cultures if difficult. If the patient is first seen in the community setting intramuscular antibiotics should be given straight away.

The following causes are common and easily reversed and should never be forgotten.

- **Hypoglycaemia**: if there is any suspicion, administer IV glucose without delay (with thiamine if alcoholic/malnourished).
- **Opiate overdose**: this is suggested by bradypnoea and small, equal, sluggishly reactive pupils. Naloxone rapidly reverses the coma. Administer slowly if heroin addict as withdrawal crises can occur.

- **Benzodiazepine overdose**: flumazenil can be used (caution if unknown ingestion or mixed overdoses as it can trigger seizures).
- **Hypoxia or hypercapnia**: opening the airway, administering oxygen and appropriate ventilation can reverse this.

Phase 2 management (2–6 hours)

- **General measures**: keep the patient nil by mouth, catheterize the bladder and measure urine output, keep the patient well hydrated. Nasogastric feeding can be initiated later.
- **Review diagnosis**: the cause of coma should be becoming clear by now.
- **Consider lumbar puncture**: provided that there are no contraindications, as occult meningoencephalitis subtle SAH may be detected.
- **Discuss with neurosurgeon**: all head injury patients with depressed level of consciousness should be discussed with a neurosurgeon even if the CT scan does not show any major abnormality.
- **Hepatic coma**: it should be remembered that hepatic coma can be improved by administering lactulose, neomycin, treating precipitants, steroids in some cases. Transplant may need to be considered.
- **Cerebral oedema**: treatment of cerebral oedema may be required. Options include: head elevation, hyperventilation, mannitol, hypertonic saline, steroids (dexamethasone usually), surgical decompression.

Ongoing management

- **Good supportive treatment**: is the key in ongoing management, especially for drug overdoses.
- If the initial work-up proves inconclusive consider rarer conditions such as cerebral vasculitis, exotic infections, etc.
- In patients with irreversible causes of coma where recovery is thought unlikely, e.g. massive intracranial bleeds, appropriate palliation should be initiated.
- Organ donation should be considered in appropriate patients: especially those with brain stem death.

Other aspects of treatment

- **Many intracranial pathologies can cause seizures**: these should be treated aggressively as seizure activity increases secondary brain injury. Appropriate treatment for seizures provoked by structural lesions is benzodiazepines and phenytoin. Steroids may help reduce oedema around tumours/abscesses. Treatment of seizures caused by overdoses is complex and varied, consult Toxbase for details.
- Supportive care is important in patients with ongoing coma.
- Adequate nutrition should be initiated.
- **Prevention of VTE, pressure sores, and aspiration pneumonia is important**.

Patient safety tips

- ✔ **Initial resuscitation irrespective of final diagnosis**: it is important to remember that initial resuscitation takes priority over precise diagnosis.
- ✔ **Common reversible causes should never be missed**.
- ✔ **Prevention of deterioration and death centres on adequate neurological monitoring**: in those who are at risk of deterioration.

Coma

Leo Flower is a 38-year-old man who is admitted having been found collapsed in the street. On admission to the emergency department resuscitation suite, it is clear that he is deteriorating fast as he was able to talk using intelligible words to the ambulance crew when they arrived at the scene of the collapse.

On examination he is opening eyes to pain, there are occasional unintelligible words and there is movement to pain only. His BP is 156/98 mmHg, pulse is 112 regular, temperature is 37.2 °C, respiratory rate is 18. Neurological examination reveals a dilated left pupil that is sluggishly responsive to a bright light with no afferent pupil reflex.

Witnesses later corroborate the story that he was hit on the head by an object that was thrown at him as he left a bar in the city centre.

This assessment will be based around a discussion on the management of coma with reference to above scenario.

		Self	Peer	Peer /tutor	Tutor
Background	• Coma is a common medical emergency with which all medical personnel should be able to deal with. This condition has a myriad of causes but a relatively small number of causes account for the majority of cases seen in hospital. It should be stressed that dealing with immediate complications of coma often takes precedence over the exact diagnosis, which can be made later.	☐	☐	☐	☐
Diagnosis	Coma is a severe depression in the level of consciousness characterized by unresponsiveness to external stimuli:	☐	☐	☐	☐
	• Components of GCS	☐	☐	☐	☐
	• Score <8/15	☐	☐	☐	☐
	• Late stage of many conditions	☐	☐	☐	☐
	• What is this patient's GCS score.	☐	☐	☐	☐
	•	☐	☐	☐	☐
Causes of coma	What are the likely diagnoses in this patient?				
	• With neck stiffness: meningitis, encephalitis, SAH	☐	☐	☐	☐
	• Vascular, e.g. stroke, venous thrombosis, shock, vasculitis, hypertensive encephalopathy	☐	☐	☐	☐
	• Metabolic, e.g. hypoglycaemia, liver/kidney failure, electrolyte imbalance	☐	☐	☐	☐
	• Drug/toxin, e.g. opiate, benzodiazepine, alcohol, carbon monoxide poisoning	☐	☐	☐	☐
	• Structural subdural/extradural haematoma, tumour, abscess, obstructive hydrocephalus	☐	☐	☐	☐
	• Other: status epilepticus, psychogenic coma	☐	☐	☐	☐
	•	☐	☐	☐	☐
Phase 1 initial management (first hour)	• Clinically: history (emphasis on drug history, psychiatric and social history, past medical history, accurate drug history), examination as per ABCDE. Focus on identifying potential causes	☐	☐	☐	☐
	• Initiate management. airway adjuncts, checks blood sugar, IV access	☐	☐	☐	☐
	• May require intubation for airway protection	☐	☐	☐	☐
	• Investigations: FBC, U&Es, glucose, LFTs, bone, CRP, INR, ECG, ABGs, urinalysis, chest X-ray, CT/MRI brain	☐	☐	☐	☐
	• Treat easily reversed causes: hypoglycaemia, opiates, benzodiazepines, hypoxia/hypercarbia	☐	☐	☐	☐
	• Consider blood culture, TFTs, cortisol, paracetamol and salicylate, ethanol, serum/urine drug screen, lumbar puncture, blood film for malarial parasite, pregnancy test, arterial ammonia level, autoimmune screen, EEG	☐	☐	☐	☐
	• More intensive monitoring: ICU/HDU?	☐	☐	☐	☐
	• Start antibiotics if meningitis suspected	☐	☐	☐	☐
	•	☐	☐	☐	☐
Phase 2 management (2–6 hours)	• Keep the patient nil by mouth	☐	☐	☐	☐
	• Catheterize the bladder and measure urine output	☐	☐	☐	☐
	• Keep the patient well hydrated. NG feeding can be initiated later	☐	☐	☐	☐
	• If still uncertain a lumbar puncture should be performed	☐	☐	☐	☐
	• Discussion with neurosurgeon	☐	☐	☐	☐
	• Treatment of cerebral oedema may be required	☐	☐	☐	☐
	•	☐	☐	☐	☐

Phase 3 ongoing management	• Good supportive treatment is the key in ongoing management. Especially for drug overdoses	☐	☐	☐	☐
	• If the initial work-up proves inconclusive consider rarer conditions such as cerebral vasculitis, exotic infections, etc.	☐	☐	☐	☐
	• In patients with irreversible causes of coma where recovery is thought unlikely, e.g. massive intracranial bleeds, appropriate palliation should be initiated	☐	☐	☐	☐
	• In appropriate patients with brain stem death the issue of organ donation should be considered	☐	☐	☐	☐
	•	☐	☐	☐	☐
Other aspects of treatment	• Treatment of seizures	☐	☐	☐	☐
	• Supportive care is important in patients with ongoing coma	☐	☐	☐	☐
	• Adequate nutrition should be initiated	☐	☐	☐	☐
	• Prevention of DVT, pressure sores, and aspiration pneumonia is important	☐	☐	☐	☐
	• Knowledge of brainstem death and organ donation and awareness of medicolegal aspects	☐	☐	☐	☐
	•	☐	☐	☐	☐
Complications	• Mortality and morbidity can be high in those with persistent non-traumatic and non-metabolic coma	☐	☐	☐	☐
	• Patients unresponsive for a prolonged time are said to be in a persistent vegetative state	☐	☐	☐	☐
	•	☐	☐	☐	☐
Patient safety tips	• Importance of ABC management	☐	☐	☐	☐
	• Adequate monitoring of those at risk of neurological deterioration	☐	☐	☐	☐
	•	☐	☐	☐	☐
Clinical note writing and handover	• Adequate neurological observations in patients at risk of deterioration	☐	☐	☐	☐
	•	☐	☐	☐	☐

			U B S E	U B S E	U B S E	U B S E
Self-assessed as at least borderline:	Signature:	Date:				
Peer-assessed as ready for tutor assessment:	Signature:	Date:	U B S E	U B S E	U B S E	U B S E
Tutor-assessed as satisfactory:	Signature:	Date:	U B S E	U B S E	U B S E	U B S E

Notes

11.12 Stroke and transient ischaemic attack

Background

Despite being a largely preventable and treatable disease, stroke is the third leading cause of death in the industrialized world after heart disease and cancer. In the UK, stroke accounts for 11% of all deaths annually. More than 900 000 people in England are currently suffering the consequences of this condition, with half of them dependent on others for help with daily activities. Stroke is therefore the leading cause of serious disability in adults. Stroke is an acute focal or global impairment of brain function resulting from impairment of cerebral circulation that lasts for more than 24 hours. Stroke can be broadly classified as either ischaemic (85%) or haemorrhagic (10–15%) in nature.

A transient ischaemic attack (TIA) causes sudden focal loss of neurological function that resolves completely in less than 24 hours. TIAs are important predictors of subsequent infarcts. Within 5 years of a single TIA, 30% of patients have a stroke (10% within one year) and 15% have a myocardial infarction. It is vital therefore that patients diagnosed with a TIA are seen early by a specialist to ensure optimum management of any modifiable risk factors and to prevent disease progression.

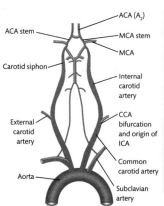

The cerebral circulation can be affected by emboli arising from the more proximal circulation (aortic valve, arch of the aorta, carotid arteries, vertebral and basilar arteries) or thrombosis can occur *in situ*.

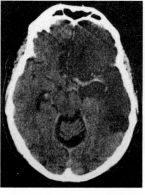

Urgent CT scan in a stroke patient is needed to diagnosis a thrombotic stroke and exclude haemorrhagic strokes. Thrombotic strokes may be amenable to treatment by thrombolysis if diagnosis is made within 1–3 hours of onset of stroke.

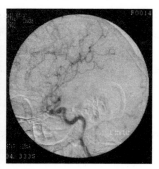

Cerebral angiography will help define the precise site of the cerebral infarction. Sometimes these lesions are amenable to treatment, for example, stenosis of the external carotid artery.

Figure 11.17 Images in stroke.

Diagnosis

The clinical presentation of stroke depends on the cortical areas damaged by vascular insult. A working knowledge of the vascular territories and functional anatomy of the brain is necessary to interpret focal neurology and approximate the location of the lesion.

A bewildering array of stroke syndromes have been characterized, but the Oxford Community Stroke Project (OCSP) or Bamford classification provides a relatively simple method of categorizing stroke subtypes. Having been in use for nearly 20 years, this classification has the added benefit that considerable data are now available regarding the complications and prognosis of these stroke subgroups, allowing the development of targeted management strategies. The most common symptom of stroke is hemiparesis. The next most common symptom is aphasia.

The OCSP classification

419

11.12
**Stroke and
transient
ischaemic attack**

The last letter of the acronym can be S, I, or H. These represent the terms syndrome (used before imaging when pathogenesis is uncertain), ischaemia, and haemorrhage, respectively. Therefore clinically a patient with stroke may be deemed to have TACS (total anterior circulatory stroke). If computed tomography (CT) of the head shows this to be haemorrhagic then it is termed TACH (total anterior circulatory stroke: haemorrhagic).

Total anterior circulatory stroke (TACS)

- Hemiparesis (ipsilateral motor and or sensory deficit of at least two areas of face, arms, legs)
- *Plus* homonymous hemianopia
- *Plus* higher cerebral dysfunction (dysphasia, neglect, apraxia, dyscalculia, visuospatial problems).

In the presence of impaired consciousness, higher cerebral function and visual fields deficits are assumed.

Partial anterior circulatory stroke (PACS)

- Two of the three components of TAC process
- *Or* isolated cortical dysfunction such as dysphasia
- *Or* motor/sensory loss more limited than for LAC pathology

Lacunar stroke (LACS)

- Pure motor or pure sensory deficit affecting two of face, arm or leg
- *Or* sensorimotor stroke, stroke (basal ganglia and internal capsule)
- *Or* ataxic hemiparesis (cerebellar-type ataxia with ipsilateral pyramidal signs (motor signs due to internal capsule or pons dysfunction)
- *Or* dysarthria plus clumsy hand syndrome
- *Or* acute onset movement disorder (hemichorea, hemiballismus due to basal ganglia dysfunction)

Posterior circulatory stroke (POCS)

- Cranial nerve deficit with contralateral hemiparesis or sensory deficit,
- *Or* bilateral stroke
- *Or* isolated cerebellar stroke
- *Or* disorders of conjugate eye movement
- *Or* isolated homonymous hemianopia

ROSIER scale (Recognition Of Stroke In the Emergency Room)

This enables clinical staff to differentiate between stroke patients and other conditions:

- Has there been loss of consciousness or syncope? Yes minus 1, no zero.
- Has there been seizure activity? Yes minus 1, no zero.
- Is there a *new acute* onset (or on awakening from sleep)?
  - Asymmetric facial weakness: Yes plus 1, no zero
  - Asymmetric arm weakness: Yes plus 1, no zero
  - Asymmetric leg weakness: Yes plus 1, no zero
  - Speech disturbance: Yes plus 1, no zero
  - Visual field defect: Yes plus 1, no zero.
- **Total score**: Stroke likely if score greater than 0. In many cases an urgent CT head will be needed to consider thrombolysis.

ABCD² scale for TIA assessment

The ROSIER scale is not suitable for patients with suspected TIA with no neurological signs when seen. This assessment assists in the identification of patients with a high or low risk of early disabling stroke.

- **A**ge is 60 years or older: 1 point
- **B**lood pressure >140/90 mmHg: 1 point
- **C**linical features: 1 point each unilateral weakness or speech disturbance without weakness or other suitable feature. Maximum 2 points
- **D**uration: >60 minutes (2 points), 10–60 minutes (1 point), <10 minutes (0 points)
- **D**iabetes mellitus: 1 point
- **Total score**: (total score 0–7). High-risk patients (6 or 7 points) have an 8.1% 2-day recurrent stroke risk. High-risk TIA patients (scoring 4 or more on ABCD² score) should be seen at a TIA clinic for review, urgent investigation, and initiation of secondary prevention.

Any patient with more than one episode in the last week is at a greater than 30% risk of stroke within a week and should be admitted for investigation and review by a consultant stroke physician.

Causes of stroke

- **Cardioembolism (30%)**: atrial fibrillation, myocardial infarction, prosthetic heart valves, cardiac surgery, cardioversion, infectious endocarditis, paradoxical embolism.
- **Atherothrombosis (20%)**: rupture of atherosclerotic plaques causes thrombosis in the carotid, vertebrobasilar and cerebral arteries, often proximal to major branches.
- **Lacunar (20%)**: caused by occlusion of deep penetrating arterial branches, especially the lenticostriate braches of the middle cerebral artery (MCA) that supply the internal capsule. Infarct is usually a result of microatheroma, lipohyalinosis, and fibrinoid necrosis secondary to hypertension.
- **Other ischaemic/cryptogenic (15–20%)**: sudden BP decrease >40 mmHg, venous sinus thrombosis, vasculitis, thrombophilia, carotid artery dissection, giant cell arteritis.
- **Haemorrhagic (10–15%)**: hypertension, trauma, rupture of saccular or berry aneurysm, arteriovenous malformation rupture.

Management

Phase 1 initial management (first hour)

- **Clinical history and examination**: history and examination with collateral information if possible. Use validated tool or clinical history and examination to establish diagnosis.
- **If onset of symptoms <3 hours, patient is a candidate for thrombolysis**: Arrange for urgent head CT using local protocol. Patient may need emergency transfer to suitable stroke facility.
- **Consider differential diagnoses**: especially subdural bleed, migraine, Todd's paresis (post epilepsy), trauma, drug overdose.
- **Evaluate risk factors**: age, hypertension, smoking, diabetes mellitus, heart disease, hyperlipidaemia, increased clotting, alcoholism.
- **Look for evidence of ischaemic pathology**: history of TIA/stroke, atrial fibrillation, carotid bruit, peripheral vascular disease, heart murmurs, endocarditis, myocardial infarction.
- **Look for evidence of haemorrhagic pathology**: history of hypertension, anticoagulation with warfarin, meningism, severe headache, reduced conscious level.

Investigations

- FBC, U&Es, lipids, coagulation, ESR (to exclude giant cell arteritis), random blood glucose.

- ECG, CXR.
- Brain imaging should be done immediately (<1 hour) if the following apply:
  ○ Patient meets criteria for thrombolysis
  ○ On anticoagulant therapy
  ○ Known bleeding tendency
  ○ GCS <13
  ○ Unexplained progressive or fluctuating symptoms
  ○ Papilloedema, nuchal rigidity, or fever
  ○ Severe headache at stroke onset
- **Consider**: blood cultures for endocarditis, sickle cell tests, syphilis serology.

Treatment

- **Stabilize and resuscitate patient** as necessary using ABCDE approach. Airway protection needed in many cases.
- **Exclude hypoglycaemia**.
- **Check criteria for thrombolysis**: a stroke specialist may recommend alteplase (tissue plasminogen activator) 0.9 mg/kg (up to a maximum of 90 mg) as an IV infusion over 60 minutes; 10% of the dose should be given as a bolus initially.
- If patient does not meet criteria for thrombolysis, establish nature of stroke and treat accordingly.
- **For ischaemic stroke**: give 300 mg aspirin unless contraindicated.
- **For haemorrhagic stroke**: reverse anticoagulation and refer to neurosurgeon for consideration of decompressive craniectomy.
- **Control physiological parameters**: to prevent expansion of stroke penumbra.
- **Hydrate, prevent hyperthermia (>37.2 °C), control BP if hypertensive emergency, given oxygen only if saturations <95%, blood sugar 4–11 mmol/L.**

Phase 2 management (2–6 hours)

- **Admit to a specialist stroke unit as soon as possible**: evidence suggests that it is all the aspects of care that a stroke unit provide that reduces morbidity and mortality and not the geographical location *per se*.
- **Assess swallowing**: before giving oral food, fluid or medication. All patients should have an early swallow assessment and insertion of an NG tube if necessary to prevent aspiration.
- Screen patient for malnutrition and consider nutritional supplementation.
- Turn regularly and keep dry to avoid pressure sores.

Phase 3 ongoing management

- **Specialist feeding strategies**: for malnourished patients and those at risk of aspiration. Some patients may require a percutaneous endoscopic gastrostomy (PEG) tube.
- **Rehabilitation**: with input from physiotherapy, speech and language therapy (SALT) and occupational therapy.
- **Medical management of risk factors prior to discharge**: cholesterol lowering drugs, BP control, dietary advice, antiplatelet treatment, lifestyle advice (especially smoking, weight, fresh fruit and vegetables, and physical activity). Optimizing control of diabetes.
- **Consider assessment of carotid arteries**.

Other aspects of treatment

- **TIA treatment**: if neurological symptoms have fully resolved within 24 hours, the patient should be treated for TIA. Give aspirin 300 mg and provide best medical treatment with cholesterol lowering therapy, blood pressure management and smoking cessation advice. Assess risk of subsequent stroke using ABCD^2 score.

○ Score <4, specialist assessment and investigation within 1 week.

○ Score ≥4, specialist assessment and investigation within 24 hours.

● **Neuroimaging**: if vascular territory or pathology uncertain, perform diffusion-weighted MRI. This should be done within 7 days ideally but will depend on local services.

● **Carotid stenosis**: if greater than 70%, the patient may be a candidate for carotid endarterectomy. Refer to suitable surgeon. If symptomatic stenosis of 70–90% according to European Carotid Surgery Trial criteria, patient should undergo carotid intervention.

Complications

● **Aspiration pneumonia**: 40% of patients with stroke will have difficulties with swallowing. Aspiration pneumonia is a common stroke complication that has a significant mortality. All stroke patients should have a swallowing assessment soon after presentation and oral intake should be modified accordingly. In high-risk patients, an NG tube may be passed to prevent aspiration.

● **Pressure sores**: frequently result from immobility. Patients should be kept dry and turned regularly to prevent their occurrence. Good nursing is vital in this regard. Catheter insertion may be beneficial in some cases.

● **Psychological complications of stroke**: should not be underestimated. The burden of stroke on patients and their carers is considerable, and physicians should be alert for evidence of depression or substance misuse in these groups.

Patient safety tips

✔ **CT head urgently**: this is to identify patients who are amenable to treatment with thrombolysis for their thrombotic stroke. Disability is significantly reduced if given within the first 3 hours after onset of stroke

✔ **Meticulous attention to key aspects of general care**: safe swallowing, pressure sores, VTE prophylaxis, and treatment of secondary complications, psychological review.

✔ **Ensure post-stroke management bundle**: most patients will need to be on a combination of diuretic (indapamide has the most specific evidence), ACE inhibitor, and a statin. Antiplatelet treatment in most cases will be aspirin with dipyridamole, clopidogrel can also be used but there is less specific evidence available for it. It is estimated that strokes can be reduced by a third with these measures in the first 5 years after a stroke. If the patient had atrial fibrillation, consider for warfarin or a direct thrombin inhibitor.

Student name:	Medical school:	Year:

Stroke and TIA

Sir James Chettam is a hypertensive gentleman with a 30-pack year smoking history, who drinks 30 units of alcohol a week. His father had a myocardial infarction aged 53. He is admitted with slurred speech, weakness and diminished sensation in his left arm and leg. This lasted 18 hours during which there was no diminishing of consciousness.

This assessment will be based around a discussion on the management of stroke and TIA with reference to above scenario.

		Self	Peer	Peer/tutor	Tutor
What is the OCSP classification in relation to strokes? What does the above patient have?	• **Total anterior circulatory stroke (TACS)**: hemiparesis + homonymous hemianopia + higher cerebral dysfunction (dysphasia etc.)	☐	☐	☐	☐
	• **Partial anterior circulatory stroke (PASC)**: two of TACS or isolated cortical dysfunction or motor/sensory loss more limited than for LAC pathology	☐	☐	☐	☐
	• **Lacunar stroke (LACS)**: pure motor or pure sensory deficit affecting two of face, arm or leg or sensorimotor stroke or ataxic hemiparesis or dysarthria plus clumsy hand syndrome or acute onset movement disorder	☐	☐	☐	☐
	• **Posterior circulatory stroke (POCS)**: cranial nerve deficit with contralateral hemiparesis or sensory deficit *or* bilateral stroke *or* isolated cerebellar stroke *or* disorders of conjugate eye movement *or* isolated homonymous hemianopia	☐	☐	☐	☐
What is the ABCD^2 scale for TIA Assessment?	For severity of TIA and future stroke risk: **A**ge ≥60, **B**P >140/90, **C**linical features, **D**uration, **D**iabetes mellitus	☐	☐	☐	☐
What the main causes of stroke?	• **Cardioembolism**: AF, MI, prosthetic valves, cardioversion, endocarditis	☐	☐	☐	☐
	• **Atherothrombosis**: atheromatous rupture in carotid, vertebrobasilar, and cerebral arteries	☐	☐	☐	☐
	• **Lacunar**: microatheroma, lipohyalinosis, and fibrinoid necrosis secondary to hypertension	☐	☐	☐	☐
	• **Other ischaemic/cryptogenic**: BP drop, venous thrombosis, vasculitis, thrombophilia, carotid artery dissection, giant cell arteritis	☐	☐	☐	☐
	• **Haemorrhagic**: hypertension, trauma, rupture of aneurysm, arteriovenous malformation	☐	☐	☐	☐
What are the main aspects of phase 1 initial management (first hour)?	• **Clinic history and examination**: history and examination with collateral information	☐	☐	☐	☐
	• **If onset of symptoms <3 hours, patient is a candidate for thrombolysis**: urgent head CT	☐	☐	☐	☐
	• **Consider differential diagnoses**: subdural bleed, migraine, Todd's paresis, trauma, drugs	☐	☐	☐	☐
	• **Evaluate risk factors**: CVD risk factors, increased clotting, alcoholism	☐	☐	☐	☐
	• **Evidence of ischaemic cause**: TIA/stroke, atrial fibrillation, carotid bruit, PVD, endocarditis, myocardial infarction	☐	☐	☐	☐
	• **Evidence of haemorrhagic cause**: hypertension, warfarin, meningism, severe headache	☐	☐	☐	☐
	• **Investigations**: bloods, ECG, CXR, CT head	☐	☐	☐	☐
	• **Treatment**:	☐	☐	☐	☐
	○ **Stabilize and resuscitate patient** as necessary using ABCDE approach				
	○ **Exclude hypoglycaemia**				
	○ **Check criteria for thrombolysis**				
	○ **For ischaemic stroke**: give 300 mg aspirin unless contraindicated				
	○ **For haemorrhagic stroke**: reverse anticoagulation and refer to neurosurgeon				
	○ **Control physiological parameters**: to prevent expansion of stroke penumbra				
	○ Hydrate, prevent hyperthermia (>37.2 °C), control BP if hypertensive emergency, given oxygen only if saturations <95%, blood sugar 4–11 mmol/L				
What are the main aspects of phase 2 management (2–6 hours)?	• **Admit to a specialist stroke unit as soon as possible**	☐	☐	☐	☐
	• **Assess swallowing**	☐	☐	☐	☐
What are the main aspects of phase 3 ongoing management?	• **Specialist feeding strategies**: for malnourished patients and those at risk of aspiration	☐	☐	☐	☐
	• **Rehabilitation**: Physiotherapy, SALT, and occupational therapy	☐	☐	☐	☐
	• Medical management of risk factors prior to discharge	☐	☐	☐	☐
	• Consider assessment of carotid arteries	☐	☐	☐	☐
What are the main avoidable complications?	• **Aspiration pneumonia and pressure sores**	☐	☐	☐	☐
What are the key patient safety tips in relation to stroke care?	• **CT head urgently**: to identify patients amenable to thrombolysis	☐	☐	☐	☐
	• **Meticulous attention to key aspects of general care**: swallowing, pressure sores, VTE	☐	☐	☐	☐
	• **Ensure post stroke management bundle**: diuretic, ACE inhibitor, statin, antiplatelet treatment	☐	☐	☐	☐

Self-assessed as at least borderline:	Signature:	Date:	U B S E	U B S E	U B S E	U B S E
Peer-assessed as ready for tutor assessment:	Signature:	Date:	U B S E	U B S E	U B S E	U B S E
Tutor-assessed as satisfactory:	Signature:	Date:	U B S E	U B S E	U B S E	U B S E

Notes

11.13 Diabetes emergencies: diabetic ketoacidosis, hyperosmolar hyperglycaemic syndrome, and hypoglycaemia

Background

Diabetes emergencies are common and in many cases avoidable. While meticulous attention is needed in the early management of all diabetes emergencies, the same care should be given to patients (and or carer) education to reduce the chances of the diabetes emergency from happening again. In UK, the 'Think Glucose' campaign by the National Institute for Innovation and Improvement, has helped to refocus our attention on the safe management of inpatients with diabetes irrespective of the reason for admission. It must be remembered that, on average, a person with diabetes stays in hospital 2 days longer than a person without diabetes and the same condition. Better in-hospital diabetes management would reduce this excess length of stay with as significant saving of resources, especially as 1 in 7 of all adult beds in UK are occupied by a person with diabetes.

Diabetic ketoacidosis

This common but serious clinical emergency has considerable morbidity and mortality attached to it. It is a mistake to assume that DKA only occurs in patients with type 1 diabetes only. Around 40% of cases occur in type 2 diabetes. Meticulous attention to assessment and especially rates of fluid infusion and electrolyte levels is needed to reduce complications.

Diagnosis

History of virtually any illness in a patient with diabetes mellitus. Classical symptoms will include recent infection, nausea, vomiting, abdominal pain, loss of consciousness. Presentation can be to an emergency surgical unit.

- Glucose >11 mmol/L and venous pH <7.3 or arterial <7.28.
- Low HCO_3 (less than 15 mmol/L).
- Capillary ketone levels >3 or urinary ketones > or equal ++.
- High anion gap acidosis (anion gap = $[K^+ + Na^+] - [Cl^- + HCO_3^-]$ (normal range = 8–12, in DKA >15 mmol/L, often 20–25 mmol/L).

Causes of DKA

- **Lack of insulin**: missed dose.
- **Intercurrent illness**: especially infection (e.g. UTI, chest infection), myocardial infarction (often silent), renal disease, pancreatitis, stroke, addisonian crisis.
- **Stress**: physical or emotional.
- **Other similar disorders**: lactic acidosis, uraemia, rhabdomyolysis, salicylate, glycol, methanol, formaldehyde, toluene, paraldehyde.

The DKA component of this chapter is adapted from the Joint British Diabetes Societies Guidelines (2010).

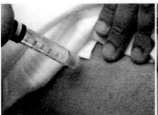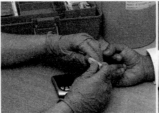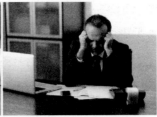

Insulin omission, accidental or otherwise, is the commonest cause of hyperglycaemia which if not corrected quickly, can in susceptible patients lead to DKA.

Hypoglycaemia must be managed aggressively. In most cases the patient is able to help themselves alone, help is needed from another person in more serious hypos and parenteral treatment in severe hypoglycaemia.

Physical or emotional stress can lead to adrenergic surges resulting in hyperglycaemia and insulin resistance. Patient must be advised on how to manage their diabetes during illnesss and times of increased stress.

Figure 11.18 Images in diabetes emergencies. Right © Aldo Murillo/iStockphoto.

Management

Phase 1 initial management (first hour)

- **Clinically** – history, examination focus on respiratory rate, temp, BP, pulse, oxygen saturations, GCS, MEWS. VTE assessment.
- **Investigations** – random blood sugar, venous bicarbonate, U&Es, ABG only if the patient is hypoxic (saturations <94%).
- **Consider** – urine and blood cultures, CXR, ECG if patient older than 30.
- **Fixed rate insulin infusion**: 0.1 unit/kg/hour of soluble insulin.
- **Monitoring**: hourly capillary glucose (and ketones if available), venous bicarbonate and potassium at 60 minutes then 2-hourly.
- **More intensive monitoring** – continuous cardiac monitoring, CVP, catheter, NG tube.
- Monitor bedside blood glucose and ketones.
- **If systolic <90 mmHg**: give 1000 mL 0.9% saline over 15–30 minutes. Next litre over 1–2 hours.
- **If systolic ≥90 mmHg**: give 1000 mL 0.9% saline in 1 hour.
- Two IV lines required.
- Potassium should be added if below 5 mmol/L.
- Consider ITU support if patient remains unstable.

Phase 2 management (2–6 hours)

- Continue insulin and fluids as above until – venous pH >7.3, bicarbonate >18 mmol/L and capillary ketones <0.3 mmol/L.
- Continue long-acting subcutaneous insulin analogues that patient is already taking.
- When the blood glucose <14 mmol/L use 5% glucose instead of 0.9% saline (expected drop 3–5 mmol/L/h.
- Continue IV 0.9% saline according to fluid balance. A total of 3 L in first 4 hours is reasonable.
- Continue to monitor vital signs, U&Es, and bedside monitoring of blood ketones and blood glucose hourly.
- Potassium very likely to be required for IV fluids.

Phase 3 ongoing management

- Fluids according to BP, urine output and U&E results.
- Continue to monitor vital signs, U&Es, and bedside monitoring of blood ketones and blood glucose 2 hourly
- When ketones <0.3 mmol/L, blood sugar <15 mmol/L, pH >7.3, venous bicarbonate >20 mmol/L, subcutaneous insulin can be commenced provided patient is now eating and drinking.

- At 12 hours check venous pH, bicarbonate, potassium, ketones and a laboratory glucose.
- Inform local diabetes team as soon as patient is admitted and to be reviewed ASAP.
- Stopping sliding scale:
  - ○ If previous history of diabetes change back to previous regimen, give insulin 20–30 minutes before stopping sliding scale (with meal)
  - ○ If newly diagnosed, calculate 24-hour insulin requirement and reduce by 20%
  - ○ Twice daily regimen = two-thirds of calculated insulin dose such as NovoMix® 30 before breakfast and one-third before evening meals.
  - ○ Basal bolus regimen: calculate amount of insulin required in 24 hours, give 50% of this as long-acting analogue at bedtime. Divide remaining 50% by 3 and give this dose before each meal as short-acting insulin. These percentages will depend on local insulin preferences and protocols.

Other aspects of treatment

- High-risk patients should have an NG tube to avoid aspiration (common cause of death).
- Catheter to ensure fluid balance (remember continued diuresis worsens dehydration).
- Check urine for ketones on each voiding, or 2 hourly if patient has a urinary catheter.
- Look for infection and treat vigorously.
- Remember silent myocardial infarction.
- High mortality in elderly with multi-organ disease (risk of hyperosmolar state).
- Convert to patient's normal treatment once eating and drinking.
- Intravenous insulin must overlap with the patients own subcutaneous insulin by 20–30 minutes, otherwise DKA can be precipitated.
- Low-dose heparin prophylaxis should be considered – (usually enoxaparin 40 mg subcutaneously once daily.

Complications

- Death unfortunately is still reported to occur in 1–5% of cases; in many cases this will be due to cerebral oedema or hypokalaemia.
- Morbidity and mortality can also be due to the underlying precipitating cause, e.g. chest infection with septicaemia.

Hyperosmolar hyperglycaemic syndrome

Hyperosmolar hyperglycaemic syndrome (HHS) is an acute metabolic complication of type 2 diabetes usually encountered in elderly patients. It was previously known as hyperosmolar non-ketotic hyperglycaemia. It is characterized by gradual development of very severe hyperglycaemia leading to dehydration, renal impairment, and hyperosmolality. Significant acidosis and ketonuria are absent. Patients with undiagnosed diabetes can present with HHS for the first time. Precipitating factors include infections such as pneumonia, stroke, silent myocardial infarction, and drugs (e.g. high-dose corticosteroids or thiazide diuretics). There is an increased risk of thromboembolism with HHS. Mortality is much higher than that of DKA.

HHS should be suspected in patients with very high blood glucose (>35 mmol/L) and mental status changes (acute confusion, drowsiness, and coma). There is invariably renal impairment. Serum osmolality should be measured in such patients to confirm the diagnosis.

Treatment of HHS

Treatment consists of:

- Rehydration and electrolyte replacement (usually with 0.9% saline *or* 0.45% normal saline when serum sodium >150 mmol/L)
- Continuous IV insulin infusion

- Prophylactic anticoagulation
- Treatment of precipitating factors (e.g. antibiotics for pneumonia).

- Prophylactic anticoagulation
- Treatment of precipitating factors (e.g. antibiotics for pneumonia).

hypotensive patients not responding to fluid replacement and those with a pH less than or equal to 6.8, H^+ 159 nmol/L .No further correction necessary after urine output established (>30 mL/hour).

✔ **Continuation of long-acting subcutaneous insulin**: This is recommended as this will allow a small amount of insulin to be present at all times and reduce hepatic gluconeogenesis.

✔ **Communicate diagnosis and changes** in diabetes care accurately and in a timely fashion to the primary care team.

✔ **Refer patients to specialist diabetes care using guidelines below**: as with all guidelines, use professional judgement in individual patients and circumstances

---

Box 11.4 Who to refer for specialist advice from the hospital diabetes care team (adapted from the National Institute for Innovation and Improvement 'Think Glucose' Campaign)

Note: Use professional judgement in individual patients and circumstances, for guidance only

Referral not usually required

- Mild, self-treated hypoglycaemia
- Transient hyperglycaemia
- Simple educational need
- Routine dietetic advice
- Well-controlled diabetes
- Good self-management skills
- Routine diabetes care

Referral may be required

- IV insulin infusion with good control
- Nil by mouth for greater than 24 hours post surgery
- Significant diabetes educational need
- Persistent hyperglycaemia
- Possible new diagnosis of diabetes
- Transient or stress hyperglycaemia
- Poor wound healing
- Steroid therapy

Always refer

- Admission for urgent or major elective surgical procedure
- ACS
- DKA/HHS
- Severe hypoglycaemia
- Sepsis or vomiting
- Impaired consciousness
- Previous problems with diabetes as inpatient
- IV insulin with glucose levels uncontrolled
- IV insulin for greater than 48 hours
- Parenteral or direct enteral nutrition
- Foot ulceration
- Newly diagnosed diabetes (type 1 or 2)
- Patient request

Diabetic ketoacidosis

Sharon Rock is a 54-year-old and works as an actor. She has an extremely busy schedule that she had difficulty managing. She is called to go out of town on an assignment. After a late night party she is found collapsed in her hotel bedroom by her assistant. She is taken to the local emergency department. Her usual medications are basal bolus regimen using a long-acting insulin analogue and one short-acting analogue injection before each meal. Her results on admission are as follows:

pH 7 .45–7.35	PaO$_2$ 10.5–13.5 kPa	PaCO$_2$ 4.7–6.0 kPa	HCO$_3^-$ 22–28 mmol/L	● Temperature 37.1 °C
pH 7.08	PaO$_2$ 13.9	PaCO$_2$ 2.8	HCO$_3^-$ 11.2	● Heart rate 124/min
				● Respiratory rate 28
				● Glucose level: 44.8

This assessment will be based around a discussion on the management of DKA with reference to above scenario.

		Self	Peer	Peer/tutor	Tutor
What is the most likely diagnosis and precipitating cause in the above patient?	●	☐	☐	☐	☐
How is the diagnosis of DKA made?	Look out for condition especially if recent infection, nausea, vomiting, acute abdominal pain, loss of consciousness.				
	● Glucose >11 mmol/L, venous pH <7.3 or arterial <7.28	☐	☐	☐	☐
	● Low HCO$_3$ (less than 15 mmol/L), capillary or urinary ketones raised	☐	☐	☐	☐
	● High anion gap acidosis (>15): anion gap = [K$^+$ + Na$^+$] – [Cl + HCO$_3^-$]	☐	☐	☐	☐
	●	☐	☐	☐	☐
What are the main causes of DKA?	● Lack of insulin: missed dose, UTI, chest infection, myocardial infarction (often silent), renal disease, pancreatitis, stroke, stress (physical/mental), addisonian crisis	☐	☐	☐	☐
	● Other similar disorders: lactic acidosis, uraemia, rhabdomyolysis, salicylate, glycol, methanol, formaldehyde, toluene, paraldehyde	☐	☐	☐	☐
	●	☐	☐	☐	☐
What are the main aspects of phase 1 initial management (first hour)?	● Clinically: history, examination focus on respiratory rate, temperature, BP, pulse, oxygen saturations, GCS, MEWS. VTE assessment	☐	☐	☐	☐
	● Investigations: random blood sugar, venous bicarb, U&Es, ABG only if the patient is hypoxic (saturations <94%)	☐	☐	☐	☐
	● Consider: blood and urine culture, CXR, ECG if patient older than 30	☐	☐	☐	☐
	● More intensive monitoring: continuous cardiac monitoring, CVP, catheter, NG tube	☐	☐	☐	☐
	● Fixed rate insulin, and monitor bedside blood glucose and ketones	☐	☐	☐	☐
	● 0.9% saline IV	☐	☐	☐	☐
	● Potassium should be added if below 5 mmol/L	☐	☐	☐	☐
	●	☐	☐	☐	☐
What are the main aspects of phase 2 management (2–6 hours)?	● Continue insulin and fluids as above until – venous pH >7.3, bicarbonate >18 mmol/L and capillary ketones <0.3 mmol/L	☐	☐	☐	☐
	● Continue long-acting subcutaneous insulin analogues that patient already taking	☐	☐	☐	☐
	● When glucose <14 mmol/L use 5% glucose instead of 0.9% saline (expected drop 3–5 mmol/L/h)	☐	☐	☐	☐
	● Continue IV 0.9% saline according to fluid balance	☐	☐	☐	☐
	● Monitor vital signs, U&Es, and bedside blood ketones and blood glucose hourly	☐	☐	☐	☐
	●	☐	☐	☐	☐
What are the main aspects of phase 3 ongoing management?	● Fluids as above.	☐	☐	☐	☐
	● Continue to monitor vital signs, U&Es, and bedside monitoring of blood ketones and blood glucose 2 hourly.	☐	☐	☐	☐
	● When ketones <0.3 mmol/L, blood sugar <15 mmol/L and venous bicarbonate >20 mmol/L, subcutaneous insulin can be commenced provided patient is now eating and drinking	☐	☐	☐	☐
	● Inform local diabetes team as soon as patient is admitted and to be reviewed ASAP	☐	☐	☐	☐
	● If previous history diabetes, change back to previous regimen, give insulin 20–30 minutes before stopping sliding scale (with meal)	☐	☐	☐	☐
	● If newly diagnosed, calculate 24-hour insulin requirement and reduce by 20%	☐	☐	☐	☐
	● Twice daily regimen = two-thirds of calculated insulin dose as NovoMix® 30 before breakfast and one-third before evening meals	☐	☐	☐	☐
	● Basal bolus regimen ≈16% short-acting before each meal and 50% as long-acting at night	☐	☐	☐	☐
	●	☐	☐	☐	☐

What are the other main aspects of treatment?	• High-risk patients should have a NG tube to avoid aspiration (common cause of death)	☐	☐	☐	☐
	• Catheter to ensure fluid balance (remember continued diuresis worsens dehydration)	☐	☐	☐	☐
	• Check urine for ketones on each voiding, or two hourly if patient has a urinary catheter	☐	☐	☐	☐
	• Look for infection and treat vigorously, remember silent myocardial infarction	☐	☐	☐	☐
	• High mortality in elderly with multi-organ disease (risk of hyperosmolar state)	☐	☐	☐	☐
	• Convert to patient's normal treatment once eating and drinking	☐	☐	☐	☐
	• IV insulin must overlap with the patient's own subcutaneous insulin by 20–30 minutes, otherwise DKA can be precipitated.	☐	☐	☐	☐
	• Low-dose heparin should be considered for VTE prophylaxis	☐	☐	☐	☐
	•	☐	☐	☐	☐
What are the main complications of DKA?	• Death, often due to cerebral oedema or hypokalaemia.	☐	☐	☐	☐
	• Morbidity and mortality can be due to the underlying precipitating cause, e.g. sepsis	☐	☐	☐	☐
	•	☐	☐	☐	☐
What are the main patient safety tips in relation to DKA or any diabetes emergency care?	• **Fluid balance**: too little and renal dysfunction precipitated, too much and cardiac failure precipitated	☐	☐	☐	☐
	• **Potassium levels**: ECG monitor, after first litre fluid replacement use 20 mmol K^+ per litre infusate, unless K^+ >5.4. Recheck U&Es 1–2 hours after starting IV fluids, titrate K^+ accordingly, e.g. 20–40 mmol/L. Hypokalaemia is a common cause of death	☐	☐	☐	☐
	• **Subcutaneous heparin**: to prevent VTE	☐	☐	☐	☐
	• **Insulin overlap**: when transferring patient back to normal insulin, continue IV insulin for at least 20 minutes to give the soluble fast-acting insulin to get into the blood stream	☐	☐	☐	☐
	• **Bicarbonate infusion**: no need in almost all cases: promotes intracellular acidosis, increases hypokalaemia, and cerebral oedema	☐	☐	☐	☐
	• **Continuation of long-acting subcutaneous insulin**: This is recommended as this will allow a small amount of insulin to be present at all times and reduce hepatic gluconeogenesis	☐	☐	☐	☐
	• **Refer to diabetes specialist team**: if needed accorded to clinical need or consulting 'Think Glucose' guideline	☐	☐	☐	☐
	•	☐	☐	☐	☐
Clinical note writing and handover	Stress that patient's clinical state and electrolytes must be reviewed regularly	☐	☐	☐	☐
	•	☐	☐	☐	☐

				U B S E	U B S E	U B S E	U B S E
Self-assessed as at least borderline:	Signature:	Date:					
Peer-assessed as ready for tutor assessment:	Signature:	Date:					
Tutor-assessed as satisfactory:	Signature:	Date:					

Notes

11.14 Headache

Background

Headache is one of the commonest symptoms for which patients seek medical attention. One in five of the general population will suffer a headache severe enough to consult a doctor. It is very important to bear in mind and exclude the rare but devastating causes of headache. These are subarachnoid haemorrhage and meningitis in recent onset severe headache and temporal arteritis in sub-acute progressive headache in the elderly.

The common misconceptions about headache relate to brain tumour and high blood pressure. Brain tumours usually manifest as seizure and focal neurological deficit (such as hemiparesis) related to the part of brain affected by tumour. It is very unusual for a space-occupying lesion to cause headache without other symptoms and signs. It is not wise to attribute uncontrolled systemic hypertension as the cause of headache, unless the diastolic blood pressure is more than 100 mmHg and other causes have been excluded.

Diagnosis

The majority of patients with headache will have normal physical examination. The diagnosis of the cause of headache therefore depends entirely on detailed history taking and an understanding of the characteristics of various headaches. The most important clinical clue lies in the duration of headache and its pattern (acute, recurrent, progressive, and chronic). A recent onset severe headache might be due to a serious cause such as subarachnoid haemorrhage or meningitis, whereas headache lasting for years is unlikely to be anything serious.

Causes of headache

The International Headache Society classifies headache as primary and secondary. Primary headaches are those in which headache and its features are the disorder itself, as compared with secondary headaches caused by another disorder such as meningitis and subarachnoid haemorrhage.

Common causes of headache (in order of frequency):

- **Primary**
  - Tension headache
  - Migraine
  - Cluster headache
- **Secondary**
  - Systemic infection (such as flu)
  - Head injury
  - Subarachnoid haemorrhage and meningitis
  - Temporal arteritis (in older people)
  - Brain tumour (very rare as the only symptom) or cerebral metastases

Subarachnoid haemorrhage

- Sudden onset (within seconds) severe ('worst ever') headache, with or without loss of consciousness, often described as a 'thunder-clap' headache.
- Usually occipital in location, but could be anywhere in the head.
- Look for reduced conscious level, neck stiffness and focal neurological deficit (remember examination can be normal).

- Urgent CT scan of the brain, and if CT scan normal, followed by lumbar puncture at least 12 hours later for CSF xanthochromia.
- Urgent referral to neurosurgical unit, if subarachnoid haemorrhage confirmed.
- Usually caused by an aneurysm or arteriovenous malformation, which require neurosurgical intervention.

Meningitis

- Recent onset (hours to days) headache associated with fever and neck stiffness
- Suspect meningococcal septicaemia, if associated with typical non-blanching rash (usually seen in the legs), and start antibiotics without any delay (do not wait for test results!).
- Perform urgent CT scan of the brain followed by lumbar puncture.
- High neutrophil count with low glucose level in CSF indicates bacterial meningitis, while a high lymphocyte count with normal glucose level is typical of viral meningitis.
- Suspect tuberculosis meningitis in patients (particularly immigrants from high prevalence areas) with headache of few weeks duration and CSF findings of high lymphocytes and low glucose.
- Start antibiotics as per local antibiotic protocol/microbiology advice (usually ceftriaxone 2 g daily ± amoxicillin 2 g 4 hourly) for bacterial meningitis.
- Seek expert advice in non-bacterial meningitis.

Temporal arteritis

- Subacute (weeks to months) progressive headache in people older than 50 years of age.
- Can be associated with symptoms of polymyalgia rheumatica such as myalgia and stiffness.
- Look for inflamed and tender temporal arteries.
- **High risk of progression to permanent blindness, if untreated**.
- Do urgent ESR (elevated in most patients but can be normal) and start high-dose prednisolone (60–80 mg).
- Arrange temporal artery biopsy as soon as possible.

Migraine

- Common cause of recurrent debilitating headache (twice as common in women).
- Often unilateral, temporal, and pulsating headache, associated with nausea, vomiting, photophobia, and phonophobia.
- Can be preceded by aura such as visual phenomena or speech and sensory disturbances.
- Acute attacks treated with analgesics, antiemetics, and triptans (5-hydroxytryptamine [5-HT] agonists).
- People with more than two attacks a month can be treated with prophylactic medication such as β-blockers.
- Remember more than one type of headache can occur in the same person (people with a history of migraine can also develop subarachnoid haemorrhage)

Tension headache

- Bilateral tight band-like discomfort, builds up slowly, and either episodic or chronic (lasting days to months).
- No clear association with tension and this type of headache.
- Not associated with nausea, vomiting, photophobia, and phonophobia (unlike migraine).
- Treatment is with simple analgesics.
- Amitriptyline useful in the chronic form.

Cluster headache

- Unilateral, usually retro-orbital severe pain occurring at the same time of the day for the duration of the cluster followed by pain-free interval.
- Three times more common in men than women.
- Associated with watering of the eye or nasal congestion on the same side as the headache.
- Acute episodes treated with high-flow (10–12 L) high concentration oxygen (100%) or 6 mg subcutaneous sumatriptan.
- Verapamil and less commonly lithium used to prevent acute episodes.

Other causes of headache/facial pain

Acute angle-closure/glaucoma

Severe eye pain with redness in the eye and moderately dilated fixed pupil. Urgent diagnosis with tonometry and treatment.

Acute sinusitis

Pain and tenderness over the sinuses with a history of preceding upper respiratory viral illness. Antibiotics will usually help.

Trigeminal neuralgia

Frequent, unilateral, severe, and short-lasting (minutes) pain. Often in the distribution of maxillary and mandibular divisions of trigeminal nerve.

Carotid or vertebral artery dissections

Headache and other signs such as Horner's syndrome. Neck pain also prominent feature. MRI for diagnosis.

Venous sinus thrombosis

Elusive diagnosis as headache can be non-specific. MRI is the preferred imaging modality.

Pituitary apoplexy

Sudden severe headache with collapse (secondary adrenal insufficiency) and diplopia (visual loss [pituitary mass effect]).

Hypertensive emergencies

Headache worse on waking and improves throughout the day. Headache is bilateral and occipital.

Patient safety tips

- ✔ **Careful full history and detailed examination**.
- ✔ **Watch out for Cushing's reflex**: this is the triad of hypertension, bradycardia and irregular respiration in the setting of raised intracranial pressure.
- ✔ **CT head or MRI head**: essential in ruling out treatable causes, especially sub-arachnoid haemorrhage. If the diagnosis remains plausible, consider LP for CSF blood/xanthochromia.

Student name:	Medical school:	Year:

Headache

This assessment will be based around a discussion of headaches.

		Self	Peer	Peer/tutor	Tutor
Background	• Common presentation in both primary and secondary care. Tension headache and migraine are common causes. Clinical examination is normal in most patients with headache and diagnosis is made entirely on detailed history. Meningitis and subarachnoid haemorrhage are serious life-threatening causes of headache.	☐	☐	☐	☐
	•	☐	☐	☐	☐
Diagnosis	• History – onset and duration of headache: instantaneous (within seconds), acute (minutes to hours), subacute (days to weeks) and chronic (months to years)	☐	☐	☐	☐
	• Pattern – constant, intermittent, progressive	☐	☐	☐	☐
	• Aggravating and relieving factors	☐	☐	☐	☐
	• Associated symptoms: loss of consciousness at onset of headache, fever, stiff neck, photophobia, phonophobia, flashing lights, and other visual phenomenon, nausea and vomiting	☐	☐	☐	☐
	• People over 50 years of age: pain and stiffness in proximal muscles, jaw claudication and pain on combing hair	☐	☐	☐	☐
	• Other neurological symptoms: seizure, weakness of limbs, and bladder and bowel disturbance	☐	☐	☐	☐
	• Examination: Full neurological examination including fundoscopy for papilloedema and neck stiffness	☐	☐	☐	☐
	• Palpation of temporal arteries in people over 50	☐	☐	☐	☐
	• Cushing's reflex: bradycardia, hypertension, reduced respiration	☐	☐	☐	☐
	•	☐	☐	☐	☐
Causes of headache	• Tension headache, migraine	☐	☐	☐	☐
	• Space occupying lesions, e.g. primary brain tumour or metastases	☐	☐	☐	☐
	• Cluster headache	☐	☐	☐	☐
	• Subarachnoid haemorrhage	☐	☐	☐	☐
	• Meningitis	☐	☐	☐	☐
	• Temporal arteritis (in over 50s)	☐	☐	☐	☐
	• Acute angle-closure glaucoma	☐	☐	☐	☐
	•				
Investigations	• Routine full blood count and U&Es	☐	☐	☐	☐
	• Urgent CT scan of head – if subarachnoid haemorrhage is suspected followed by lumbar puncture 12 hours later (if CT negative)	☐	☐	☐	☐
	• Urgent CT head followed by lumbar puncture if meningitis is suspected (remember to start antibiotics before any tests in suspected meningococcal septicaemia); also CRP and blood cultures	☐	☐	☐	☐
	• ESR in suspected temporal arteritis	☐	☐	☐	☐
	•	☐	☐	☐	☐
Treatment	• *Bacterial meningitis*: IV antibiotics (as per local antibiotic guidelines)	☐	☐	☐	☐
	• *Subarachnoid haemorrhage*: Urgent neurosurgical referral and nimodipine 60 mg four hourly	☐	☐	☐	☐
	• *Temporal arteritis*: high dose prednisolone (60–80 mg daily)	☐	☐	☐	☐
	• *Migraine*: analgesics, antiemetics and triptans for acute episodes. Consider preventative treatment for recurrent episodes	☐	☐	☐	☐
	• *Tension headache*: simple analgesics and reassurance. Consider amitriptyline in chronic form	☐	☐	☐	☐
	•	☐	☐	☐	☐

		Self	Peer	Peer/tutor	Tutor
Self-assessed as at least borderline:	Signature:	Date:	U B S E	U B S E	U B S E	U B S E
Peer-assessed as ready for tutor assessment:	Signature:	Date:	U B S E	U B S E	U B S E	U B S E
Tutor-assessed as satisfactory:	Signature:	Date:	U B S E	U B S E	U B S E	U B S E

Notes

11.15 Management of the multi-trauma patient

Background

Trauma is the leading cause of death in young individuals and is a significant world health issue. By 2020, injury may advance to become the second or third leading cause of death in all age groups. Since the introduction of the ATLS guidelines, there have been significant improvements in the care of the injured patient. The systematic ABCDE approach enables rapid initial assessment, primary management, stabilization, and transfer to a specialist trauma centre if necessary.

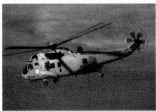
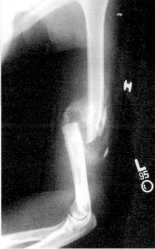
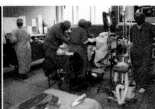

Whether your patient arrives dramatically by helicopter or ambulance, the management is the same. ABCDE approach captures the key aspects of life-saving management.

It is highly likely that multiple systems have been affected. A meticulous secondary survey is essential to define all the injuries and conditions that need to be treated.

Teamwork is even more important in managing the multi-trauma patient. Care needs to be coordinated, immediate and focused on the clinical needs of the patient, which will often change dramatically from one moment to the next.

Figure 11.19 Images in management of the multi-trauma patient. Left © Photolibrary; middle from Bill Rhodes, licensed under Creative Commons.

Diagnosis

The conventional approach of history and examination is inappropriate for patients with life-threatening injuries. There are three fundamental principles upon which ATLS management is based:

1 Treat the greatest threat to life first.

2 Commence indicated treatment without waiting to establish definitive diagnosis.

3 Do not delay evaluation of the patient in order to gain a detailed history.

Causes of multi-trauma

There are a myriad of causes of multi-trauma: all relate to physical or chemical or biological trauma. The list is vast and is as long as the imagination. The main causes encountered in clinical practice are: motor vehicle collisions, falls, burns, machinery, drowning, chemical injuries, electrical injuries, crime-weapons (including firearms, knives, blunt instruments of violence). War and natural disasters such as earthquakes, flooding and tsunamis occur sporadically but have devastating effects on communities, often due to trauma.

Management

Phase 1 initial management (first hour)

Primary survey

The aim of the primary survey is to identify life-threatening conditions and institute treatment. Although it is described as a sequence, in practice assessment of these parameters occurs simultaneously (Table 11.9).

Table 11.9 The ABCDE technique

		Assessment	Treatment	Monitoring
A	**A**irway maintenance with cervical spine protection	Look for agitation/obtundation/foreign bodies Listen for abnormal sounds Feel for location of trachea Is the GCS <8?	Chin lift Jaw thrust Airway adjuncts – oropharyngeal nasopharyngeal laryngeal mask airway definitive airway	
B	**B**reathing and ventilation	Look for symmetrical movement of chest/laboured breathing Listen for movement of air on both sides	Oxygen Bag-valve-face mask Ventilator-assisted Treat life-threatening conditions	Respiratory rate Pulse oximetry End-tidal carbon dioxide
C	**C**irculation with haemorrhage control	Look for cutaneous vasoconstriction, obvious sites of haemorrhage, evidence of trauma to upper torso Feel for temperature	Gain IV access Commence IV fluid therapy, preferably warmed or blood if available Control at sites of active haemorrhage Treat life-threatening non-haemorrhagic conditions	Heart rate Capillary refill Blood pressure Pulse pressure Mental status Urine output
D	**D**isability/neurologic status	Determine level of consciousness (AVPU) Perform brief neurological examination – pupil response, best motor function, degree of sensation	Fluid resuscitation Oxygenation	GCS/pupil response Blood glucose
E	**E**xposure/environmental control	Undress patient and perform head to toe examination	See secondary survey	

Life-threatening injuries that need to be addressed in primary survey include:

- **Tension pneumothorax** – air enters pleural space but cannot escape (one-way valve effect), causing mediastinal shift with compression of opposite lung and reduced venous return. Immediately insert large calibre needle (16 F) into second intercostal space, mid-clavicular line, followed by chest drain.
- **Open pneumothorax** – a large defect of the chest wall which is two thirds diameter of trachea causing air to flow preferentially into the chest rather than the trachea ('sucking' chest wound). Place a sterile occlusive dressing over the defect and seal with tape on three sides creating a flutter type valve. Place chest drain at site remote from wound.

- **Flail chest** – occurs with two or more rib fractures in two or more places producing a segment of the chest wall that moves paradoxically in comparison to the rest of the chest wall. Pay close attention to oxygenation, fluid resuscitation, and pain control to prevent compounding underlying lung injury.
- **Massive haemothorax** – defined as more than 1500 mL of blood or more than one-third of the patient's circulating volume in the chest cavity. Insert large-bore chest drain and replace blood loss with IV fluids or blood if available. Contact cardiothoracic team for early thoracotomy.
- **Cardiac tamponade** – pericardial effusion that compromises cardiac contractility resulting in hypotension, elevated venous pressure with distended neck veins, and muffled heart sounds. Perform pericardiocentesis and continue fluid resuscitation.

Investigations

- Cross-match
- ABGs
- ECG
- X-rays – chest/pelvis/cervical spine (trauma series)

If there are signs of shock, suspect:

- Tension pneumothorax or cardiac tamponade if patient does not respond to aggressive fluid resuscitation and there is evidence of injury to the upper torso.
- Neurogenic shock if there is no tachycardia or cutaneous vasoconstriction with evidence of possible spinal injury.

Phase 2 management (2–6 hours)

- Obtain a detailed history from patient, family, or ambulance crew
- Obtain history of injury-producing event
- Perform secondary survey consisting of head to toe examination to exclude any other injuries.

Secondary survey

- Head and skull
- Maxillofacial and intraoral
- Neck
- Chest
- Abdomen including back
- Perineum/rectum/vagina
- Musculoskeletal
- Neurologic examination

Perform log roll with cervical spine immobilization to look for spinal injury and if there is no evidence or injury, remove spinal board as early as possible.

Catheterize if there is no evidence of pelvic injury.

Consider NG tube insertion if there is no evidence of maxillofacial injury.

Further investigations

- Extremity X-rays
- Ultrasound
- CT head/chest/abdomen/pelvis
- Endoscopy
- Obtain early specialist input from neurosurgery/cardiothoracic/general/orthopaedic surgery as appropriate
- Involve obstetric or paediatric team if patient is pregnant or a child

- If injuries exceed capability of the institution, arrange transfer to a hospital with necessary facilities
- Do not delay transfer of patient as this can increase mortality.

Phase 3 ongoing management

- Monitor vital signs including urine output, if any deterioration, reassess using above ABCDE algorithm.
- Continue fluid resuscitation; if there is transient or no response, look for occult haemorrhage.
- Consider insertion of central line and arterial line for invasive monitoring.

Other aspects of treatment

- Give adequate analgesia.
- Stabilize any pelvic injury by internal rotation of the legs and use of a sling wrapped around the pelvis.
- Consider tetanus prophylaxis if patient has any open fractures or penetrating injury.
- Only use antibiotics for open fractures after consultation with a surgeon.
- Consider mannitol infusion after consultation with neurosurgeon if severe brain injury or sudden deterioration in GCS.
- Discuss events with patient's family and inform them of treatment plan.
- Arrange appropriate equipment and staff for safe transfer of patient.

Complications

- Death from traumatic injury occurs in three time periods from time of injury:
  - Immediate death due to apnoea from severe brain/high spinal cord injury or rupture of heart/aorta/large blood vessels.
  - Early deaths within minutes to several hours from extradural/subdural haemorrhage or injuries associated with large blood loss such as ruptured spleen, haemothorax or laceration in liver.
  - Late deaths several days to weeks after injury from sepsis and multiple organ dysfunction.
- Disability from severe head injury or spinal cord injury
- Morbidity from permanent end-organ dysfunction due to direct injury or from hypovolaemic shock and reduced tissue perfusion

Patient safety tips

✔ **Rapid initial assessment**: ABCDE approach enables systematic approach that can be conducted quickly and enables early intervention for life-threatening injury.

✔ **Do not delay transfer**: patient outcome is directly related to time from injury to institution of definitive care.

✔ **Talk to other specialities early**: it is important to involve other specialist teams that can provide definitive surgical care.

✔ **Trauma team**: this usually consists of a team leader, nurse, anaesthetist and doctors from other specialities including orthopaedics, general surgery, and the emergency department.

✔ **Clear instructions, delegate, communicate effectively**: the approach to a trauma patient requires the team leader to give instructions that will optimize the role of each member and enable them to work together effectively.

Trauma (ATLS)

M. Mawmsey (76 Kensington Avenue, Farnborough, CL4 8HG; date of birth 5 September 1970, hospital number GE49583759, A&E department) was thrown from his horse onto a fence while riding through the Warwickshire countryside. He has just arrived into the emergency department via ambulance, having sustained serious facial and head injuries and severe trauma to the chest and possibly abdomen. His left leg is broken.

This assessment will be based around a discussion on the management of trauma with reference to above scenario.

		Self	Peer	Peer /tutor	Tutor
Background	Leading cause of death in young. ATLS guidelines describe a systematic ABCDE approach, enabling rapid initial assessment, primary management, stabilization and transfer to a specialist trauma centre if necessary.	☐	☐	☐	☐
	•	☐	☐	☐	☐
Diagnosis	Conventional history and examination is inappropriate. Instead, follow the three principles:				
	• Treat the greatest threat to life first	☐	☐	☐	☐
	• Commence indicated treatment without waiting to establish definitive diagnosis	☐	☐	☐	☐
	• Do not delay evaluation of the patient in order to gain a detailed history	☐	☐	☐	☐
	•	☐	☐	☐	☐
Causes of trauma	• The causes of trauma are multiple, but include multi-vehicle accidents, falls, burns (heat, electrical, chemical), drowning, and weapons including firearms and knives	☐	☐	☐	☐
	• Trauma can be blunt or penetrating	☐	☐	☐	☐
	•	☐	☐	☐	☐
Phase 1 initial management (first hour)	• Follow the ABCDE algorithm to identify life-threatening conditions and commence treatment	☐	☐	☐	☐
	• **A**irway maintenance with cervical spine protection:	☐	☐	☐	☐
	○ Look for agitation/obtundation/foreign bodies, listen for abnormal sounds, palpate trachea location. Assess GCS. Treat with chin lift, jaw thrust, add airway adjuncts to form a definitive airway				
	• **B**reathing and ventilation:	☐	☐	☐	☐
	○ Look for symmetrical chest movement and laboured breathing, listen for air movement bilaterally. Give oxygen, using bag-valve-face mask and ventilator if necessary. Monitor respiratory rate, pulse oximetry and end-tidal carbon dioxide				
	• **C**irculation with haemorrhage control:	☐	☐	☐	☐
	○ Look for cutaneous vasoconstriction, obvious sites of haemorrhage, evidence of trauma to upper torso. Feel for temperature. Gain IV access and commence IV fluid therapy, preferably warmed or blood if available. Control active haemorrhage and treat life threatening non-haemorrhagic conditions. Monitor heart rate, capillary refill, blood pressure, pulse pressure, mental status and urine output				
	• **D**isability/neurologic status	☐	☐	☐	☐
	○ Determine level of consciousness (AVPU), brief neurological examination – pupil response, best motor function, degree of sensation. Give fluid resuscitation and ensure adequate oxygenation. Monitor GCS/pupil response and blood glucose.				
	• **E**xposure/environmental control	☐	☐	☐	☐
	○ Undress patient and perform head to toe examination				
	• Look for and treat life threatening injuries:	☐	☐	☐	☐
	○ Tension pneumothorax. Immediately insert large calibre needle (16 F) into second intercostal space, mid-clavicular line, followed by chest drain				
	○ Open pneumothorax. Place a sterile occlusive dressing over the defect and seal with tape on 3 sides creating a flutter type valve. Place chest drain at site remote from wound.				
	○ Flail chest. Pay close attention to oxygenation, fluid resuscitation and pain control to prevent compounding underlying lung injury				
	○ Massive haemothorax. Insert large-bore chest drain and replace blood loss with IV fluids or blood if available. Contact cardio-thoracic team for early thoracotomy.				
	○ Cardiac tamponade. Perform pericardiocentesis and continue fluid resuscitation.				
	• Investigations: Cross-match, ABG, ECG, trauma series X-rays (chest/pelvis/cervical spine), consider DPL/FAST scan.	☐	☐	☐	☐
	• If there are signs of shock, suspect tension pneumothorax or cardiac tamponade (if patient does not respond to aggressive fluid resuscitation and there is evidence of injury to the upper torso) or neurogenic shock (if there is no tachycardia or cutaneous vasoconstriction with evidence of possible spinal injury).	☐	☐	☐	☐
	•	☐	☐	☐	☐

Phase 2 management (2–6 hours)	● Obtain a detailed history from patient, family, or ambulance crew	☐	☐	☐	☐
	● Obtain history of injury-producing event	☐	☐	☐	☐
	● Perform secondary survey consisting of head to toe examination to exclude any other injuries, including: head and skull, maxillofacial and intra-oral, neck, chest, abdomen including back, perineum/rectum/vagina, musculoskeletal, neurological examination	☐	☐	☐	☐
	● Log roll with cervical spine immobilization to look for spinal injury. If there is no evidence or injury, remove spinal board as early as possible	☐	☐	☐	☐
	● Catheterize if there is no evidence of pelvic injury	☐	☐	☐	☐
	● Consider NG tube insertion if there is no evidence of maxillofacial injury	☐	☐	☐	☐
	● Relevant further investigations: extremity X-rays, ultrasound, CT head/chest/abdomen/pelvis, endoscopy	☐	☐	☐	☐
	● Obtain early specialist input from neurosurgery/cardiothoracic/general/orthopaedic surgery as appropriate	☐	☐	☐	☐
	● Involve obstetric or paediatric team if patient is pregnant or a child	☐	☐	☐	☐
	● If injuries exceed capability of the institution, arrange transfer to a hospital with necessary facilities. Do not delay transfer	☐	☐	☐	☐
	●	☐	☐	☐	☐
Phase 3 ongoing management	● Monitor vital signs including urine output, if any deterioration, reassess using ABCDE algorithm	☐	☐	☐	☐
	● Continue fluid resuscitation; if there is transient or no response, look for occult haemorrhage	☐	☐	☐	☐
	● Consider insertion of central line and arterial line for invasive monitoring	☐	☐	☐	☐
	●	☐	☐	☐	☐
Other aspects of treatment	● Provide adequate analgesia	☐	☐	☐	☐
	● Stabilize pelvic injuries	☐	☐	☐	☐
	● Consider tetanus prophylaxis for open fractures or penetrating injuries	☐	☐	☐	☐
	● Consult a surgeon before using antibiotics for open fractures	☐	☐	☐	☐
	● Consult with neurosurgeon for mannitol infusion if severe brain injury or sudden deterioration in GCS	☐	☐	☐	☐
	● Discuss events with patient's family and inform them of treatment plan	☐	☐	☐	☐
	● Arrange appropriate equipment and staff for safe patient transfer	☐	☐	☐	☐
	●	☐	☐	☐	☐
Complications	● Death occurs in three time periods from time of injury:	☐	☐	☐	☐
	1 Immediate (apnoea and cardiac or major vessel rupture)				
	2 Minutes to hours (extradural/subdural haemorrhage or injuries associated with large blood loss such as ruptured spleen, haemothorax or liver laceration)				
	3 Days to weeks (sepsis and multiple organ dysfunction).				
	● Disability arises from severe head or spinal cord injury.	☐	☐	☐	☐
	● Morbidity from permanent end-organ dysfunction due to direct injury or hypovolaemic shock and ischaemia	☐	☐	☐	☐
	●	☐	☐	☐	☐
Patient safety tips	● Rapid initial ABCDE assessment saves lives	☐	☐	☐	☐
	● Do not delay transfer	☐	☐	☐	☐
	● Involve other specialities early	☐	☐	☐	☐
	● Clear instructions, delegate, communicate effectively	☐	☐	☐	☐
	● Team leader to optimize the role of each member and enable team to work together effectively	☐	☐	☐	☐
	●	☐	☐	☐	☐
Clinical note writing and handover	Transfer to another hospital may be required if injuries exceed capability of the institution. Do not delay transfer as this can increase mortality. Obtain specialist input early	☐	☐	☐	☐
	●	☐	☐	☐	☐

	Signature:	Date:				
Self-assessed as at least borderline:	Signature:	Date:	U B S E	U B S E	U B S E	U B S E
Peer-assessed as ready for tutor assessment:	Signature:	Date:	U B S E	U B S E	U B S E	U B S E
Tutor-assessed as satisfactory:	Signature:	Date:	U B S E	U B S E	U B S E	U B S E

Notes

Suite 4 Professional skills

Unit 12 Public health: health promotion and health inequalities

12.1 Reducing health inequalities

Background

Each clinical encounter should be seen as a potential opportunity to influence the future health of the patient that you are seeing. In many cases there will also be the chance to have a discussion with the family, relatives or carer or even the community in relation to the clinical situation, for example risk of diabetes. It may for example be opportune, if sensitivities allow, to discuss smoking cessation with a family after a patient has been admitted with community-acquired pneumonia in a patient with chronic obstructive pulmonary disease. Health promotion can equally be called 'ill health prevention'. Clinicians working in the acute and urgent sectors in healthcare sometimes need persuading that 'ill health prevention' skills are just as important as acute care skills such as leading a cardiac arrest team. These skills have potential to improve morbidity and mortality, albeit in a different temporal axis – the future.

The clinical encounter can therefore be deconstructed into the following three strands – a *triple helix* of intertwining stories or agendas that should always take place.

- **Patient's story and agenda**: clearly the whole clinical encounter must revolve around the issues that have been presented. A thorough clinical history and examination, together with a specific exploration of the patient's ideas, concerns and expectations will allow full elucidation of the clinical context. Often the patient's carers, family and other advocates will help with this process.

- **Professional agenda**: as clinicians we relish the diagnosis and outlining a care plan that works. Ultimately we want patients to get better or be helped in some way with their clinical problem. This must be individualized to each patient, evidence-based, ideally, and safely delivered to a competent standard.

- **Public health and reducing health inequalities agenda**: this component is often glossed over in the busy humdrum of everyday clinical practice. Just a few minutes dedicated to this can potentially reap many future benefits for your patient, and their family and community.

This section will review practical aspects of reducing health inequalities and then focus on the key aspects of health psychology that help develop clinical skills to reduce health inequalities. The following section on health promotion and ill-health risk assessment relies on principles and skills learnt from this section.

Health inequalities

"It is easier to build strong children than to repair broken men."
Frederick Douglass (US Social Reformer and Statesman, 1818–95)

When we talk about health inequalities we need to consider what determines good health and what we mean by this? Firstly, health is more than absence of disease. It is about a sense of wellbeing. It is also about how much control we have over our lives, including the personal, social, and material assets available to us to make health promoting choices and changes for good health.

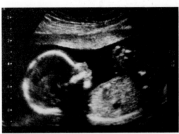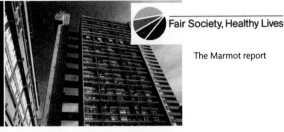

Fair Society, Healthy Lives

The Marmot report

The 'fetal housing' is increasingly recognized as being vital to future well being. Many cardiovascular diseases, diabetes, and learning difficulties have their origins in poor feto-maternal nutrition and factors such as maternal smoking and nutrition.

Poorer quality social housing itself can have an impact on life expectancy through low expectations of life being manifest in behaviours leading to future health risk such as smoking, low levels of physical activity and low educational achievement.

Figure 12.1 Images in reducing health inequalities. Left © Isabelle Limbach/iStockphoto; middle © Photodisc; right © The Marmot Review 2011

Health inequalities, at the simplest level, can be defined as the differences in the health status of one group of people compared with another. It is generally accepted that society should govern itself such that the better health status achieved in any specific group is later enjoyed by the whole society. There are marked differences in health between people from different social and economic situations, which are partly explained by their circumstances such as disposable income, educational achievement, the kind of housing in which they live, and ease of access to transport. The differences in health can be measured in terms of both ill health and disease (morbidity) and death (mortality).

Health inequalities can be described by geographical area, for example comparing people living in one local authority or neighbourhood with another. As well as geographical differences in health indicators, there are other dimensions of health inequalities such as age, gender, ethnicity, disability, socioeconomic position, legal status, and institutionalization. We cannot eliminate all the differences that may exist between different groups but we do want to focus on those differences that are avoidable, unnecessary, and unjust. For example, differences in health outcomes relating to differences in income or socioeconomic position may be considered to be unfair and unjust. Such differences that are unfair and unjust are sometimes more correctly referred to as health 'inequities'. However, the term inequalities is used as this is a more familiar term than inequities.

Key facts

- **Life expectancy**: varies significantly with socioeconomic deprivation. People in the poorest areas live an average of 7 years less than those living in the richest areas. If everyone enjoyed the same health as university graduates, then there would be an estimated 200 000 fewer deaths in England.

- **Inequalities start in childhood**: what happens in early childhood including in the womb, has lifelong effects on many aspects of health and wellbeing from obesity, heart disease, cognitive development, educational attainment, mental health, and eventual economic status.

- **Social support and connections**: have a significant impact on health and health inequalities. These links that connect people to their communities can be a source of resilience and act as a buffer against particular risks of poor health.

- **Ill health prevention and promoting health is important**: Differences in smoking prevalence is the single most important contributor to inequalities in avoidable deaths between different socioeconomic groups.

Fair Society, Healthy Lives, a strategic review of health inequalities in England by Sir Michael Marmot published in 2010 makes recommendations around six policy objectives for tackling health inequalities:

- Give every child the best start in life
- Enable all children, young people, and adults to maximize their capabilities and have control over their lives
- Create fair employment and good work for all
- Ensure healthy standard of living for all
- Create and develop healthy and sustainable places and communities
- Strengthen the role and impact of ill health prevention.

What can a clinician do?

All healthcare systems, and particularly the National Health Service (NHS), need to play their part in ensuring everything that its clinicians do enhances individual and community resources to maximize good health. Furthermore, for the NHS to fully realize its role as a 'health' service rather than 'sickness' service, every clinician can actively consider the opportunity to promote health **at every encounter** with a patient. All clinicians should make it their professional business to address this in their daily encounters with patients.

Key actions for a clinician are to:

- **Be knowledgeable about the wider social determinants of health and health inequalities**: and how these impact on an individual's health and wellbeing.

- **Ensure active consideration of the social and economic influences**: when giving clinical advice and support to a patient, these may impact on their ability to respond to treatment, advice, and behavioural change (see Figure 12.2).

- **Make every contact with a patient count as an opportunity to promote health**: such as advice and support for stopping smoking, promoting physical activity, and healthy weight and diet.

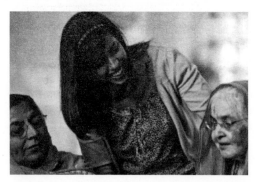

Figure 12.2 Healthcare should be individualized to the patient. Health education and promotion is often effective at the community level especially if culturally sensitive. © Xavier Arnau/iStockphoto

Health psychology skills in reducing health inequalities

Recent developments, for example *A Core Curriculum for Psychology on Undergraduate Medical Education* and *Tomorrows Doctors: incorporating Psychological Principles and Knowledge to Medical Practice*, stress some of the following key aspects of health psychology in relation to daily clinical practice.

The bio-psychosocial approach: understanding the interaction between physical, psychological, and social processes

Health and illness are determined by a combination of biological, psychological, and social factors.

The bio-psychosocial model draws on the mind/body interaction, where the person is seen as a whole. In addition to biological factors, psychosocial factors include cognitions, emotions and behaviours, social values of health and illness, culture and ethnicity, and social class. In a clinical setting, assessment and treatment should incorporate attitudes and beliefs, behaviour change, and coping strategies.

Psychological factors in health and illness: health behaviour and beliefs, illness behaviour and beliefs, illness cognitions

Health beliefs and illness representations will influence a patient's decisions to engage in changing behaviours and concord with treatment plans. The 'health belief model' highlights how core beliefs including perceived susceptibility, severity, benefits and barriers to behaviour change directly influence whether a patient engages in behaviour change. Attitudes and self efficacy (the belief that one has the ability, skills, and confidence) are also important contributions (theory of planned behaviour). Illness cognitions include a patient's own 'common sense' belief about their illness and generate a general understanding, coping framework, and appraisal. Five key elements are identity, perceived cause of illness, time line, consequences and curability, and controllability.

- **The doctor–patient relationship and decision making**

The doctor–patient relationship is fundamental in determining process and outcomes. Patient-centred communication is the eliciting of patients' ideas, concerns, and expectations (ICE). A biopsychosocial approach facilitates patient participation during the consultation. Verbal and non-verbal communication skills are important within patient-centred communication, improving patient satisfaction, patient recall, and adherence to treatment. Shared decision making is also improved by tailoring advice, informing patients, and discussing treatment options which again lead to better patient outcomes.

- **Chronic illness (long-term conditions)**

Understanding psychological and social factors are crucial to the self-management of chronic illness and diseases. Illness perceptions, health beliefs, and cognitions such as fear, anxiety, self efficacy, and catastrophizing will impact on management and coping strategies. Screening for co-morbidities such as depression, offering psychological interventions and patient education are important features.

- **Addiction – psychological interventions aimed at behaviour change**

Recognizing and screening for addiction is an important clinical skill. As discussed above it is crucial to consider the beliefs, perceptions, and cognitions of the patient before working on a treatment plan. The Prochaska and DiClemente transtheoretical model of behaviour change provides a framework for the process of behaviour change and maintenance. How successful a patient is in behaviour change is determined by stage progression (pre-contemplation, contemplation, preparation, action, and maintenance). Psychological interventions help assess the patient as well as motivate them to progress through the each stage.

Student name:	Medical school:	Year:

Reducing health inequalities

This assessment will be based around a discussion of two patients describing their life experiences and general principles in relation to reducing health inequalities and health psychology skills.

Charles

Baby — Born to affluent parents - will live 10 years longer than Mark

10 — Enjoying a good life, lots of opportunity to play sport

20 — At university with 10 x A* at GCSE. Plays rugby and eats a healthy diet

45 — Fit and healthy businessman, manages stress by playing squash

60 — Retired early to spend time with his grandchildren and travel

Mark

Baby — One of teenage conceptions. Will live 10 years less than Charles

10 — Growing up in poverty

20 — Left school with no qualifications, casual labourer, drinks, smokes and takes drugs

45 — Weighs 18 stone, has high cholesterol, type 2 diabetes

60 — Died from massive stroke

NHS North West SHA

		Self	Peer	Peer /tutor	Tutor
How can the clinical encounter be deconstructed into the three main agendas of clinical care?	• Patient's story and agenda	☐	☐	☐	☐
	• Professional agenda	☐	☐	☐	☐
	• Public health and reducing health inequalities agenda	☐	☐	☐	☐
	•	☐	☐	☐	☐
In the scenario about Mark presented above what key interventions may have helped reduce the life expectancy by around 10 years?	•	☐	☐	☐	☐
What are the six policy objectives for tackling health inequalities in Fair Society, Health Lives, the strategic review of health inequalities in England 2010, by Sir Michael Marmot?	• Give every child the best start in life	☐	☐	☐	☐
	• Enable all children, young people, and adults to maximize capabilities and control over their lives	☐	☐	☐	☐
	• Create fair employment and good work for all	☐	☐	☐	☐
	• Ensure healthy standard of living for all	☐	☐	☐	☐
	• Create and develop healthy and sustainable places and communities	☐	☐	☐	☐
	• Strengthen the role and impact of ill health prevention	☐	☐	☐	☐
	•	☐	☐	☐	☐
What are the key actions to consider in every clinical encounter?	• Be aware of the wider social determinants of health and health inequalities and how these impact on an individual's health and wellbeing	☐	☐	☐	☐
	• Ensure when giving clinical advice and support, there is active consideration of the social and economic influences which may impact on their ability to respond to treatment	☐	☐	☐	☐
	• Make every contact with a patient count as an opportunity to promote health, such as advice and support for stopping smoking, promoting physical activity, and healthy weight and diet	☐	☐	☐	☐
	•	☐	☐	☐	☐
What are the key aspects of health psychology that apply in relation to daily clinical practice?	• **Biopsychosocial approach**: interaction between physical, psychological, and social processes	☐	☐	☐	☐
	• **Psychological factors in health and illness**: health and illness behaviour and beliefs	☐	☐	☐	☐
	• **Doctor–patient relationship and decision making**: patient-centred, exploring ICE	☐	☐	☐	☐
	• **Long-term conditions: chronic illness**: promote self management of chronic illness	☐	☐	☐	☐
	• **Addiction – psychological interventions**: recognizing, screening for, and treating addiction	☐	☐	☐	☐
	•	☐	☐	☐	☐

				U B S E	U B S E	U B S E	U B S E
Self-assessed as at least borderline:	Signature:		Date:				
Peer-assessed as ready for tutor assessment:	Signature:		Date:				
Tutor-assessed as satisfactory:	Signature:		Date:				

Notes

12.2 Health promotion and behavioural change

Background

The burden of mortality, morbidity, and disability attributable to long-term conditions (non-communicable and chronic disease) is rapidly increasing and poses a significant strain on healthcare resources. Many are associated with nutritional transitions from traditional high-fibre, low-fat diets to Westernized energy-dense, high-fat diets, accompanied by reductions in physical activity and an increase in high-risk activities, particularly smoking and unprotected sex. Evidence strongly suggests that the majority of long-term conditions may be preventable before the age of 75 years. The Inter-Heart Study reported that 90% of the risk of myocardial infarction was due to abnormal lipids, smoking, hypertension, diabetes, abdominal obesity, psychosocial factors, reduced consumption of fruits and vegetables, alcohol and reduced physical activity. Approximately 80% of heart disease, stroke, and type 2 diabetes cases and over 33% of cancers could be prevented by eliminating tobacco and excessive alcohol consumption, maintaining a healthy diet and being physically active. These risk factors have been declared by the World Health Organization (WHO) as the main shared risk factors in the development of long-term conditions including cancers. WHO has devised a 5-year action plan (2008–2013) for the global strategy for the prevention and control of non-communicable diseases, which aims to prevent and control cardiovascular diseases, cancers, chronic respiratory diseases, and diabetes. One of the six objectives of this plan is to 'promote interventions to reduce the main shared modifiable risk factors for non-communicable diseases: tobacco use, unhealthy diets, physical inactivity and harmful use of alcohol'.

Patient-focused interventions require patients to be actively involved in the process of securing appropriate, effective, and safe healthcare, and aim to ensure a more personalized service. Patient-focused interventions are commonly aimed at improving health literacy, clinical decision making, self-care, patient safety, access to health advice, better experience of care, and health service development. Clinicians need to be expert at recognizing risk factors that compromise future health and in behavioural change.

The HEALTH (Helping Everyone Achieve Long Term Health) concept

The HEALTH passport (Figure 12.3) is a patient hand-held record designed to allow assessment of risk to long-term health through a consideration of the 10 most important risk factors. It is a public domain tool that can be printed locally. The idea was developed following an in-depth review of existing clinical research into long-term conditions and their prevention. From this evidence base, the modifiable risk factors stated on the HEALTH passport were identified. The concept of the HEALTH passport is based on the progression from an evidence base, to a Health CHAT (Comprehensive Health Assessment Talk) and finally to providing an individualized action plan. The ideas can remind us to think about health promotion in every clinical encounter. Other patient-specific health promotion factors should be added by the healthcare professional.

The HEALTH passport identifies the 10 most important modifiable risk factors for achieving long-term health under the 4 ABCD headings:

- **Advice**: not to smoke, normal weight, physically active, consume five portions of fruit and vegetables daily, avoid alcohol and drug misuse, safe sexual behaviour, 'five-a-day' programme for mental wellbeing.
- **Blood pressure (BP)**: undergo regular BP monitoring and treatment if indicated.
- **Cholesterol check**: know your cholesterol (especially >40 years) and have treatment if indicated.
- **Diabetes** prevention or good control.

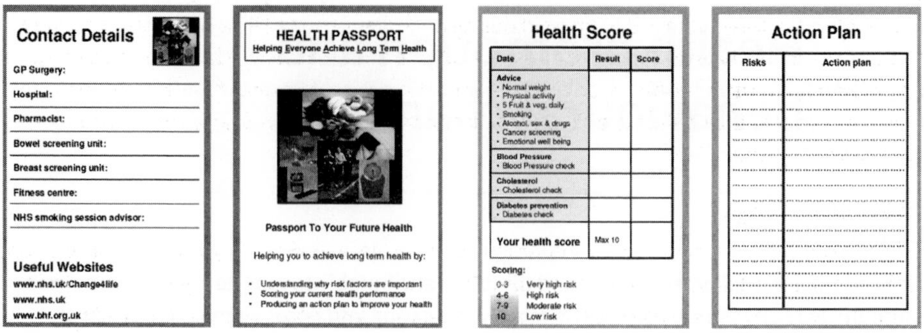

The HEALTH passport is an evidence-based approach to risk assessing individuals with respect to their future health. It is estimated that these 10 risk factors account for around 75% of all LTC, including cancer, before the age of 75 years.

The individual is assessed and a personalized action plan constructed according to the individual's desire for optimizing future health and local available resources to help change behaviour.

Figure 12.3 The HEALTH passport.

Aspects in relation to improving or maintaining good mental health are worthy of further detail.

In 2008, the New Economics Foundation was commissioned by the UK Government's Foresight Project on Mental Capital and Well-being to review the work of over 400 scientists from across the world. The aim was to identify a set of evidence-based actions to improve wellbeing and mental health. The overall conclusion was that five simple steps could be incorporated into daily life that can benefit mental health. This can contribute to a more productive and fulfilling life.

The 'five-a-day' programme for mental wellbeing (akin to the five-a-day fruit and vegetables daily) encourages people to:

● **Connect**: developing relationships with family, friends, colleagues, and neighbours to enrich your life and bring you support.

● **Be active**: sports, hobbies such as gardening or dancing, or just a daily stroll will make you feel good and maintain mobility and fitness. Outdoor activities with nature may have added benefit.

● **Be curious and live in the moment**: noting the beauty of everyday moments as well as the unusual and reflecting on them helps you to appreciate what matters to you. Trying to pick one positive moment from every day is a useful exercise.

● **Learn something new**: the challenge and satisfaction of this brings fun and improves confidence: e.g. cooking, DIY (be careful!), fixing a bike, learning an instrument, computer use, reading new things, swimming

● **Give**: A bit of philanthropy – helping friends and strangers – links your happiness to a wider community and is very rewarding. Such voluntary work or charity can be local, national or international of course.

The HEALTH passport aims to improve health literacy by providing patients with the evidence as to why they should consider modifying risk factors for long-term conditions accompanied by the evidence for the benefits of change. By increasing patient awareness, understanding, and health ownership through engaging patients in their healthcare, it is hoped that concordance with lifestyle interventions will be greatly improved, increasing the efficacy of healthcare services and reducing the burden of long-term conditions. Generally, two facts are given about each risk factor, followed by what can be done to address the risk if applicable.

As patients often forget things that are said during consultations, the HEALTH passport provides a simple record of what was discussed and agreed for the future review, which may be carried out personally or with a health coach or another healthcare professional. A further section is provided to record the contact details of local healthcare services, fitness centres, and other physical activity amenities.

Behavioural change

All health promotion requires the commitment, knowledge, and ability of the individual to adopt significant lifestyle changes in order to modify the current risk factors affecting their long-term health. Behavioural change models such as that proposed by Prochaska and DiClemente demonstrate the processes which must be undertaken to enable such a change in behaviour:

1   **Pre-contemplation**: no intent to change behaviour. ? unaware change is needed or possible.

2   **Contemplation**: considering but not committed to taking action.

3   **Preparation**: intention to change, minor behaviour such as collecting information, and deciding when change should take place.

4   **Action**: change of behaviour occurs.

5   **Maintenance**: maintain new behaviour.

6   **Relapse**: returning to old behaviours, abandoning the new changes but often potential to restart above cycle again towards permanent change. Smokers will relapse many times before cessation.

Prochaska and DiClemente noted that this is a cyclical process involving both progress and relapse and affected by social, cultural, ethical, spiritual, resource, political, and legal factors. As individuals progress through the stages at their own rate, the patient should decide when a stage is completed and when to progress to the next stage in order to achieve stable, long-term change. It is, therefore, essential for the patient to take control of their lifestyle choices, with the support of their healthcare professional. Other theories of behavioural change further support the evidence for self-efficacy, motivation, and need for patient-led interventions when implementing behavioural change.

A health promotion implementation algorithm and a very short model for discussing specific risk factors is shown in Figures 12.4 and 12.5, respectively. In the algorithm it is assumed that the HEALTH passport or similar approach has been used and the person has scored 7 out of 10.

Patient safety

One should not immediately assume that all the main aspects of health promotion would be entirely risk-free. As always, the advice should be individualized to the patient, making sure that it is safe, culturally appropriate, and likely to be of distinct benefit to the patient. Potential pitfalls include:

✔ **Calorie restriction**: in a patient on insulin or sulfonylureas. Treatment should be adjusted to account for the high risk of hypoglycaemia.

✔ **Physical activity**: a sudden increase may be hazardous in unstable angina, severe osteo-arthritis. Remember one person's 2 km walk is another person's marathon!

✔ **Five portions of fruit and vegetables daily**: this includes fruit juices which often have in excess of 10% sugars which can worsen glycaemic control in diabetes.

✔ **Smoking cessation**: will always benefit the patient, but watch out for worsening of asthma initially, in all cases easily treated by advising on augmenting treatment if needed.

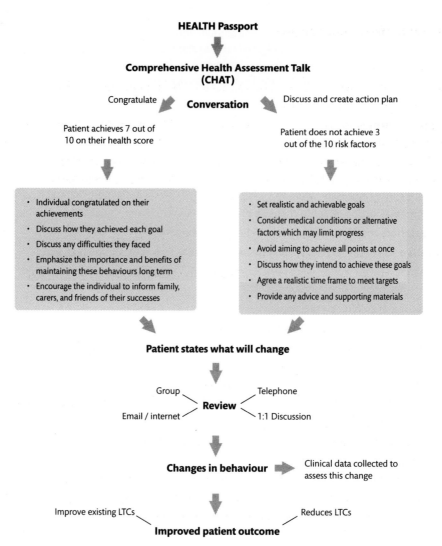

Figure 12.4 HEALTH promotion implementation algorithm.

3-Minute Behaviour Change Model

What stage is the patient:	
Pre-contemplation	What do you think about smoking?
Contemplation Preparation Action Maintenance (Relapse)	Do you really think that you can give up smoking ?
Conviction? Confidence?	How confident are you that you will be able to give up smoking?

Figure 12.5 A schematic representation of the 3-minute behaviour change model in action, using the Health Passport Approach.

HEALTH passport: facts and action plan

Advice:

Physical activity

- Regular exercise can reduce the risk of becoming obese or developing diabetes by 50%.
- Weight-bearing exercise reduces osteoporosis and fracture risk.

   Exercising for 30 minutes, five times a week, reduces the risk of heart disease and stroke.

5 Fruit and vegetables daily

- Reduces risk of heart disease (20%), stroke (11%), cancer and reduces symptoms of asthma.
- Nutrients in fruit and vegetables support bone health and reduce the risk of osteoporosis.

   Aim to eat 400 g of fruit and vegetables daily; fresh, canned, frozen, dried, juice all count.

Normal weight

- Being overweight increases your risk of diabetes, breast and colon cancer, stroke and heart disease.
- If overweight, 5% weight loss reduces diabetes risk by 50% and reduces blood pressure.

   Try to reduce your fat, sugar, and carbohydrate intake and increase physical activity.

Smoking

- Smokers have a 15 times increased risk of lung cancer.
- On average, smokers die 10 years earlier than non-smokers.

   1 in 6 people successfully stop smoking with nicotine replacement therapy.

Alcohol, sex, and drugs

- Heavy drinkers have increased risk of liver cirrhosis (×13), stroke, dementia.
- 61 863 men and 61 155 women diagnosed with *Chlamydia* in the UK in 2008. Practise safe sex!
- Drug use is linked to anxiety, depression, and psychosis.

   Drink responsibly; maximum 2 units per day for women, 3 for men.

Cancer screening

- Cervical screening prevents 6000 women dying of cervical cancer per year in UK
- Up to 1 in 6 colon cancer deaths can be prevented with bowel screening.

   Be aware of signs and symptoms of cancer and attend screening session.

Emotional wellbeing

- Aerobic and strength exercises can reduce anxiety, stress, and mild to moderate depression.
- Insomnia leads to increased risk of a psychiatric disorder.

   Every day try to be physically active, connect with family, friends, and neighbours, learn a new skill, help others and positively reflect on one aspect of the day.

Blood pressure

- A blood pressure of 140/90 mmHg or higher increases the risk of heart attacks and stroke.
- Improving your diet and increasing physical activity reduces high blood pressure in over-weight individuals.

   Reduce salt intake to 5 g per day, exercise and get your blood pressure checked regularly

Cholesterol

- Too much cholesterol can cause blockages in the arteries leading to heart attacks and stroke.
- Statins (cholesterol lowering drugs) can reduce heart disease and strokes by 33%.

   Aim for a cholesterol of below 5 mmol/L or below 4 mmol/L in heart disease, stroke, or diabetes patients.

Diabetes prevention and control

- Men who smoke 40 cigarettes a day are 45% more likely to develop diabetes than non-smokers.
- People aged over 45 years or with a waist circumference above 94 cm (men) or 80 cm (women), a family history of diabetes or history of high blood pressure or heart disease are at greater risk.

   4 in 5 cases of type 2 diabetes below the age of 65 can be prevented by weight management, exercise, and a healthy diet.

Student name: Medical school: Year:

Health promotion and reducing health inequalities

Please consider the following case history and advise on various aspects of health promotion and reducing health inequalities.

Hetty Sorrel (Inglenook Cottage, On Bede Farm End, Adamtown, hospital number GE69351, Lewes Ward) was admitted because of nausea, vomiting, and increasing cough and wheeze. She is known to have asthma and lives in a small privately rented flat with damp and fungal blackening of the bathroom and bedroom walls. She smokes 15 cigarettes a day and has around 2 pints of cider per day. She is not tolerating any oral fluids or food at all. Her blood β-human chorionic gonadotrophin is positive. She is 28 years old. Her investigations on admission were as follows:

Hb 9.8 g/dL Potassium B_{12} 122 ng/dL
Folate 3.2 µmol/dL 3.1 mmol/L

		Self	Peer	Peer /tutor	Tutor
What are the main health promotion factors that can be identified in the above scenario?	• Smoking: details to calculate pack years of smoking	☐	☐	☐	☐
	• Excess alcohol, quantifies in units	☐	☐	☐	☐
	• Asks about the other potential risk to future health	☐	☐	☐	☐
	•	☐	☐	☐	☐
What does the data show, how would you interpret it and what diagnoses can be made?	• Patient is pregnant with hyperemesis gravidarum	☐	☐	☐	☐
	• Potassium level is low	☐	☐	☐	☐
	• There is anaemia with low B_{12}	☐	☐	☐	☐
	•	☐	☐	☐	☐
What additional factors should be considered to address health inequalities/ health promotion	• Dietary history: note results	☐	☐	☐	☐
	• Fungal growth due to damp, may worsen asthma, ? contact council	☐	☐	☐	☐
	• Potassium is low ? low intake of fruit ? hyperemesis or both	☐	☐	☐	☐
	•	☐	☐	☐	☐
State the 10 main aspects of health promotion in relation to the HEALTH passport concept	• **Advice**:	☐	☐	☐	☐
	○ Not to smoke	☐	☐	☐	☐
	○ Normal weight	☐	☐	☐	☐
	○ Physical activity	☐	☐	☐	☐
	○ Consume five portions of fruit and vegetables daily	☐	☐	☐	☐
	○ Avoid alcohol and drug misuse	☐	☐	☐	☐
	○ Safe sexual behaviour	☐	☐	☐	☐
	○ Mental wellbeing programme	☐	☐	☐	☐
	• **BP**: undergo regular BP monitoring and treatment if indicated	☐	☐	☐	☐
	• **Cholesterol check**: knowing your cholesterol and treatment if indicated	☐	☐	☐	☐
	• **Diabetes**: prevention or good control	☐	☐	☐	☐
	•	☐	☐	☐	☐
States the components of the 'five-a-day' programme for mental wellbeing	• **Connect**: developing relationships to enrich your life and bring you support.	☐	☐	☐	☐
	• **Be active**: sports, hobbies, daily stroll, outdoor activities with nature	☐	☐	☐	☐
	• **Be curious and live in the moment**: see beauty, reflect, positive moments.	☐	☐	☐	☐
	• **Learn something new**: challenge and satisfaction improves confidence (is fun)	☐	☐	☐	☐
	• **Give**: philanthropy: voluntary work/charity; local, national or international	☐	☐	☐	☐
	•	☐	☐	☐	☐
Please role play a consultation in relation to one health promotion issue using the Prochaska and DiClemente model of behavioural change	• Pre-contemplation→	☐	☐	☐	☐
	• Contemplation →	☐	☐	☐	☐
	• Preparation →	☐	☐	☐	☐
	• Action→	☐	☐	☐	☐
	• Maintenance	☐	☐	☐	☐
	•	☐	☐	☐	☐

				U B S E	U B S E	U B S E	U B S E
Self-assessed as at least borderline:	Signature:		Date:	U B S E	U B S E	U B S E	U B S E
Peer-assessed as ready for tutor assessment:	Signature:		Date:	U B S E	U B S E	U B S E	U B S E
Tutor-assessed as satisfactory:	Signature:		Date:	U B S E	U B S E	U B S E	U B S E

Notes

Unit 13 Prescribing

13.1 Background and the legal prescription

Background

The sanction to prescribe drugs is a defining characteristic of doctors and other clinicians such as pharmacists, nurses, dentists and veterinary surgeons. There are many more dimensions to prescribing than the writing of the prescription alone. There are specific skills in relation to prescribing drugs that documents such as *Tomorrow's Doctors* (2009) emphasize.

- **Ensuring patient safety, clinical effectiveness, evidence-based practice, and cost-efficiency**: these are over-arching principles that apply to activities in relation to the use of drugs.
- **Establishing an accurate drug history**: specific doses should be recorded. All prescribed and non-prescribed drugs, including complementary medications and illicit drug use, should be stated.
- **Allergies**: to any drugs must be recorded together with the nature of the allergy, i.e. rash, anaphylaxis along with drug intolerances.
- **Ability to plan therapy for common indications**.
- **Write safe and legal prescriptions**: manually or electronically.
- **Calculate appropriate drug doses**: for the individual patient taking into account factors such as weight, age, renal function, ethnicity, pregnancy.
- **Clinically monitor the outcomes of prescribing**: in relation to biochemistry and change in clinical state and drug levels, for example, treatment of hypertension or epilepsy.
- **Choose an appropriate route of administration of drug**: for the clinical condition and patient preference.
- **Involve the patient in drug choices where appropriate**: prescribing should always take place within a clinical culture that promotes patient education.
- **Self-management**: by the patient based on patient education, care planning, and drug information.
- **Ability to access reliable and safe information about drugs**.
- **Ability to detect and report significant drug reactions**: both locally and nationally.
- **Ability to manage patient-individualized factors in relation to concordance with treatment**.

Full use should be made of local formularies as these reflect local professional practice. These protocols are also usually widely known, liable to be cost-effective, and safer to follow; however, remember that formularies are not set in stone and remain changeable to the clinical needs of the patient, introduction of new medications and devices, changing costs of medications, and changing professional guidance. The latter is especially relevant in relation to national guidelines such as those from the National Institute for Health and Clinical Excellence (NICE) or the Royal Colleges.

Aims

The aims of this unit are to:

- Promote and aid good prescribing techniques with a special focus on patient safety and evidence-based practice
- Increase knowledge of prescribing in common clinical situations.

Objectives

The objectives of this unit are to:

- Learn the practical aspects of safe prescribing
- Increase knowledge of commonly used drugs
- Learn how to prescribe intravenous (IV) fluids
- Increase awareness of safe prescribing in pregnancy to prevent fetal malformations
- Increase awareness of medications with a narrow therapeutic range
- Increase awareness of routes of administration.

Clinical prescribing

Medicines should be prescribed only when they are necessary, and in all cases the benefit of administering the medicine should be considered in relation to the risk involved. This is particularly important during pregnancy when the risk to both mother and fetus must be considered. There are often specific changes that are needed for prescribing in the elderly and within other disease states such as liver and renal failure. Extensive use of the UK *British National Formulary* (BNF) has been made in creating this unit. In UK, the BNF, both the printed version and electronic version, remains the single most valuable tool in safe prescribing and should be used extensively in daily clinical practice.

It is important to discuss treatment options carefully with the patient to enable them to make an informed decision about taking prescribed medications. The patient should be helped in distinguishing the side effects of prescribed drugs from the effects of the medical disorder. If the beneficial effects of the medicine are likely to be delayed, the patient should be advised of this. This is particularly important in relation to the treatment of depression, when there can be little or no beneficial effect for several weeks. Patients should also receive advice about how to discontinue medications safely (such as β-blockers).

The prescriber and the patient should agree on desirable health outcomes and on the strategy for achieving them ('concordance'). The prescriber should be sensitive to religious, cultural, and personal beliefs that can affect patients' acceptance of medicines. For example, some patients will not want animal products such as gelatine capsules and prefer tablets or liquid forms of the medication. On the other hand, heparin, although often of porcine origin, is acceptable to all communities because of its use in preventing serious illness. Given a life or death situation, certain communities may be open to accepting medication they would ordinarily reject. Prescribers should, sensitively, obtain a full drug history from the patient to include any over-the-counter (OTC) or illegal drugs which should be taken into account when further prescriptions are made. Alternative treatments, including herbal, homeopathic, Chinese, Indian Ayurvedic and other medication should be listed in a drug history if possible. These often have powerful therapeutic or unwanted effects. Occasionally they also contain unknown amounts of standard treatments such as steroids and oral hypo-glycaemic agents.

Generic names of drugs should be used in prescribing. This will enable any suitable product to be dispensed, thereby saving delay to the patient and sometimes expense to the health service. The only exception is where bioavailability problems are so important that the patient should always receive the same brand (in such cases, the brand name and/or the manufacturer should be stated).

Prescribers should advise patients if treatment is likely to affect their ability to drive a motor vehicle (e.g. insulin, other hypoglycaemic agents). This applies especially to drugs with sedative effects; patients should be warned that these effects are increased by alcohol.

Prescription writing

The legal prescription

It is absolutely essential to include in all prescriptions:

- **Full name and address of the patient**: state allergies on inpatient drug chart and the type of reaction, e.g. rash, anaphylaxis, intolerance.
- **Age or date of birth** of the patient should be stated. State age if < 12 years.
- **Legible text**: printed or written legibly in black ink or otherwise so as to be indelible.
- **Dated and signed by the prescriber**: the prescriber's name should be given under the signature in most cases.
- **Drug details**: clearly state for each drug: dose, strength, route, and frequency. Do not abbreviate drug names.
- If amending the prescription draw a line through the incorrect part and initial and date the change and re-prescribe. Consider stating form of medication.
- All of the above rules are adapted for electronic prescribing and close attention must be paid to the local protocol. Electronic prescribing allows all of the above to be performed without the use of ink.

Please note the following important safety points:

- Avoid decimal points, e.g. 3 mg, not 3.0 mg (which may be misconstrued as 30 mg)
- Quantities of 1 gram or more should be written as 1 g, 2.5 g.
- Quantities less than 1 gram should be written in milligrams, e.g. 500 mg, not 0.5 g.
- Quantities less than 1 mg should be written in micrograms, e.g. 100 micrograms, not 0.1 mg.
- When decimals are unavoidable a zero should be written in front of the decimal point where there is no other figure, e.g. 0.5 mL, not .5 mL.
- Use of the decimal point is acceptable to express a range, e.g. 0.5 to 1 g.
- 'Micrograms' and 'nanograms' should not be abbreviated. Similarly 'units' should not be abbreviated. 4 U of insulin has been interpreted as 40 units, resulting in an unnecessary intensive care unit (ICU) admission.

Latin and other useful abbreviations

Use of abbreviations should be kept to a minimum. However, Latin abbreviations are often useful when prescribing and writing a drug history. Table 13.1 shows a list of Latin terms and abbreviations in common medical usage and other useful abbreviations.

Table 13.1 Abbreviations

Latin abbreviations used in prescribing	Other useful abbreviations
od: *omni die* (every day)	**ACE-I**: angiotensin-converting enzyme inhibitor
bd: *bis die* (twice daily)	**ARB or A$_2$-blocker**: angiotensin receptor blocker
tds: *ter die sumendum* (to be taken three times daily)	**BMI**: body mass index
qds: *quater die sumendum* (to be taken four times daily)	**e/c**: enteric-coated
	g/r: gastro-resistant
prn: *pro re nata* (when required)	**f/c**: film-coated
stat: immediately	**HRT**: hormone replacement therapy
om: *omni mane* (every morning)	**IM**: intramuscular
on: *omni nocte* (every night) or nocte	**INR**: international normalized ratio
	IV: intravenous
ac: *ante cibum* (before food)	**MAOI**: monoamine-oxidase inhibitor
pc: *post cibum* (after food)	**max.**: maximum
pr: *per rectum*	**mr**: modified-release
po: *per os* (by mouth)	**NICE**: National Institute for Health and Clinical Excellence
	NSAID: non-steroidal anti-inflammatory drug
	rINN: recommended International Non-proprietary Name
	SC: subcutaneous
	SSRI: selective serotonin reuptake inhibitor

Prescribing examples

As an absolute minimum, for each drug that you prescribe, you should know:

- the **rINN**
- **Additional instructions**: e.g. before meals
- **Dose**: e.g. x mg, 1–2 drops
- **Route**: e.g. oral IM, IV, pr, sc
- **Form**: e.g. capsule, tablet, liquid, suppositories
- **Frequency**: e.g. od, bd, tds, qds
- **Start date**: essential as certain drugs, e.g. warfarin, might start on day 3 after admission
- **Indications and contraindications**
- **Drug class and mechanism of action**
- **Common major side effects, contraindications**

Prescription notes

- All prescriptions must be clearly legible using black ink ideally in block capitals.
- Use approved, generic names and metric doses, i.e. do not write as 2 tabs (of 250 mg) but as 500 mg.
- Only use common and accepted abbreviations: e.g. od, bd, tds, qds.
- Special instructions are often very important e.g. nocte only, pre-meals, fasting.

Example 1 Furosemide

rINN			**Indications**
Furosemide		0600	Cardiac failure, intravenously especially in the acute setting
Additional instructions			**Drug class and mechanism of action**
Watch out for marked diuresis		0800	Class: loop diuretic
			MOA: stimulates excretion of water and sodium chloride
Dose	**Route**	1200	by blocking the NKCC-2 (Na⁺K⁺Cl⁻ channel) in the
50 mg	IV		ascending loop of Henle. Also mild veno-dilator reducing
		1400	pre-load to the heart.
Frequency	**Start date**		**Major side-effects and contraindications**
od	26/02/2011	1800	Major SE: hypokalaemia (therefore cramps and lethargy),
			hypomagnesaemia, gout by urate retention
Signature		2200	Contraindications: hypovolaemia, severe hypokalaemia,
			anuria

Example 2 Carbimazole

rINN			**Indications**
Carbimazole		0600	Hyperthyroidism
Additional instructions		0800	**Drug class and mechanism of action**
			Class: Anti-thyroid (thyroid peroxidase)
		1200	MOA: Prevents TPO (thyroid peroxidase) from coupling
			and iodinating tyrosine residues on thyroglobulin and
Dose	**Route**	1400	hence reduces production of T3 and T4
40 mg	PO		
Frequency	**Start date**	1800	**Major side-effects and contraindications**
od	26/02/2011		Major SE: Bone marrow suppression (neutropenia and
		2200	agranulocytosis) rare; rash common
Signature			Contraindications: severe blood disorders.

Example 3 Tropicamide

rINN			**Indications**
Tropicamide 1%		0600	Examination of fundus
Additional instructions		0800	**Drug class and mechanism of action**
			Class: Mydriatics and cycloplegics
		1200	MOA: dilate the pupil and paralyse the ciliary muscle
Dose	**Route**	1400	
2 drops	both eyes topical		
Frequency	**Start date**	1800	**Major side-effects and contraindications**
stat	26/02/2011		Transient stinging, blurred vision
		2200	
Signature			

Example 4 Lamotrigine

rINN
Lamotrigine

Additional instructions

Dose   **Route**
100 mg   PO

Frequency   **Start date**
BD   26/02/2011

Signature

0600

0800

1200

1400

1800

2200

Indications
Monotherapy and adjunctive treatment of partial seizures and primary & secondarily generalized tonic clonic seizures

Drug class and mechanism of action
Class: antiepileptic
MOA: modulates voltage gated sodium channels (theory)

Major side-effects and contraindications
Major SE: serious skin reactions (Stevens Johnson and toxic epidermal necrolysis); hypersensitivity syndrome; blood disorders e.g. aplastic anaemia, pancytopenia

The legal prescription

Fred Vincie, a 63-year-old, semi-retired plumber, has long-standing chronic obstructive pulmonary disease (COPD). He developed a chest infection on return from holiday to Thailand and had 3 days of oral penicillin V, 500 mg qds, with some improvement. He has nausea and vomiting. You discuss the case with the locum registrar on call. He advises you to write up his current medications and change the oral penicillin to IV co-amoxiclav (a decision later reversed by the consultant on the ward round).

Use a standard hospital drug chart or prescription pad (paper or electronic).

Please write out the following nine drugs:

- Paracetamol 1 g qds
- Simvastatin 40 mg nocte
- Ramipril 10 mg od
- Salbutamol 100 micrograms inhaler qds
- Oxygen 40% continuously
- 2 glycerin suppositories nocte
- Enoxaparin SC 40 mg at 6 pm
- 1% hydrocortisone cream to left hand bd
- Co-amoxiclav 1.2 g IV tds

		Self	Peer	Peer /tutor	Tutor
Understands indications, drug class and mechanism of action of each of these drugs	**Paracetamol**: pain relief, simple analgesic, cyclo-oxygenase (COX)-3 inhibitor acting centrally in thalamus (still theory)	☐	☐	☐	☐
	Simvastatin: lowers total cholesterol (especially low-density lipoprotein [LDL]), HMG-CoA reductase inhibitor	☐	☐	☐	☐
	Ramipril: lowers blood pressure, offers renal protection, cardiovascular disease (CVD) reduction, ACE-I	☐	☐	☐	☐
	Salbutamol: asthma, COPD, β_2-agonist bronchodilator	☐	☐	☐	☐
	Oxygen: vital gas, aerobic tissue respiration	☐	☐	☐	☐
	Glycerin suppositories: constipation, lubricant, increased contraction	☐	☐	☐	☐
	Enoxaparin: venous thromboembolism (VTE) prophylaxis, fractionated heparin acting in intrinsic clotting pathway	☐	☐	☐	☐
	Hydrocortisone cream: dermatitis, mild steroid with glucocorticoid anti-inflammatory action	☐	☐	☐	☐
	Co-amoxiclav: infections such as chest infection, β-lactam antibiotic blocking bacterial wall mucopeptide with clavulanic acid (bacterial β-lactamase inhibitor)	☐	☐	☐	☐
	●	☐	☐	☐	☐
	●	☐	☐	☐	☐
	●	☐	☐	☐	☐
	●	☐	☐	☐	☐
States common and major side effects for each of the drugs	**Paracetamol**: constipation, liver toxicity in overdose or liver failure only	☐	☐	☐	☐
	Simvastatin: myalgia, headaches, rarely abnormal liver function, very rarely rhabdomyolysis	☐	☐	☐	☐
	Ramipril: cough (dry irritating), hyperkalaemia, hypotension	☐	☐	☐	☐
	Salbutamol: tachycardia, anxiety (especially nebulizer)	☐	☐	☐	☐
	Oxygen: if patient has hypoxic drive to ventilation – apnoea and reduced respiration can result	☐	☐	☐	☐
	Glycerin suppositories: local irritation, embarrassment as pr medication	☐	☐	☐	☐
	Enoxaparin: rash, local infection	☐	☐	☐	☐
	Hydrocortisone cream: prolonged use associated with thinning of skin	☐	☐	☐	☐
	Co-amoxiclav: allergic reaction, *Clostridium difficile* infection as co-amoxiclav is a broad-spectrum antibiotic	☐	☐	☐	☐
	●	☐	☐	☐	☐
	●	☐	☐	☐	☐
	●	☐	☐	☐	☐
	●	☐	☐	☐	☐
Understands common abbreviations in Latin	**od** = *omni die* (every day)	☐	☐	☐	☐
	bd = *bis die* (twice daily)	☐	☐	☐	☐
	tds = *ter die sumendum* (to be taken three times daily)	☐	☐	☐	☐
	prn = *pro re nata* (when required)	☐	☐	☐	☐
	qds = *quater die sumendum* (to be taken four times daily)	☐	☐	☐	☐
	pr = *per rectum* (through the rectum)	☐	☐	☐	☐
	stat = immediately	☐	☐	☐	☐
	po = *per os* (by mouth)	☐	☐	☐	☐
	●	☐	☐	☐	☐
	●	☐	☐	☐	☐
	●	☐	☐	☐	☐
	●	☐	☐	☐	☐

Understands common abbreviations in English					
	• **ACE-I**: angiotensin-converting enzyme inhibitor	☐	☐	☐	☐
	• **BMI**: body mass index	☐	☐	☐	☐
	• **NICE**: National Institute for Health and Clinical Excellence **e/c**: enteric-coated	☐	☐	☐	☐
	• **rINN**: recommended International Non-proprietary Name	☐	☐	☐	☐
	• **f/c**: film-coated	☐	☐	☐	☐
	• **HRT**: hormone replacement therapy	☐	☐	☐	☐
	• **g/r**: gastro-resistant	☐	☐	☐	☐
	• **INR**: international normalized ratio	☐	☐	☐	☐
	• **IM**: intramuscular	☐	☐	☐	☐
	• **MAOI**: monoamine-oxidase inhibitor	☐	☐	☐	☐
	• **IV**: intravenous	☐	☐	☐	☐
	• **NSAID**: non-steroidal anti-inflammatory drug	☐	☐	☐	☐
	• **SC**: subcutaneous	☐	☐	☐	☐
	• **SSRI**: selective serotonin reuptake inhibitor	☐	☐	☐	☐
	• **max.**: maximum	☐	☐	☐	☐
	• **mr**: modified-release	☐	☐	☐	☐
	• **HMG Co-A reductase-I**: hydroxyl-methyl-glutaryl Co-A reductase inhibitor	☐	☐	☐	☐
	•	☐	☐	☐	☐
	•	☐	☐	☐	☐
	•	☐	☐	☐	☐
Legal prescription requirements demonstrated in all prescriptions					
	• **Full name and address of the patient, age or date of birth**	☐	☐	☐	☐
	• **Legible text, dated and signed by the prescriber**: prescriber's name under signature	☐	☐	☐	☐
	• **Drug details**: clearly state for each drug: dose, strength, route, and frequency	☐	☐	☐	☐
	• **State allergies**	☐	☐	☐	☐
	• If amending the prescription: draws line through the incorrect part, initials, dates	☐	☐	☐	☐
	•	☐	☐	☐	☐
	•	☐	☐	☐	☐
Seeks help as appropriate					
	• Consults BNF for correctness of prescribing	☐	☐	☐	☐
	• Checks local clinical guidelines for informing correct choice of drugs	☐	☐	☐	☐
	• Seeks expert help if needed from, for example clinical pharmacist, nurse, or doctor	☐	☐	☐	☐
	•	☐	☐	☐	☐
Post-procedure management and professionalism					
	• Documents changes to prescribing in notes and any specific requirements such as monitoring for urea and electrolytes (U&Es)	☐	☐	☐	☐
	• Allows enough time to concentrate on task and complete task efficiently and competently	☐	☐	☐	☐
	•	☐	☐	☐	☐
Explanation to patient					
	• Explains changes in prescription to patients including indications and main side-effects	☐	☐	☐	☐
	• Allows patient opportunity to ask about medications	☐	☐	☐	☐
	•	☐	☐	☐	☐

			U B S E	U B S E	U B S E	U B S E
Self-assessed as at least borderline:	Signature:	Date:				
Peer-assessed as ready for tutor assessment:	Signature:	Date:				
Tutor-assessed as satisfactory:	Signature:	Date:				

Notes

13.2 Ensuring patient safety

Background

Prescribed medicines are the commonest clinical intervention in most clinical specialties. There are specific considerations in relation to prescribing that will help ensure the highest standards of patient safety. Patient-specific education is probably the single most important factor that requires clinical attention. A patient who is a passive recipient of care is far more likely to come to harm, and indeed not benefit from treatment, than a well-informed patient. The National Patient Safety Agency (NPSA) has shown that children and those patients who are allergic to certain medicines are potentially more vulnerable to patient safety incidents than other groups.

Within the National Health Service (NHS), the NPSA defines a patient safety incident as:

> Any unintended or unexpected incident which could have or did lead to harm for one or more patients receiving NHS-funded healthcare.

Medication errors are classified as patient safety incidents and can happen at any stage of the process from prescribing to administration. As prescribers, it is important to acknowledge that prescribing has the potential to do both harm and good, and therefore care and diligence is required.

The NPSA has produced a seven-step plan to reduce medication errors – five of these are particularly relevant to prescribers:

1 Increase reporting and learning from medication incidents

2 Implement NPSA safer medication practice recommendations

3 Improve skills and competencies

4 Minimize dosing errors

5 Document patients' medicine allergy status.

This unit will use examples from recent clinical practice to illustrate various aspects of patient safety when prescribing.

Ensuring patient safety in prescribing

The following are points that aid NPSA recommendations as well as highlight common problems.

Reporting of side effects

This is still rarely done. Each copy of the BNF has a yellow card report that can be filled out and sent on to the Medicines and Healthcare products Regulatory Agency (MHRA). This is in the event of a side-effect that needs reporting. A useful summary of side-effects in relation to the drug that you reported is then forwarded back to the department. It is the concerted reporting of side-effects that often leads to the discontinuation of a drug from the national formulary and from marketing authorizations. A good example of this is the withdrawal of rimonabant. This was a centrally acting cannabinoid CB1 receptor antagonist that was originally licensed and extensively promoted for obesity. However, it was found to increase the risk of suicidal ideation and depression significantly and thus withdrawn. Shared learning is thus critical to improving drug safety.

Monitoring of medications

Many medications either require monitoring in the early stages of prescribing or require interval monitoring continuously.

- **ACE-I**: in many cases U&Es, particularly the potassium and creatinine, should be known prior to starting treatment and creatinine should be rechecked 7–10 days after initiation of an ACE-I or dose change. If there is hyperkalaemia or a creatinine rise by more than 20% and a fall in estimated glomerular filtration rate (eGFR) of 15%, treatment needs to be stopped in most cases or an urgent review conducted by an expert clinician. The reason for this is often renal artery stenosis. ACE-Is reduce the levels of aldosterone which results in the retention of potassium. Creatinine increase may be attributed to a blunted ability of the preglomerular circulation to vasodilate following normalization of blood pressure, leading to hypoperfusion of the kidneys.

- **NSAIDs**: examples include ibuprofen and naproxen. If patients are on these treatments, constant review is required. They are very effective usually for arthritic pain and for general pain relief. There are significant interactions with ACE-I (in that decreased renal perfusion can be caused by ACE-I and addition of an NSAID adds to the underperfusion). NSAIDs may also antagonize the hypotensive effect of ACE-I (prostaglandins are thought to be involved in the hypotensive effect of ACE-Is) and NSAIDs inhibit prostaglandin synthesis, There is also a significant risk of gastrointestinal tract haemorrhage.

- **Insulin treatment**: a fine balance needs to be struck between the need for good glycaemic control (and a low HbA_{1c}%) and hypoglycaemia. Mild hypoglycaemia (glucose <4 mmol/L, with the patient able to help themselves out of the problem) is generally not a problem. Severe hypoglycaemia (low glucose with the patient requiring the help of a third party to help them out of a hypoglycaemic attack) can be life-threatening or result in severe disability, including stroke and poor cognition.

- **Therapeutic monitoring**: some drugs require specific drug monitoring of levels if they have a narrow therapeutic index. The divide between treatment and toxicity can be quite slim. For example, for vancomycin, a reduction in efficacy because of an interaction can sometimes be just as harmful as an increase. Patients taking warfarin who are given rifampicin need more warfarin to maintain adequate anticoagulation. Other drugs that require close monitoring include lithium and digoxin.

- **Monitoring drug effects**: if a drug has been prescribed for a specific reason, e.g. management of hypertension then it is important to ensure that there is monitoring of the clinical outcome intended (the blood pressure). For example, monitor blood pressure and pulse when prescribing β-blockers. Monitoring hypoglycaemia when insulin and sulfonylureas are prescribed.

Checking for significant drug reactions

An interaction is said to occur when the effects of one drug are changed by the presence of another drug, herbal medicine, food, drink, or by some environmental chemical agent. For example, β-blockers and diltiazem lead to an increased risk of atrioventricular (AV) block. NSAIDs co-prescribed with aspirin increase the risk of bleeding due to the antiplatelet effect of aspirin. Prescribing benzodiazepines with opioids can have an additive effect causing psychomotor impairment, restlessness, reduced alertness.

Calculation errors

Some drugs need to be prescribed based on body surface area or actual body weight. It is therefore important to ensure accurate calculations are completed otherwise the final dose may be subtherapeutic or higher than required and possibly cause adverse effects. For example, cyclophosphamide in certain chemotherapy regimens is prescribed as per body surface area, i.e. 750 mg/m^2. Dose of enoxaparin as a treatment for pulmonary embolism is based on the patient's weight as per 1.5 mg/kg.

Patient education

Any new medications should be fully explained to the patient as this will promote concordance. If patients are more empowered regarding their drug treatments, general management may improve. For example, an explanation of initiating antibiotics advising why they have been given, advising about possible gastrointestinal upset may ensure that the patient is more likely to complete the given course than if they were not made aware of the importance of the treatment and possible adverse effects.

Polypharmacy review

Many patients will benefit from a review of their medication, particularly with respect to effectiveness, safety, and concordance. A good example of this is the consideration of stopping warfarin in patients with falls. Warfarin may well have been started more than 5 years ago in a patient with atrial fibrillation. In a patient with recurrent falls the risks of cerebral haemorrhage and bleeding at other sites and the difficulty with monitoring of the INR may result in a clinical decision to stop warfarin and use aspirin instead. Other important considerations include: stopping antiepileptic treatment in a patient having had a single fit many years ago, side-effect treatment pairs (NSAIDs and proton pump inhibitors [PPIs]), and reviewing long-term antidepressants. Antiepileptic medications should only be stopped after senior expert advice.

A polypharmacy review can also be helpful in investigating why medication has not been taken, e.g. blood pressure raised and patient has stopped taking ACE-I due to side-effect of cough. This could then be replaced with an angiotensin II antagonist.

Not asking for help

One of the most important clinical skills is realizing when you do not know. If you are unsure of what you are prescribing, or why, or whether it is safe or not – pause. Consult the BNF; ask for help from someone who might know, such as a doctor colleague or nurse, clinical pharmacist, or more senior help from the supervising clinician. Always prescribe within the limitations of your knowledge, skills, and experience. The junior doctor who prescribed sildenafil 100 mg od at 6 pm for a patient admitted for community-acquired pneumonia, was a little embarrassed when the mistake was pointed out on a ward round!

Illegible handwriting

This can cause harmful errors in administration if the person administering the medication deciphers the handwritten prescription incorrectly. Also it can result in non-administration of the drug if the person is unable to decipher what is written.

Dosing

Care should also be taken with writing appropriate doses, e.g. a patient was prescribed 1 g of diazepam for anxiety, not half a 2 mg tablet, that is, 1 mg. Be aware of maximum and minimum doses, e.g. bisoprolol was prescribed at a dose of 75 mg once in the morning by a senior house officer. The maximum dose for this drug is 20 mg/day.

Inadequate drug knowledge

Be aware of what you are prescribing and ensure it prescribed correctly. For example, indapamide (diuretic) was prescribed twice as both the generic form and via the brand name on a drug chart. The patient was prescribed the indapamide 2.5 mg in the morning but the brand name at night.

Poor history taking

This can be a sole cause of mismanagement of a patient's condition and potentially lead to readmissions. In some hospitals as many as 30% of patients have incomplete or incorrect medicines recorded on admission although this may have reduced since the introduction of NICE guidance. It is important to establish current therapy, as inaccuracies can lead to error which can be detrimental to patient care. A comprehensive drug history will rely on the patient, carers/family, GP records, hospital records and pharmacists. It is important to ask about OTC (over the counter) drugs, inhalers, complementary therapies, recreational drugs, etc. Some medications should not be stopped abruptly and regular medications may affect newly prescribed treatments. There is a potential for increased drug interactions and an increased length of hospital stay. A patient was admitted for shortness of breath attributed to heart failure and was started on bisoprolol 2.5 mg daily. An inaccurate drug history led to a reduction in this medication as the patient was previously taking bisoprolol 7.5 mg daily pre-admission and was consequently discharged on 2.5 mg daily.

Prescribing in pregnancy

All prescribers should be extremely careful about prescribing in pregnancy and more importantly in the pre-conception and first 12 weeks of pregnancy. Prescription of certain drugs in the first trimester leads to significant fetal malformations. All women of reproductive potential should be counselled with respect to medication in pregnancy. A balance needs to be struck between the risk to the mother and child due to the underlying condition and the risk of using medication. Many drugs pass into breast milk, however, it is the quantity of drug passing through that governs whether it is safe for the newborn. In all cases the BNF or specialist literature should be consulted for the latest advice. Only a few drugs are listed in Table 13.2 to illustrate those that are safe and those that are risky.

Table 13.2 Drugs in pregnancy

Drugs unsafe in pregnancy especially first trimester and conception	Drugs safe in pregnancy
Oral anticonvulsants: all such agents such as phenytoin, valproate, carbamazepine, lamotrigine should be reviewed prior to conception and if continued give folic acid 5 mg daily preconception and throughout pregnancy to reduce risk of neural tube defects	**Hypertension**: best managed for the 9 months of pregnancy with methyldopa, labetalol, or a calcium-channel blocker such as slow-release nifedipine (do not use short-acting agents)
ACE-I, angiotensin II receptor blockers, statins: major renal, neural and cardiac fetal malformations have been reported. These agents must be stopped or substituted	**Thyroxine and propylthiouracil**: are safe in pregnancy
β-blockers: pure β-blockers such as atenolol cause intrauterine growth retardation in direct proportion to length of time used	**Steroids and inhalers**: for asthma, all appear to be safe
Carbimazole: rare but characteristic side-effect of aplasia cutis – switch to propylthiouracil pre-conception or as soon as possible thereafter	**Metformin and all standard insulins**: appear to be safe. Some clinics will only use the older non-analogue insulins until full safety data are available
Trimethoprim: unsafe potential for inducing folate deficiency	**B$_{12}$, iron supplementation also safe**
	Penicillins are safe
	Low-molecular-weight and other heparins: no concerns reported since these drugs do not cross the placenta

Unsafe practices

Table 13.3 lists 31 causes of drug error and unsafe practice encountered in clinical practice, particularly in the professional practice of a junior doctor. This is not an exclusive list and draws on local experience and some highly publicized national cases. The recently published EQUIP study by the General Medical Council (GMC) showed a prescribing error rate of 8.4% among newly qualified first-year doctors. Only 40% of the errors were judged to be minor.

Box 13.1 Definitions

- **Adverse drug event (ADE)**: a medical occurrence temporarily associated with the use of a medicinal product, but not necessarily causally related.
- **Adverse drug reaction (ADR)**: a response to a drug which is unintended, and which occurs in doses normally used in humans, for the prophylaxis, diagnosis, and treatment of disease, or for the modification of physiological states
- **Unexpected adverse reaction**: a reaction which is not consistent with the applicable product information or the characteristics of the drug.
- **Side-effect**: an unintended effect occurring at normal doses related to the pharmacological properties of the medicine.
- **Serious adverse event or reaction**: any untoward medical occurrence that occurs at any dose which is life-threatening or results in death, requires inpatient hospitalization or prolongs current hospital stay or results in persistent significant disability or incapacity. Often called suspected unexpected serious adverse reactions (SUSAR).
- **Medication error**: any error in the prescribing, dispensing, or administration of a drug, irrespective of whether such errors lead to an adverse consequences or not.

Table 13.3 Common prescribing concerns compromising patient safety

1 **Illegibility**: common drugs can be misinterpreted when drugs are illegible, e.g. chlorphenamine may be misinterpreted as chlorpromazine

2 **Wrong dose, omitted, or delayed medicine**: Warfarin dosing or omission can be critical. Delays in insulin can often precipitate diabetic ketoacidosis

3 **Digoxin and furosemide**: hypokalaemia is often encountered with potassium-losing diuretics such as furosemide. Hypokalaemia increases risk of arrhythmias

4 **Amiodarone and digoxin**: co-prescribing of amiodarone increases the level of digoxin when first added. Digoxin dose should be halved

5 **Incomplete drug histories**: drugs such as NSAIDs and other OTC drugs are often omitted. Patients will often miss out non-oral medications such as inhalers, eye drops. Include herbal and homeopathic remedies. Cases: Chinese herbal medicines causing arrhythmias, evening primrose oil or St John's wort interactions with anticoagulants

6 **Penicillin allergies**: there are several antibiotics, for example 'co-amoxiclav' that actually have a penicillin base structure and equally precipitate the allergic reaction

7 **Not recording the allergy or intolerance**: it is important to be clear whether there is an allergy or intolerance or minor side-effect. Statins may cause mild myalgia but most patients will be happy to continue on treatment because of the CVD benefits if informed

8 **Tramadol and SSRI**: SSRIs such as fluoxetine interact with tramadol by reducing the seizure threshold

9 **Lactulose prn use**: this drug takes between 24 and 48 hours to be effective. Prescribing on a prn basis will negate its effects by increasing the time to act

10 **Not stating frequency of medication or maximum dose for prn**: for paracetamol, even on the prn side of the prescription chart, your intentions must be clearly stated. For example, paracetamol 1 g prn, at least 4 hourly, maximum qds. This is more crucial for drugs such as antipsychotics used for treating short-term agitation and anxiety.

11 **Wrong dose of LMWH for VTE prophylaxis**: dose must be reduced in poor renal function and bleeding diatheses.

12 **SSRI and risk of bleeding**: this is especially the case if the admission is for a gastrointestinal bleed

13 **Insulin units**: prescribed as units and not whole numbers: e.g. 6 Units can be mistakenly read as 60 units. It is better just to write the whole number alone

14 **Furosemide and bumetanide co-prescribed**: both are potassium-losing diuretics and life-threatening hypokalaemia can result

15 **Proton-pump inhibitor and H$_2$ antagonist co-prescribed**: Proton-pump inhibitors such as omeprazole or lansoprazole have similar therapeutic effects to H$_2$ antagonists such as ranitidine

16 **Statins and antibiotics**: certain antibiotics, e.g. erythromycin, can increase the risk of myopathy with most statins. Co-prescription should be avoided where possible especially if antibiotics are for long-term use. In this case a statin which does not interact should be prescribed

17 **Warfarin and antibiotics**: some antibiotics will affect the INR by either increasing or decreasing it, and as such additional monitoring may be required to ensure the range remains within therapeutic indices

18 **Controlled-drug prescriptions that are illegal**: certain strong opioids such as morphine are classified under the Medicines Act as Schedule 2 controlled drugs. As such their possession, and supply, is under strict regulations, which includes prescribing requirements

19 **Deviation from drug formulary**: this may sound trivial but if, for example, the specific ACE-I is not on the hospital or local formulary, this will result in a delay to the patient's treatment commencing. The drugs not on the formulary are often more expensive

20 **Tramadol prescribed in epilepsy:** tramadol can reduce the seizure threshold, therefore should not be used in patients with a history of epilepsy as it can increase risk of seizures

21 **Co-codamol and tramadol co-prescribed**: the higher strength of co-codamol (30/500) is equipotent to tramadol. Co-prescription does not offer any additional analgesia yet increases the opioid side-effects

22 **Clexane dose incorrect due to guessing weight or miscalculation**: this can lead to inappropriate anticoagulant treatment leading to an even higher risk of re-thrombosis

23 **GFR not calculated for gentamicin or tobramycin use**: drugs such as aminoglycosides have a narrow therapeutic index and their frequency of administration is based on renal function. If creatinine clearance is low then the dose interval may not necessarily be the conventional once or twice daily. If an appropriate GFR is not calculated, this risks renal and oto-toxicity

24 **Accurate time of paracetamol overdose**: not determined for correct and timely use of *N*-acetylcysteine risking longer accumulation of paracetamol within the body.

25 **Isosorbide mononitrate (ISMN) slow-release prescribed bd**: ISMN should be prescribed as a long-acting formulation od. Unless there is a period of at least 10 hours with very low levels of nitrate the phenomenon of nitrate tachyphylaxis (tolerance) occurs and there will be little or no benefit in prescribing the drug

26 **Not considering the full 'bundle' of drugs**: for explanation to patient certain conditions at discharge: a common example is the omission, e.g. glyceryl trinitrate, in a patient with acute coronary syndrome

27 **Inappropriate use of abbreviations**: AZT can be confused for both azathioprine and zidovudine

28 **Expensive drugs**: used instead of drugs with a similar evidence base but more economic to use: simvastatin is now only 2% of its initial price now that it is available as a generic drug.

Rare but associated with significant morbidity and mortality

29 **Intrathecal injection of cytotoxic agents**: errors in dosing have a proven record of mortality. Always check the correct dose for the routes whether oral, IV, IM, or intrathecal.

30 **Wrong patient's drugs prescribed**: always ensure an accurate drug history is taken and ensure you prescribe the right drug for the right person.

31 **Allergy**: never prescribe a penicillin or related antibiotic to a patient who previously experienced a severe adverse reaction to it, e.g. anaphylaxis. Such administration could endanger life

Student name:	Medical school:	Year:

Ensuring patient safety

Joseph Lister, a 56-year-old man with type 2 diabetes mellitus and atrial fibrillation, is admitted for arthroscopy to his left knee for severe pain and a suspected meniscus tear. He recently had a urinary tract infection (UTI) with left-sided loin pain. The consultant microbiologist suggests that a single dose of gentamicin is given to ensure that the UTI does not flare up during the admission.

He admits that he has been feeling suicidal since he started rimonabant for weight loss.

Use a standard hospital drug chart or prescription pad (paper or electronic).

Please write out the following nine drugs:

- Lisinopril 20 mg od
- Ibuprofen 400 mg tds
- Glargine insulin 40 units nocte
- Gentamicin (use specific chart if available)
- Warfarin 5 mg od at 6 pm for 2 days as loading doses (use specific warfarin chart)
- Bisoprolol 5 mg od
- Diltiazem SR 120 mg od
- Temazepam 10 mg nocte
- Morphine as slow-release formulation 20 mg bd

		Self	Peer	Peer /tutor	Tutor
Understands indications, drug class and mechanism of action of each of the drugs	**Lisinopril**: lower blood pressure, renal protection, CVD reduction, ACE-I,	☐	☐	☐	☐
	Ibuprofen: osteoarthritis knee, NSAID	☐	☐	☐	☐
	Glargine insulin: type 2 diabetes, long-acting analogue insulin	☐	☐	☐	☐
	Gentamicin: aminoglycoside antibiotic, these agents interrupt protein synthesis by inhibiting t-RNA and m-RNA at the ribosomal level	☐	☐	☐	☐
	Warfarin: atrial fibrillation, coumarin anticoagulant, interferes with vitamin K metabolism	☐	☐	☐	☐
	Bisoprolol: β-blocker, usually for cardiac failure, post-acute coronary syndrome, hypertension	☐	☐	☐	☐
	Diltiazem: atrial fibrillation, non-dihydropyridine calcium-channel blocker, blocks plateau phase of action potential	☐	☐	☐	☐
	Temazepam: hypnotic to help sleep pattern, benzodiazepine (schedule 3, CD status), other agents preferred	☐	☐	☐	☐
	Morphine: as MST: pain relief, opioid	☐	☐	☐	☐
	●	☐	☐	☐	☐
	●	☐	☐	☐	☐
Understands monitoring requirements, common side effects for the drugs listed above	**Lisinopril**: cough (dry irritating), hyperkalaemia, hypotension	☐	☐	☐	☐
	Ibuprofen: check U&Es, may worsen congestive cardiac failure (CCF), side effects: gastrointestinal bleed	☐	☐	☐	☐
	Glargine insulin: regular glucose monitor, adjust dose to avoid hypoglycaemia	☐	☐	☐	☐
	Gentamicin: gentamicin levels, nephrotoxicity, ototoxicity	☐	☐	☐	☐
	Warfarin: regular INR, full blood count (FBC) if bleed suspected, watch out for bleeding side effects	☐	☐	☐	☐
	Bisoprolol: titrate dose to reduce symptoms of CCF and side effects such as bradycardia	☐	☐	☐	☐
	Diltiazem: avoid co-prescription with β-blockers where possible. Risk of AV block; monitor clinical state and heart rate	☐	☐	☐	☐
	Temazepam: monitor for evidence of excessive sedation	☐	☐	☐	☐
	Morphine as MST: monitor for constipation, respiratory rate, sedation	☐	☐	☐	☐
	●	☐	☐	☐	☐
Understands the national MHRA reporting system for adverse side effects of drug	Shows location of the yellow card in the BNF	☐	☐	☐	☐
	Discusses the requirements of the report: age, sex, co-morbidities in the patient, description of the side-effect, concurrent medications	☐	☐	☐	☐
	●	☐	☐	☐	☐
Demonstrates ability to take a comprehensive drug history including allergies	At least six drugs documented	☐	☐	☐	☐
	rINN used, dose stated, route stated, indication stated	☐	☐	☐	☐
	Enquires about medication often forgotten by patient, e.g. inhalers and topical agents	☐	☐	☐	☐
	Enquires about OTC and alternative medications	☐	☐	☐	☐
	Allergy history, penicillin allergy excluded	☐	☐	☐	☐
	●	☐	☐	☐	☐
	●	☐	☐	☐	☐
Legal prescription requirements demonstrated in all prescriptions	Full name, address, DOB or age, allergies, legible, signed and dated, no abbreviations, rINN names	☐	☐	☐	☐
	●	☐	☐	☐	☐

Able to discuss at least 10 common prescribing concerns	For example:				
	● Illegibility, wrong dose, incomplete drug history, not recording allergies	☐	☐	☐	☐
	● Not stating frequency of medication, insulin doses	☐	☐	☐	☐
	● Digoxin and furosemide or hypokalaemia, amiodarone and digoxin	☐	☐	☐	☐
	● Statins and erythromycin	☐	☐	☐	☐
	● Prescribing in pregnancy	☐	☐	☐	☐
	●	☐	☐	☐	☐
	●	☐	☐	☐	☐
	●	☐	☐	☐	☐
Seeks help as appropriate	● Consults BNF for correctness of prescribing	☐	☐	☐	☐
	● Checks local clinical guidelines for informing correct choice of drugs	☐	☐	☐	☐
	● Seeks expert help if needed from, for example, clinical pharmacist, nurse, or doctor	☐	☐	☐	☐
	●	☐	☐	☐	☐
Post-procedure management and professionalism	● Documents changes to prescribing in notes and any specific requirements such as monitoring for U&Es	☐	☐	☐	☐
	● Allows enough time to concentrate on task and complete task efficiently and competently	☐	☐	☐	☐
	●	☐	☐	☐	☐
Explanation to patient	● Explains changes in prescription to patients including indications and main side effects	☐	☐	☐	☐
	● Allows patient opportunity to ask about medications	☐	☐	☐	☐
	● Use one drug as example to test	☐	☐	☐	☐
	●	☐	☐	☐	☐

Self-assessed as at least borderline:	Signature:	Date:	U B S E	U B S E	U B S E	U B S E
Peer-assessed as ready for tutor assessment:	Signature:	Date:	U B S E	U B S E	U B S E	U B S E
Tutor-assessed as satisfactory:	Signature:	Date:	U B S E	U B S E	U B S E	U B S E

Notes

13.3 Common prescribing bundles

Background

Unpublished work concludes that most clinicians prescribe fewer than 100 medications 90% of the time. It is therefore far more important, especially in terms of patient safety, to know how to prescribe a smaller number of drugs well, than to know a little about a large range of drugs that you may not have the opportunity to prescribe in clinical practice. The best example of a prescribing bundle, or a short list of medications to consider for a specific clinical problem, is the Liverpool Care Pathway in palliative care, which will be discussed in another section.

The aim of this section is to provide prescribing bundles for common clinical situations such as pain, hypertension, and need for sedation and antibiotic use.

Pain

The World Health Organization (WHO) analgesic ladder (Figure 13.1) recommends a practical three-stage stepwise pharmacological approach to pain management (see also Table 13.4).

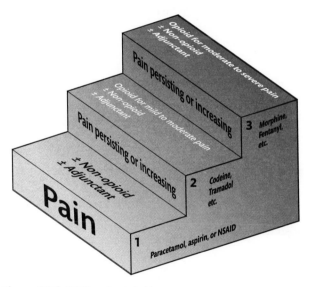

Figure 13.1 WHO analgesic ladder.

Table 13.4 Pain classification and analgesia

WHO pain classification	Type of analgesia	Examples
1: Mild	Non-opioid ± adjunctant	Paracetamol Aspirin (rarely used) NSAID
2: Mild to moderate	Opioid ± non-opioid ± adjunctant	Codeine Tramadol
3: Moderate to severe	Opioid ± non-opioid ± adjunctant	Morphine Fentanyl

Pain prescribing notes:

- **Paracetamol**: is very safe at the recommended doses for the short- and medium-term relief of pain. Aspirin can be difficult to tolerate at analgesic doses.
- **NSAIDs**: usually very effective although often cause side effects. This includes gastrointestinal upset, possibly causing bleeding, and with long-term use fluid retention and worsening of cardiac failure and hypertension.
- **NSAIDs in combination with paracetamol**: can often be as effective as mild opioids with fewer side effects, especially post operatively.
- **Opioid prescribing route**: it is important to consider the most appropriate route according to patient needs and side effects: oral, SC injection or infusion or a patch.
- **WHO ladder**: may be too simplistic for some forms of pain such as neuropathic and chronic pain. Other agents such as amitriptyline, nortriptyline and gabapentin may be needed for neuropathy. Carbamazepine is useful in neuralgia. Naproxen is often very efficacious in bone pain. Expert advice from a Pain Clinic is often indicated.

Hypertension

Lifestyle interventions: can reduce blood pressure and should always be discussed with the patient. Interventions include: normalizing weight, increasing physical activity if the current activity undertaken is less than recommended, reducing any excess alcohol consumption, smoking cessation, reducing caffeine intake and reducing salt consumption if excessive to prevailing guidelines.

Drug therapy: reduces the risk of CVD disease and death (Figure 13.2). Pharmacological therapy is offered to:

- Patients with persistent high blood pressure of 160/100 mmHg or more
- Patients with persistent blood pressure above 140/90 mmHg and raised CVD risk (10-year risk of cardiovascular disease of at least 20%, existing CVD or target organ damage)

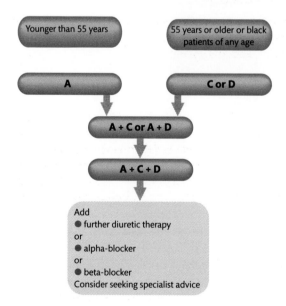

Abbreviations

A = ACE inhibitor (consider angiotensin-II receptor antagonist if ACE-I intolerant)
C = calcium-channel blocker
D = thiazide-type diuretic

Black patients are those of African or Caribbean descent, and not mixed race, Asian or Chinese patients

Figure 13.2 NICE and British Hypertension Society guidelines for hypertension (2006).

- Patients with diabetes mellitus with blood pressure above 140/90 or above 130/70 with diabetes complications such as retinopathy or nephropathy or any CVD
- The usual target blood pressure is <149/90, <130/80 in patients with diabetes and at least one microvascular or macrovascular complication.

Hypertension prescribing notes:

- **Teratogenic drugs**: ACE-Is (e.g. ramipril, lisinopril, perindopril), angiotensin II receptor blockers (e.g. losartan, irbesartan, candesartan) and statins (e.g. simvastatin, atorvastatin, rosuvastatin) are highly teratogenic (15% risk of severe physical malformations) and should never be used in women of reproductive potential. This must be explained to the patient and effective contraception ensured.
- **Type 1 or type 2 diabetes mellitus**: for these patients, ACE-Is are often used first line for their renal, retinal, and CVD protective properties.
- **Potassium and sodium levels**: significant side effects are often encountered with hyperkalaemia and the use of ACE-Is and angiotensin II receptor blockers. Hypokalaemia and hyponatraemia are important side effects of potassium-losing diuretics such as bendroflumethiazide, indapamide, and furosemide. Mg^{2+} loss can also be a significant problem with diuretics.

Lipid-lowering

- **Current recommendations**: are that all patients with established CVD or diabetes mellitus should be considered for statin treatment. For other patients, total cholesterol above 6 mmol/L or family history of CVD or cardiovascular risk greater than 20% over 10 years should trigger consideration of treatment with statins. The choice should be based on cost of prescribing and the side effects. Evidence-based doses should be used where possible, e.g. simvastatin 40 mg rather than lower, possibly ineffective, doses.
- **NICE targets for established CVD**: Total cholesterol ≤4.0 mmol/L and LDL ≤2.0 mmol/L. Other important considerations include the secondary lipid targets: HDL cholesterol ≥1.0 for males and ≥1.2 for females, triglycerides <2.0 mmol/L.
- **Non-pharmacological measures as well as pharmacological interventions**: both should be advocated to improve lipid profiles. Other pharmacological measures include ezetimibe, a cholesterol absorption inhibitor, nicotinic acid, and fibrates.

Nausea, vomiting, dyspepsia

- **Nausea and vomiting**: drugs used vary in their efficacy depending on the cause. Generally all the drugs have a greater effect on vomiting than nausea. Drugs include antihistamines such as cyclizine, antimuscarinics such as hyoscine hydrobromide, and dopamine antagonists such as metoclopramide, domperidone, and prochlorperazine. The side effects of prochlorperazine are similar to metoclopramide in that they can cause extrapyramidal side effects. Drugs such as these should be avoided in patients with parkinsonism, as they will exacerbate the patient's existing condition. Domperidone, however, does not cross the blood–brain barrier and therefore avoids the dystonic reactions seen with other dopamine antagonists.
- **Gastro-oesophageal reflux disease (GORD and peptic ulcer disease)**: patients may complain of heartburn, oesophagitis, acid reflux, or epigastric pain. It is important to be aware of red flag symptoms such as dysphagia, pain on swallowing, weight loss, melaena, coffee grounds in vomitus, or haematemesis. Several drugs can also exacerbate GORD such as NSAIDs affecting the mucosal lining, and others affecting sphincter tone such as nitrates, theophylline, and antimuscarinics such as hyoscine. Antacids and lifestyle modifications are usually first line management for symptomatic relief. It is worth noting that aluminium-containing antacids can cause constipation and magnesium-containing antacids can exert a laxative effect. Risks of accumulation of aluminium and magnesium are increased in renal failure and can result in neurological side-effects. Management with H_2 antagonists, e.g. ranitidine, and PPIs e.g. omeprazole can improve symptoms. PPIs are generally more effective.

Constipation

- **Common problem**: can cause general distress and confusion if there is long-standing constipation. There can be 'overflow diarrhoea', which must not be mistaken for other forms of diarrhoea. If untreated, constipation can lead to impaction, rectal bleeding, and anal fissures. Some drugs can cause constipation, such as opioids, some antidepressants (tricyclics), and antimuscarinic drugs. Care should be taken to review existing medications before initiating further treatment. Agents to manage constipation: bulk forming (e.g. ispaghula husk), stimulants (e.g. senna), faecal softeners (e.g. glycerin suppositories), osmotic laxatives (e.g. macrogols, lactulose, and phosphate enemas).

Antibiotic and antiviral prescribing

Hospitals and larger general practice units will have their own antibiotic policy. Table 13.5 lists the commonly used antibiotics for specific clinical conditions and the organism(s) that are being targeted. Antibiotic use undoubtedly saves lives and reduces morbidity, however, injudicious prescribing leads to both microbial resistance and opportunistic infections such as with *C. difficile*. The inappropriate use of certain antibiotics or having a longer course of antibiotics than needed clinically can often lead to severe *C. difficile* diarrhoea and pseudomembranous colitis, with its associated increased risk of mortality. On the other hand, antibiotic prophylaxis is required in certain conditions such as:

- Meningitis due to *Neisseria meningitidis*: rifampicin or ciprofloxacin
- Meningitis due to *Haemophilus influenzae*: rifampicin
- Recurrent UTIs: e.g. *Proteus mirabilis*: trimethoprim

Sleep sedation and agitation

- **Insomnia**: is a disturbance of normal sleep patterns and can arise in hospitals due to the disruption to the patient's normal sleeping routine. Short-term hypnotics may be prescribed, during inpatient stay on a prn basis only. Other causes should be considered: is the patient on an SSRI administered in the evening? When is the last dose of steroid being administered? Both of these may cause insomnia. Is the patient on any other medication that causes central nervous system (CNS) excitation? Ideally the patient should be advised to try relaxation techniques and avoid caffeine containing drinks pre bed. Hypnotics such as zopiclone and zolpidem are widely used to induce sleep. However, their effects can be long-lasting compared with the shorter-acting benzodiazepines such as temazepam. It is important to ensure that patients are not discharged home on such medicines as there is risk of continuation addiction.

- **Rapid tranquillization**: may be used in patients who are aggressive or agitated, and may be given to prevent the patient from behaving violently or presenting a danger to both themselves and others. Those showing signs of confusion should have a mini-mental state examination and a physical examination should also be carried out to rule out any organic cause. Tranquillization should only be carried out if the risks of not treating outweigh the risks of acute pharmacological management. De-escalation strategies should be implemented first line in order to calm down an escalating situation. Drugs used are lorazepam and haloperidol, however, antipsychotics should not be used in patients at risk of extrapyramidal effects, or with pre-existing cardiac disease or any other contraindications. Lorazepam may be given first line in a dose of 1–2 mg orally or IM. The dose may be repeated after 30 minutes. The maximum dose should be 4 mg in 24 hours. If there is a degree of psychosis (hallucinations, delusions, or aggression) then haloperidol may be considered first line or added to lorazepam in a dose of 5 or 10 mg orally or IM which may be repeated after 30 minutes. The maximum dose should be no more than 15 mg in 24 hours. Local dosing advice for lorazepam and haloperidol may be different from that stated here.

Table 13.5 Clinical conditions

Clinical condition	Common microbes	Commonly used specific treatments
Community-acquired pneumonia	*Streptococcus pneumoniae* *Haemophilus influenzae* *Moraxella catarrhalis*	Penicillins Co-amoxiclav as resistance often seen with amoxicillin and second-generation cephalosporins
Atypical pneumonia	*Legionella pneumophila* *Mycoplasma pneumoniae* *Chlamydia pneumoniae* or *psittaci* *Coxiella burnettii*	Erythromycin Clarithromycin
Pneumonia in immune compromise	*Staphylococcus aureus* *Klebsiella* spp. *Pseudomonas aeruginosa*	Erythromycin
Aspiration pneumonia	Anaerobic infection, *Fusobacterium* spp.	Co-amoxiclav, metronidazole
Cellulitis	*Streptococcus pyogenes* (group A) *Staphylococcus aureus* *Streptococcus epidermidis* Group B streptococcus	Penicillin V or amoxicillin and flucloxacillin
Cholecystitis	*Klebsiella* spp.	Cephalosporins, gentamicin
Diverticulitis	Mixed gut flora	Cephalosporins, metronidazole
Urinary tract infection	*Proteus mirabilis* *Escherichia coli*	Trimethoprim, nitrofurantoin, cephalosporins
Gastroenteritis: general	*Bacillus cereus* *Escherichia coli* O157 VTEC *Salmonella* *Shigella* *Campylobacter*	Usually no treatment required: erythromycin for severe cases of *Campylobacter* infection
Antibiotic-associated diarrhoea	*Clostridium difficile*	Metronidazole, vancomycin
MRSA infection	*Staphylococcus aureus* (meticillin-resistant)	Locally determined by cultures
Peptic ulcer disease	*Helicobacter pylori*	Metronidazole, clarithromycin, amoxicillin
Meningitis	*Neisseria meningitidis* *Haemophilus influenzae*	Benzylpenicillin, ceftriaxone
Dental abscess		Amoxicillin and/or metronidazole
Chlamydia	*Chlamydia* spp.	Doxycycline, macrolides
Gonorrhoea	*Neisseria gonorrhoeae*	Third generation cephalosporin
Syphilis	*Treponema pallidum*	Long-acting penicillins
Tuberculosis	*Mycobacterium tuberculosis*	Rifampicin, pyrazinamide, isoniazid
Viral encephalitis	Herpes simplex virus	Aciclovir
Influenza	Influenza A, B	Oseltamivir, zanamivir (only according to current National Guidelines)

Student name:	Medical school:	Year:

Common prescribing bundles

Use a standard hospital drug chart or prescription pad (paper or electronic).

Please write out two drugs for each of the following common prescribing bundles:

			Self	Peer	Peer /tutor	Tutor
• Pain • Blood pressure • Lipid lowering	• Nausea, vomiting, dyspepsia • Constipation • Antibiotics for community-acquired pneumonia	• Antibiotics for peptic ulcer disease • Sleep sedation and agitation				

			Self	Peer	Peer /tutor	Tutor
Understands indications, drug class and mechanism of action of each of the above drugs			☐	☐	☐	☐
Understands common side effects for the drugs chosen above			☐	☐	☐	☐
Legal prescription requirements demonstrated in all prescriptions	• Full name, address, DOB or age, allergies, legible, signed and dated, no abbreviations, rINN names •		☐	☐	☐	☐

Is able to complete the gaps in the table of clinical conditions, common microbes, and specific treatment according to local protocols	Clinical condition	Common microbes	Commonly used specific treatments	☐	☐	☐	☐
	Community-acquired pneumonia	*Streptococcus pneumoniae* *Haemophilus influenzae* *Moraxella catarrhalis*					
	Atypical pneumonia		Erythromycin clarithromycin				
	Cellulitis	*Streptococcus pyogenes* (Group A) *Staphylococcus aureus* *Streptococcus epidermidis,* Group B streptococcus					
	Urinary tract infection		Trimethoprim, nitrofurantoin, cephalosporins				
	Antibiotic-associated diarrhoea						
	Meningitis						
	Viral encephalitis						
	Influenza						

		Self	Peer	Peer /tutor	Tutor
Understands specific safety issues	• In relation to prolonged use of broad-spectrum antibiotics and risk of *C. difficile* infection •	☐	☐	☐	☐
Seeks help as appropriate	• Consults BNF for correctness of prescribing • Checks local clinical guidelines for informing correct choice of drugs • Seeks expert help if needed from, for example, clinical pharmacist, nurse, or doctor •	☐	☐	☐	☐
Post-procedure management and professionalism	• Documents changes to prescribing in notes and any specific requirements such as monitoring for U&Es • Allows enough time to concentrate on task and complete task efficiently and competently •	☐	☐	☐	☐
Explanation to patient	• Explains changes in prescription to patients including indications and main side-effects • Allows patient opportunity to ask about medications • Use one drug as example to test	☐	☐	☐	☐

Self-assessed as at least borderline:	Signature:	Date:	U B S E	U B S E	U B S E	U B S E
Peer-assessed as ready for tutor assessment:	Signature:	Date:	U B S E	U B S E	U B S E	U B S E
Tutor-assessed as satisfactory:	Signature:	Date:	U B S E	U B S E	U B S E	U B S E

Notes

13.4 Drug prescription charts

Background

A patient's drug chart is instrumental in their care and is a key document during their hospital stay.

The drug chart should be critically examined on a daily basis on the ward. It will always be useful to take account of currently prescribed and recently given drugs when assessing an ill patient on the wards in any circumstance.

A drug chart has several functions:

- It provides instructions to staff members dispensing medicines
- It provides colleagues with accurate information regarding medication given
- It serves as a legal document, which can be examined in court. (Both the Medical Defence Union and Medical Protection Society have case studies on their websites that highlight the cost of medication errors.)

Several studies now indicate that the error rate in prescribing on drug charts for inpatients is in the order of 25%. These errors commonly include missing off drugs that have been used long term, wrong doses, wrong routes of administration, and duplication of prescription.

This section is designed to help you acquire the skills necessary, using a systematic approach, to complete the drugs chart correctly, efficiently, and safely. Writing out drug charts is an important skill, which will be utilized on a daily basis at every level of your clinical career.

Prescribing principles

Key principles, indeed legal requirements, have been covered above. The patients should be identified by name, address, date of birth, and age. In most cases the hospital number or other patient identification number should also be included. The BNF advises that all prescriptions should be written legibly in indelible ink. There are some accepted abbreviations (a list can be found in the BNF), but for the majority of medications, the quantities, and instructions should be written out fully. Avoid the unnecessary use of decimal points and ensure that correct units are used.

Sequence

Documentation and preparation

Absolutely ensure that you are writing the prescription chart for the patient intended. Check the identity of the patient and take a full and accurate drug history with special attention to any allergies and potential drug interactions. Each entry should be dated and signed by the doctor. Remember, that when writing a drug chart, the local trust policy and BNF should be nearby and consulted if necessary. Do not be afraid to look up or even check the appropriate dose for each treatment you prescribe. Triangulating the information with a colleague may also be useful. The final responsibility rests with the prescribing clinician (Figure 13.3).

Explanation and consent

In many cases, the drug prescription should be discussed with the patient. Promote patient education by talking to the patient and allowing meaningful dialogue for the patient in relation to the management generally to cover prescribed drugs as well.

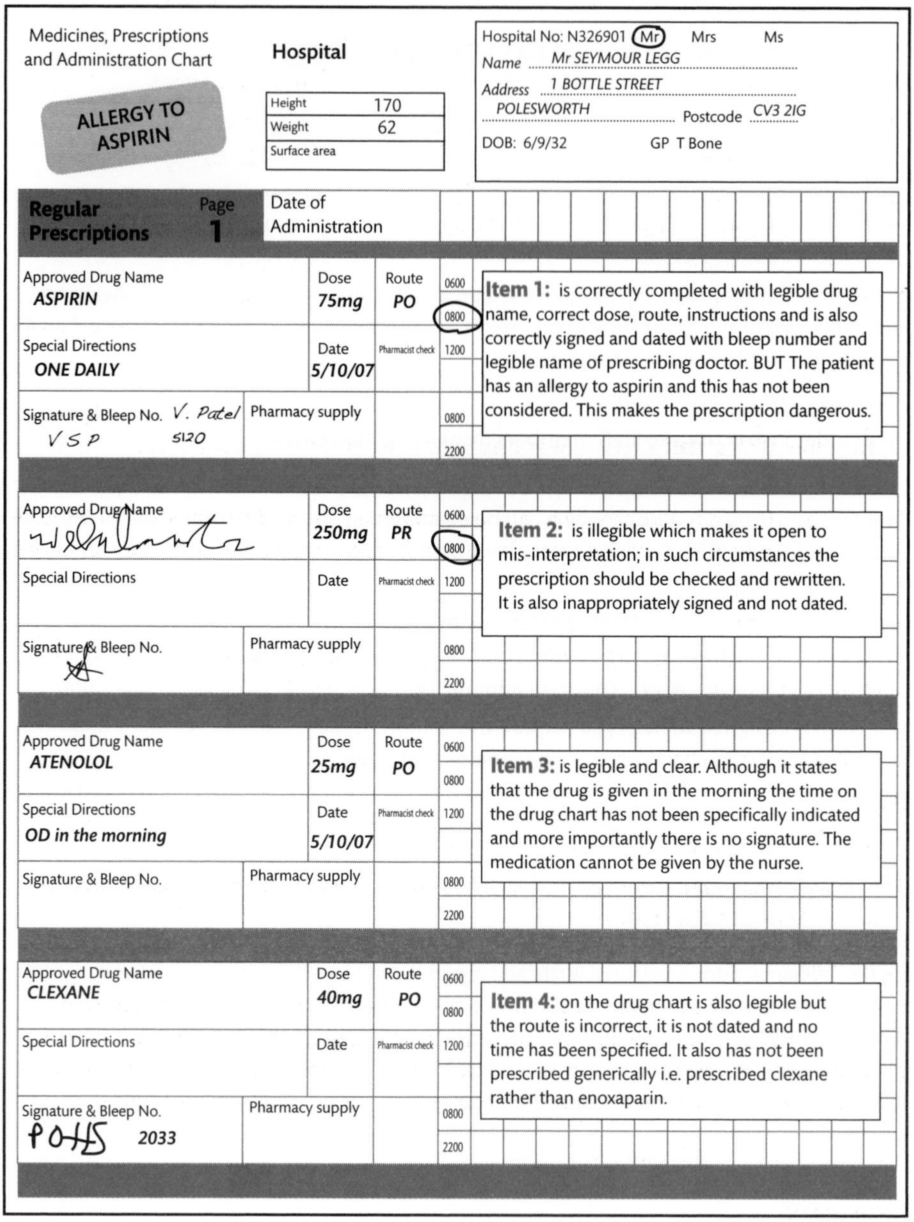

Figure 13.3 Common mistakes on a drug chart.

Writing the prescription chart

For each drug, ensure you know its correct spelling, correct dose, correct indication in the patient you are prescribing for, its class and mechanism of action, side effects and key interactions. Table 3.6 offers a reminder of common abbreviations that can be used.

Note: 'micrograms' and 'units' should not be abbreviated

Insulin – write as numbers alone e.g. Glargine 8 nocte or as 8 units. _Do not_ use 8 U (because 8 U might be mistaken for <u>80</u> units). There are reported cases in the medico-legal literature of this leading to ITU admission and significant morbidity such as stroke.

Post-protocol management

Explain the main treatments to the patient or carer in some cases. Use patient information sources to facilitate patient understanding of the need and effects of the medication including potential side effects.

Table 13.6 Common abbreviations

od	Once daily	tds	Three times daily
bd	Twice daily	qds	Four times daily
om	Every morning	stat	Immediately
on	Every night	prn	When required
IM	Intramuscular	IV	Intravenous
SC	Subcutaneous	mL	Millilitre
g	Gram	mg	Milligram

Professionalism

Communicate important and relevant changes in treatment to the nursing staff, clinical pharmacists, and other clinical staff. Certain drugs may need to be ordered from pharmacy.

A clinician must also monitor the effects of the medications prescribed. If an adverse event that is anything other than commonly known is ever noted, ensure that an adverse reaction form (yellow form found at the back of the BNF) is completed. Certain drugs will require drug level monitoring.

Patient safety and clinical governance tips

In view of the many potential and real errors in relation to prescribing, a specific section in this unit has been dedicated to this. See Section 13.2.

Writing a drug chart

Patient details

● Name, date of birth, address. State age if < 12 years

These are legal requirements. In addition, include hospital number, ward, consultant, and the general practitioner (GP) details.

Allergy box

This must be completed. If patient has no allergies write 'No Known Allergies'. Only use the abbreviation NKA if it is an accepted local policy. If possible, detail the nature of the allergy. Some patients will state an allergy to aspirin when they actually suffer from mild heartburn. But in the event of a stroke, a clinical decision can be made to initiate aspirin with concomitant PPI.

Outpatient or general practice prescription

Patient details

● Name, date of birth, address

These are legal requirements. In addition, include hospital number, ward, consultant, and GP details.

Prescription

Example:

Aciclovir 200 mg tablets

200 mg orally *FIVE* times a day for 5 days

Supply 25 tablets

[No more items on this prescription]

Doctor's signature (Address, GMC number if dispensed in the community)

The vast majority of GP prescriptions are now processed electronically in UK, but prescriptions are often handwritten in emergencies or in outpatients in hospitals.

The name of the drug is followed by its precise dose, timing, and length of treatment. What you wish to be supplied should also be stated.

Student name:	Medical school:	Year:

Drug prescription charts

Use a standard hospital drug chart or prescription pad (paper or electronic) to write out a drug chart for:

Mr Peter Farebrother (222b Holmes Road, Carlton, CL2 9SV; date of birth 2 March 1948, hospital number GE11235813, Lydgate Ward) has no known allergies except to plasters, which cause redness. He weighs 78 kg and is admitted because of swelling of the left calf and haemoptysis. He is known to have asthma, hypertension, back pain due to osteoarthritis, and has recently developed conjunctivitis. His medications from general practice were as follows:

Salbutamol inhaler 100 micrograms – two puffs, four times a day via a volumatic device	*Chloramphenicol 0.5% – 1 drop in each eye every 4 hours*	*Fluticasone 50 micrograms inhaler – two puffs, twice a day via volumatic device*
Aspirin 75 mg once daily	*Co-codamol 30/500 – two tablets, four times a day*	*Ramipril 10 mg od*

After the ward round, your consultant, Dr Kohner, wants the following medications prescribed for possible pneumonia and deep vein thrombosis (DVT) or pulmonary embolism pending further investigation.

Amoxicillin – 500 mg three times a day intravenously	*Clarithromycin – 500 mg twice a day intravenously*	*Enoxaparin – 1.5 mg/kg subcutaneously once a day*

In addition to the above, please prescribe a laxative, paracetamol prn and a PPI.

		Self	Peer	Peer/tutor	Tutor
Understands indications, drug class and mechanism of action of each of these drugs	• Salbutamol, chloramphenicol, fluticasone, aspirin, co-codamol, ramipril, amoxicillin, clarithromycin, enoxaparin, laxative, paracetamol, PPI •	☐ ☐	☐ ☐	☐ ☐	☐ ☐
States common and major side effects for each of these drugs	• Salbutamol, chloramphenicol, fluticasone, aspirin, co-codamol, ramipril, amoxicillin, clarithromycin, enoxaparin, laxative, paracetamol, PPI •	☐ ☐	☐ ☐	☐ ☐	☐ ☐
Legal prescription requirements demonstrated in all prescriptions	• Full name and address of the patient • Age or date of birth • State allergies • Text: printed or written legibly in black ink (with correct spelling) • Dated and signed by the prescriber • Clearly states for each drug: dose, strength, route, and frequency • Generic name of drug and no abbreviations in this part • If amending the prescription, draws a line through the incorrect part and initials and dates the change • Prescriber's name under signature (ideally) •	☐ ☐ ☐ ☐ ☐ ☐ ☐ ☐ ☐ ☐	☐ ☐ ☐ ☐ ☐ ☐ ☐ ☐ ☐ ☐	☐ ☐ ☐ ☐ ☐ ☐ ☐ ☐ ☐ ☐	☐ ☐ ☐ ☐ ☐ ☐ ☐ ☐ ☐ ☐
Additional drug chart completion requirements	• Hospital number • Location: hospital and ward stated correctly • Patient weight stated correctly • Your bleep number • Consultant name identified •	☐ ☐ ☐ ☐ ☐ ☐	☐ ☐ ☐ ☐ ☐ ☐	☐ ☐ ☐ ☐ ☐ ☐	☐ ☐ ☐ ☐ ☐ ☐
Seeks help as appropriate	• Consults BNF for correctness of prescribing • Checks local clinical guidelines for informing correct choice of drugs • Seeks expert help if needed from, for example, clinical pharmacist, nurse, or doctor •	☐ ☐ ☐ ☐	☐ ☐ ☐ ☐	☐ ☐ ☐ ☐	☐ ☐ ☐ ☐
Post-procedure management and professionalism	• Documents changes to prescribing in notes and any specific requirements such as monitoring for U&Es • Allows enough time to concentrate on task and completes task efficiently and competently •	☐ ☐ ☐	☐ ☐ ☐	☐ ☐ ☐	☐ ☐ ☐
Explanation to patient	• Explains changes in prescription to patients including indications and main side-effects • Allows patient opportunity to ask about medications •	☐ ☐ ☐	☐ ☐ ☐	☐ ☐ ☐	☐ ☐ ☐

				Self	Peer	Peer/tutor	Tutor
Self-assessed as at least borderline:	Signature:		Date:	U B S E	U B S E	U B S E	U B S E
Peer-assessed as ready for tutor assessment:	Signature:		Date:	U B S E	U B S E	U B S E	U B S E
Tutor-assessed as satisfactory:	Signature:		Date:	U B S E	U B S E	U B S E	U B S E

Notes

13.5 Prescribing controlled drugs

Background

Controlled drugs are commonly prescribed for a variety of clinical indications including pain relief, insomnia, cardiac failure, and end of life care. In UK, the Misuse of Drugs Act 1971 regulates dangerous or harmful drugs by designating these as controlled drugs. These drugs are subject to tighter measures relating to possession, supply, manufacturing, import, and export. Controlled drugs may be used within medicine as legislated by the Misuse of Drugs Regulations 2001 and later amendments and revisions. Only points pertinent to prescribing these drugs at a junior clinician level will be covered in this section. In the 2001 legislation, the drugs were separated again into five schedules based upon differing levels of control.

Schedule 1 – Controlled drug licence

- These drugs may not be used for medicinal purposes. Their production and possession is limited, in the public interest to purposes of research or other special purposes.
- **Examples are cannabis, LSD (lysergic acid diethylamide).**
- Medical practitioners and pharmacists need a special licence issued by the Home Office to possess or supply these drugs.

Schedule 2 – Registered controlled drugs: prescription-only medicines (POMs)

- Includes the opiates, and major stimulants.
- **Examples are diamorphine (heroin), morphine, pethidine, remifentanil, secobarbital, glutethimide, amfetamine, cocaine.**
- A pharmacist may supply these drugs to a patient only on the authority of a prescription issued by a practitioner, i.e. a doctor. These drugs may only be administered to a patient by a doctor or dentist or any person acting in accordance with the directions of a doctor or dentist.
- According to the new legislation, prescriptions do not have to be handwritten. Apart from the prescriber's signature, the entire prescription including the date, may be computer generated. In practice, within hospitals that do not have electronic prescribing, a handwritten prescription with appropriate requirements (see below) is necessary.

Controlled drugs are kept in a locked safe, cupboard, or room, which is constructed and maintained in accordance with the Misuse of Drugs (safe custody) Regulations 1973. Safe custody requirements are stringent and must be strictly adhered to: on wards controlled drugs are kept in a locked controlled drugs cupboard. The nurse in charge of the ward will be in charge of the keys for accessing this cupboard.

- All these controlled drugs have to be entered into a register. The total amount put into the controlled drugs cabinet will be recorded. All controlled drugs prescribed and dispensed will also be recorded to keep an accurate input–output record, i.e. balance.
- Prescriptions are valid for 28 days only.

Schedule 3 Non-registered controlled drugs (POMs)

- Includes the barbiturates (except secobarbital) and a number of minor stimulants which are less likely to be abused than those listed in Schedule 2.
- **Examples include temazepam, midazolam, and buprenorphine**.
- **Safe custody requirements (i.e. store in a locked controlled drugs cupboard) are still necessary for these drugs except phenobarbital.**
- Prescription writing requirements apply to this class of controlled drug.

Schedule 4 Mainly benzodiazepines and hormonal agents (POMs)

- **Part 1**: **Benzodiazepines and zolpidem** (except temazepam and midazolam, which are Schedule 3).
- **Part 2**: **Androgenic and anabolic steroids (e.g. testosterone), human chorionic gonadotrophin (hCG), somatotropin, and somatropin**.
- There is no restriction on the possession when it is part of a medicinal product. Specific controlled drugs prescription writing requirements or safe custody requirements do not apply.
- Prescriptions are only valid for 28 days.

Schedule 5 Controlled drugs in low-strength preparations

- These are preparations of controlled drugs which are present in medicinal products in low strength.
- **Examples include codeine, pholcodine, and morphine**.
- Therefore, exempt from virtually all controlled drugs requirements other than that invoices must be kept for a minimum of 2 years as for all controlled drugs.
- Prescriptions are valid for 6 months.

Prescriptions for controlled drugs

- The 2005 amendment to the Misuse of Drugs Regulations 2001 removed the prior requirement that controlled drugs prescriptions had to be written in the prescriber's own handwriting. Now, controlled drugs prescriptions can be typewritten, handwritten, or computer printed. **Only the signature of the prescriber has to be handwritten**. It remains good practice to write the prescriber's name, easily legible, next to the signature.
- The 2006 amendments included:
  - Patients or other people collecting medicines on their behalf must sign for them
  - A prescription for Schedule 2, 3, and 4 controlled drugs to be valid for 28 days only
  - Strong recommendation that the maximum quantity be limited to 30 days for prescriptions of Schedule 2, 3, and 4 controlled drugs.
  - Professional guidance that doctors should prescribe controlled drugs for themselves or family members only in rare, clearly documented, exceptional circumstances.
- Doctors are only able to prescribe diamorphine and cocaine to substance misusers for the treatment of addiction if they hold a licence issued by the Home Office.

Writing the prescription

- Prescription must contain the following:
  - Patient's NHS number and hospital number
  - Patient's full name, address and age or date of birth
  - Name and form of the drug, even if only one form exists (e.g. tablet, solution, patch)
  - Strength of the preparation
  - Dose to be taken and when (how often)
  - Total quantity of the preparation, or the number of dose units, to be supplied in both **words and figures**
  - Handwritten signature of the prescriber
  - Write the prescriber's name, easily legible, next to the signature.
- The prescriber should sign any script changes.

- A pharmacist is not allowed to dispense a controlled drug, unless all the information required by law is given on the prescription; conversely it is also illegal to issue an unauthorized prescription.

Example of a controlled drugs GP prescription

There are three sections to a controlled drugs prescription:

6 **Patient details**
   - Name, address, date of birth
   - Hospital number/unique identifier

7 **Prescription**
   - Drug name and form
   - Total quantity in numbers and words
   - Dosage and mode of administration
   - Indication of the end of prescription

8 **Doctor details**
   - Name, signature, date, address
   - Contact number, not a legal requirement but good practice.

For further information, the BNF has a section regarding controlled drugs and Figure 13.4 shows an example of a controlled drug prescription.

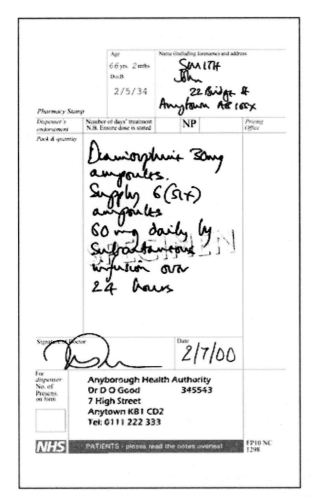

Figure 13.4 Example of a controlled drug prescription.

Student name:	Medical school:	Year:

Controlled drug prescribing

Use a standard discharge letter prescription chart (paper or electronic) to write out the following drugs:

- 30 mg bd of modified release morphine for 14 days
- 120 mL of Oramorph (100 mg/5mL) 5 mg 4 hourly qds

for the following patient:

Mrs Tanita Hermann (222b Holmes Road, Carlton, CL2 9SV; date of birth 12 August 1953, hospital number GE31853211, Dorothea Ward), who has carcinoma of breast with metastatic deposits to her spine. She has been reviewed by the pain consultant and the above medications were advised. She has no known allergies. She weighs 72 kg.

		Self	Peer	Peer /tutor	Tutor
Understands indications, drug class and mechanism of action of each of these drugs	• Modified release morphine • Oramorph (several strengths available) •	☐ ☐ ☐	☐ ☐ ☐	☐ ☐ ☐	☐ ☐ ☐
States common and major side effects for each of these drugs	• Modified release morphine • Oramorph (several strengths available) •	☐ ☐ ☐	☐ ☐ ☐	☐ ☐ ☐	☐ ☐ ☐
Legal prescription requirements demonstrated in all prescriptions	• Full name and address of the patient • Age or date of birth • Hospital number/unique identifier • Text: printed or written legibly in black ink (with correct spelling) • Drug name and form • Total quantity in numbers and words • Dosage and mode of administration • Indication of the end of prescription • Dated and signed by the prescriber • Name of prescriber, address, and contact number •	☐ ☐ ☐ ☐ ☐ ☐ ☐ ☐ ☐ ☐ ☐	☐ ☐ ☐ ☐ ☐ ☐ ☐ ☐ ☐ ☐ ☐	☐ ☐ ☐ ☐ ☐ ☐ ☐ ☐ ☐ ☐ ☐	☐ ☐ ☐ ☐ ☐ ☐ ☐ ☐ ☐ ☐ ☐
Seeks help as appropriate	• Consults BNF for correctness of prescribing • Checks local clinical guidelines for informing correct choice of drugs • Seeks expert help if needed from, for example, clinical pharmacist, nurse, or doctor •	☐ ☐ ☐ ☐	☐ ☐ ☐ ☐	☐ ☐ ☐ ☐	☐ ☐ ☐ ☐
Post-procedure management and professionalism	• Documents changes to prescribing in notes and any specific requirements • Allows enough time to concentrate on task and complete task efficiently and competently •	☐ ☐ ☐	☐ ☐ ☐	☐ ☐ ☐	☐ ☐ ☐
Explanation to patient	• Explains changes in prescription to patients including indications and main side effects • Allows patient opportunity to ask about medications •	☐ ☐ ☐	☐ ☐ ☐	☐ ☐ ☐	☐ ☐ ☐

				Self	Peer	Peer /tutor	Tutor
Self-assessed as at least borderline:	Signature:		Date:	U B S E	U B S E	U B S E	U B S E
Peer-assessed as ready for tutor assessment:	Signature:		Date:	U B S E	U B S E	U B S E	U B S E
Tutor-assessed as satisfactory:	Signature:		Date:	U B S E	U B S E	U B S E	U B S E

Notes

Reference: Patient Net 2010 (EMIS)

13.6 Prescribing intravenous fluids

Background

A regular request on the wards is to write up IV fluids for a patient. Deciding what fluids to give, when to give them, and how much to give are the three things that have to be considered carefully before writing up any fluids. Appropriate management of fluid and electrolyte therapy is essential to protect organ function. Improper fluid and electrolyte management leads to increased morbidity, duration of hospital stay, and mortality. Correct fluid management requires an understanding of normal physiology of water and electrolytes as well as body fluid compartments.

Clinical indications

A patient's fluid output needs to be matched with an adequate input. On average, a healthy adult will require ~3 L of fluid in through food and drink to match the ~3 L that will be lost through urine output and other insensible losses. In addition to 3 L of fluid that a patient should take, s/he will need approx 100 mmol of sodium (Na^+) and 70 mmol of potassium (K^+).

However, if a patient is unable to take any fluid orally or intake is poor, then supplementation may be necessary. Fluid replacement is intended to correct acute losses or maintain homeostasis, or both.

Parenteral fluids are usually given by the IV route; however, in some cases the subcutaneous route may be necessary when venous access is a problem.

Physiological principles

Fluid compartments

Total body water (TBW) is distributed between the intracellular fluid (ICF) and the extracellular fluid (ECF) compartments (Figure 13.5). Interstitial fluid is mostly found in tissues adjacent to the microvascular circulation. Transcellular fluid (e.g. peritoneal, pleural, synovial fluid) is extracellular in nature and considered as a part of interstitial volume (1% of TBW). It may vary from 1 L to 10 L with larger volumes occurring in diseased states (e.g. bowel obstruction or cirrhosis with ascites). It also depends on age (highest in neonates and least in elderly) and gender (higher in male than female due to higher fat content in female).

Extracellular
Blood/plasma: 5% bodyweight
3.5 L

Extracellular
Interstitial fluid: 15% bodyweight
10.5 L

Intracellular
40% bodyweight
28 L

Total 42 L, 60% bodyweight

70 kg person

Daily water balance in health

'Input':
Ingested fluid (1300 mL)
Solid food (800 mL)
Water of metabolism (400 mL)
=
Output
900 ml (0.5 mL/kg/hr from skin and lungs)
Losses from urine (1500 mL) and faeces (100 mL).

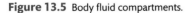

Figure 13.5 Body fluid compartments.

Electrolyte and water distribution

Distribution and movement of water between the intracellular and interstitial spaces is governed by the osmotic forces created by the differences in non-diffusible solute concentrations. The cell membrane separating the fluid compartments is selective and allows the free passage of water but not solutes, unless there is osmolar difference between compartments. In contrast the capillary endothelium is non-selective and freely permeable to both water and ions; plasma and interstitial fluids have similar solute compositions. Therefore, the major determinant of water flux is plasma protein concentration.

Regulation of ECF volume and composition

The volume of ECF is mainly determined by the amount of Na$^+$ that it contains. Thirst and antidiuretic hormone (ADH) control the intake and excretion of water, respectively. The electrolyte composition of urine is largely determined by the renal mechanisms, in particular the renin–angiotensin–aldosterone system, which increases the sodium reabsorption. Water is needed to eliminate the daily solute load and to replace daily insensible fluid loss.

Electrolyte balance and clinical implications

Sodium

Sodium is the principal cation of the ECF. Total body sodium content is 4000 mmol/70 kg with a normal ECF (serum) concentration of 134–145 mmol/L. Daily ingestion has a wide range (50–300 mmol). Normothermic extrarenal losses are minimal (~10 mmol/day).

Hypernatraemia (serum sodium >145 mmol/L) can be caused by excessive administration of sodium salts (chloride or bicarbonate), water depletion, and excess sodium and loss of water. Hypernatraemia usually produces symptoms if the serum sodium exceeds 155–160 mmol/L. It can lead to pyrexia, restlessness, irritability, drowsiness, lethargy, confusion, and coma. Convulsions are uncommon. Treatment depends on the cause. For pure water depletion, water administration or if IV fluid is required, 5% dextrose or hypotonic saline are often used. As rapid correction can lead on to cerebral oedema, the change in serum sodium should usually be no greater than 2 mmol/L per hour, and usually no more than 12 mmol/L in 24 hours.

The symptoms in hyponatraemia depend on the cause (Table 13.7), magnitude, and rapidity of onset. Acute symptomatic hyponatraemia is a medical emergency corrected by treating the underlying cause. The aim of treatment is to raise plasma concentration to 125 mmol/L gradually over a period of no less than 12 hours or by no greater than 2 mmol/L per hour (whichever is slower). Rapid correction of hyponatraemia using hypertonic saline may produce central pontine myelinosis and is a common cause of death in children and young adults due to overzealous correction of hyponatraemia or hyperglycaemia. The rate of correction is usually no more than 12 mmol/L in 24 hours.

Table 13.7 Some causes of hyponatraemia (sodium <135 mmol/L)

Misleading result	Water retention	Water retention and salt depletion
Hyperlipidaemia	Renal failure	Post-operative, post-trauma, or patients with excess fluid losses given inappropriate replacement
Hyperproteinaemia	Hepatic failure	Diuretic excess
Hyperglycaemia	Cardiac failure	Adrenocortical failure
Excess mannitol, glycine, etc.	Syndrome of inappropriate secretion of ADH	Hypothyroidism
	Psychogenic polydipsia	

Potassium

Potassium is the principal intracellular cation and accordingly (along with its anion) fulfils the role of the ICF osmotic provider. It also plays a major role in the functioning of excitable tissues (e.g. muscle and nerve) and is responsible for the resting membrane potential.

Total body potassium is 3500 mmol/70 kg, 90% of which is intracellular. The potassium load must be cleared rapidly from ECF. Some of the causes of hypokalaemia (serum potassium <3.5 mmol/L) are mentioned in the Table 13.8. Hypokalaemia may produce muscle weakness, hypotonicity, paralytic ileus, rhabdomyolysis, and even coma. Treatment includes potassium supplements and treatment of the underlying condition. IV administration of potassium should usually not exceed 10–20 mmol/h and plasma potassium should be monitored at 1–4-hourly intervals.

Table 13.8 Main causes of hypokalaemia and ECG changes

Less intake	Abnormal losses	Compartmental shift
Inadequate dietary intake	**Gastrointestinal**: vomiting, nasogastric aspiration diarrhoea, fistula loss	Alkalosis
	Renal: diuretics, steroids Cushing's and Conn's syndromes	Insulin
		Sympathomimetic agents such as salbutamol

Possible ECG changes: ventricular tachycardia, long PR interval, T wave inversion, prominent U waves.

Table 13.9 Some causes of hyperkalaemia

Collection abnormalities	Excessive intake	Decreased renal excretion	Compartmental shift
Haemolysis	**Exogenous**: Oral or IV Massive blood transfusion	Drugs Spironolactone, ACE-I, etc.	Acidosis
	Endogenous: Burns Rhabdomyolysis	Renal failure	Insulin deficiency
		Addison's disease	Suxamethonium

Possible ECG changes: T wave peaking, P wave flattening, long PR interval, QRS complex widening, deep S wave. Cardiac arrhythmias may be life-threatening, especially a sine wave ECG pattern deteriorating to asystole at K+ 7 mmol/L or greater.

Some of the causes of hyperkalaemia (serum potassium >5 mmol/L) are given in Table 13.9. Treatment is directed at the underlying cause but may include dialysis. Immediate treatment is necessary if plasma concentration exceeds 7 mmol/L or if there are serious electrocardiographic (ECG) abnormalities. Treatment options include calcium chloride or gluconate (antagonizes cardiac effects of hyperkalaemia, effect short lived), glucose with insulin, sodium bicarbonate, Calcium Resonium® (exchange resin per rectum) and peritoneal or haemodialysis.

Calcium

Although almost all (99%) of the total body calcium (1000 g) is present in the bone, a small but significant quantity of ECF ionized calcium is important for many cellular activities including neuromuscular impulse formation, contractile functions, and clotting. Clinical features of reduced serum ionized calcium include tetany, cramps, mental changes, decrease in cardiac output, and prolonged QT interval on the ECG. The treatment is with oral calcium and vitamin D and, if severe, supplemental IV calcium. Clinical features of hypercalcaemia include nausea, vomiting, pancreatitis, polyuria, polydipsia, muscular weakness, mental disturbance, and ectopic calcification. Urgent treatment is required before investigation if severe hypercalcaemia exists.

Treatment includes rehydration followed by induced diuresis to increase renal calcium loss, and specific agents such as biphosphonates and steroids.

Magnesium

Magnesium is primarily an intracellular ion which acts as a metallo-coenzyme in numerous phosphate transfer reactions. It has a critical role in the transfer, storage, and utilization of energy. Normal plasma concentration is 0.70–0.95 mmol/L. Hypomagnesaemia can result from decreased intake or increased loss. Clinical features include neurological signs of confusion, irritability, delirium tremors, convulsion, and tachyarrhythmias. Hypomagnesaemia is often associated with resistant hypokalaemia and hypocalcaemia. Treatment consists of IV magnesium sulphate. A typical regimen is: Day 1: give 0.5 mmol/kg then 0.25 mmol/kg for the next 4 days, up to a maximum of 160 mmol in 5 days.

Hypermagnesaemia is often associated with excessive administration of magnesium salts or conventional doses of magnesium in the presence of renal failure. Clinical features include drowsiness, hyporeflexia, coma, vasodilatation, hypotension, respiratory arrest, conduction abnormalities and asystole. IV calcium may be used for rapidly treating the cardiac conduction defects but definitive treatment may require dialysis.

Box 13.2 Some causes of hypomagnesaemia

Gastrointestinal disorders
- Malabsorption
- Gastrointestinal fistulae
- Diarrhoea
- Parenteral nutrition

Alcoholism

Endocrine diseases
- Hyperparathyroidism
- Hyperthyroidism
- Conn's syndrome

Renal diseases
- Renal tubular acidosis
- Diuretic phase of acute tubular necrosis

Drugs
- Aminoglycosides
- Diuretic therapy
- Cisplatinum

Losses from abdominal organs

Gastrointestinal losses

Clinical effects of fluid loss from the gastrointestinal tract are largely determined by the volume and composition of the fluid. Pure gastric fluid loss (e.g. from vomiting, nasogastric suction) results in water, sodium, hydrogen ion, potassium, and chloride depletion. Hence hypokalaemic hypochloraemic metabolic alkalosis, hypotension, and dehydration develop if the sodium, potassium, and chloride losses are not correctly replaced.

Pancreatic and biliary fluid losses

Examples include pancreatic and biliary fistula. These may result in hyperchloraemic acidosis with hypokalaemia, hypotension, and dehydration if the losses of bicarbonate, potassium, and saline are inadequately replaced.

Intestinal losses

This can happen in diarrhoea, intestinal fistula, ileostomy, and ileus, and result in hypokalaemia, hypotension, and dehydration if the saline and potassium losses are not replaced.

Prescribing IV fluids

There are two major categories of IV fluids – colloids and crystalloids. Crystalloids are solutions containing small molecules in water (e.g. sodium chloride 0.9%, glucose 5%, Hartmann's solution) which pass freely between intravascular and interstitial compartments.

Hartmann's solution is physiologically closer to plasma in terms of chloride ions and sodium content. Colloids are composed of larger molecules that are retained initially within the blood as the molecules are too big to diffuse easily through blood vessels into other compartments. Examples include the gelatines, starches and dextrans, e.g. Gelofusine, Voluven. They are mainly used to maintain or increase plasma volume, particularly during shock or trauma.

Clinical assessment

Before prescribing IV fluid replacement (Table 13.10) carry out an assessment of fluid balance charts, weight, blood pressure, capillary refill time, and skin turgor. Choosing an appropriate fluid depends on the type of fluid loss, patient's renal and cardiac function, and electrolyte levels. A patient with healthy kidneys and no co-morbidities who requires fluid replacement for homeostasis may have a combination regimen with a glucose base followed by a saline-based fluid. In general recommendations to meet maintenance requirements, an adult should receive 50–100 mmol sodium per day, 40–80 mmol potassium per day in 1.5–2 L of water via oral, enteral, or parenteral routes. Additional 500 mL may be given to cover insensible losses. This may be given as a combination dextrose-saline infusion, however, this combination is not recommended for long-term maintenance as it has a lower content of sodium and larger volumes would need to be administered. It is important to encourage oral nutrition and fluids as soon as possible to prevent gut stasis. IV infusions should be discontinued as soon as possible. Table 13.11 shows some examples.

Table 13.10 Commonly prescribed fluids with their constituents

Fluid (1 L)	Na$^+$ (mmol/L)	K$^+$ (mmol/L)	Cl$^-$ (mmol/L)	Additional information
5% Dextrose	0	0	0	
Dextrose-saline	30	0	30	4% dextrose, 0.18% saline
0.9% Saline	154	0	150	Can be given subcutaneously over 12 hours if venous access is a problem
Hartmann's	131	5	111	+Lactate, HCO_3^-, Ca^{2+} (2 mmol/L)
Gelofusine	154	0.4	125	

Table 13.11 Two alternative regimens for giving IV fluids (not for children, elderly patients, or those with heart or liver failure)

Regimen 1 (each litre given over 8 hours)	Regimen 2 (each litre given over 8 hours)
Dextrose-saline 1 L + 20 mmol K$^+$ **Dextrose-saline 1 L + 20 mmol K$^+$** **Dextrose-saline 1 L + 20 mmol K$^+$**	**5% Dextrose 1 L + 20 mmol K$^+$** **0.9% Saline + 20 mmol K+** **5% Dextrose 1 L + 20 mmol K$^+$**
Total sodium = 90 mmol Total potassium = 60 mmol Total fluid = 3 L Total dextrose = 120 g	Total sodium = 154 mmol Total potassium = 60 mmol Total fluid = 3 L Total dextrose = 100 g

The standard regimens can be increased if a patient is:

- Dehydrated
- Shocked
- Has additional losses, e.g. during theatre, burns, surgical drains, etc.

If a patient has liver or heart failure avoid sodium loads, use 5% dextrose.

Patient safety tips

✔ Chart the patient's fluid losses and input deficit and replace this.

✔ Aim for a urine output minimum of 0.5 mL/kg per hour.

✔ Measure U&Es regularly if the patient is unwell, attention especially to the potassium level.

✔ Start oral fluids as early possible.

✔ Potassium (K^+) via a peripheral line should never exceed 10–20 mmol/L per hour on general wards. Under specialist advice, for example, in the ICU, higher concentrations are given with extreme caution, and ECG monitoring.

✔ 5% dextrose may deteriorate glycaemic control in patients with diabetes.

✔ Distinct potential for harm is shown in Box 13.3. The common main problem is that of precipitating cardiac failure or worsening it in a patient with stable cardiac failure. There are also the multiple problems in relation to the IV cannula itself especially in relation to bacteraemia (particular issue if due to MRSA), septicaemia, and local cellulitis. Other dangers of fluid replacement include hypernatraemia, hyperchloraemia, and hyperkalaemia if fluids are given with additional potassium. It is therefore important to monitor the patient both clinically and biochemically for hyper/hypovolaemia and electrolyte imbalances.

Box 13.3 Signs of insufficient fluid and fluid overload

Signs of insufficient fluid prescription/hypovolaemia

- Headache
- Dry mucous membranes
- Prolonged capillary refill
- Absent jugular venous pressure (JVP) on lying flat
- Postural hypotension
- Poor urine output/dark urine
- Reduced skin turgor
- Raised urea, haematocrit
- Fast pulse

Signs of fluid overload

- Dyspnoea
- Orthopnoea/paroxysmal nocturnal dyspnoea
- Cough ± white frothy sputum
- Raised JVP and respiratory rate
- Oedema
- Bibasal crepitations
- Gallop rhythm (third heart sound)
- Pulmonary oedema on chest radiograph
- ECG – myocardial infarction/left ventricular hypertrophy

Documentation and preparation

An example prescription for maintenance IV fluids is given below.

Date	Fluid	Route	Additives	Volume	Rate	Signature
26/2/10	5% Dextrose	IV	20 mmol Potassium	1 L	8hrs	GSmith
26/2/10	0.9% Saline	IV	20 mmol Potassium	1 L	8hrs	GSmith
26/2/10	5% Dextrose	IV	20 mmol Potassium	1 L	8hrs	GSmith

Or

Date	Fluid	Route	Additives	Volume	Rate	Signature
26/2/10	Dextrose-Saline	IV	20 mmol Potassium	1 L	8hrs	GSmith
26/2/10	Dextrose-Saline	IV	20 mmol Potassium	1 L	8hrs	GSmith
26/2/10	Dextrose-Saline	IV	20 mmol Potassium	1 L	8hrs	GSmith

Explanation and consent

Clearly explain to patient why the IV fluids are being given. Explain specific aspects of the treatment such as care of the IV cannula and looking out for extravasation of the IV fluids, pain, and cellulitis. Indicate to the patient how long treatment is likely to continue for.

IV fluid rota protocol

- Ensure that the patient's name, hospital number, allergy status, ward, and date of birth and address are at the top of the fluid rota.
- Assess the patient, giving your examination findings and the indications for IV fluids in the patient's hospital notes.
- Prescribe the patient fluids – either maintenance fluids as shown in the example, or a quantity that will improve their clinical condition without overloading them.
- Ensure that handwriting is legible.
- Ensure that the patient has IV access.

It is appropriate to give fluid challenges to patients who have low blood pressure or low urine output. A bolus of 500 mL (or 250 mL in the elderly) of a colloid (Gelofusine) or 0.9% saline can be given over 30 minutes. If the blood pressure or urine output improves this suggests that hypovolaemia was the cause and the volume of IV infusion can be increased or further fluid challenges may be given.

Post-protocol management

Document in the notes.

Professionalism

Discuss management plans with nursing and other appropriate healthcare professionals such as the dietician and speech and language therapist where appropriate.

Student name:	Medical school:	Year:

IV fluid prescription charts

Use a standard hospital IV fluid prescription chart (paper or electronic) to write out an IV fluid prescription for the following patient:

Mr John Raffles (Shire Inn, 17 Dexter Close, Bosworth, BW3 3XL; date of birth 24 July 1938, hospital number GE3587356, Tolstoy Ward) has been admitted because of nausea, vomiting, epigastric pain. He is known to have abused alcohol in the past and has a history of peptic ulcer disease. He is not on any medication currently apart from bendroflumethiazide 2.5 mg daily for hypertension. He is not tolerating any oral fluids at all. His investigations on admission were as follows:

Sodium 142 mmol/L	Potassium 3.1 mmol/L	Urea 13.2 mmol/L
Creatinine 146 µmol/L	Calcium 1.83 mmol/L	Amylase 788 U/L

Columns: Self | Peer | Peer /tutor | Tutor

Interprets data correctly
- This is a patient with pancreatitis ☐ ☐ ☐ ☐
- Low potassium due to vomiting and/or thiazide diuretic treatment ☐ ☐ ☐ ☐
- Raised urea and creatinine due to dehydration ☐ ☐ ☐ ☐
- Low calcium due to raised lipase causing saponification of triglycerides ☐ ☐ ☐ ☐
- Raised amylase indicating pancreatitis ☐ ☐ ☐ ☐
- ☐ ☐ ☐ ☐

States indications and need for IV fluid therapy
- Patient not eating/drinking ☐ ☐ ☐ ☐
- Potassium level dangerously low ☐ ☐ ☐ ☐
- Bendroflumethiazide to be stopped and reviewed if needed later ☐ ☐ ☐ ☐
- Checks for fluid overload ☐ ☐ ☐ ☐
- ☐ ☐ ☐ ☐

Legal prescription requirements
- Full name and address of the patient ☐ ☐ ☐ ☐
- Age or date of birth ☐ ☐ ☐ ☐
- Text: printed or written legibly in black ink (with correct spelling) ☐ ☐ ☐ ☐
- Dated and signed by the prescriber ☐ ☐ ☐ ☐
- Clearly state for each drug: dose, strength, route, and frequency ☐ ☐ ☐ ☐
- Only very common abbreviations used ☐ ☐ ☐ ☐
- If amending the prescription, draws a line through the incorrect part and initials and dates the change ☐ ☐ ☐ ☐
- Prescriber's name under signature (ideally) ☐ ☐ ☐ ☐
- ☐ ☐ ☐ ☐

Additional IV fluid completion requirements in most cases
- Hospital number ☐ ☐ ☐ ☐
- Location: hospital (yours) and ward stated correctly ☐ ☐ ☐ ☐
- Your bleep number ☐ ☐ ☐ ☐
- Consultant name identified ☐ ☐ ☐ ☐
- Allergies if any ☐ ☐ ☐ ☐
- ☐ ☐ ☐ ☐

Prescribes IV fluids correctly
- ☐ ☐ ☐ ☐

Seeks help as appropriate
- Consults BNF for correctness of prescribing ☐ ☐ ☐ ☐
- Checks local clinical guidelines for informing correct choice of IV fluids ☐ ☐ ☐ ☐
- Seeks expert help if needed from, for example, clinical pharmacist, nurse, or doctor ☐ ☐ ☐ ☐
- ☐ ☐ ☐ ☐

Post-procedure management and professionalism
- Documents IV fluid therapy in notes and any specific requirements such as monitoring for cardiac failure and U&E checks ☐ ☐ ☐ ☐
- Allows enough time to concentrate on task and complete task efficiently and competently ☐ ☐ ☐ ☐
- ☐ ☐ ☐ ☐

Explanation to patient
- Explains reason for treatment to patient and main side effects ☐ ☐ ☐ ☐
- Allows patient opportunity to ask about treatment ☐ ☐ ☐ ☐
- ☐ ☐ ☐ ☐

	Signature:	Date:	U B S E	U B S E	U B S E	U B S E
Self-assessed as at least borderline:						
Peer-assessed as ready for tutor assessment:	Signature:	Date:	U B S E	U B S E	U B S E	U B S E
Tutor-assessed as satisfactory:	Signature:	Date:	U B S E	U B S E	U B S E	U B S E

Notes

13.7 Anticoagulation prescribing

Background

In clinical practice anticoagulants are commonly prescribed. Serious complications are associated with both over-treatment and under-treatment using these agents. This class of drugs is over-represented in prescribing error surveys and NPSA alerts. The latter cites anticoagulants as 'one of the classes of medicines most frequently identified as causing preventable harm and admission to hospital'. The agency's advice is that:

- Staff should be adequately trained
- Written procedures and clinical protocols should be updated to ensure they reflect safe and current practice
- Anticoagulant services conduct an annual clinical audit based on NPSA safety indicators
- Patients prescribed anticoagulants receive appropriate information
- Safe practice for prescribers and pharmacists is promoted to check that the INR is monitored regularly and that the INR level is safe before issuing or dispensing repeat prescriptions for oral anticoagulants
- Safe practice for prescribers co-prescribing one or more clinically significant interacting medicines for patients already on oral anticoagulants is promoted
- Additional INR testing with the anticoagulation service informed, should be undertaken when a potentially interacting medication is prescribed.

Clinical indications

VTE is common and there is the need for treatment of the DVT or pulmonary embolism and prevention of these two conditions. The NICE guidelines on VTE prophylaxis state that around 25 000 patients suffer from VTE and that preventive measures could reduce the risk by at least 90%. It has been suggested that as many as 50% of patients undergoing orthopaedic surgery may have subsequent DVT, and this figure is about 20% within patients admitted for general medicine who do not receive appropriate anticoagulation.

Indications for anticoagulation

- Treatment of DVT or pulmonary embolism
- VTE thromboprophylaxis (see Section 11.9)
- Patients with atrial fibrillation to prevent stroke and transient ischaemic attacks
- Patients with recurrent VTE due to thrombophilia (such as factor V Leiden abnormality, prothrombin variant, protein S deficiency, protein C deficiency and antithrombin deficiency, antiphospholipid syndrome. These are often familial).
- Patients with dilated cardiomyopathies or some prosthetic heart valves (non-tissue valves).

Prescribing principles

The two main types of anticoagulants are warfarin and heparin. Warfarin is mainly used for long-term treatment/prophylaxis and heparin is used for short-term management or when there is a requirement for quick reversal of anticoagulation.

Heparin

Heparin acts by inhibition of factor Xa in the coagulation pathway. There are two types of heparin, low-molecular-weight (LMWH) and unfractionated (UFH). Heparin is used in DVT/pulmonary embolism prophylaxis and therapy, and also in acute coronary syndromes/myocardial infarction therapy. UFH should be considered as a first dose bolus in massive PE or where rapid reversal of effect may be needed. Otherwise LMWH should be used (equally efficacious and safe and easier to use). UFH therapy is guided by the APTTr (activated partial thromboplastin time ratio). Conventional heparin has a shorter half-life and is eliminated by both the liver and kidneys. LMWH is predominantly renally excreted and has a longer predictable half-life, which allows a more predictable dose response than UFH. This caters for once or twice daily dosing regimens with a fixed dose, also without the need for continuous laboratory monitoring as is the case with APTT monitoring with UFH.

The major side effect of any form of heparin is the risk of haemorrhage. This risk increases in those with heart or liver disease, renal disease due to decreased metabolism, and in those with general disability. Heparin may cause thrombocytopenia and, in the long-term, osteoporosis. Thrombocytopenia can occur within the first few days of treatment or after days or weeks of treatment. LMWH is less likely to cause thrombocytopenia than UFH.

The prescription of LMWH (e.g. enoxaparin 20–40 mg/24h SC) for patients as prophylaxis for DVT/pulmonary embolism is common, and as such needs to be remembered! Other important doses are therapeutic doses for DVT/pulmonary embolism (e.g. enoxaparin 1.5 mg/kg/24h SC) and acute coronary syndromes/myocardial infarction (enoxaparin 1 mg/kg/12h SC). Weighing the patient is essential so that doses can be given accurately.

Warfarin

Warfarin is the most widely used anticoagulant. It acts by interfering with vitamin K metabolism. It is given orally and is rapidly and completely absorbed. It is metabolized by the liver and has an average half-life of about 40 hours. This means it can take about a week of administration to reach steady state. An initial loading dose is therefore given. The major adverse effect of warfarin is haemorrhage and thus monitoring is crucial. It is essential therefore to ensure the appropriate doses are prescribed to avoid over-anticoagulation.

Warfarin therapy is usually commenced once a patient's need for it is confirmed, any contraindications assessed, and a drug history elicited. A drug history is essential as warfarin metabolism is affected by a variety of other drugs and compounds. Warfarin dosing is guided by the INR, which is a ratio of the patient's prothrombin time to a standard. As warfarin is a vitamin K antagonist it increases the INR. In most cases (atrial fibrillation, DVT, pulmonary embolism) an INR of 2.5 (between 2 and 3) is the target, in some cases an INR of 3.5 (between 3 and 4) is necessary (e.g. in those with recurrent thromboembolic events, prosthetic cardiac valves, and grafts).

If a patient is on a heparin when starting warfarin, the heparin is continued until the INR is within the desired target range.

Drug interactions with warfarin

- **Increase INR** – alcohol, amiodarone, cimetidine, simvastatin, NSAIDs
- **Decrease INR** – carbamazepine, phenytoin, rifampicin, oestrogens.

Contraindications (Table 13.12)

Table 13.12 Indications/contraindications for anticoagulation

	Indications	Contraindications
Heparin	DVT, pulmonary embolism, myocardial infarction, acute coronary syndromes, pre/post-operative, haemodialysis acute peripheral arterial occlusion	Haemophilia, active gastroduodenal ulcer, thrombocytopenia, allergy, recent major trauma/haemorrhagic cerebrovascular accident (CVA)
Warfarin	DVT, pulmonary embolism, atrial fibrillation, prosthetic heart valves	Recent haemorrhagic CVA, hypertension (severe) pregnancy, active gastroduodenal ulcer, cerebral artery thrombosis, liver failure, risk of falls or non-compliance

Adapted from the *Oxford Handbook for the Foundation Programme*.

New agents

Recently there have been newer drugs available which may be used for prophylaxis against VTE. These include a direct thrombin inhibitor called dabigatran and a direct inhibitor of activated factor X called rivaroxaban. Dosing is dependent on both age and renal function. The common side effect for both of these drugs as for most anticoagulants is haemorrhage, and patients should be monitored for signs of bleeding or anaemia.

Adverse effects

As for all anticoagulants bleeding is a major complication. Treatment with warfarin for atrial fibrillation in the elderly should be reviewed, especially if there is evidence of falls and safe anticoagulant becomes difficult or not needed. Heparin in addition can cause thrombocytopenia; occasional monitoring should be undertaken, and it is vital when there are additional symptoms such as easy bruising.

Patient safety and clinical governance tips

✔ **Timing of anticoagulant**: ensure patient is prescribed or advised to take warfarin at the same time each day (Figure 13.6).

✔ **Counsel patient to avoid any changes in habits**: such as sudden changes in alcohol consumption, or starting vitamin K supplements. Certain dietary factors such as cranberries (or their juice) can affect the INR.

✔ **New medications especially antibiotics**: advise patient to always ensure new medicines prescribed do not interact with warfarin and so to check with the pharmacist when collecting the medicines. The anticoagulation team will be able to advise on increased monitoring if needed.

✔ **Duration of treatment**: ensure patient is aware of likely duration of anticoagulant therapy to avoid dangerous prolongation of treatment.

✔ **Reversal of anticoagulant effect**: heparin can be reversed with protamine and warfarin with vitamin K. Clearly reversal needs to be considered if there is serious gastrointestinal or especially intracerebral bleeding. There is an inherent danger in reversing anticoagulation as well, for example, doing this in a patient with a prosthetic valve may result in catastrophic clotting within the heart.

ANTICOAGULANT THERAPY

HOSPITAL	NAME		HOSPITAL No.
University	JOHN SMITH		N12345

WARD	ADDRESS		
Ward 2C	Ivy Cottage, Newtown, NW5, J12		

CONSULTANT	DATE OF BIRTH		AGE	SEX
Dr JJ	12/5/40		67	M

DIAGNOSIS AF	LENGTH OF A/C THERAPY REQUIRED 2 – 3

ANTICOAGULANT HEPARIN						ANTICOAGULANT WARFARIN OR DINDEVAN					
THERAPUTIC RANGE REQUIRED 1.5 – 2.5						THERAPUTIC RANGE REQUIRED ( ) to complete see over					
DATE	P.T.T. RATIO	DOSAGE (L)/24HRS	NEXT TEST DUE	DRS SIG	ADMIN BY	DATE	P.T.T. RATIO	DOSAGE (mg)	NEXT TEST DUE	DRS SIG	ADMIN BY
						1/3	1.2	10mg	2/3	AB	CD
						2/3	1.7	10mg	3/3	AB	CD
						3/3	2.1	5mg	4/3	AB	CD
						4/3	2.6	4.5mg	5/3	AB	CD
						5/3	2.5	4.5mg	2/3	AB	CD
						6/3	2.5	4.5mg	3/3	AB	CD
						7/3	2.5				

Usual treatment

- If the INR >5, always omit warfarin until INR<5.
- If INR >8 give the patient Vitamin K
- If bleeding: give Vitamin K 5mg IV stat and 2-4 units IV.
- Seek senior help and discuss with haematologist. It may be necessary to consider giving clotting factors (II, VII, IX or X).
- Withhold warfarin until INR<5

Figure 13.6 Anticoagulation chart: local example.

Prescription: This is a standard inpatient anticoagulation therapy card. As with any other prescription: patient name, date of birth, address and hospital number should be written on it.

Diagnosis: should be clearly stated. Especially important if the on-call team have to assess and dose the patient's warfarin.

Warfarin dosing: Ensure the latest INR value is known. If this is recent enough then a recommendation on the warfarin dose can be made. In the example; the patient had four days of warfarin loading (10mg, 10mg, 5mg). The maintenance warfarin dose is 4.5mg daily. The appropriate dose for 7/3 would be 4.5mg.

If INR varies from previous values then a warfarin dose adjustment is needed:
- If the INR increases to 2.7 it would be safe to continue with 4.5mg until recheck soon or alternatively, decrease the dose by 0.5mg to 4mg
- If the INR decreases to 2.3 it would be safe to continue with 4.5mg until recheck soon or alternatively increase the dose by 0.5 mg to 5mg.

Student name:	Medical school:		Year:

Drug prescription charts

Use a standard hospital drug chart or warfarin prescription chart (paper or electronic) to write out a prescription for:

Mrs Celia Brooke (16 Eliot Way, Hill Top Farm, Coveaton, CV9 9XL; date of birth 12 September 1958, hospital number GE73685813, Elizabeth Ward), who has no known allergies except penicillin. She weighs 78 kg and presented with a swollen, tender, and painful left calf muscle and chest pain. She is diagnosed as having DVT and pulmonary embolism clinically. She has just returned from Australia on a long-haul flight throughout which she slept most of the time. Initially she is started on a LMWH. After a few days (and after confirming the diagnosis) she is commenced on warfarin.

She later develops symptoms and signs leading to a diagnosis of pneumonia. As she has an allergy to penicillin she is started on clarithromycin.

		Self	Peer	Peer /tutor	Tutor
Understands indications, drug class and mechanism of action of these drugs	● Warfarin, LMWH	☐	☐	☐	☐
States common and major side effects for each of these drugs	● Warfarin, LMWH	☐	☐	☐	☐
Heparin prescription	● How much heparin does this patient need and which route?	☐	☐	☐	☐
	● Prescribes the appropriate treatment dose, i.e. tinzaparin 175 units/kg od, enoxaparin 1.5 mg/kg od	☐	☐	☐	☐
	● How long does the patient need the heparin for?	☐	☐	☐	☐
Warfarin prescription	● How long will this patient need warfarin for?	☐	☐	☐	☐
	● How does clarithromycin affect the INR?	☐	☐	☐	☐
	● What should happen to the warfarin dose?	☐	☐	☐	☐
	● What would you do if the INR was 6.2 on 6 mg warfarin?	☐	☐	☐	☐
	● What would you do if the INR was 1.3 on 6 mg warfarin?	☐	☐	☐	☐
		☐	☐	☐	☐
Legal prescription requirements demonstrated in all prescriptions	● Full name and address of the patient	☐	☐	☐	☐
	● Age or date of birth	☐	☐	☐	☐
	● State allergies	☐	☐	☐	☐
	● Text: printed or written legibly in black ink (with correct spelling)	☐	☐	☐	☐
	● Dated and signed by the prescriber	☐	☐	☐	☐
	● Clearly state for each drug: dose, strength, route, and frequency	☐	☐	☐	☐
	● Generic name of drug and no abbreviations in this part	☐	☐	☐	☐
	● If amending the prescription draw a line through the incorrect part and initial and date the change	☐	☐	☐	☐
	● Prescriber's name under signature (ideally)	☐	☐	☐	☐
Additional drug chart completion requirements	● Hospital number	☐	☐	☐	☐
	● Location: hospital (yours) and ward stated correctly	☐	☐	☐	☐
	● Patient weight stated correctly	☐	☐	☐	☐
	● Your bleep number	☐	☐	☐	☐
	● Consultant name identified	☐	☐	☐	☐
Seeks help as appropriate	● Consults BNF for correctness of prescribing	☐	☐	☐	☐
	● Checks local clinical guidelines for information if needed	☐	☐	☐	☐
	● Seeks expert help if needed from, for example, clinical pharmacist, nurse, or doctor	☐	☐	☐	☐
Post-procedure management and professionalism	● Documents changes to prescribing in notes and any specific requirements such as monitoring for INR, FBC	☐	☐	☐	☐
	● Allows enough time to concentrate on task and complete task efficiently and competently	☐	☐	☐	☐
Explanation to patient	● Explains changes in prescription to patients including indication and main side effects	☐	☐	☐	☐
	● Allows patient opportunity to ask about medications	☐	☐	☐	☐

			Self	Peer	Peer/tutor	Tutor
Self-assessed as at least borderline:	Signature:	Date:	U B S E	U B S E	U B S E	U B S E
Peer-assessed as ready for tutor assessment:	Signature:	Date:	U B S E	U B S E	U B S E	U B S E
Tutor-assessed as satisfactory:	Signature:	Date:	U B S E	U B S E	U B S E	U B S E

Notes

13.8 Safe use of insulin

Background

Insulin has far more than its fair share of patient safety alerts. The use of insulin in clinical practice is thought to be complex and the special domain of specialized diabetes teams. In reality, 1 in 6 hospital inpatient beds are occupied by patients with diabetes mellitus, and of these, at least a third are expected to be on insulin.

There are several clinical encounters when insulin use is central to the patient's management. This includes:

- **Diabetes type 1**: all patients will be on insulin
- **Diabetes type 2**: many patients will be on oral hypoglycaemic agents and may be on insulin
- **Hyperglycaemia**: defined by clinical condition. In ICU protocols the glucose target is around 4–8 mmol/L. In coronary care the target is usually 4–11 mmol/L
- **Pregnancy**: many patients with gestational diabetes will be on insulin with normalization of the glucose level after delivery such that the insulin can be stopped
- **Management of hyperkalaemia**: an insulin bolus is often indicated together with calcium gluconate, glucose bolus, salbutamol nebulizer, Calcium Resonium®.

Specific management of patients in relation to incretin-mimetics such as exenatide and liraglutide will not be covered in this section. In most cases of acute illness these agents will be stopped, temporarily, until the acute condition has stabilized. Expert advice should be sought.

This chapter will focus on the management of hyperglycaemia in emergency settings only.

Action of insulin

Human insulin is a 51-amino-acid peptide hormone that is normally produced in the pancreatic β cells. Insulin is released after stimulation by glucose or protein. It is the main hormone responsible for the regulation of hyperglycaemia and its action can be seen as physiologically opposite to the actions of the pancreatic α cell hormone, glucagon. Insulin is an anabolic hormone, and its main actions at the cellular level are:

- Increased glyconeogenesis – promote the conversion of glucose to glycogen mainly in the liver and muscle tissue. This directly reduces plasma glucose levels
- Increased fatty acid synthesis and esterification of fatty acids
- Decreased proteolysis and increased amino acid uptake
- Decreased lipolysis and decreased gluconeogenesis
- Increased potassium uptake: intracellular potassium uptake lowers plasma potassium levels.

In patients with diabetes mellitus, there is hyperglycaemia due to either autoimmune destruction of pancreatic β cells (type 1 diabetes mellitus) or resistance to insulin action and eventual pancreatic β cell dysfunction (type 2 diabetes mellitus). Chronic hyperglycaemia, together with concomitant conditions such as hypertension, dyslipidaemia, and microalbuminuria, results in complications that include: coronary artery disease, cerebrovascular disease, peripheral vascular disease, diabetic retinopathy, diabetic nephropathy, and diabetic neuropathy. Insulin replacement, by subcutaneous injection, is essential to restore normoglycaemia in all patients with type 1 diabetes and many with type 2 diabetes. Many patients, with or without diabetes, will additionally require specialized insulin regimens to manage hyperglycaemia.

There are also animal insulins available of pork or beef origin. These are rarely used nowadays but some patients may be taking them due to lack of hypoglycaemia and allergies with human or analogue insulins.

Table 13.13 Commonly used insulins

	Onset of action and duration profiles

Short-acting insulin

- **Human insulin**:
  - ○ Examples: Actrapid, Humulin S
- **Clinical notes**: these need to be injected 20–30 minutes before the meal. Due to their duration of action being less than 6 hours, overnight insulin cover is usually needed with a longer-acting insulin. The duration of action increases risk of hypoglycaemia in between meals in some patients. Patients often need to snack between meals. These insulins are also used intravenously

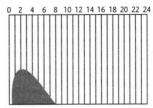

Onset: within 30 minutes
Maximum effect: 1–3 hours
Duration: 8 hours

- **Rapid-acting analogue insulin**:
  - ○ Examples: Lispro (Humalog), Aspart (Novo-rapid), Glulisine (Apidra)
- **Clinical notes**: these agents differ from human insulin by two amino acids. The property of the insulin is altered such that it does not form hexamers. There is more rapid absorption into the blood stream after SC injection. The shorter duration of action reduces the risk of hypoglycaemia in between meals in some patients. Overnight insulin cover is usually needed with a longer-acting insulin

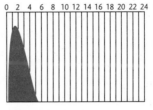

Onset: 10–20 minutes
Maximum effect: 1–3 hours
Duration: 3–5 hours

Intermediate-acting insulin

- **NPH Human insulin isophane**:
  - ○ Examples: Insulatard, Humulin I
- **Clinical notes**: neutral protamine Hagedorn insulin. The protamine component delays absorption of the human insulin. Although long duration of action, absorption is more erratic and less predictable than long-acting analogue insulin. These insulins are cloudy. There is also a zinc insulin which is combined with bovine insulin and is even longer-acting than Insulatard but is rarely used.

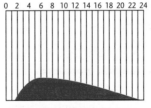

Onset: within 1.5 hours
Maximum effect: 4–12 hours
Duration: up to 24 hours

Long-acting analogue insulins

- **Analogue insulins**:
  - ○ Examples: Insulin Glargine (Lantus) and Insulin Detemir (Levemir)
- **Clinical notes**: these agents differ from human insulin by two amino-acids. The property of the insulin is altered such that there is slower rapid absorption into the blood stream after SC injection. The long duration of action reduces the risk of lack of insulin, and reduces the risk of diabetic ketoacidosis

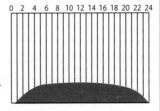

Onset: 1 hour
Duration: 24 hours

Table 13.13 (Continued)

	Onset of action and duration profiles

Common insulin regimens

- **Once-daily medium or long-acting insulin**: usually overnight or od in morning
- **BD pre-mixed insulin**: These insulins are a mixture of short and medium-acting insulin. If given before breakfast, the short-acting insulin covers this meal and the medium-acting insulin covers lunch. The evening meal insulin would cover the evening meal (short-acting) and overnight (medium-acting). The short-acting insulin can be human recombinant or short-acting analogue.
  ○ Examples: Novomix 30 (30% aspart, 70% isophane), Humalog Mix 25 (25% lispro, 75% isophane), Humulin M3
- **Basal-bolus regimen**: the main idea is to give a short-acting insulin with each meal and a long-acting insulin to provide background insulin all the time.
  ○ Examples: any of the analogue short-acting insulins with Glargine or Detemir

Premixed insulin

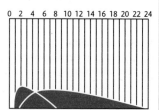

Onset: within 30 minutes
Maximum effect: 2–8 hours
Duration: 24 hours

Sliding scale insulin regimen

An insulin sliding scale involves IV administration of a human short-acting insulin to maintain near normoglycaemia with a particular emphasis on preventing hypoglycaemia and hyperglycaemia greater than a pre-specified level. Blood glucose levels are monitored using bedside, finger-prick capillary glucose levels. The rate of infusion of insulin is adjusted according to the glucose level. Glucose levels will be checked every 15 minutes, 30 minutes, or 1–2 hourly, depending on the clinical necessity. ***IV insulin only has a half-life of minutes***. It is therefore essential that an insulin regimen does not fail due to a blocked cannula or syringe driver failure for any longer than 10–15 minutes, otherwise the process of diabetic ketoacidosis (DKA) can start.

Indications

- **DKA and hyperosmolar hyperglycaemic state (HHS)**.
- **Surgical procedures** complicated by hyperglycaemia (emergency and elective). Many surgical units use the GIK regimen (see below).
- **Surgical patients with diabetes** waiting for surgical procedures.
- **Patients who have sustained a major vascular event**: acute coronary syndromes (DIGAMI protocol is used).
- **Post CVA**: in cases of persistent hyperglycaemia, use sliding of scale insulin is advised (hyperglycaemia in acute stroke conditions is an adverse prognostic factor).
- **Refractory or highly fluctuating hyperglycaemia**: in any acute clinical condition, especially sepsis.

Preparing insulin for a sliding scale regimen

- Prepare a 50 mL syringe with 49.5 mL of 0.9% sodium chloride for injection. Attention to asepsis with respect to the infusate.
- Add 50 units of short-acting (soluble) insulin to the syringe.
- The total volume is now 50 mL (insulin is 100 units per mL).
- 1 mL of infusate will now have 1 unit of insulin per mL.
- Label syringe: name of patient, date of birth, hospital number, contents (e.g. 'soluble insulin 50 units in 0.9% NaCl, 50 mL volume').

- Set up syringe driver and set appropriate alarms.
- Measure capillary blood glucose level and document on chart.
- Start insulin IV at dose according to local sliding scale.
- Check glucose levels according to clinical need. Usually hourly, then 2-hourly when stable.
- IV insulin prepared has an expiry time of 24 hours, therefore a new syringe should be prepared daily if not used up.
- It is normally not necessary to discontinue the patient's long-acting insulin (e.g. glargine or detemir) when they are on IV sliding scale insulin.

How to use IV sliding scale insulin

All hospitals will have their own sliding scale regimen that has been adopted into local guidelines. Table 13.14 should only be used as an example to understand these skills. Local protocols, accepted by local senior clinicians, should be used at all times.

Set alarms, on the syringe driver, to detect cessation of infusion and 1 hour prior to anticipated time of syringe becoming empty.

Adjust infusion as follows: Check glucose levels every 15 minutes, 30 minutes, or 1–2 hourly, dependent on the clinical necessity. More frequent testing until glucose levels within the target range.

Table 13.14	IV Sliding scale insulin (units per hour)				
Glucose in mmol/L	Low glucose scale	Standard scale A	Higher glucose scale	Individualized scale 1	Individualized scale 2
<2.5	*Stop insulin and review: treat hypoglycaemia*				
2.6–3.9	0	0.5	0.5		
4.0–6.9	0.5	1.0	2.0		
7.0–10.9	1.0	2.0	3.0		
11.0–14.9	2.0	3.0	4.0		
15.0–19.9	3.0	4.0	6.0		
20.0+	4.0	6.0	8.0		

- Start with scale A
- Review appropriateness of scale according to clinical need, usually every 4 hours
- If glucose levels are greater than 11.0 mmol/L step up insulin to higher glucose scale
- If glucose remains low, less than 4.0 mmol/L, step down insulin to lower glucose scale
- If these three standard scales do not control the glucose level seek advice and create individual scale and write in appropriate doses of insulin
- Anticipate potassium levels to drop due to the insulin infusion: check at least twice daily initially then daily.

It is very likely that a medical review will be sought if the glucose levels remain less than 4 mmol/L or greater than 17 mmol/L for even a short period of time.

Think very carefully about discontinuing insulin in all patients particularly those with type 1 diabetes. Discontinuing insulin even for a short period of time can precipitate DKA or HHS. If glucose levels have dropped to less than 4 mmol/L on the insulin sliding scale, it would be better to continue small amounts of insulin and add an IV infusion such as:

- 5% dextrose with 40 mmol/L potassium, or
- Dextrose-saline with 40 mmol/L potassium.

Encourage normal food intake, if not contraindicated clinically, as soon as possible.

Discontinuing sliding scale insulin

Some patients will be able to discontinue insulin altogether. Many, and all who were on insulin prior to the use of the sliding scale, will continue on insulin.

Once the patient is clinically stable and eating and drinking, safe transition from sliding scale insulin to oral agents or insulin can take place.

Insulin

It is essential to continue the IV sliding scale insulin for 30 minutes after starting SC insulin.

Change to SC insulin is recommended using the method below:

- Calculate total sliding scale insulin over last 24 hours = X
- From total X subtract 10% if on insulin prior to admission OR subtract 20% if not previously on insulin = Y
- Common regimens:
  - **Premixed insulin regimen (two daily injections of insulin)**: 60% of Y morning (pre-breakfast) and 40% of Y evening (pre-evening meal).
  - **Basal-bolus regimen (four daily injections of insulin)**: 25% of Y as basal injection usually pre-bed, and three injections of 25% of Y of bolus insulin. The bolus is given before each main meal.
  - **Patients' usual regimen**: In most cases, patients previously on insulin may wish to continue on their previous insulin regimen.

There are many nuances in the above protocol that are specific to local diabetes teams. These must be used at all times. One recent idea is the continuance of the basal insulin when patients are admitted, realizing that the sliding scale insulin dose will need to be adjusted downwards. In patients with normal peripheral perfusion, SC sliding scale insulin with a fast-acting analogue may give equally good glycaemic control. This is effectively the idea of using an 'insulin pump' regimen and may be easier and safer to manage in inpatients.

Oral agents

- **Metformin**: When recommencing metformin, restart only if the patient is clinically stable:
  - Renal function is stable with a creatinine <140 μmol/L without dehydration
  - Cardiac failure, liver failure, and sepsis excluded
  - Radiological imaging with IV contrast agents not anticipated
- **Sulphonylureas**: such as gliclazide, often need to be started at a lower dose than usual for the patient due to lower calorie intake. As the patient's intake improves, the usual dose can be used. Dose adjustment may also be needed for residual renal function.
- **Thiazolidinediones ('glitazones')**: As above but must be reviewed and usually stopped in any patient with cardiac failure.
- **DPP IV inhibitors ('gliptins')**: Restart after senior advice. These are new agents, and it must be clear that the underlying hospital admission is not due to these agents.

Criticisms of sliding scale insulin regimens

Theoretically, a sliding scale insulin regime would provide excellent glycaemic control as it is based on measuring a glucose value and treating it. However:

- Accurate monitoring: can be difficult when needing hourly monitoring. This is uncomfortable for the patient and will disrupt the normal sleep pattern. Nursing input is also extensive and may not always be available.

- Standard regimens do not always work: individualizing treatment requires a high level of expertise which may be difficult to access in a timely fashion.
- IV is needed: if the IV fails for even 15–30 minutes the type 1 diabetes patient or the insulin-dependent type 2 diabetes patient can decompensate into DKA.
- Glucose focus: can lead to less stress being placed on potassium, sodium, renal, and arterial blood gas abnormalities.

Alternatives or modifications, to the classic sliding scale regimen, such as continuing with the basal insulin and using a lower insulin dose sliding scale, would help. It is likely that SC sliding scales with basal insulin will be increasingly used in the future.

Insulin use in acute coronary syndromes: The DIGAMI protocol

The DIGAMI protocol (Diabetes Mellitus, Insulin Glucose Infusion in Acute Myocardial Infarction) has been adopted by many coronary care services. A randomized controlled trial showed that an insulin-glucose infusion followed by intensive SC insulin in patients with diabetes improves long-term survival. The effect seen at 1 year continues for at least 3.5 years, with an absolute reduction in mortality of 11%. This means that one life is saved for every nine patients treated using this regimen. This is a treatment effect greater than aspirin or thrombolysis post myocardial infarction. The effect was most apparent in patients who had not previously received insulin treatment. There are many hypotheses for the mechanism of the beneficial effect. It may just be the effect of insulin driving glucose and oxygen into ischaemic myocardial cells and either preventing cell death or arrhythmias. Hypoglycaemia must be avoided otherwise mortality is increased.

Criteria for insulin infusion for first 48 hours following myocardial infarction:

- All patients with pre-existing diabetes
- Blood glucose above 11 mmol/L on admission (confirm by laboratory sample).

Cardiac criteria

- Suspected or confirmed myocardial infarction on ECG changes.
- LVF secondary to probable myocardial infarction.

DIGAMI protocol

Stage 1 (for at least 24 hours):

Infusion:

- 500 mL 5% glucose with 80 units soluble insulin: 1 unit of insulin/6 mL infusate
- Start with 30 mL/h (5 units insulin per hour)
- Check blood glucose after 15 minutes, 30 minutes then hourly. Adjust infusion according to protocol below (or local adaptation)
- Aim for blood glucose 7–10 mmol/L
- Recheck blood glucose every 2 hours, or 1 hour if infusion rate changed
- If blood glucose <11 mmol/L after 10 pm, consider reducing infusion rate by 50% overnight.

Note: serum potassium (K^+) to be measured at entry to coronary care unit or ward and then again at 6 hours, 12 hours, and 24 hours. Hypokalaemia (and hyperkalaemia) can cause life-threatening cardiac arrhythmias.

Specific changes to infusion according to glucose levels (Table 13.15)

The changes below should be considered around 2 hours after setting up the infusion. Hypoglycaemia should be treated urgently at all times.

Table 13.15 Changes to infusion according to glucose levels

Blood glucose	Action
>15 mmol/L	• Give 4–8 units of insulin by IV bolus • Increase rate by 6 mL/h (1 unit insulin per hour)
11–14.9 mmol/L	• Increase infusion rate by 3 mL/h (0.5 unit insulin per hour)
7–10.9 mmol/L	• Leave infusion rate unchanged
4–6.9 mmol/L	• Decrease infusion rate by 6 mL/h (1 unit insulin per hour)
Hypoglycaemia <4 mmol/L	• Stop infusion for 15 minutes. • If patient has symptoms/signs of hypoglycaemia then give 30 mL of 20% glucose intravenously • Check glucose every 15 minutes until glucose is >7 mmol/L • The infusion is restarted with an infusion rate decreased by 6 mL/h (1 unit insulin per hour) when blood glucose is >7 mmol/L

Stage 2

The original DIGAMI protocol advised the insulin-glucose infusion for at least 24 hours followed by multi-dose insulin treatment, for at least 3 months, to keep glucose levels in between 4 and 11 mmol/L. This can be achieved by any suitable regimen such as:

- **Premixed insulin regimen (2 daily injections of insulin):**
- **Basal-bolus regimen (4 daily injections of insulin):**

GIK regimen: peri-operative and operative surgical regimen

A variation of the insulin sliding scale is the GIK regimen also known as the GKI or Alberti regimen. This consists of an infusion of <u>G</u>lucose, <u>I</u>nsulin and <u>K</u>$^+$. This regimen corrects for the absolute or relative hypokalaemia that is liable to occur when insulin is given. The GIK regimen is less likely to result in hypokalaemia. GIK is often the regimen of choice for surgical patients but can also be used whenever a sliding scale is indicated.

Surgical patients: insulin treated

Pre-operative

- Optimize blood glucose control, aiming for fasting blood glucose concentrations between 4 and 7 mmol/L and in most cases an HbA$_{1c}$% <8. Poor glycaemia compromises recovery from surgery and especially wound healing. There is also increased risk of VTE. Surgery may need to be delayed if control is poor.
- Check for complications of diabetes which may complicate management (cardiac, renal, peripheral neuropathy, proliferative retinopathy).
- Patients on long-acting insulins such as glargine or detemir. Continue with this but the amount of insulin added to the standard GIK bag may need to be reduced.

GIK Infusion peri and post operatively

All diabetes patients on insulin should be managed by use of the GIK regimen. Aim for glucose levels 4–10 mmol/L.

Standard 500 mL GIK infusion bag: consists of 500 mL of 10% dextrose with 10 mmol potassium chloride and 16 units of soluble insulin added. The potassium concentration is therefore 20 mmol/L. The insulin should be added to the 500 mL 10% dextrose bag using a syringe with a longer >3 cm detachable needle, i.e. blue or green needle. This is because the standard shorter subcutaneous insulin needle may leave the insulin highly concentrated at the injection port. The bag once prepared must be well mixed and connected to the volumetric infusion device for an accurately timed infusion rate.

Post operatively, the blood glucose may be checked 2-hourly if stable. The GIK infusion is continued until the patient is able to eat normally. Oral fluids and light diet can continue on the GIK regimen (Table 13.6).

Continue the GIK infusion for 30–60 minutes after giving the first dose of SC insulin to minimize chances of insulin deficiency to occur.

U&Es should be checked daily, hyponatraemia may develop with prolonged use of GIK especially in the presence of renal failure. If sodium is less than 130 mmol/L, the infusion regimen is changed to 20% dextrose with double the concentration of soluble insulin and potassium. This regimen should also be used if fluid overload is likely to be a problem (e.g. CCF).

Post operative:

Change to insulin therapy using guidelines for sliding scale use above.

Table 13.16 GIK regimen		
Standard rate: 80 mL/h	**Insulin added to 500 mL bag of 10% dextrose**	**Potassium dose in GIK regimens**
Standard	16 units of soluble insulin added	500 mL of 10% dextrose with 10 mmol potassium chloride and potassium concentration is therefore 20 mmol/L.
Obesity, insulin resistant, uncontrolled hyperglycaemia on above	20 units of soluble insulin added	
Thin, usual insulin dose low	12 units of soluble insulin added	
Patients with renal failure (creatinine above 150 μmol/L). Infuse 500 mL over 12 hours	12 units of soluble insulin added	**No potassium to be added** **Monitor U&Es bd then od**
Hyperglycaemia or hypoglycaemia: Units of insulin added to GIK bags can be adjusted by 4 units upwards if uncontrolled hyperglycaemia or downwards if hypoglycaemia.		

Surgical patients: not on insulin

Pre-operative

- Optimize blood glucose control and check for complications of diabetes as above.
- Long-acting sulphonylureas such as glibenclamide can cause hypoglycaemia especially in the elderly and those with poor renal functions. These should be changed to short-acting agents such as gliclazide or tolbutamide at least several days prior to surgery.
- Metformin should be stopped and for 24 hours post-operatively.

Peri-operative

- **If glucose control is acceptable** (glucose levels under 11 mmol/L). Simply omit the oral hypoglycaemic agent(s) on the day of surgery. Monitor blood glucose concentrations 1 or 2 hourly and avoid infusion of glucose and lactate containing fluids (Hartmann's, dextrose saline, dextrose). When the patient is able to eat and drink, the oral agents are restarted as advised above.

- **If the blood glucose control is poor** (fasting over 11 mmol/L). Manage using GIK regimen as above for insulin-treated patients. For these individuals, it is often necessary to use SC insulin temporarily or more permanently once they are able to eat.

Insulin pump therapy

Increasingly more and more patients with type 1 diabetes are being placed on insulin pump therapy to ensure tight glycaemic control. Insulin pump therapy is actually more accurately called continuous SC insulin infusion. The pump is a small device worn outside the body, which continuously delivers insulin into the body through a very thin tube that is attached to a cannula inserted under the skin. The insulin can be delivered at a set rate throughout the day, which can be increased when needed, for example, at meal times. Current guidelines suggest that sliding scale insulin regimens and GIK regimens would apply equally well to these patients. However, in many cases, it will be possible to continue with insulin pump alone with appropriate changes in doses. This will especially apply to more minor procedures and less severe illness.

Patient education

Self-management by the patient is central to good clinical care of all long-term conditions. It is particularly critical in conditions such as diabetes, exemplified by complex insulin regimens, home blood glucose monitoring, and insulin dose adjustment. In many cases the expert diabetes team will be required to help with this task. Ideally a care plan should be provided in written form and it should be made clear to the patient whom they should contact if their diabetes control deteriorates for reasons of hypoglycaemia or hyperglycaemia. Timely advice is likely to reduce admissions for hypoglycaemia, DKA, and HHS. As with all patient education the right balance needs to be struck between complexity of medical terms and concepts and simplicity. It is always important to check that understanding has taken place and that the patient is better equipped to deal with their conditions and its treatment and monitoring.

Patient safety tips

- ✔ **Ensure high quality patient education and understanding**: this includes ensuring concordance with treatment, regular meals, home blood glucose monitoring and diary, insulin dose adjustment, how to treat hypoglycaemia, insulin injection site rotation, watching out for concomitant illness particularly sepsis, who to contact if needed
- ✔ **Sliding scales, GIK regimens and DIGAMI protocols**: all need to be individualized to the patient if the standard protocol does not achieve outcomes intended such as tight glycaemic control.
- ✔ **Hypokalaemia**: it is easy to forget that intravenous insulin will drive potassium into cells and the resulting hypokalaemia can generate life-threatening arrhythmias. Check potassium levels often and correct hypokalaemia (and hyperkalaemia) meticulously.
- ✔ **Hyponatraemia**: can result as a consequence of the reliance on 10% dextrose as the infusate in the GIK regimen. Check U&Es regularly and watch out for confusion which is often an initial presenting compliant or concern noted by a number of healthcare professionals.

Safe use of insulin

Mrs Millicent Tweedie (Eccles Court, Bosworth, BW3 4CD; date of birth 6 December 1958, hospital number GE1235813, Joyce Ward) has been admitted for routine laparoscopic cholecystectomy. Due to adhesions from previous episodes of cholecystitis and pancreatitis, open surgery for cholecystectomy became necessary. She usually takes metformin 500 mg tds and gliclazide 160 mg bd. Previously when a glitazone was tried she developed peripheral oedema and mild congestive cardiac failure. She works as a nurse and has variable shift patterns. Her glycaemic control prior to surgery was less than optimal with an HbA$_{1c}$ of 9.2% (89 mmol/mol). Her admission glucose level is 12.4 mmol/L and 2 hours prior to surgery it is 13.6 mmol/L.

This assessment will focus on insulin and its use in patients such as outlined in the clinical vignette.

		Self	Peer	Peer /tutor	Tutor
What are the main indications for use of insulin? Why will it be considered in this case?	● Type 1 diabetes mellitus, type 2 diabetes mellitus on insulin, hyperglycaemia in acute setting uncontrolled on usual treatment, hyperglycaemia in pregnancy, management of hyperkalaemia	☐	☐	☐	☐
	●	☐	☐	☐	☐
What are the main actions of insulin?	● Increased glycogenogenesis, increased fatty acid synthesis and esterification of fatty acids, decreased proteolysis and increased amino acid uptake, decreased lipolysis and decreased gluconeogenesis, increased potassium uptake (subsequent hypokalemia can result)	☐	☐	☐	☐
	●	☐	☐	☐	☐
For each of the following insulin types, please give a locally used example, its onset of action, duration profile and clinical use	● Human short-acting insulin, analogue short-acting insulin, intermediate-acting insulin, long-acting insulin, pre-mixed insulins	☐	☐	☐	☐
	●	☐	☐	☐	☐
What common insulin regimens have you encountered in local clinical practice?	● ?od, ?bd, ?qds	☐	☐	☐	☐
	●	☐	☐	☐	☐
If this patient needed to be transferred onto insulin long term, which regimen would suit her best in your opinion and why?	● Ask patient about preferences. A bd regime or qds regime may be used. Once daily insulin is unlikely to work	☐	☐	☐	☐
	●	☐	☐	☐	☐
How can this patient's glycaemic control be optimized prior to surgery?	● GIK regimen or sliding scale insulin (immediately pre and post surgery)	☐	☐	☐	☐
	●	☐	☐	☐	☐
What are the main indications for a sliding scale insulin regimen?	● DKA, HHS, surgical procedures complicated by hyperglycaemia (emergency and elective). Many surgical units use the GIK regimen, major vascular event: acute coronary syndromes (DIGAMI protocol is used), post CVA, refractory or highly fluctuating hyperglycaemia: in any acute clinical condition especially sepsis	☐	☐	☐	☐
	●	☐	☐	☐	☐
How is insulin prepared for a sliding scale regimen?	● 50 mL syringe with 49.5 mL of 0.9% NaCl for injection	☐	☐	☐	☐
	● Add 50 units of short-acting (soluble) insulin. 1 mL of infusate will now have 1 unit of insulin per mL	☐	☐	☐	☐
	● Label syringe: name of patient, date of birth, hospital number and contents	☐	☐	☐	☐
	● Set up syringe driver and set appropriate alarms	☐	☐	☐	☐
	● Measure capillary blood glucose level and document on chart	☐	☐	☐	☐
	● Start insulin IV at dose according to local sliding scale. Check glucose levels according to clinical need and adjust insulin dose. Usually hourly, then 2-hourly when stable	☐	☐	☐	☐
	● IV insulin prepared has an expiry time of 24 hours, therefore a new syringe should be prepared daily if not used up	☐	☐	☐	☐
	●	☐	☐	☐	☐

This patient is reviewed by the diabetes care team and insulin treatment on discharge is recommended. The patient decides that a bd regimen would suit her best initially. She has required 50 units of insulin in the previous 24 hours and now she is eating and drinking normally. What dose of a pre-mixed insulin would you recommend?	• 50 units minus 20% = 40 units; 60% am, 40% pm therefore 24 units pre-breakfast and 16 units pre evening meal	☐	☐	☐	☐
	•	☐	☐	☐	☐
What are the main factors to consider before restarting metformin?	• The patient must be clinically stable: renal function stable with a creatinine of <140 µmol/L without dehydration, cardiac failure, liver failure and sepsis excluded, radiological imaging with IV contrast agents not anticipated	☐	☐	☐	☐
	•	☐	☐	☐	☐
What are the main aspects in relation to patient safety and safe use of insulin?	• Always monitor and treat high and low glucose levels diligently. Patients can rapidly decompensate if hypoglycaemia is any time longer than a few minutes or hyperglycaemia is untreated (leads to DKA, HHS, worsening sepsis and the failures)	☐	☐	☐	☐
	• Ensure high-quality patient education and understanding	☐	☐	☐	☐
	• Sliding scales, GIK regimens and DIGAMI protocols: all need to be individualized to the patient if the standard protocol does not achieve outcomes intended, such as tight glycaemic control	☐	☐	☐	☐
	• Hypokalaemia: this can generate life-threatening arrhythmias. Check potassium levels often and correct hypokalaemia (and hyperkalaemia) meticulously.	☐	☐	☐	☐
	• Hyponatraemia: can result due to 10% dextrose in the GIK regime. Check U&Es regularly and watch out for confusion (common initial symptom)	☐	☐	☐	☐
	•	☐	☐	☐	☐

Self-assessed as at least borderline:	Signature:	Date:	U B S E	U B S E	U B S E	U B S E
Peer-assessed as ready for tutor assessment:	Signature:	Date:	U B S E	U B S E	U B S E	U B S E
Tutor-assessed as satisfactory:	Signature:	Date:	U B S E	U B S E	U B S E	U B S E

Notes

Unit 14 **Certificates and forms**

14.1 **Consent**

....

Background

Every interaction between a healthcare worker and a patient can only be carried out if the patient gives consent. There are three types of consent: implied, verbal, and written. Written consent is important for several reasons. If the process is carried out correctly, a patient will be given all the information regarding any procedure they are about to undertake including the benefits and potential risks. They must be able to understand what they are being told, and will subsequently make an informed choice as to whether or not they wish to have the procedure.

In obtaining written consent, there is also physical evidence that the patient has given consent as the document once completed by the doctor requires the patient's signature.

....

Clinical indications

The issue of consent must be addressed in each and every clinical encounter.

Professional principles

A reminder of the four bioethical principles that apply in relation to consent is always useful.

- **Autonomy**: respect for the individual and their right to make individualized decisions for their own health and management of their illnesses. This also implies that a plurality of options must be presented where possible.
- **Beneficence**: acting in and to the benefit of the patient. Difficult to define, avoid vague concepts and labelling such as 'poor quality of life'.
- **Non-maleficence**: central to all ideas relating to patient safety and historically a fundamental principle of clinical care expressed as *primum non nocere* – first do no harm.
- **Justice**: the principle of fairness, indeed kindness to the individual patient. The context of the wider community and society must also be considered.

From the above, in practical terms arise the key criteria for assessing competence that must be assessed against for valid consent. These are enshrined in the Mental Capacity Act (2005):

- The patient must be deemed competent to give consent
- The patient must not be forced or coerced by any means to give consent
- The patient must understand and believe the information given
- The patient must be able to deliberate about the matter under discussion especially in relation to choices.

Patients are considered to be competent adults over the age of 18 unless a mental or physical illness or condition precludes this. In between the ages of 16 and 18, patients are treated as adults but clinical decisions and consent can be over-ridden by legal representatives or those with parental responsibility. Similarly patients under the age of 16 can be deemed able to give consent if the above three criteria are met. The two principles established into law by the Gillick case (1985) were:

- If a child has sufficient understanding to give consent, then the right of a legal guardian, including parents, to give or withhold consent to treatment is no longer needed. The child is then deemed to be 'Gillick competent'

- The treating doctor or other clinician is able to ascertain whether the child is 'Gillick competent'.

If a patient is deemed not to have the capacity or competence to give valid consent for the decision in hand, then this 'capacity for consent' must be assessed and recorded.

Informed consent can only be taken having established the patient is *competent*: that is they have the *capacity* to understand the information and retain it long enough to process it and make an informed decision. If the patient is confused (e.g. sepsis), or critically ill and unable to communicate (e.g. head injury or major trauma), the procedure should be performed if the doctor responsible for the patient deems it to be in the patient's best interests.

Confidentiality and data protection

Issues of confidentiality often arise in relation to consent, for example, people phoning into a ward to enquire about a family member or a friend. It is important to determine what information the patient does and does not want disclosing, otherwise a breach of confidentiality can arise. A useful general rule is that you must never discuss a patient with anyone unless there is a clear professional reason to do so and you are confident that the information will be treated equally professionally. Similarly we as healthcare workers must exercise considerable caution when discussing our work with other members of the public including our close friends and family. Any discussion of patients that will breach confidentiality must be avoided. Even discussion of patients at an educational meeting must comply with the very highest standards of confidentiality by, for example, only using the most basic of demographic details such that the patient can never be directly identified. It is also our duty to protect the access to clinical notes and data such that the above rules are addressed.

There are, however, several scenarios when we are obligated to give information about a patient where there is an actual breach of confidentiality from the perspective of the individual patient. This is because there is a now a greater need to serve the wider community and society. In almost all cases the matter should be discussed with the patient and the precise facts revealed stated and why the information needs to be shared. Examples include:

- **Requirement of the law**: criminal investigation including determining details of road traffic accidents
- **Potential for serious harm to patients or others**: especially in relation to child abuse, domestic violence, driving safety (for example in dementia, epilepsy or recurrent hypoglycaemia)
- **Statutory obligation**: registration of birth, deaths, and marriages
- **Registration of infectious disease**
- **Reasons of national security**
- **Reporting of significant side effects**: clinical cases that could potentially improve the care of others.

Contraindications

You should not obtain consent if you are not familiar with the procedure with respect to its details including indications, how it is carried out, and complications. The General Medical Council's guidance on consent states that it is not essential that you have the ability to perform the procedure for which consent is required. In some cases you may be able to provide only part of the information that is needed. This preparation will at least assist the final process of formally signing off the consent by a more experienced senior colleague.

Sequence for consent for surgical procedure

Documentation and preparation

The Department of Health consent form (entitled 'Patient agreement to investigation or treatment') (Figure 14.1)

Patient identifier/label

George Eliot Hospital **NHS**
NHS Trust

ConsentForm3
Patient/parental agreement to investigation or treatment
(procedures where consciousness not impaired)

Name of Procedure
(include brief explanation if medical term not clear)

Statement of health professional (to be filled in by health professional with appropriate knowledge of proposed procedure, as specified in consent policy)

I have explained the procedure to the patient/parent. In particular, I have explained:
The intended benefits ....

Serious or frequently occurring risks..........

I have also discussed what the procedure is likely to involve, the benefits and risks of any available alternative treatments (including no treatment) and any particular concerns of those involved.

☐ The following leaflet/tape has been provided ....

Signed.......... Date..........

Name (PRINT).......... JobTitle..........

Statement of interpreter (where appropriate)
I have interpreted the information above to the patient/parent to the best of my ability and in a way in which I believe s/he/they can understand.

Signed .... Date.......... Name(PRINT)..........

Statement of patient/person with parental responsibility for patient
I agree to the procedure described above.
I understand that you cannot give me a guarantee that a particular person will perform the procedure.
The person will, however, have appropriate experience.
I understand that the procedure will/willnot involve local anaesthesia.

Signature.......... Date..........

Name(PRINT).......... Relationship to patient..........

Confirmation of consent (to be completed by a health professional when the patient is admitted for the procedure, if the patient/parent has signed the form in advance)

I have confirmed that the patient/parent has no further questions and wishes the procedure to go ahead.
Signature.......... Date..........

Name(PRINT) .... JobTitle..........

Copy accepted by patient/parent: yes/no (please ring)

YELLOW COPY: CASE NOTES WHITE COPY: PATIENT/PARENT

- Patient details (name, date of birth, address, hospital number)
- Name of proposed procedure or course of treatment
  - Name of procedure
  - Brief details outlining/explaining procedure
- Statement of health professional (benefits and risks)
  - Benefits and potential risks of procedure
  - Any extra procedure(s) that may be necessary during main procedure
  - Type of anaesthesia to be used (if any)
  - Extra details (leaflets, telephone numbers)
- Statement of patient
  - Understanding of details given by health professional
  - Agreement to procedure
  - Signed and dated by patient
- Confirmation of consent (signed and dated by the healthcare professional)

Figure 14.1 Consent form example.

Explanation and consent

Introduce yourself clearly to the patient. Consent can be withdrawn at any time by the patient and they should be made aware of this. Written consent, using the above format, is used widely for a variety of both surgical and medical procedures. Verbal consent is appropriate when asking a patient if you can take a history from them or examine them. Implied consent is appropriate when you ask a patient something, e.g. to check their blood pressure, and they extend their arm out to you without any verbal response.

Protocol

In addition to consent, an important issue is that of capacity. In some cases there is a question of whether the patient understands what they is being told and is unable to make an informed decision; this concern is high in the elderly and psychiatric patients. Similar issues arise in under-18s, especially with parents or guardians being involved with their care. The Department of Health has published guidelines on consent ('Good practice in consent implementation guide: consent to examination or treatment'). The Mental Health Act may be needed in certain cases and senior help needed together with the involvement of a social worker.

Formal documentation

The most important feature relating to consent is documentation. Appropriate consent should always be obtained, but ensure that it is all documented in the patient notes. If it is not documented, and the patient denies ever giving consent, then any examination/procedure that has been carried out could result in criminal proceedings against you.

In summary

- Identify yourself and role in the procedure
- Explain why the procedure needs to be done and by whom
- Possible alternatives
- What the procedure entails, use simple diagrams, information leaflets, and similar
- Risks, discomforts, and complications
- Ask permission using open questions
- Check understanding and permission obtained by getting the patient to explain back to you and consenting verbally
- Invite any additional questions, address concerns
- Obtain written consent if needed and close.

Post-protocol management

Clearly document in the notes that consent has been obtained and file the consent file into the notes so that you know for sure that it is there when needed – often minutes before a patient is anaesthetized.

Professionalism

The importance of obtaining consent to high standards is critical to good clinical care and ensure that the patient is fully informed and thus greatly reducing the potential for litigation. In many cases you will remain responsible for the care of the patient you have consented. Ensure that you address the effects of the anaesthetic, especially tiredness. You will also need to look out for the specific complications of the surgery but especially for generic complications such as sepsis, deep vein thrombosis, pulmonary embolism, and bleeding.

Adverse effects

Not obtaining valid consent and carrying out a procedure is at worst an assault on the body of the patient. It will be for the clinician to decide, taking into account current medical practice, whether implied, verbal, or written consent is needed.

Patient safety and clinical governance tips

- ✔ **Consent taking**: this opportunity should also be used to clarify in your mind what the procedure is that is being undertaken and its clinical indication. This will add an extra safety layer to ensuring that, for example, the right operation is carried out on the right limb.
- ✔ **Complications**: specifically remind yourself of and look out for any complications.
- ✔ **Best interests of the patient**: if the patient cannot give consent, act in the patient's best interest in an emergency with life saving and stabilization being the key priority. Clearly, expert advice should always be sought if needed.
- ✔ **Consider conducting a clinical audit on consent**.

Student name:	Medical school:	Year:

Consent

Please consent Mr(s) Lesley Longton (date of birth 13 July 1947, hospital number RLTN400078), for an elective pleural biopsy. There has been a persistent pleural effusion and the biopsy will be performed under local anaesthesia. Please role play with the assessor as subject. Please fill in a local version of the consent form.

Further information: The intended benefits of the procedure are to determine the cause of the patient's effusion or any abnormality of the pleura. The risks associated are pneumothorax, fall in blood pressure during the procedure due to stimulation of the nerves. The procedure has been discussed with patient, including alternative treatment or no treatment and no particular concerns were noted. A booklet giving more information regarding the procedure, pre- and post-procedure plan, contact telephone number of the respiratory unit for further information and support has been given to the patient. The patient is literate, does not need an interpreter, and has no advance directive/living will.

		Self	Peer	Peer /tutor	Tutor
Patient details	• First name	☐	☐	☐	☐
	• Surname	☐	☐	☐	☐
	• Date of birth	☐	☐	☐	☐
	• Responsible health professional	☐	☐	☐	☐
	• Job title	☐	☐	☐	☐
	• NHS no. or other identifier	☐	☐	☐	☐
	• Sex of the patient	☐	☐	☐	☐
	• Documents any special requirements	☐	☐	☐	☐
	•	☐	☐	☐	☐
Procedure	• Name of the procedure	☐	☐	☐	☐
	• Brief explanation if medical term is not clear	☐	☐	☐	☐
	•	☐	☐	☐	☐
Intended benefits and risks	• Intended benefits	☐	☐	☐	☐
	• Potential risks	☐	☐	☐	☐
	• Potential additional procedures	☐	☐	☐	☐
	•	☐	☐	☐	☐
Anaesthesia	• Use of anaesthesia	☐	☐	☐	☐
	•	☐	☐	☐	☐
Clinician details	• Signature of the consenting clinician	☐	☐	☐	☐
	• Name of consenting clinician in print	☐	☐	☐	☐
	• Job title	☐	☐	☐	☐
	• Date	☐	☐	☐	☐
	• Contact details	☐	☐	☐	☐
	•	☐	☐	☐	☐
Patients details	• Patient's signature is documented	☐	☐	☐	☐
	• Patient's name is printed	☐	☐	☐	☐
	• Date of consent	☐	☐	☐	☐
	•	☐	☐	☐	☐
Notes	• Checks for any advance directives/ living wills	☐	☐	☐	☐
	•	☐	☐	☐	☐
What are the general complications of surgery	• General complications: tiredness, low mood, infection, deep vein thrombosis, pulmonary embolism, bleeding	☐	☐	☐	☐
	• Endoscopy: perforation of viscus, hoarse voice (upper gastrointestinal endoscopy)	☐	☐	☐	☐
	• Colonic surgery: constipations, ileus, anastomotic leaks, stoma problems,	☐	☐	☐	☐
	• Breast surgery: early arm oedema with more permanent lymphoedema	☐	☐	☐	☐
	• Thyroid surgery: hoarse voice, tracheal obstruction due to bleed in pre-tracheal fascia, low calcium state	☐	☐	☐	☐
	• Prostatectomy/cystoscopy: urine retention, urethral stricture, UTI, urinary incontinence	☐	☐	☐	☐
	•	☐	☐	☐	☐

				Self	Peer	Peer/tutor	Tutor
Self-assessed as at least borderline:	Signature:	Date:		U B S E	U B S E	U B S E	U B S E
Peer-assessed as ready for tutor assessment:	Signature:	Date:		U B S E	U B S E	U B S E	U B S E
Tutor-assessed as satisfactory:	Signature:	Date:		U B S E	U B S E	U B S E	U B S E

Notes

14.2 Blood forms and requesting samples

Background

Blood investigations are an important part of a patient's workup. Blood samples are usually sent to the labs for analysis with an attached form identifying the patient and the tests required. If the forms are not filled out correctly then important results will be missed and management decisions may not be made. All healthcare systems operate in environments characterized by limited resources: financial, functional, and staffing. Overloading an already stretched laboratory with unnecessary requests is wasteful both in terms of human resources and financially. All requests for laboratory investigation should be clinically indicated, but on the other hand do not miss asking for any investigations that are necessary.

Clinical indications

Almost 100% of patients admitted to hospital will have blood tests. The majority of patients seen in general practice or clinics elsewhere will have had or have tests regularly. There many examples of specific tests that need special attention. Important examples of this are the monitoring of the international normalized ratio (INR) regularly in the dosage of warfarin, and the monitoring of antibiotic levels in gentamicin and vancomycin levels. If levels are not measured in the administration of these drugs, then patient safety will be compromised.

Professional principles

There are several departments that analyse blood in the hospital and other external analysing companies provide support for more specific tests, but remember to order the basic tests before pursuing the more complex ones. Do not be tempted to tick a few too many boxes when requesting blood tests. Is it really necessary to request to request C reactive protein and INR in all patients at admission? There should a clear link between the diagnoses that you are considering and the tests requested.

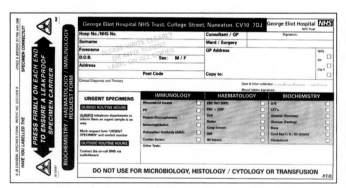

Blood sampling forms usually list the common tests that can be requested from the main pathology departments: haematology, biochemistry and immunology as shown here. The microbiology request form is often a different form. Ensure that you know what the above tests are and when they are indicated.

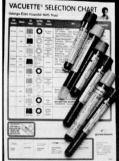

Blood sampling bottles have an array of additives such as EDTA, citrate such that the sample is presented optimally for analysis. It is essential to use the correct bottle for the test- there is usually a chart to help.

Figure 14.2 Images in blood forms and requesting samples.

Contraindications

Unnecessary blood tests are of particular disservice to patients with bleeding diatheses. Check carefully as to the need for investigations. Determine whether the tests can be done on a single sample at a specified time.

Sequence

Documentation and preparation

There are three areas to complete on the form:

- **Patient identification**: ensures that correct results are given for the correct patient
  - ○ Name, address, date of birth, hospital number
  - ○ Named consultant, location in the hospital, doctor's signature
  - ○ Date and time of sample, blood-taker's signature.
- **Brief background**: provides the indication to the laboratory, so any specific abnormalities can be reported in its clinical context. This part is often inadequately filled in. Please consider the question: if the result is abnormal, will the clinical biochemist or haematologist or immunologist be able to determine what may be happening to the patient and therefore be triggered into contacting the appropriate clinician urgently.
  - ○ Current diagnosis, relevant co-morbidities
  - ○ Relevant therapy (e.g. warfarin, antibiotics, etc).
- **Be specific about the requested test**. Do not write TFTs (thyroid function tests) if all you need is the thyroid-stimulating hormone (TSH) or you actually do need the free T_4 only in a patient with hypopituitarism.
  - ○ Tick the box of the test you require
  - ○ Additional tests can be written in the space provided.

Explanation and consent

Venepuncture should have a verbal consent at least and it is good practice to inform the patient in advance that a blood test is going to be done.

Post procedure

Make a record of the tests ordered and when they were ordered in the patient's notes. Once completed, ensure that sample tubes are labelled correctly, attached to the request form, secured carefully to ensure that there are no spillages, and send to the relevant departments. Some blood will need to be rushed to the laboratory for freezing, spinning down or urgent analysis.

Professionalism

Care to ensure that only necessary investigations are requested is re-emphasized. Be sure to inform patients about the blood tests and their need.

Key points

- Blood forms are not only used for blood samples! Other body fluids can also be sent for analysis including sputum, urine, faeces, cerebrospinal fluid, joint aspirate, pleural fluid, peritoneal fluid, and also swabs from any site.
- Many hospitals have at least two pathology forms. One for haematology/biochemistry/ immunology and one for microbiology. This may vary between hospitals and other areas of clinical practice.
- Ideally if a patient identification label is available, it should be used, but be aware that some forms may be in triplicate so ensure you label each copy. Never use a patient identification

label to label blood samples for cross-match or grouping of blood. These sample bottles must always be hand-written.

● Avoid any unnecessary tests.

Adverse effects

Venepuncture has its set of complications as detailed elsewhere in the book. Also think about adverse effects on healthcare finances due to inappropriate or unnecessary tests.

Patient safety and clinical governance tips

✔ **Appropriate testing**: many aspects have been covered above. Conducting a clinical audit on blood test requesting, how quickly and efficiently are abnormal results acted upon, and treatment given may be important areas of clinical care to consider.

✔ **Abnormal results**: a very important point is that abnormal results must be acted upon urgently in most cases and follow-up of the tests arranged. Management should be clearly documented in the clinical notes. Tabulation of results is often helpful, for example, serial urea and electrolytes (U&Es) in a patients with hyperkalaemia and raised creatinine and urea. Another example, would be the haemoglobin, platelets and INR in a patients with a gastro-intestinal bleed due to warfarin therapy.

✔ **Serial blood forms or 'bundles of tests'** are often needed, especially in the examples above. A few further commonly encountered examples are given in Box 14.1 (it is assumed that all patients will have day 1 U&Es, glucose and a full blood count [FBC] with differentials).

Box 14.1 Commonly used investigations for common conditions

● **Acute myocardial infarction**: troponin T for confirmation, baseline lipid profile – total cholesterol, low-density lipoprotein (LDL), high-density lipoprotein (HDL), triglycerides – and glucose, serial cardiac enzymes (now unusual), U&Es especially if angiotensin enzyme-converting inhibitors are being used

● **Renal failure**: baseline FBC, calcium, serial U&Es

● **Diabetes in any patient**: HbA1c (% or mmol/L), U&Es, lipid profile, B_{12}/folate if on metformin

● **Cardiac failure**: U&Es, TSH, FT_4

● **Liver failure**: U&Es, FBC, liver function tests, INR

● **Anaemia**: B_{12}/folate, Fe, ferritin, faecal occult blood

● **Warfarin initiation**: daily INR for 7 days or until stable on treatment dose.

● **Total parental nutrition** (not always total!): daily U&Es (watch K+), thrice weekly liver function tests (LFTs), calcium, phosphate, alkaline phosphate, weekly magnesium, FBC, consider zinc.

● **Postoperative patients**: Daily FBC, U&Es until stable, then usually alternate days.

Student name:	Medical school:	Year:

Blood forms

Mrs Beatrice Tyler has been admitted to hospital with severe abdominal pain. Her date of birth is 17-3-29. Her address is 346 Nagcole Street, Nunford. You conclude that this is an exacerbation of her pre-existing pancreatitis. She is known to have type 2 diabetes mellitus. She is pyrexial. You have been asked to do some 'standard' blood tests by the registrar on duty.

Please pick or write in appropriate tests that need to be requested for this patient and fill in the appropriate forms correctly.

		Self	Peer	Peer /tutor	Tutor
Fills blood forms in appropriately	**Patient details**:				
	• Name	☐	☐	☐	☐
	• Address	☐	☐	☐	☐
	• Date of birth	☐	☐	☐	☐
	• Hospital number	☐	☐	☐	☐
	Administration details				
	• Consultant name	☐	☐	☐	☐
	• Signature of the doctor ordering test	☐	☐	☐	☐
	• Time when sample was taken	☐	☐	☐	☐
	• Date when sample was taken	☐	☐	☐	☐
	• Blood-taker's signature	☐	☐	☐	☐
	Clinical details				
	• Current diagnosis	☐	☐	☐	☐
	• Relevant co-morbidities	☐	☐	☐	☐
	•	☐	☐	☐	☐
Requests investigations as below	**Biochemistry**				
	• **Urea, creatinine, Na+, K+**: assess renal function and electrolytes	☐	☐	☐	☐
	• **LFTs**: to assess liver disease secondary to pancreatitis	☐	☐	☐	☐
	• **Calcium**: ? low due to raised lipase	☐	☐	☐	☐
	• **Amylase level**: current state of elevation, then to monitor response to treatment	☐	☐	☐	☐
	• **Glucose level**: plasma sample will be more accurate than bedside testing	☐	☐	☐	☐
	• **HbA1c%**: indicates glycaemic control over the previous 2 months	☐	☐	☐	☐
	• **Lipid profile**: hypertriglyceridaemia can make pancreatitis worse or precipitate attack	☐	☐	☐	☐
	Haematology				
	• **FBC with differential**: ? infection with neutrophilia ? anaemia	☐	☐	☐	☐
	• **G&S**: consider this not essential if diagnosis clear.	☐	☐	☐	☐
	Microbiology				
	• **Blood cultures**: ? bacterial septicaemia	☐	☐	☐	☐
	•	☐	☐	☐	☐
Seeks help as appropriate	• Considers seeking expert help: e.g. the Medical Laboratory Scientific Officer (MLSO), clinical biochemist, clinical haematologist	☐	☐	☐	☐
	•	☐	☐	☐	☐
Professionalism	• Writes legibly	☐	☐	☐	☐
	• Documents requests in notes	☐	☐	☐	☐
	• Plans follow-up of results	☐	☐	☐	☐
	• Discusses requests with biochemistry, haematology department as per local protocols	☐	☐	☐	☐
	•	☐	☐	☐	☐
Explanation to patient	• Explains requests to patient as appropriate as part of management plan	☐	☐	☐	☐
	• Allows patient opportunity to ask questions	☐	☐	☐	☐
	•	☐	☐	☐	☐

		Self	Peer	Peer/tutor	Tutor
Self-assessed as at least borderline:	Signature:	Date:	U B / S E	U B / S E	U B / S E	U B / S E
Peer-assessed as ready for tutor assessment:	Signature:	Date:	U B / S E	U B / S E	U B / S E	U B / S E
Tutor-assessed as satisfactory:	Signature:	Date:	U B / S E	U B / S E	U B / S E	U B / S E

Notes

14.3 Clinical coding

Background

Every time a patient is admitted, a clinical diagnoses form is inserted into the patient's notes. In the UK, this is the KMR or Kohner Medical Record. The completion of this form is important as it has four purposes:

1. **It is a clinical *aide-memoire* for the clinical diagnoses and procedures undertaken by the patient**
2. **To calculate standardized mortality rate (SMR) and morbidity indices**
3. **Allocate the patient to the appropriate healthcare resource group for calculating cost**
4. **Clinical audit.**

Clinical indications

The details that need to be entered on the forms are the current diagnoses, co-morbidities, and any procedures and/or treatments that the patient has received. The Charlson Index contains around 20 categories of co-morbidity. These co-morbidities are defined using the *International Classification of Diseases* (ICD)-10 diagnoses code. Each category has a weighted index score, taken from the original Charlson paper, which is based on the adjusted risk of 1-year mortality. The overall co-morbidity score reflects the cumulative increased likelihood of 1-year mortality; the higher the score, the more severe the burden of co-morbidity.

It is useful to get started on clinical coding as soon as possible and, especially, to fill it in during daily ward rounds. It is particularly useful for a clinician who is new to the patient, to have a comprehensive list of diagnoses to look at quickly before reading the more detailed clinical notes. The clinical coding sheet (Figure 14.3) is often the first page of the clinical notes that is looked at in a cardiac arrest situation and it should not be blank!

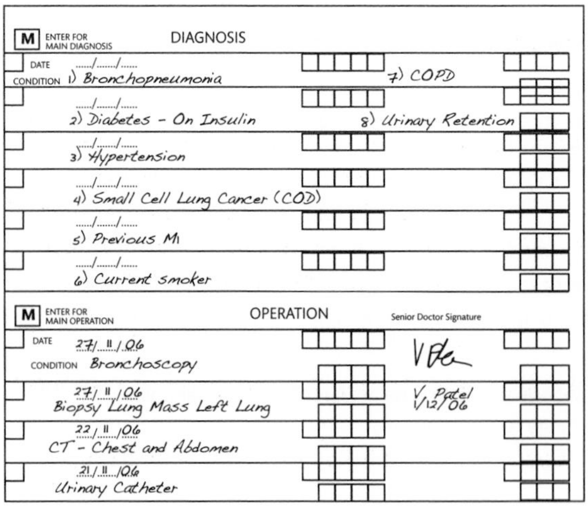
M ENTER FOR MAIN DIAGNOSIS — DIAGNOSIS
DATE ....../....../......
CONDITION 1) Bronchopneumonia
7) COPD
2) Diabetes – On Insulin
8) Urinary Retention
3) Hypertension
4) Small Cell Lung Cancer (COD)
5) Previous MI
6) Current smoker
M ENTER FOR MAIN OPERATION — OPERATION — Senior Doctor Signature
DATE 27/11/06
CONDITION Bronchoscopy
27/11/06
Biopsy Lung Mass Left Lung
V. Patel 1/12/06
22/11/06
CT – Chest and Abdomen
21/11/06
Urinary Catheter

Clinical diagnoses: Hypertension, Liver Disease, Renal Failure
Endocrine (Diabetes, Thyroid)
Respiratory (Asthma, COPD)
Thromboembolic (PE, DVT)
Cardiac (AF, Valve Disease, CCF, IHD)
Vascular (CVA, TIA, Stroke)
Smoker, Ex-Smoker
Procedures: CT/MRI scan
Catheterization, Nasogastric Tube
Endoscopy/Bronchoscopy/Colonoscopy
Costly drugs, e.g.Chemo, Thrombolysis, etc.
Subcutaneous Injections (insulin, enoxaparin)

Figure 14.3 Clinical coding form and important co-morbidities.

Professional principles

The Charlson list of diagnoses is a useful check list in the overall clinical assessment of your patient. The more diagnoses the patient has the greater the complexity of the management of the patient overall in most cases, and this may highlight the need for more senior clinical intervention and general vigilance. Completion of the KMR forms allows rapid collation of statistics regarding patient mortality and morbidity. It also ensures that the hospital gets paid for the care it gives. Taking this into account, in the case of community-acquired pneumonia, an 85-year-old patient with several other conditions will require more resources and a longer hospital stay compared with a 25-year-old patient with community-acquired pneumonia. These ideas can also be an interesting backdrop to learning and teaching within a multidisciplinary team.

The clinical coding department will always be helpful in resolving your queries and will often have training for clinical staff. All entries have to be signed off by a senior, but if in doubt about anything note it down and discuss with senior.

Contraindications

Accuracy in filling in the form is a professional duty as well. Be careful that what you placed on the form is accurate, otherwise the potential for investigation does exist. There are strict rules on what can and cannot be written into the record. 'Probable' diagnoses are acceptable but 'possible' are not. Clearly, senior opinion will be helpful is there is any doubt.

Sequence

Documentation and preparation

The form will have all the patient details (name, address, date of birth, hospital number, date of admission, next of kin details and general practitioner [GP] details). These details may be printed onto the clinical coding sheet when the patient is admitted.

Diagnosis list

The current diagnosis and all active co-morbidities need to be noted down. The primary diagnosis should be highlighted with an 'M or Main' next to it. In the event of patient death 'COD' should be noted next to the primary cause (COD = cause of death).

Procedures, operations, and specific treatments

In this section all procedures, treatments, investigations should be noted down, including transports to and from other hospitals. Each clinical coding will advise on what needs to be included for each clinical area. Blood transfusion should always be recoded.

Explanation and consent

This is rarely an issue. The potential does exist for certain very sensitive diagnoses to be omitted from the record by the expressed wish of the patient. However, this is rare and needs to be discouraged as the data are used nationally as part of the public health dataset for a large variety of reasons including incidence and prevalence data for various illnesses. If these were not recorded, then patients with these conditions are likely to be under-represented in resource allocation.

Summary protocol

Use a black ballpoint pen and press hard to allow writing to appear on the duplicate copy sheet as well!

- **Fully complete the KMR 1**. This must be signed off (with a printed name as well) with the grade of the doctor stated.
- **Identify primary diagnosis**. Must be indicated by the letter 'M' or 'Main'. This is to prevent errors of coding, where the first diagnoses, e.g. syncope is coded as primary diagnosis which is then assumed to be the cause of death in national datasets for calculating mortality statistics by hospital. In reality the patient may have been admitted with syncope due to lung cancer with cerebral metastases. Identify cause of death as 'COD' after the relevant diagnosis. This is *not* necessarily the main diagnosis.

- **Identify all co-morbidities**. These are important for determining resources required and risk associated with the patient's condition.
- **Identify all main procedures and investigations**. Including transports, injections and operations.
- If in doubt: **Write it in!** (and discuss with seniors).

Post-protocol management

Many hospitals undertaken regular clinical audits on various criteria including accuracy of recoding clinical diagnoses, procedures, investigations. The single most important criterion is: has an attempt been made to complete it?

Professionalism

Filling in the clinical coding form is often seen as a low priority task. For all the reasons above please give it the professional time it deserves and you will find that it actually helps you overall in the day-to-day management of your patient, especially as the co-morbidities become part of your expert system to identify the patients with co-morbidities who are at highest risk of more serious illness, greater length of stay, and death.

Patient safety and clinical governance tips

- ✔ **Omission of important diagnoses**: This can, potentially, have serious implications, if for example an important diagnosis such as type 2 diabetes is omitted. It then becomes more likely that this is not mentioned at any clinical handover, on the discharge letter or bought to attention when the patient is readmitted and previous notes briefly reviewed.
- ✔ **Healthcare resources**: although, clinicians often have an aversion to finer aspects of health economics, leaving out diagnoses can result in allocation of significant lower financial resources to the hospital and possibly lower clinical standards of care arising from this. Several reports indicate that the resources allocation can be reduced by around 10%, purely because of poor standards of clinical coding. Even in a small UK hospital with a £100 million budget, this is £10 million.
- ✔ **Reputation of the clinical institute**: A study in *The Lancet* indicated attention to clinical coding was one of the main factors in reducing one particular hospital's SMR from over 125 (suggesting 25% more deaths at this hospital than expected) to less than 100 (average expected).

Clinical coding form

Please complete the clinical coding form for the following person:

Mr Jakin (date of birth 13 December 1929) was admitted from Eliot Residential Home with shortness of breath and confusion. He was referred by his GP, Dr Johnson (of The Surgery, High Street) who was concerned because of the patient's previous pulmonary emboli. Mr Jakin has had type 2 diabetes for many years and has developed an ulcer on his foot.

His daughter presented a list of Mr Jakin's medication to the junior doctors (below). She explained that her dad's memory had been deteriorating over some time, but had become much worse over the past week in addition to the confusion. A computed tomography (CT) scan was performed and showed changes consistent with age as well as evidence of cerebral atrophy and old infarctions suggesting vascular dementia.

Mr Jakin was started on antibiotics for pneumonia and was catheterized due to poor urine output. His blood results showed that his renal function was greatly impaired. Due to his arthritis causing immobility, he was given prophylactic enoxaparin. He was declared medically fit for discharge a week later, but his discharge was unfortunately delayed. His daughter did, however, keep his spirits up by taking him outside for a cigarette every day.'

Mr Jenkins's medications:

- Amlodipine
- Ramipril
- Glyceryl trinitrate spray
- Warfarin
- Thyroxine
- Insulin
- Zoladex
- Omeprazole
- Co-codamol.

		Self	Peer	Peer /tutor	Tutor
Patient details	Name	☐	☐	☐	☐
	Address	☐	☐	☐	☐
	Date of birth	☐	☐	☐	☐
	Hospital number	☐	☐	☐	☐
	GP details	☐	☐	☐	☐
	Next of kin details	☐	☐	☐	☐
	Admission date	☐	☐	☐	☐
	Named consultant	☐	☐	☐	☐
		☐	☐	☐	☐
Diagnosis	Current admission diagnosis	☐	☐	☐	☐
	Co-morbidities	☐	☐	☐	☐
	Main diagnosis indicated	☐	☐	☐	☐
	Cause of death indicated if relevant	☐	☐	☐	☐
	Signed *and* dated by senior clinician	☐	☐	☐	☐
		☐	☐	☐	☐
Operations	Investigations	☐	☐	☐	☐
	Treatments	☐	☐	☐	☐
	Procedures	☐	☐	☐	☐
	Operations	☐	☐	☐	☐
	Transports	☐	☐	☐	☐
	All entries dated	☐	☐	☐	☐
	Signed *and* dated by senior clinician	☐	☐	☐	☐
		☐	☐	☐	☐
Legibility	All entries legible	☐	☐	☐	☐
	No abbreviations	☐	☐	☐	☐
		☐	☐	☐	☐

	Signature:	Date:	Self	Peer	Peer/tutor	Tutor
Self-assessed as at least borderline:			U B S E	U B S E	U B S E	U B S E
Peer-assessed as ready for tutor assessment:			U B S E	U B S E	U B S E	U B S E
Tutor-assessed as satisfactory:			U B S E	U B S E	U B S E	U B S E

Notes

14.4 Infectious disease notification

Background

Notification of infectious diseases is essential to protecting the health of the public. There is a legal requirement for medical practitioners to notify infectious diseases in a suitable time frame to allow investigation by the relevant public health agency. This activity may allow prevention of further cases. Furthermore, notification allows data collection regarding success of vaccination schedules or areas requiring further investigation. The Health Protection (Notification) Regulations 2010 have updated the obligations of medical practitioners to notify conditions causing a risk to the general public.

Clinical indications

Table 14.1 lists infectious diseases that need to be notified. The microorganism responsible and a possible or an actual clinical scenario is given. Most are based on real clinical cases we have treated or read about!

Table 14.1 Infectious diseases that need to be notified

Infectious disease: *organism(s)*	Typical clinical scenario
Most common	
Tuberculosis *Mycobacterium tuberculosis*	Indian subcontinent-born man with chronic cough, weight loss, sweats
Scarlet fever or severe streptococcal infection *Streptococcus pyogenes (Group A streptococcus)*	A 5-year-old boy develops sore throat and fever, followed by a widespread erythematous rash A young woman with type 1 diabetes develops necrotizing fasciitis on her leg
Meningitis: *Neisseria meningitidis Haemophilus influenzae, Streptococcus pneumoniae Listeria monocytogenes*	Unwell student with severe headache, photophobia, and pyrexia
Meningococcal septicaemia *Neisseria meningitidis*	Listless, floppy child with petechial, non-blanching rash
Food poisoning ***Toxin-borne****: Bacillus cereus, Staphylococcus aureus,* ***Infection****: Campylobacter, Salmonella, Shigella, Escherichia coli O157*	A couple with vomiting and diarrhoea 6 hours after a shared take-away Chinese meal with rice Thirty five guests at a wedding with diarrhoea and abdominal pain 3 days after the event
Acute encephalitis *Herpes simplex virus (HSV) 1 or 2*	Previously well man, now drowsy, confused, with headache, fever, and a seizure
Legionnaire's disease *Legionella pneumophila*	A central heating engineer suffers an atypical pneumonia
Acute infectious hepatitis *Hepatitis A, B, C, or E viruses*	A young man with lethargy, vomiting, anorexia, becomes clinically jaundiced
Malaria *Plasmodium falciparum, vivax, ovale, malariae, knowlesi*	Traveller returning from endemic area with rigors, fever, headaches, vomiting. Did not bother with antimalarial prophylaxis

Table 14.1 *(Continued.)*

Infectious disease: *organism(s)*	Typical clinical scenario
Typhoid or paratyphoid fever *Salmonella typhi, S. paratyphi*	Returned traveller from India has high fever, prostration, and headache
Less common	
Dysentry *(amoebic or bacterial)* *Entamoeba histolyticum, Shigella dysenteriae*	A returned traveller has fever and bloody diarrhoea
Haemolytic uraemic syndrome *(HUS)* *Escherichia coli O157*	After a farm visit, a 7-year-old child develops bloody diarrhoea, and is hospitalized due to acute renal failure
Leptospirosis *Leptospira spp.*	A surgeon exploring rivers in Borneo presents with jaundice and renal failure 1 week after having 'flu'
Measles *Measles virus*	A non-immunized child becomes unwell with cough and widespread maculopapular rash
Mumps *Mumps virus*	A student develops swollen painful parotid glands
Ophthalmia neonatorum *Neisseria gonorrhoeae* *Chlamydia trachomatis*	A newborn baby develops purulent conjunctivitis in the first week of life
Rubella *Rubella virus*	A pregnant 18-year-old woman from a travelling family has joint pain, maculopapular rash, and malaise
Tetanus *Clostridium tetani*	A gardener cut his foot with a spade, now has a weak foot and 'tight' jaw
Botulism *Clostridium botulinum*	A man develops blurred vision, dysphagia and dysarthria, then descending symmetrical weakness
Whooping cough *Bordetella pertussis*	A 6-year-old girl with respiratory tract infection develops paroxysmal fits of coughing, then vomits

Rare in the UK, significant travel history or of historical interest

Anthrax *Bacillus anthracis*	Sheep leather worker from abroad with pustule, dark eschar on shoulder
Brucellosis *Brucella melitensis*	A Greek shepherd suffering from fever and sweats
Cholera *Vibrio cholerae*	Many people in a refugee camp with profuse watery diarrhoea, causing severe dehydration
Diphtheria *Corynebacterium diphtheriae*	A Russian boy has sore throat, fever, and dysphagia. Examination shows a membrane on the tonsils
Viral haemorrhagic fever *Ebola, Marburg, Lassa viruses*	Unwell UN soldier airlifted back from rural Democratic Republic of Congo, acutely unwell with petechiae and bruising
Leprosy *Mycobacterium leprae*	Nepalese man has hypopigmented skin lesions and peripheral neuropathy
Plague *Yersinia pestis*	A traveller in Mongolia develops fever, rigors, and painful, much-enlarged groin lymph nodes

Table 14.1 (Continued.)	
Infectious disease: *organism(s)*	Typical clinical scenario
Acute poliomyelitis *Poliovirus*	A girl in rural Nigeria has acute viral meningitis and weakness of one leg follows
Rabies *Rabies virus*	A traveller is bitten by a wild dog in Morocco. A month later he becomes aggressive and confused
Relapsing fever *Borrelia spp.*	A traveller to Peru has an acute febrile illness, which abruptly terminates. A week later it recurs
SARS *SARS coronavirus*	An outbreak of very severe respiratory illness occurs in a hotel in Hong Kong
Smallpox *Smallpox virus*	Smallpox has been successfully eradicated. Last reported case was in a laboratory scientist
Typhus *Rickettsia prowazekii, R. typhi*	A traveller to Ethiopia develops a maculopapular rash with fever and headache
Yellow fever *Yellow fever virus*	A conservationist in Panama becomes unwell with headache, fever, back pain, jaundice, haematemesis

Professional principles

- **Legal obligation**: there is a legal obligation on all registered medical practitioners to notify the specific infectious diseases listed above, or any other condition that may pose a risk to the general public (including non-infectious agents, e.g. radiation, chemical contamination), whether a patient is alive or deceased. If the doctor does not personally notify the conditions, then, he or she should know that notification has already been or will actually be done by another doctor. There has been a serious degree of under-reporting of communicable diseases by doctors.

- **Notify on clinical suspicion**: doctors should notify cases based upon clinical suspicion and not wait for laboratory confirmation, as this may take considerable time and delay public health measures (weeks in the case of tuberculosis). Where a case may have acute implications for health, there is a need to contact the appropriate authority urgently by telephone, then follow with a hard copy. In either case, paper notification should take place within 72 hours of diagnosis. The local health protection unit (part of the Health Protection Agency) is normally the contact for acute notifications; hospital switchboards usually have contact details and the details are on the HPA website. There is an on-call officer for acute problems overnight.

- **Microbiology laboratories weekly returns**: all cases of reportable microorganisms are reported to the HPA on a weekly basis. Human immunodeficiency virus (HIV) and sexually transmitted infections are not notifiable (to protect patient confidentiality) but genitourinary medicine clinics notify the case load in relation to specific sexually transmitted diseases. Suspected cases of Creutzfeldt–Jakob Disease (CJD) should be notified directly to the National CJD Surveillance Unit.

The infectious diseases notification form results in the specific condition, patient's name, and address being notified to the Proper Officer of the local authority for action on prevention of further cases. Local authority powers are considerable in this regard and can include isolation of an infectious person or in the case of food-producing establishments, improvement orders or even closure.

Sequence

Explanation and consent

Explain to the patient that the suspected condition may have public health implications. The patient may require isolation or special measures within the healthcare setting, in which case, this should be explained; the infection control team may have patient literature or further information.

Consent is not needed as this is a statutory duty with a focus on protecting the wider public.

Documentation and preparation

There are multiple fields to complete on the form. Sufficient detail should be given. Ensure the form is filled as comprehensively as possible and returned within an appropriate time frame.

- Date of notification.
- Details of notifying doctor: name and contact details.
- Patient demographics: name, date of birth, gender, ethnicity, address, and contact telephone number. Current address should be provided if not the same as home address, (e.g. boarding school, prison etc). The 10-digit NHS number is requested.
- The notifiable condition: nature of condition, date of onset, date of diagnosis, date of death (if appropriate).
- Further information as appropriate, e.g. occupation, contact details of workplace or school, history of foreign travel.

Clinical note

Make a record of the notification in the patient notes. This would includes all the details given in the infectious disease notification.

Protocol

Consider whether there is a need to notify urgently by phone, e.g. acute presentation, specific risks to others, readily transmissible source or if there is a public health intervention that can prevent further cases.

Post-protocol management

Once completed, ensure that the form is sent to the correct place.

Professionalism

Ensure that appropriate infection control precautions are carried out and the infection control team are aware if there is a risk to other patients (e.g. tuberculosis, meningitis, group A streptococcus infection, diarrhoea, contagious viral conditions)

Patient safety and clinical governance tips

There are some specific conditions that require a tailored approach in the community or hospital to prevent spread, for example:

✔ **Meningitis**: prophylactic antibiotics may be required for close contacts where meningococcal or *Haemophilus influenzae* type B infection is suspected. The public health team will assess which contacts require this.

✔ **Tuberculosis**: a specialist tuberculosis team will perform contact-tracing in the community. Contacts may be screened for tuberculosis (e.g. Mantoux test, chest X-ray, interferon-based assays) and if appropriate will be monitored or offered antibiotic prophylaxis or therapy.

✔ **Watch out for rare conditions**: Although a lot of the conditions are rare they do occur. Detailed history is important to ascertain many of these conditions and to keep an open mind when treating pyrexia of unknown origin or if your patient is not improving.

Student name:	Medical school:	Year:

Infectious disease notification

John Master (55 Crick Lane, Nunhampton; date of birth 10 November 2005, hospital number A98765, NHS number 9998765432) became drowsy and increasingly unwell at Sunnyside School, and is rushed to the Emergency Department, where he is found to have a stiff neck, aversion to light, and a non-blanching rash on his trunk.

The paediatric consultant asks you to 'ensure that public health are aware'. Consider your next steps and fill in the appropriate forms.

		Self	Peer	Peer /tutor	Tutor
Explanation and consent	● Consent not necessary	☐	☐	☐	☐
	● Explanation of role of notification	☐	☐	☐	☐
	●	☐	☐	☐	☐
Patient details	● Name	☐	☐	☐	☐
	● Address	☐	☐	☐	☐
	● Date of birth	☐	☐	☐	☐
	● NHS number	☐	☐	☐	☐
	●	☐	☐	☐	☐
Admin details	● Date of notification and onset	☐	☐	☐	☐
	● Contact details of notifying doctor	☐	☐	☐	☐
	●	☐	☐	☐	☐
Brief background	● Appropriate diagnosis on form	☐	☐	☐	☐
	● Recognize that this requires urgent telephone notification	☐	☐	☐	☐
	● Notifying school name as an additional factor	☐	☐	☐	☐
	●	☐	☐	☐	☐
Language	● Legible handwriting	☐	☐	☐	☐
	●	☐	☐	☐	☐
Professionalism	● Ensure form is correct and sent off	☐	☐	☐	☐
	● Telephone to warn agencies of case	☐	☐	☐	☐
	●	☐	☐	☐	☐

Self-assessed as at least borderline:	Signature:	Date:	U B S E	U B S E	U B S E	U B S E
Peer-assessed as ready for tutor assessment:	Signature:	Date:	U B S E	U B S E	U B S E	U B S E
Tutor-assessed as satisfactory:	Signature:	Date:	U B S E	U B S E	U B S E	U B S E

Notes

14.5 Death certificates

Background

The death of a loved one is a difficult time that causes much pain and sadness. To make a difficult period as easy as possible, procedures after death should be hastened, and carried out efficiently and correctly. The clinician should express and display the highest professional standards possible especially in relation to dealing with family members and friends of the deceased patient. The bereavement service will be invaluable to family members and friends. Clinicians may also need support from the bereavement service, especially with patients such as deaths in children and other close patients.

Confirmation of death

It is a professional duty to examine the patient who has died to clinically confirm death. There are many instances, anecdotally and in the medical literature, where patients were revived in the mortuary! This can be avoided by verifying and confirming death as follows:

- Fixed pupils that are unresponsive to a bright light
- No respiratory effort or breath sounds (auscultation over trachea and anterior upper chest)
- No pulses: check carotids, radials, brachials
- No heart sounds (listen over usual apex position, 30–60 seconds)
- No response to sternal rub/supra-orbital pressure (painful stimuli)
- Retinal examination, occasionally undertaken, would reveal discontinuous clots in retinal veins.

If a patient was known to you and you are going to do the death certificate then it will be useful to start by establishing the cause of death. Also check for the presence of a pacemaker, this is easier to check in a patient who has recently died rather than in the mortuary.

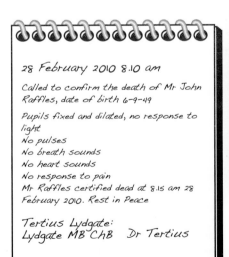

28 February 2010 8.10 am

Called to confirm the death of Mr John Raffles, date of birth 6-9-49

Pupils fixed and dilated, no response to light
No pulses
No breath sounds
No heart sounds
No response to pain
Mr Raffles certified dead at 8.15 am 28 February 2010. Rest in Peace

Tertius Lydgate:
Lydgate MB ChB   Dr Tertius

Clinical Note to Confirm Death may be written as above

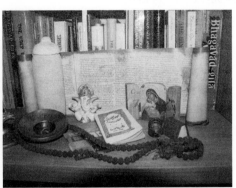

Religious Paraphernalia of Christianity, Islam, Hinduism, Buddhism, Sikhism and Judaism.

Figure 14.4 Images in death certification.

Professional principles

There are important aspects in relation to the removal of the body and its eventual final state dependent on the specific religion, if any. The standard secular choice is a straightforward burial or cremation after the body has been removed to the mortuary and funeral arrangements have been made. The following notes are for general guidance only and each death should be treated as an individual case. Specific religious wishes are best discussed with the multi-faith chaplaincy service that now operates in most hospitals in UK. It is also best to clarify wishes with regards to post-mortem and or organ donation on an individual basis with the next of kin.

- **Christianity**
  - Several variations in relation to final moments and care after death depending on the denomination.
  - A priest may be required to offer last rites if death imminent.
  - Final state: burial or cremation.
- **Islam**
  - If death imminent inform family.
  - Family will wish to be with deceased to offer last rites and prepare body after death.
  - Prompt burial imperative, hence try to complete death certificate as soon as possible.
- **Judaism**
  - Body prepared and washed prior to burial by family.
  - If no family contact local hospital rabbi or local Hebrew burial society or Jewish community.
  - Prompt burial imperative, hence try to complete death certificate as soon as possible.
- **Hinduism**
  - Various rituals according to specific denomination.
  - Hindu priest to be contacted to perform last rites.
  - Cremation usually.
- **Sikhism**
  - Family may wish to perform last rites and prepare body.
  - Cremation usual but stillborn/miscarriages are buried.
  - Endeavour to complete relevant documentation for cremation as soon as possible.
- **Buddhism**
  - Advisable not to remove body before monk/sister arrives.
  - Cremation common.
- **Jehovah's Witnesses**
  - No ceremonial rites.
  - Usual preparation appropriate.

Death certification

The death certificate is completed by a doctor and is given to the family who then need to register the death with the registrar of births and deaths. This will then allow the family to hold a funeral and arrange burial or cremation. For a death certificate to be legally valid, the doctor completing and signing the form, must have seen the patient alive in the last 14 days before death. Once the death certificate has been completed, it has to be delivered to the registrar within 5 days (England, Wales, Northern Ireland but within 8 days in Scotland).

The pad of the *Medical Certificates of Cause of Death* has guidance at the beginning that will help you complete the certificate, but remember that you can always ask a colleague who knew the patient better to help you complete the certificate. To get it correct is absolutely vital, because once given to the family, any errors may hold up proceedings and will cause the family distress.

Referring to the coroner

There are many reasons why a death needs to be discussed with the coroner. In reality the discussion takes place between the doctor and the coroner's officer (a police officer). The following should be discussed with the coroner's office.

- Death suspicious in any way: potential murder, recent assault
- Unknown cause of death
- Patient not seen by certifying doctor in the last 14 days
- All deaths within 24 hours of admission to hospital
- All deaths in relation to surgery or anaesthesia or any medical treatment
- Death due to road traffic accident, other accidents, trauma, industrial injury
- Death due to violence, neglect, abortion, suicide or poisoning (including alcohol)
- Deaths in legal custody
- Death in any cases where issue of negligence has been raised
- Death due to industrial injury or employment.

The coroner can decide on one of three options: allow the death certificate to be issued concordant with the discussion; order a post-mortem to be held; or hold a coroner's inquest to establish cause of death.

Sequence

Documentation and preparation

The most crucial part of the death certificate is the 'cause of death' section. There are four parts: I(a), I(b), I(c), and II. The direct cause of death is given in I(a) with intermediate and underlying cause of death given in parts I(b) and I(c), respectively. Any co-morbidity that may have contributed to death should be noted in part II. *Abbreviations should not be used on the death certificate.* It is crucial that you read through the clinical notes thoroughly. Important facts may emerge, for example, the stroke that led to the bronchopneumonia as the cause of death was due to a cerebral tumour not cerebral atherosclerosis.

Specific terms

There are many terms that imply mode of dying rather than cause of death. When filling out the cause of death section, ask yourself 'why did that happen?' For example, renal failure is an acceptable term but unacceptable as the sole cause of death. However, if I(a) is renal failure, I(b) is glomerulonephritis and I(c) is Goodpasture's disease, then not only has a cause of death been given but a background has been given as well. Other such examples of terms implying mode of dying rather than cause of death include asphyxia, exhaustion, organ failure, shock, and cardiac arrest.

Counterfoil and notice to informant

In addition to the actual certificate, there are two other sections to complete. The counterfoil is kept with the certificate book and provides the hospital with proof of issue of certificate. The Notice to Informant is given along with the certificate to the deceased's relative whose duty it is to deliver the certificate to the registrar. No additional information is needed to complete these parts of the certificate.

Filling in of the death certificate

- **Name of the deceased**: should be given in full, as should the place of death. The dates should also be given in full, e.g. '**seventh** day of **August 2011**'. Clearly, this must be within the previous 14 days prior to death.

- **Indication of whether death referred to the coroner**: a death is usually referred to the coroner for a post-mortem if the cause of death is unknown, suspicious, violent, unnatural, occupational, if there has been recent surgery or other procedure that could have caused death, and several other reasons.

- **Cause of death**: the most important part of the certificate, this section contains the cause of death, underlying causes and additional co-morbidities. For example, the cause of death might have: I(a) intracerebral haemorrhage caused by I(b) cerebral metastases, which were a result of I(c) squamous cell carcinoma of the lung. In part II, diabetes type 2 was a significant co-morbidity.

- **Interval between onset of condition and death**: this is often left blank but can add clarity of diagnosis of deceased's illness and death. This section is also useful for clinical research and audit.

- **Answer whether there is any suspicion of occupation related death**: A large number of industrial workers are exposed to materials that could lead to respiratory problems and general poisoning. There is a long list of known associations. Such deaths need to be referred to the coroner.

Signature

By signing this document, you are testifying that all the information given on the certificate is given to the best of your knowledge. In addition to your signature, print your name in block capitals, give your qualifications (e.g. MB ChB) and give the date. For residence, give the address of the hospital as a 'care of' address. Your personal residence does not need to written down in this public record.

Post-protocol management

The certificate is supplied to the next of kin or representative in a sealed envelope. State that the certificate needs to be delivered to the registrar within the stipulated time. It may be useful to discuss the diagnoses on the certificate to allay anxieties and reduces queries in the future. Please remember that the registrar will copy your diagnoses onto the eventual official death certificate. The next of kin will have one copy with additional copies made, if paid for.

Professionalism

Timely attention to this duty will really help the family. Be sure, as always, to minimize errors that would result in the certificate being unacceptable. It is essential that the patient's GP is informed as soon as possible. Consider the need for a post-mortem.

Professional tips

- ✔ **Discuss cause of death with senior clinician**: in almost all cases, the junior clinician should discuss the cause of death of a patient with the responsible senior clinician.

- ✔ **Coroner's officer**: if there is any doubt as to the cause of death or there is a need to consider a post-mortem, discuss the case with the Coroner's office as soon as possible.

- ✔ **Sources of help**: the bereavement team, social worker and nursing staff will be of great help if needed.

Student name:	Medical school:	Year:

Death certificates

Please complete this patient's death certificate

Mr Vibhuti Banerjee was a 77-year-old man who presented with left-sided weakness. During his current stay at Central University Hospital he developed symptoms of pneumonia after having seizures and subsequently died this morning. He had had several myocardial infarctions in the past and was known to have type 2 diabetes mellitus. As his junior doctor, you last saw him 2 days ago. Please complete his death certificate using a real or facsimile of the local death certificate form.

		Self	Peer	Peer /tutor	Tutor
Checks patient notes	● Confirms that patient has been certified correctly	☐	☐	☐	☐
	●	☐	☐	☐	☐
Fills in patient details and last time seen alive	● Name of deceased	☐	☐	☐	☐
	● Age of deceased	☐	☐	☐	☐
	● Date of death	☐	☐	☐	☐
	● Place of death	☐	☐	☐	☐
	● 'Last seen alive by me' filled correctly	☐	☐	☐	☐
	●	☐	☐	☐	☐
Post-mortem	● Appropriate number circled	☐	☐	☐	☐
	●	☐	☐	☐	☐
Seen after death	● Appropriate letter circled	☐	☐	☐	☐
	●	☐	☐	☐	☐
Cause of death	● Section Ia filled correctly	☐	☐	☐	☐
	● Section Ib filled correctly	☐	☐	☐	☐
	● Section Ic filled correctly	☐	☐	☐	☐
	● Section II filled correctly	☐	☐	☐	☐
	●	☐	☐	☐	☐
Employment related death	● Employment-related disease box ticked if appropriate	☐	☐	☐	☐
	●	☐	☐	☐	☐
Doctor details filled in correctly	● Doctor's signature/printed name	☐	☐	☐	☐
	● Qualification	☐	☐	☐	☐
	● Residence	☐	☐	☐	☐
	● Date	☐	☐	☐	☐
	● Consultant	☐	☐	☐	☐
	●	☐	☐	☐	☐
Completion	● Counterfoil completed appropriately	☐	☐	☐	☐
	● Notice to informant completed appropriately	☐	☐	☐	☐
	●	☐	☐	☐	☐
Language	● Handwriting legible	☐	☐	☐	☐
	● Spelling correct	☐	☐	☐	☐
	●	☐	☐	☐	☐
Awareness/Questions	● Difference between mode and cause of death	☐	☐	☐	☐
	● Knowledge of when to refer to coroner	☐	☐	☐	☐
	●	☐	☐	☐	☐

				Self	Peer	Peer/tutor	Tutor
Self-assessed as at least borderline:	Signature:	Date:		U B S E	U B S E	U B S E	U B S E
Peer-assessed as ready for tutor assessment:	Signature:	Date:		U B S E	U B S E	U B S E	U B S E
Tutor-assessed as satisfactory:	Signature:	Date:		U B S E	U B S E	U B S E	U B S E

Notes

Which of following conditions can be associated with employment and why?

- Rheumatoid arthritis
- Bladder cancer
- Pneumonia
- Mesothelioma
- Sarcoidosis
- Stroke
- Gallstones
- Systemic lupus erythematosus
- Pulmonary siderosis
- Asthma
- Farmer's lung
- Epilepsy
- Coal worker's pneumoconiosis
- Motor neurone disease
- Asbestosis

14.6 **Cremation forms**

Background

Cremation of a deceased person cannot take place unless the cause of death is definitely known and recorded appropriately. If, later on, there is any suspicion or doubt regarding the cause of death there can be no exhumation if the body has been cremated so it is vital that the cremation form is completed correctly, after the completion of the death certificate. There is a payment made for this professional duty, which must be carried out meticulously to avoid any delays to the funeral.

Professional principles

- **Two doctors independently identify the body and certify for cremation**: The first part of the form is completed by the 'registered medical practitioner who attended the deceased during their last illness'. This is most likely to be the junior doctor who has been seeing the patient on a daily basis. The second part of the form is completed by a medical practitioner who has been registered for more than 5 years and is independent of the patient and the doctor completing the first section. Incidentally, there is another section to the form that is completed by a relative of the deceased and is an application to permit cremation of the deceased. There is final part to the cremation form that is filled in by the medical referee to the local authority under whose auspices the cremation takes place.

- **Identification of the body**: a doctor is only allowed to complete the cremation form if they looked after the patient clinically and saw the patient alive and then again after death. A brief external examination confirming death is required and a specific check to ensure that there is no evidence of implants, particularly pacemakers and radioactive devices, that can explode during cremation. If a pacemakers or radio-active implant is present then this must be removed, usually by the mortuary officer.

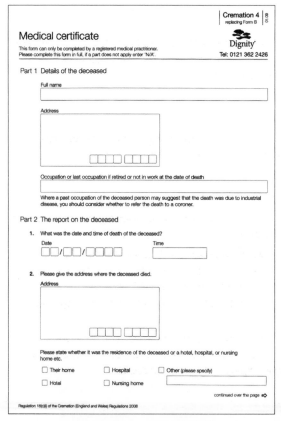

Figure 14.5 Facsimile of a cremation form.

Documentation and preparation

The questions asked on the cremation form (Figure 14.5) are designed to help rule out any untoward circumstances in relation to the death. Harold Shipman was dishonest when answering the questions on the cremation form and eventually brought to justice. Part of the evidence against him was from suspicions raised by the second certifying doctors. As a result of the investigation, Harold Shipman was identified, tried and convicted as a mass murderer.

Box 14.2 The junior doctor and the cremation form – facts established

- Time, date and place of death
- Relationship to deceased
- Any financial interests in the case?
- Attendance during illness?
- When was the deceased last seen alive?
- Referred to coroner?
- Body seen and examined after death?

- Cause of death, mode of death and duration of final illness
- Who was present at death?
- Who nursed the patient?
- Any recent operations?
- Any personal doubts about the death?
- Any suspicions?
- Has the death certificate been issued?

Key points

- The ordinary medical attendant is usually the GP; in the hospital the junior doctor would have attended the patient during their last illness.
- Cause of death should be exactly the same as that on the death certificate.
- Check with nursing staff to confirm who nursed the patient and who was with him/her when they died.
- If you have any suspicions about the death then these should be addressed before issuing the death certificate – if in doubt contact the coroner's office for advice.

Post-protocol management

The doctor completing the second medical component of the form will need to discuss the case with the doctor filling in the first part. To save time and prevent delays, the first doctor should attempt to contact the other doctor as soon as possible.

Professionalism

A delay in filling the correctly will result in a delay in the funeral and cremation taking place. Every year this happens for the simple fact that the form was not filled in on time.

Professional tips

- ✔ **Coroner's officer**: if there is any doubt as to the cause of death or there is a need to consider a post-mortem, discuss the case with the coroner's office as soon as possible.
- ✔ **Cremation of a pacemaker and some other implantable devices**: these can cause an explosion in the crematorium. Radioactive implants can cause radio-activity being released into the crematorium and atmosphere with its inherent biohazard. The clinical notes, particularly electrocardiograms, should be consulted to check whether there is a pacemaker *in situ* or not.
- ✔ **Declaration of income**: do not forget to declare any income generated, not to do so is tax evasion and could have serious repercussions on your career. Hospitals and crematoria can be asked by the tax authorities for details of payments to named doctors

Student name:	Medical school:	Year:

Cremation forms

Please complete this patient's death certificate:

Mr Vibhuti Banerjee was a 77-year-old man who presented with left-sided weakness. During his current stay at Central University Hospital he developed symptoms of pneumonia after having seizures and subsequently died this morning. He had had several myocardial infarctions in the past and was known to have type 2 diabetes mellitus. As his junior doctor, you last saw him 2 days ago. Please complete his cremation form using a real or facsimile of the local cremation form.

		Self	Peer	Peer /tutor	Tutor
Check patient's notes	Patient's death has been certified correctly	☐	☐	☐	☐
	Checks that the death certificate been issued	☐	☐	☐	☐
		☐	☐	☐	☐
Patients details	Full name	☐	☐	☐	☐
	Address	☐	☐	☐	☐
	Age	☐	☐	☐	☐
	Occupation	☐	☐	☐	☐
		☐	☐	☐	☐
Time and place of death	Date of death	☐	☐	☐	☐
	Time of death	☐	☐	☐	☐
	Place of death	☐	☐	☐	☐
		☐	☐	☐	☐
Doctor–patient encounter	Only allowed to complete the death certificate and cremation form if involved in patient's care during latest illness	☐	☐	☐	☐
	States how many days and hours before death they saw the patient	☐	☐	☐	☐
	Duration of involvement in patient's care	☐	☐	☐	☐
	Any pecuniary interests/relationships	☐	☐	☐	☐
		☐	☐	☐	☐
Cause of death	Ensures that documents same cause of death as on death certificate	☐	☐		☐
	Section Ia filled correctly	☐	☐	☐	☐
	Section Ib filled correctly	☐	☐	☐	☐
	Section Ic filled correctly	☐	☐	☐	☐
	Section II filled correctly	☐	☐	☐	☐
		☐	☐	☐	☐
Coroners	Knowledge of when to refer to coroner	☐	☐	☐	☐
		☐	☐	☐	☐
Mode of death	Aware of the difference between cause and mode of death	☐	☐	☐	☐
	Documents mode of death and time	☐	☐	☐	☐
		☐	☐	☐	☐
Pacemaker and other implants	Discussion need to ensure pacemakers and other potentially explosive or radioactive devices have been removed	☐	☐	☐	☐
		☐	☐	☐	☐
All sections filled	All sections answered	☐	☐	☐	☐
	Legible handwriting	☐	☐	☐	☐
	Correct spelling	☐	☐	☐	☐
		☐	☐	☐	☐
Doctors details	Full name	☐	☐	☐	☐
	Address	☐	☐	☐	☐
	Contact number	☐	☐	☐	☐
	Date	☐	☐	☐	☐
	Signature	☐	☐	☐	☐
		☐	☐	☐	☐

				Self	Peer	Peer/tutor	Tutor
Self-assessed as at least borderline:	Signature:	Date:		U B S E	U B S E	U B S E	U B S E
Peer-assessed as ready for tutor assessment:	Signature:	Date:		U B S E	U B S E	U B S E	U B S E
Tutor-assessed as satisfactory:	Signature:	Date:		U B S E	U B S E	U B S E	U B S E

Notes

Unit 15 Information management

15.1 Clinical notes

Background

Clinical notes represent a legal record of the management of the patient. Even more than this fact, is that the notes are of the utmost clinical importance in treating a patient safely and effectively, and ensuring that a professional record exists for purposes of follow-up, readmission, and clinical audit.

Ward round notes have a pivotal role in hospital-based care. Healthcare professionals are able to meet and develop an integrated plan of care during a ward round. Increasingly, clinical notes are becoming electronic and typed rather than handwritten. The overall principles remain unchanged.

Clinical indications

Clear, logical, legible records are required for all significant clinical encounters. A succinct and accurate record clearly improves safety and helps achieve high standards of care.

Professional principles

In medical and surgical practice, the goals of the ward round include

- Treating the patient's clinical problem
- Enhancing the quality of care
- Improving communication
- Addressing patient concerns and problems
- Planning and evaluating treatment.
- Planning discharge.

The ward round is a critical time for reviewing the initial history, examination and results, and the stage at which further treatment and investigations will be determined. However, documentation of this ward round is often inadequate, so the benefits of decision making are lost. It is also a medicolegal requirement that the patient needs to be seen regularly and an entry needs to be made in the relevant case notes. The exact interval between writing in the notes is decided by individual hospitals but common practice is daily, Monday to Friday. A clinical entry is needed if the patient is seen at any other time and always at discharge.

Three critical questions in relation to clinical notes are:

1 Are the notes an accurate and sufficient clinical record to allow continuity of care and serve as a longer-term record of events?

2 Has the over-arching need to deliver good clinical care and patient safety been addressed?

3 Would the quality of the notes both from the legibility and clinical context be defensible in an investigation including cross-examination in court?

Contents of the clinical notes is variable but ideally should have at least the following subsections, and which are clearly divided. Single-episode notes have the advantage that a shorter and smaller set of clinical notes is used. The full notes, as they include details of previous clinical care, will often be bulky and run to many hundred pages and detract from the focus on current relevant material. The previous clinical records should always be looked at with great care to ascertain relevant clinical facts for the current admission.

- **Clinical diagnosis and coding sheet**: this is usually the KMR Form in most cases in UK.
- **Clinical notes for the current admission**: often with previous clinical records notes. Ideally these should be multiprofessional.
- **Investigations**: often divided into haematology, biochemistry, radiology, etc.
- **Discharge planning**: often incorporated into daily clinical notes.
- **Discharge letter**: this could be started soon after the admission such that details are not forgotten day to day or more usually doctor to doctor.
- **Patient safety and patient information**: With respect to the former, a venous thromboembolism (VTE) risk assessment can be included or other clinical protocols such as specific antibiotic prescribing information sheets, acute coronary syndrome protocols, DKA pathway.

Documentation and preparation

As a junior doctor, you are an official spokesperson for the team through the patient's clinical notes. Mandatory requirements for entries in the notes are:

- Black ink, clearly legible
- Patient details entered on each separate page of the notes
- Date, time, and place
- Grade and name of most senior doctor present
- Approved abbreviations only
- Signature and name of person making the entry. Some hospitals stipulate writing down the GMC number as well.

Make sure that you have addressed the following every day:

- Any significant events since last note
- Vital signs: blood pressure (BP), temperature, pulse, respiratory rate, oxygen saturations, glucose levels, input/output, stool chart, medical early warning score (MEWS).
- Focused physical examination
- Investigations: blood tests and other studies such as radiology, histology, cultures
- Assessment of active problems
- VTE prophylaxis: risk assess, review need. Review drug chart
- Resuscitation status, where applicable
- Discharge planning notes.

The 'i: **SOAP-D**' format for creating a clinical note is often used and is very effective and practical:

- i: **Initial summary phrases**. The clinical entry starts with a few initial summary phrases.
- **Subjective**: this is an expression of what the patient, carer, doctor, or any other healthcare professional feels is happening. The patient may be better, or have vomiting, chest pain, ready for discharge, not safe for swallowing, etc.
- **Objective findings**: For example, observations such as how the patient looks today, standard clinical vital signs and observations (temperature, BP, pulse, respiratory rate, oxygen saturations). This can be further defined into the MEWS score if deemed clinical relevant – the latter definitely in a patient with septicaemia due to chest infection but not necessarily in a patient waiting for nursing home placement after having recovered from an urinary tract infection. This section would also include other objective findings such as chest examination, change

in function of arms and legs after stroke, decrease in circumference of a leg with cellulitis, change in area of redness, etc.

Results of any relevant investigations could also be written in. Common examples are urea and electrolytes (U&Es), haematology profile, chest X-ray result, electrocardiogram (ECG), and computed tomography (CT) head.

- **Assessment of diagnosis, progress, or prognosis**: the notes above will now allow an assessment of the patient to be formulated. For example, chest infection improving, new diagnosis to be considered ? Parkinson's disease. Statements on prognosis can also be included, e.g. patient deteriorating, likely to die from metastatic disease. This is to focus on the urgent needs specific to the patient and their condition. Discussion with the family and implementation of the Liverpool Care Pathway may be needed in the example given. It is always useful to be proactive in relation to discharge planning and a statement can be inserted here and crystallized below.

- **Plan**: this is a summary of specific actions. They are best numbered for clarity, so that they can be ticked off as they are completed. For example:

  1 Continue antibiotics IV 2 more days and discuss with microbiologist

  2 Check U&Es, FBC mane. Form left.

  3 24 hr ECG requested (Cardiac Unit phoned and request discussed)

  4 To discuss with senior doctor re need for steroids.

An addition note on the discharge plan should be added in all cases where relevant.

- **Discharge plan**: A note on the discharge plan. For example: home on Wednesday, district nursing support to be started. Nurses and family informed and happy with discharge plan. Will need blister packs for discharge medication. Now ordered.

Box 15.1 Clinical notes using the i: SOAP-D format
....

- **Initial summary**
  - ○ Marian Evans: DoB: 12-12-37
  - ○ NHS 12358132134 0915am February 2012
  - ○ Ward Round Dr Williams (Consultant) and Dr Bullen
  - ○ Patient admitted with sepsis and confusion secondary to urinary tract infection 2 days ago
- **S**:
  - ○ Patient feels much improved, no nausea, eating and drinking well
- **O**:
  - ○ Temp: 36.8 °C, BP 134/78, pulse 72 sinus rhythm,
  - ○ Urine output >500 mL last 6 hours, Intake >1000 mL. MEWS normal
  - ○ Alert orientated, no distress. Abdomen: soft, non-tender
  - ○ **Results**: 25/2/2012: Na 138, K 4.6, Urea 8.3 (previously 15.8)
  - ○ Creatinine 124 µmol/L (previously 211).
- **A**:
  - ○ Improving urinary tract infection, improving renal function
  - ○ Patient happy to be discharged back to own home today.
- **P**:
  - 1: Stop IV antibiotics
  - 2: Discharge home today on 3 days of oral trimethoprim
  - 3: Discharge letter completed and left with Staff Nurse Brookes
  - John Chapman
  - Dr John Chapman
  - House Officer bleep 2007

Explanation and consent

Explanations must be given adequately; your colleagues need to know what you were thinking or planning and what the patient or carers know. Ensure that your plan has detailed instructions so that on-call colleagues understand the plan and can carry them out safely. Be obsessive about obtaining and recording consent. Discussions with patient, family, carers, and professional healthcare staff should be accurately recorded. Express concerns from patients, family carers so these can be sorted out urgently to improve patient experience and outcome, and prevent possible future complaints. Most important of all, include the patient in all discussion about their care and allow opportunity for the patient to ask any questions or anything else.

Post-protocol management

Seek feedback from senior colleagues as to the quality of your clinical notes.

Patient safety and clinical governance tips

✔ **High standards of clinical notes**: this automatically leads to better clinical care by virtue of the fact that subjective and objective clinical data are gathered with the patient and other healthcare professionals involved. A clear assessment and management are presented with a discharge plan in mind.

✔ **Medicolegal consequences**: medicolegal consequences of poor clinical note recording have been widely documented and are a common cause of medical litigation. The low standards of clinical note-keeping often proves the clinical negligence.

✔ **Patient safety**: there can be fatal consequences of not knowing or not acting on results such as low potassium levels, high glucose levels, early sepsis, deep vein thrombosis, cardiac ischaemia and neck stiffness (meningitis). Good clinical note taking, using formats such as i-SOAP, ultimately fosters good clinical decisions and safe, effective care.

✔ **Discharge planning**: timely discharge is helpful in so many obvious ways: safer for the patient, better use of resources and by having a new patient to look after, improving your extensive clinical experience! Rarely, timely discharge will result in reducing your workload so that you can concentrate on other aspects of care such as reading, clinical audit, teaching, and research.

Student name:	Medical school:	Year:

Clinical notes

Write out clinical notes for the following patient:

Mr Mark Mawkins (date of birth 12 December 1932) has a history of type 2 diabetes mellitus, hypertension, and angina. He has been admitted with right basal pneumonia and dehydration, and is currently on intravenous (IV) antibiotics and IV fluids. It is day 3 of admission and today he is much improved with no new complaints. He is apyrexial, BP 120/60, heart rate (HR) 78/min, Oxygen saturations are 96% on room air. Input/output, in the last 24 hours has been 2200 mL/1750 mL. Cardiovascular and abdominal examination were normal and he has bronchial breathing in the right base along with some crepitations. His blood cultures were awaited and his biochemistry profile today showed Na 136 mmol/L, K 4.0 mmol/L, Urea 7.5 mmol/L, creatinine 108 μmol/L. His FBC showed Hb of 11.6 g/dL, WBC 12 × 10^9/L and platelets of 314 × 10^9/L. It is decided to change his antibiotics to oral tablets, to continue on prophylactic low-molecular-weight heparin, to stop his IV fluids but to continue to encourage oral intake. The above plan has been discussed with his family, who are happy with his improvement. He has been referred to the physiotherapist and occupational therapist to improve mobility and ensure he has adequate support at home after discharge. His tentative discharge date is 2 days from now and he will be reviewed in clinic in 6 weeks time along with a repeat chest X-ray.

		Self	Peer	Peer /tutor	Tutor
General format	• Patient details on the sheet	☐	☐	☐	☐
	• Date and time	☐	☐	☐	☐
	• Ward/location	☐	☐	☐	☐
	• Legible	☐	☐	☐	☐
	• Black ink	☐	☐	☐	☐
	• Name and grade of most senior person	☐	☐	☐	☐
	• Signature, name and bleep no at the end of note	☐	☐	☐	☐
	• Use of approved abbreviations only	☐	☐	☐	☐
	•	☐	☐	☐	☐
Initial summary phrases	• Succinct summary of admission	☐	☐	☐	☐
	• Significant past medical history	☐	☐	☐	☐
	•	☐	☐	☐	☐
Subjective	• Documents symptoms or patient's concerns	☐	☐	☐	☐
	•	☐	☐	☐	☐
Objective evidence	• Records vital signs	☐	☐	☐	☐
	• Records general condition of the patient	☐	☐	☐	☐
	• Records intake/output or blood glucose	☐	☐	☐	☐
	• Records lab results and any other investigations	☐	☐	☐	☐
	•	☐	☐	☐	☐
Assessment	• Documents progress and any significant events since last note	☐	☐	☐	☐
	• Records details of clinical examination	☐	☐	☐	☐
	• Documents diagnosis	☐	☐	☐	☐
	• Documents prognosis	☐	☐	☐	☐
	•	☐	☐	☐	☐
Plan	• Specific medical management plan documented	☐	☐	☐	☐
	• Records any changes in treatment	☐	☐	☐	☐
	• Documents discussion with family	☐	☐	☐	☐
	• Documents involvement and input of multidisciplinary team	☐	☐	☐	☐
	• Records planned discharge date	☐	☐	☐	☐
	• Records follow-up plans	☐	☐	☐	☐
	•	☐	☐	☐	☐
Doctor	• Name signed and printed	☐	☐	☐	☐
	• Bleep number	☐	☐	☐	☐
	• Rank	☐	☐	☐	☐
	•	☐	☐	☐	☐
Legibility	• Clear	☐	☐	☐	☐
	• Correct spelling	☐	☐	☐	☐
	•	☐	☐	☐	☐

			Self	Peer	Peer /tutor	Tutor
Self-assessed as at least borderline:	Signature:	Date:	U B S E	U B S E	U B S E	U B S E
Peer-assessed as ready for tutor assessment:	Signature:	Date:	U B S E	U B S E	U B S E	U B S E
Tutor-assessed as satisfactory:	Signature:	Date:	U B S E	U B S E	U B S E	U B S E

Notes

15.2 Data interpretation: blood tests

Background

Blood investigations should be ordered according to clinical need. Blood tests should be seen as testing tools to examine clinical hypotheses generated from the clinical history and examination. Competent interpretation of the results is therefore an essential prerequisite to excellent clinical care.

Clinical indications

The fundamental clinical reasons for ordering blood tests are to formulate diagnoses, *exclude* certain diagnoses, and for monitoring. Careful interpretation of the results is needed to define the best line of management for the patient, taking into account clinical urgency, co-morbidities, and clinical expertise.

Physiological and professional principles

The clinician ordering the investigations should have a clear understanding of why the tests have been ordered. There should be no such considerations such as 'routine investigations'. There must always be a distinct reason why the blood test has been ordered. Remember at worst, taking an unnecessary blood test may be akin to an injury as venepuncture is undertaken. Unnecessary blood tests will always be financially wasteful and professionally oblige the clinician to be responsible for the results and their interpretation. Meticulous attention must be paid to following up results and acting on them.

Data interpretation sequence

- **Clinical history and examination**: most results of investigations cannot be interpreted unless you have an idea of the patient's history and examination. A good example of this is a 'high' glucose level of 14.1 mmol/L in a patient you have been telephoned to review and act on. In this scenario the patient could have any of the following possibilities:
  - New diagnosis of diabetes, if classic diabetes symptoms
  - Poorly controlled known case of diabetes
  - New diagnosis of diabetic ketoacidosis (DKA) if other clinical features present
  - Stress (? sepsis) or steroid-induced single high reading.
- **Interpretation of the result in clinical context**: The following information will help with the interpretation of 50 or so common blood investigations. Other investigations, such as ECG and chest X-rays are covered elsewhere. It is a good idea to familiarize yourself with the normal ranges of the common investigations. If in doubt, ask the clinical biochemist, haematologist, or other colleagues as appropriate. Please note that normal ranges will vary from laboratory to laboratory; and be different for certain patient age and ethnic groups.

Main blood investigations and clinical notes (normal range in parentheses)

Biochemistry

- **Na^+** *(136–145 mmol/L)*: **Hyponatraemia**: causes include diuretics, IV dextrose given excessively, syndrome of inappropriate antidiuretic hormone secretion (SIADH 'anything in the head or chest'), any failure, hypothyroidism, adrenal insufficiency'. With some assays hyperlipidaemia, hyperproteinaemia, and hyperglycaemia, the Na^+ level is recorded as low (pseudohyponatraemia). **Hypernatraemia**: almost always caused by dehydration.
- **K^+** *(3.4–4.5 mmol/L)*: **Hypokalaemia**: often due to over diuresis with thiazide or loop diuretics, also IV fluids without adequate K^+ replacement, gastrointestinal losses especially

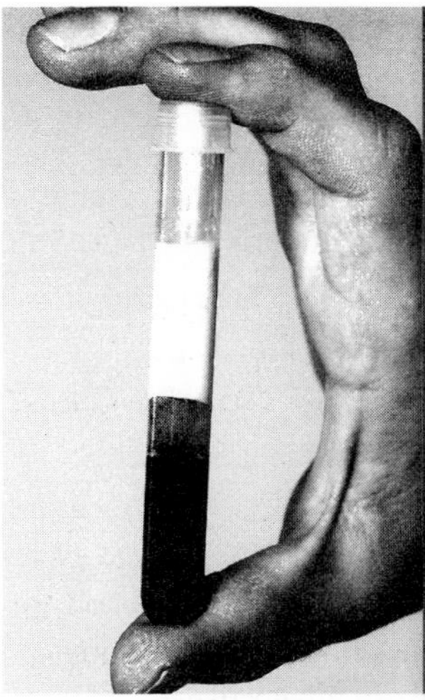

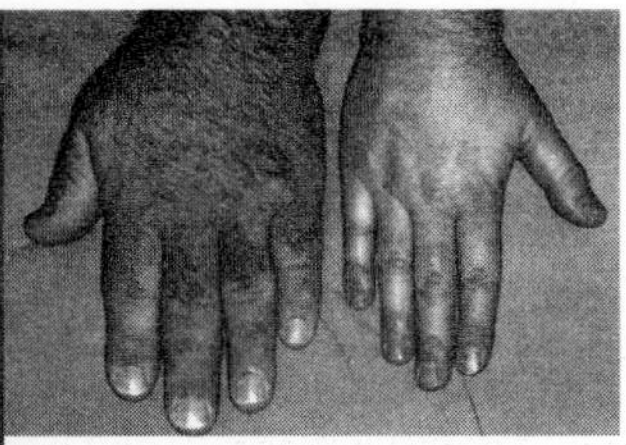

Clinical suspicion should prompt additional investigation. Here, enlarged hands and a history of changing ring size, prompted checking of the IGF-1 level and an eventual diagnosis of acromegaly (smaller normal hand for comparison)

Obviously lipaemic venous sample: this patient's cholesterol was 24.4 mmol/L with triglycerides of 78 mmol/L. Memorably both adding up to greater than 100

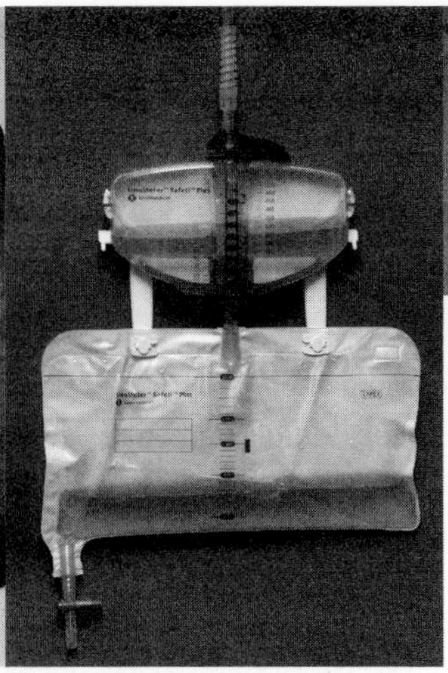

Renal output: do not forget to triangulate clinical data. The urea and creatinine results are best interpreted with other data, especially urine output, fluid intake, and even the ECG (effect of hyperkalaemia)

Figure 15.1 Images in data interpretation.

diarrhoea and vomiting, alkalosis, insulin and glucose administration, salbutamol nebulizers. **Hyperkalaemia**: metabolic acidosis, K^+-sparing diuretics (spironolactone, amiloride), acute renal failure, massive blood transfusion, adrenal insufficiency. Angiotensin-converting enzyme (ACE) inhibitors (e.g. ramipril, lisinopril) and A_2 inhibitors (e.g. losartan).

- **Urea** (*2.1–7.1 mmol/L*): **Raised**: dehydration, acute or chronic renal failure, if the creatinine alone is raised then renal failure is likely. Urea raised without raised creatinine is likely to be mainly dehydration.

- **Creatinine** (*50–90 μmol/L*): **Raised**: renal disease, acute or chronic. Rarely encountered in excess protein intake or any cause of muscle breakdown. **Low** urea and creatinine reflect low muscle mass and or poor intake of protein or liver failure.

- **Chloride** (*98–107 mmol/L*): **Raised**: plasma levels raised in fluid loss from gastrointestinal losses (small bowel fistula, diarrhoea), ureteric diversion (i.e. ileal bladder or uretero sigmoidostomy), diabetes insipidus, and also in renal failure, renal tubular acidosis, hypernatraemia or iatrogenic (drugs, e.g. acetazolamide, cholestyramine and excessive IV saline). **Low**: osmotic diuresis, e.g. DKA, hyperosmolar non-ketosis, loop diuretics, salt losing nephropathy, protracted vomiting, nasogastric suctioning. Sweat levels are elevated in cystic fibrosis.

- **Phosphate** (PO_4^{3-}) (*0.8–1.5 mmol/L*): **Raised**: decreased renal excretion due to acute or chronic renal failure, hypoparathyroidism, magnesium deficiency, acromegaly. Increased gastrointestinal absorption due to excess vitamin D intake, phosphate containing laxatives, tumoral calcinosis. Cellular shift with acidosis, i.e. DKA, respiratory or metabolic. Other conditions: rhabdomyolysis, neoplasia (lymphoma, leukaemia). **Low**: increased renal excretion due to hyperparathyroidism, Fanconi's syndrome, abnormal vitamin D metabolism. Gastrointestinal causes include dietary deficiency, long-term total parenteral nutrition (TPN), re-feeding syndrome, malabsorption, chronic alcoholism. Treatment of DKA with IV insulin causes intracellular shift. Also see under 'Bone' section.

- **Osmolality** (*275–295 mOsmol/kg*) or (*mmol/kg of solvent*): indicator of fluid balance. Measure of solute concentration in blood or urine. **Raised**: in dehydration and water loss (e.g. diabetes insipidus). **Low**: water overload (e.g. liver cirrhosis, SIADH).

- **Urate/uric acid** (*0.13–0.39 mmol/L females; 0.26–0.45 mmol/L males*): **Raised**: in gout, nephrolithiasis, uric acid nephropathy. Other causes include thiazide diuretics, excess alcohol intake, purine rich diet, increased turnover of nucleic acids (leukaemias, lymphoma, polycythaemia rubra vera, psoriasis, tumour lysis syndrome). Rare genetic causes include Lesch–Nyhan syndrome, Kelley-Seegmiller syndrome. NB: In gout urea can be normal or raised. It is a clinical diagnosis.

Liver functions tests

- **Alkaline phosphatase (ALP)** *(35–105 U/L)*: **Raised** in obstructive jaundice, or intermittent obstruction. Also raised in bone metastases, Paget's disease.
- **Alanine aminotransferase** *(5–38 U/L)*: **Raised** in hepatitic disease, commonly seen in fatty infiltration such as in metabolic syndrome, obesity or non-alcoholic steatotic hepatitis (NASH).
- **Total protein** *(60–80 g/L)*: reflects protein synthesis over the last 2 months. **Low** in chronic liver disease, nephrotic syndrome or enteropathy. **Raised**: myeloma.
- **Albumin** *(32–46 g/L)*: **Low** in recent poor nutrition (last 2 weeks) or chronic/acute liver disease.
- **Bilirubin** *(5–21 µmol/L)*: **Raised** in liver disease, especially obstructive jaundice. Raised without serious sequelae in Gilbert's disease.
- **γ-Glutamyl transpeptidase (GGT)** *(2–30 U/L)*: Raised in hepatobiliary disease, hepatic cell injury due to toxic or infectious hepatitis, alcohol- or drug-induced hepatocyte damage, cholestasis. Note other sources of GGT include renal, pancreas, and prostate, therefore not specific to liver. Useful for differentiating between liver disease and skeletal disease if ALP is raised.

Glucose

- **Glucose (random)** *(4–6 mmol/L)*: can be measured any time of the day without regard to the last meal, if greater than 11.1 mmol/L with symptoms of diabetes, then diabetes mellitus can be diagnosed. Otherwise repeat confirmatory test needed on another day.
- **Glucose (fasting)**: measured, usually overnight fast, water allowed. 7 mmol/L or more is diabetes mellitus with symptoms or test repeated on another day.

Glucose tolerance test

- **Diabetes mellitus**: fasting plasma glucose ≥7 mmol/L **or** 2h plasma glucose ≥11.1 mmol/L with symptoms, otherwise confirmatory fasting or random test needed on another day.
- **Impaired glucose tolerance (IGT)**: fasting plasma glucose <7.0 mmol/L *and* 2 h plasma glucose ≥7.9 and <11.1 mmol/L.
- **Impaired fasting glucose (IFG)**: fasting plasma glucose 6.1–6.9 mmol/L *and* 2 h plasma glucose <7.9 mmol/L.
- **Gestational diabetes**: is any abnormality of glucose handling presenting for the first time in pregnancy (on GTT fasting >5.1 mmol/L, 2 hour value >8.5 mmol/L).

Bone

- **Calcium** *(2.15–2.50 mmol/L)*: **Hypercalcaemia**: malignancy (including myeloma), hyperparathyroidism, dehydration, thiazide diuretics. **Hypocalcaemia**: consider acute hyperventilation (anxiety, pain, central lesion), total parenteral nutrition with insufficient calcium, low vitamin D, post thyroid surgery and consequent parathyroid gland damage, parathyroid surgery alone, and renal osteodystrophy (CRF).
- **Phosphate** *(0.8–1.5 mmol/L)*: **Raised** in renal osteodystrophy of chronic kidney disease. Renal retention of phosphate causes decreased serum calcium, increased parathyroid hormone (PTH) resulting in increased bone resorption. In addition raised phosphate causes a defect in vitamin D metabolism contributing to osteomalacia.
- **Alkaline phosphatase** *(35–105 U/L)*: **Raised**: bone disorders which have increased osteoblastic activity including metastases, especially (prostate adenocarcinoma), osteomalacia, Paget's disease.
- **Vitamin D** (deficient ≤10, insufficient <10–≤20, normal <20–60 µg/L). Multiple symptoms include tiredness, low mood, myalgia.

Troponin I and cardiac enzymes

- **Troponin1** *(<10 µ/L)*: best interpreted a fixed time after onset of cardiac chest time, usually 12 hours for most assays. **Raised**: cardiac myocyte damage due to myocardial infarction or myocarditis.

- **Creatine kinase (CK)** *(10–80 U/L female, 15–105 U/L male)*: Total CK is a marker of muscle damage and is **raised** in acute myocardial infarction or in skeletal muscle damage. A rise in plasma CK supports a diagnosis of an infarction though it is not diagnostic. Peak 24–48 hours.

- **CK-MB (isoenzyme)** *(4–6% of total CK)*: Heart muscle contains proportionally more CK-MB than skeletal muscle and is useful in early detection of myocardial infarction. Peak 10–24 hours.

- **Aspartate transaminase** *(8–20 U/L)*: Low specificity for any single tissue. **Raised**: cardiac damage though not diagnostic. Peak 24–48 hours.

- **Lactate dehydrogenase** *(100–190 U/L)*: Non-specific marker of cell damage. **Raised**: in myocardial infarction. Peak 48–72 hours, lung infarction as in pulmonary embolism.

- **Myoglobin** *(12–76 µg/L female, 19–92 µg/L male)*: present in both cardiac and skeletal muscle. Useful as an early marker though as it is not cardiac specific, so should be used in conjunction with other markers. Peak 2 hours.

Cholesterol/lipid profile

- **Total cholesterol** *(<5.0 mmol/L)*: **Raised** due to dietary intake, hypothyroidism, cholestasis (e.g. primary biliary cirrhosis) nephrotic syndrome, genetic disorders include familial hyper-cholesterolaemia, defective apoB gene, familial combined hyperlipidaemia.

- **Low-density lipoprotein (LDL) cholesterol** *(<4.10 mmol/L)*: **Raised**: (a) primary conditions: familial hypoalphalipoproteinaemias, ApoA1 abnormalities, Tangier's disease; (b) secondary: smoking, obesity, diabetes mellitus, metabolic syndrome, chronic renal failure, drugs (testo-sterone, β-blockers, progestogens, anabolic steroids. **Low**: abetalipoproteinaemia.

- **High-density lipoprotein (HDL) cholesterol** *(>1.0 mmol/L)*: plasma HDL is cardioprotective. **Raised** in (a) primary conditions: hyperalphalipoproteinaemia, cholesterol ester transfer protein deficiency; (b) secondary conditions: high alcohol intake, **Low**: low physical activity, type 2 diabetes.

- **Triglycerides** *(0.4–1.9 mmol/L)*: raised in obesity, high alcohol intake, diabetes mellitus, systemic lupus erythematosus (SLE), glycogen storage disorders, and with oestrogen use.

Arterial blood gases

- **Arterial blood gases (ABGs)** measure **pH** *(7.35–7.45)* *(or H$^+$ 35–45 mmol/L)*, **pCO$_2$** *(4.7–6.4 kPa)*, **pO$_2$** *(11.0–14.4 kPa)*, **base excess** *(±2)*, **Serum HCO$_3^-$** *(22–29 mmol/L)*, **O$_2$ saturations** *(95–98%)*, also to consider **anion gap, lactate** *(0.63–2.44 mmol/L)* also used to calculate anion gap, **carboxyhaemoglobin** *(1–4%)*. For interpretation, see Section 8.12.

Ferritin, total iron binding capacity (TIBC), and iron levels

- **Ferritin** *(10–120 µg/L female, 20–250 µg/L male)*, **TIBC** *(44.8–71.6 µmol/L)*, **iron levels** *(9.0–30.4 µmol/L female, 11.6–31.3 µmol/L male)*: In iron deficiency anaemia: iron is low, TIBC raised (due to increased avidity for harnessing all available Fe), ferritin is low (due to low Fe stores). Ferritin is also an acute phase reactant and is elevated in any acute inflammation/infection, pregnancy, and malignancy. A trial of iron treatment is often useful if there is doubt. **Raised** ferritin and iron, with low TIBC suggests the iron overload syndrome haemochromatosis.

Creatinine clearance

- **Creatinine clearance**: is dependent on renal blood flow and is therefore reduced in renal impairment. Serum and urine creatinine levels need to be measured and creatinine clearance calculated:

- *(Urine creatinine × urine volume)/(serum creatinine × min of duration) = (mL)/(min)*

- This value is then corrected for body surface area:

- *Creatinine clearance = ((mL)/(min)) × ((1.73 m^2)/(patient's surface area (m^2)*

- **Urine/albumin creatinine ratio (U/AC R)**: This is an useful measure of renal function in diabetic renal disease. It is measured using the first morning urine sample where practicable.

- **Microalbuminuria** is defined as: albumin:creatinine ratio >2.5 mg/mmol (men) or >3.5 mg/mmol (women) or albumin concentration >20 mg/L. Proteinuria is defined as: albumin:creatinine ratio >30 mg/mmol or albumin concentration >200 mg/L.
- **Creatine phosphokinase** (*as for CK above 30–175 IU/L*): present in cardiac and skeletal muscle, smooth muscle and in brain. **Raised**: in physical exertion, myositis, muscle injury, rhabdomyolysis, myocardial infarction, hypothyroidism, alcoholism (alcoholic myositis), statins, ciclosporin, cocaine, malignant hyperpyrexia, glycogen storage disorders.

Amylase

- **Amylase** (*<101 IU/L*): **Raised**: marked elevation in acute pancreatitis. Levels can be near normal in chronic or haemorrhagic pancreatitis. **Also raised** in severe glomerular impairment (renally excreted), DKA, perforated peptic ulcer especially if perforation into lower sac. Mild to moderate elevation with other acute abdominal presentations.

Lactate dehydrogenase

- **Lactate dehydrogenase** (**LDH**) (*200–500 IU/L*): non-specific marker of cell damage. **Raised**: in shock, hypoxia, myocardial infarction, haematological disorders (i.e. megaloblastic anaemia, acute leukaemia, lymphomas). Moderate elevation with viral hepatitis, malignancy, skeletal muscle disease, pulmonary embolism, infectious mononucleosis.

Haematology

Full blood count (FBC) with differential:

- **Haemoglobin** (**Hb**) (*13–17 g/dL*): **Low**: anaemia due to multiple clinical entities *see* Mean corpuscular volume (MCV). **Raised** in polycythaemia rubra vera, familial polycythaemia, raised altitude, congenital cardiovascular disease, smoking, renal disease, chronic obstructive pulmonary disease (COPD).
- **White cell count** (**WCC**) (*4–11 x 10⁹/L*): **Raised** with infection and haematological malignancy. **Low**: drugs, autoimmune, infection (human immunodeficiency virus [HIV], hepatitis), bone marrow failure, splenomegaly, rare genetic conditions.
- **Platelets** (*140–400 x 10⁹/L*): **Raised**: primary causes (myelofibrosis, polycythaemia rubra vera, chronic myelocytic leukaemia), secondary causes (infection, chronic inflammation, post splenectomy, malignancy). **Low** due to decreased production (cytotoxic drugs aplastic anaemia, myelodysplasia, multiple myeloma, HIV), increased consumption (autoimmune, i.e. SLE, heparin, disseminated intravascular coagulation [DIC], thrombotic thrombocytopenic purpura [TTP]), abnormal distribution (splenomegaly) or dilutional loss (massive transfusion).
- **Mean corpuscular volume** (*80–100 fL*): the MCV and a corresponding anaemia can either be **microcytic** (iron deficiency, thalassaemia, sickle cell, sideroblastic), **normocytic** (chronic disease, haemolytic, acute blood loss, bone marrow metastatic disease) or **macrocytic** (excess alcohol, B$_{12}$ or folate deficiency, excess alcohol, hypothyroidism, myelodysplasia).
- **Haematocrit** (**HCT**) (*0.4–0.5 L/L*): proportion of blood volume occupied by red and other cells. **Raised**: when Hb high or dehydration.
- **Red cell differential width** (**RDW**): This parameter provides an index of the whether the cells are all the same size or not (called anisocytosis, as in recent blood loss and increased blood production).
- **Neutrophils** (*2–7 x 10⁹/L*): **Raised** with bacterial infection, inflammation and tissue necrosis, metabolic disorders, neoplasms, acute haemorrhage/haemolysis, drugs (corticosteroids, lithium, tetracycline, chronic myeloid leukaemia, treatment with myeloid growth factors (granulocyte-colony stimulating factor [G-CSF], granulocyte macrophage-colony stimulating factor [GM-CSF]), asplenia.
- **Lymphocytes** (*1–3 x 10⁹/L*): **Raised** in acute (infectious mononucleosis, rubella, pertussis, mumps, hepatitis, cytomegalovirus (CMV), HIV, herpes simplex virus (HSV) or herpes simplex zoster) and chronic (tuberculosis, toxoplasmosis, brucellosis, syphilis) infection, chronic

lymphoid leukaemia, acute lymphoblastic leukaemia, non-Hodgkin's lymphoma. Low in immunosuppression post transplant, chemotherapy, tumours of the lymphoid system (chronic lymphocytic leukaemia and myeloma), acquired immune deficiency syndrome (AIDS), X-linked agammaglobulinaemia, aplasia of the thymus.

- **Monocytes** ($0.2-1.0 \times 10^9$/L): **Raised** in malaria, tuberculosis, typhoid, myelodysplasia. Low in autoimmune conditions (i.e. SLE), hairy cell leukaemia, and drugs (glucocorticoids, chemotherapy).

- **Eosinophils** ($0.02-0.5 \times 10^9$/L): **Raised** in allergic diseases (especially hypersensitivity reactions), in atopic individuals, parasitic diseases, dermatological conditions, vasculitis, drug sensitivity, myeloproliferative disease.

- **Basophils** ($0.01-0.1 \times 10^9$/L): **Raised** in chronic myeloid leukaemia, polycythaemia rubra vera, myxoedema, viral infection, IgE-mediated hypersensitivity reactions, inflammatory conditions, i.e. ulcerative colitis or rheumatoid arthritis, hypothyroidism. Low in thyrotoxicosis, allergic reaction, Cushing's syndrome, haemorrhage.

- **Reticulocyte count** ($20-80 \times 10^9$/L): immature red cells. **Raised** in bleeding, haemolysis, iron therapy, infection, inflammation, polycythaemia, myeloproliferative disorders, erythropoietin (EPO) therapy. **Low** in leukaemia, myeloma, lymphoma, iron/folate/B_{12} deficiency, aplastic anaemia, red cell aplasia.

- **Plasma viscosity** (<1.7) **and erythrocyte sedimentation rate** (**ESR**) ($1-14$ mm/hr): ESR **raised** with autoimmune disorders, acute and chronic infections, pregnancy, vasculitis (temporal arteritis). ESR can be raised with age alone.

- **C-reactive protein** (**CRP**) (5 mg/L): protein produced by the liver as an acute phase reactant. Non-specifically raised in inflammation and infection. Useful to monitor specific infections such as bacterial endocarditis. Low in SLE and malignancy.

- **B_{12}** ($200-800$ ng/L): B_{12} deficiency causes macrocytic megaloblastic anaemia. Causes include dietary deficiency (vegetarians, vegans) pernicious anaemia, gastrectomy, ileal disease, blind loop syndromes (bacterial overgrowth in inflammatory bowel), malabsorption, metformin treatment.

- **Folate** ($5.0-14.0$ µg/L): haematological features indistinguishable from B_{12} deficiency. Causes include dietary deficiency, increased requirements/losses (pregnancy, haemolysis, exfoliative dermatitis, renal dialysis), malabsorption, drugs (phenytoin, valproate, oral contraceptives, nitrofurantoin induce folate malabsorption) (methotrexate, trimethoprim, pentamidine all antagonize folate metabolism), alcohol.

- **International normalized ratio** (**INR**) ($1.0-1.2$): warfarin prolongs prothrombin time. INR is a measure of the ratio of patient's prothrombin time against a normal control sample. Affects the extrinsic pathway vitamin K-dependent coagulation factors. Other conditions prolonging prothrombin time include vitamin K deficiency, malabsorption, DIC, liver failure.

- **D-dimer** (<250 ng/L): breakdown product of fibrin which forms the scaffolding for blood clots to form. Plasmin cleaves fibrin to release fibrin degradation products which include D-dimer. Negative D-dimer usually excludes venous thromboembolism. **Raised**: DVT, pulmonary embolism but also affected by infection, trauma, myocardial infarction, angina, cerebrovascular accident (CVA), infection, inflammation, trauma, cancer, pregnancy, renal failure.

- **Partial thromboplastin time** (**PTT**) ($12.0-16.8$ s): measures the intrinsic pathway and tests for all clotting deficiencies except for VII and XIII. It is prolonged with use of heparin, antiphospholipid antibody (especially lupus anticoagulant), coagulation factor deficiency. Activated partial thromboplastin time (APTT) is time taken for sample to clot following addition of intrinsic pathway activator.

- **Thrombophilia screen** should include FBC, clotting screen, protein C, protein S, factor V Leiden screening test, antithrombin III, lupus anticoagulant. For arterial thrombosis add homocysteine and lipoprotein A. Ensure patient is not pregnant, on oral contraception or hormone replacement therapy (HRT), and patient should have discontinued anticoagulation for at least 1 month.

- **Fibrin degradation products**: *see* D-dimer.

Immunology

- **Rheumatoid screen** (*<15 kU/L*): Rheumatoid factor is an autoantibody **raised** in rheumatoid arthritis. It can be **raised** in Sjögren's syndrome, Felty's syndrome, systemic sclerosis, SLE, infective endocarditis, and 20% of healthy individuals over 65 years.

- **Protein electrophoresis**: used to detect presence of abnormal proteins or absence of proteins. Mainly used in diagnosis of multiple myeloma which is characterized by paraproteins (monoclonal antibodies). IgG is the most common type.

- **Immunoglobulins**: Ig antibodies are secreted by plasma cells (B lymphocytes). Five isotypes include IgA (present in mucosal membranes of the gastrointestinal, respiratory, and urinary tracts), IgD (present in bloodstream against bacterial infections), IgE (increased in parasitic infections and atopic individuals), IgG (binds to most pathogens in blood and tissues), IgM (due to size of molecule activity is limited to blood stream). Disorders characterized by amyloidosis paraproteins include multiple myeloma, e.g. Waldenström's macroglobulinaemia.

- **Anti-nuclear antibody** (*1:40*): present in autoimmune conditions SLE, rheumatoid arthritis, Sjogren's syndrome, autoimmune hepatitis, scleroderma. Up to 5% of people over 70 years may have a benign paraproteinaemia.

- **Scleroderma antibodies (Ro, La, Scl 70, RNP)**. More specific for scleroderma.

- **Coeliac screen**: check when patient is on a diet including gluten for 6 weeks. IgA anti-tissue transglutaminase antibodies (tTGAs) is the preferred investigation. Endomysial antibodies (EMAs) are used if tTGA test is not available or equivocal. If serology is positive patient should be referred for duodenal biopsy.

- **Thyroid peroxisome antibody** (**TPO**) (*<50 IU/L*): **Raised** in Hashimoto's thyroiditis, idiopathic thyroid atrophy.

- **Anti-streptolysin O**: Blood test to measure the antibodies against streptolysin O secreted by group A streptococcus. **Raised** in active streptococcal infection, bacterial endocarditis, streptococcal glomerulonephritis, rheumatic fever.

Endocrinology and diabetes

- **HbA$_{1c}$** (*<6.5%, 48 mmol/mol*): glucose binds covalently to some amino acids in the haemoglobin molecule. Gives a measure of diabetic control over 2 months. May become an international method of diagnosing diabetes mellitus.

- **Thyroid stimulating hormone** (*0.3–4.0 mU/L*) [**FT$_3$** (*2.6–6.2 pmol/L*), **FT$_4$** (*11–26 pmol/L*)]: **Raised** TSH with low FT$_4$, FT$_3$ present in hypothyroidism (Hashimoto's thyroiditis, De Quervain's thyroiditis, primary atrophic hypothyroidism). **Low** TSH with raised FT$_4$, FT$_3$ is present in hyperthyroidism (Grave's disease, multinodular goitre, toxic adenoma).

- **Prolactin** (*female <501 mU/L, male <401 mU/L*): hyperprolactinaemia leads to lethargy, reduced libido, galactorrhoea, erectile dysfunction, infertility, menstrual disturbances. Causes: pituitary tumours, PCOS, drugs, pregnancy, lactation, OCP.

- **Synacthen (tetracosactrin) test**: response to synthetic adrenocorticotropic hormone (ACTH) is measured to investigate cortisol deficiency. Serum cortisol is measured before and 30 minutes after injection of the analogue. A rise to >550 mmol/L excludes adrenal insufficiency (Addison's disease). A further sample can be obtained at 60 minutes and an additional rise of 200 mmol/L should be observed in normal subjects.

- **Cortisol** (*am 200–700 nmol/L, pm 55–250 nmol/L*): Peak in the morning and dip at night, Samples are taken at midnight to detect a loss of diurnal variation.

- **Dexamethasone suppression tests** are used to investigate Cushing's syndrome. It suppresses hypothalamic corticotrophin-releasing hormone (CRH) and pituitary ACTH.

- **Parathyroid level** (*0.8–8.5 pmol/L*): primary hyperparathyroidism is due to parathyroid gland adenoma or diffuse parathyroid gland hyperplasia. PTH excess causes hypercalcaemia and if prolonged results in bone demineralization, softening osteomalacia in adults, and rickets in children. Secondary hyperparathyroidism occurs in response to hypocalcaemia (causes include chronic renal failure, vitamin D deficiency). Hyperplastic parathyroid glands from prolonged hypocalcaemia will cause tertiary hyperparathyroidism (development of an adenoma).

- Hypoparathyroidism does not result in osteomalacia. Causes include surgical complications of thyroidectomy or parathyroidectomy, autoimmune disorder, congenital PTH resistance.
- **Testosterone** (*male 10–28 nmol/L; female <3.0 nmol/L*), **oestradiol** (*follicular phase <260 pmol/L, luteal phase 180–700 pmol/L, male <130 pmol/L*): deficiency can be primary (testicular failure *or* ovarian failure) or secondary (pituitary failure).
- **Luteinizing hormone** (**LH**) (*follicular phase 1–12 IU/L, mid-cycle 14–60 IU/L, luteal phase 1–12 IU/L, postmenopausal >16 IU/L*)/**follicle-stimulating hormone (FSH)** (*follicular phase 1–12 IU/L, mid-cycle 6–21 IU/L, luteal phase 1–12 IU/L, postmenopausal >29 IU/L*): reduced in hypopituitarism. Synthetic oestrogen and/or progestogen prevent FSH secretion thus inhibiting follicular growth and ovulation. In menopause FSH and LH increase in the absence of negative feedback. LH:FSH ratio greater than 2.0 is biochemically indicative of polycystic ovary syndrome.
- **Urinary catecholamines** (*adrenaline <200 nmol/24 h, noradrenaline <600 nmol/24 h*): **Raised**: in phaeochromocytoma; 24-hour urine is collected for analysis.
- **5HIAA**: urinary 5-hydroxy-indoleacetic acid (serotonin metabolite) excretion is raised in carcinoid syndrome.
- *β*-**human chorionic gonadotrophin (hCG)** (*<4 IU/L*): is produced by the placenta peak and is the basis of the pregnancy test. Also elevated in choriocarcinoma which develops from a hydatidiform mole. 50% of testicular teratomas secrete hCG.

Tumour markers

- **Prostate-specific antigen** (*age 40–49, <2.5 ng/mL; 50–59, <3.5; 60–69, <4.5; 70–79, <6.5*): secreted by prostate cells. **Raised**: elevated in benign prostatic hypertrophy (BPH), prostate cancer, prostate infection, digital rectal examination.
- **CA-125** (*<35 KU/L*): marker of ovarian cancer.
- **CA 19-9** (*<33 KU/L*): **Raised**: adenocarcinoma of pancreas and also colorectal and gastric carcinomas. Also raised in primary sclerosing cholangitis and useful to monitor disease activity.
- **Carcinoembryonic antigen (CEA)** (*<5 µg/L*): elevated within 60% of patients with colorectal carcinoma increases with hepatic metastasis (80–100%). Also elevated with cholangiocarcinoma.
- *α*-**Fetoprotein (AFP)** (*<9 KU/L*): marker for hepatocellular carcinoma and testicular teratomas.
- **Thyroglobulin** (*<30 ng/mL*): specific to thyroid gland. Used as a tumour marker for patients with differentiated thyroid cancer. Levels post-total thyroidectomy indicate presence of thyroid tissue. Levels may be normal or low in poorly differentiated cancer preoperatively, therefore may not be as useful for monitoring the disease in such cases.

Patient safety and clinical governance tips

- ✔ **Consent and explanation**: It is good practice to inform a patient about investigations that are conducted on them. Abnormal and normal results should be discussed as they arise. Normal results are very reassuring to patients!
- ✔ **Abnormal results**: must be acted upon urgently in most cases and follow-up of tests arranged and clearly documented in the notes
- ✔ **Track results in clinical notes**: it is often a good idea to track results such as renal function and liver in a small table in the clinical notes so that improvement or deterioration can be easily identified.
- ✔ **Seek help**: particularly important if the clinician is not sure as to how to interpret the data.
- ✔ **Explanation to patient**: an involved patient will improve safety standards. A good example is that of dysthyroid patients, who can be asked to look out for signs/symptoms of hypothyroidism or hyperthyroidism.
- ✔ **What is a test?** A test is something that is done, chosen correctly, correctly interpreted and acted on by the person who organizes it.

Data interpretation

Julie Upton, age 67, admitted because of falls and weakness down the left hand side. She has been investigated extensively for various problems including: hypertension, arthritis, weight loss.

Current medication: bendroflumethiazide 2.5 mg od, carbimazole 20 mg od

The consultant does not feel that all the investigations in the notes were clinically indicated, nevertheless the results are available!

Explain the results of Julie Upton's blood tests.

		Self	Peer	Peer /tutor	Tutor
Biochemistry: Na⁺ 124, K⁺ 3.1, Urea 14.6, Ca²⁺ 1.9, ALP 256, uric acid 0.52, glucose 14.3, total cholesterol 6.6, LDL 4.1, HDL 0.9, U/A Cr 9.9	**Hyponatraemia: Na⁺** (136-$145\,mmol/L$): diuretics most likely, note glucose level	☐	☐	☐	☐
	Hypokalaemia: K⁺ (3.4-$4.5\,mmol/L$):over diuresis with thiazide diuretics	☐	☐	☐	☐
	Urea (2.1-$7.1\,mmol/L$): **Raised**: Dehydration, over diuresis with thiazide	☐	☐	☐	☐
	Urate/uric acid (0.13-$0.39\,mmol/L$ females; 0.26-$0.45\,mmol/L$ males): **Raised**: gout, thiazide,	☐	☐	☐	☐
	ALP (35-$105\,U/L$): **Raised** ? osteomalacia, calcium low	☐	☐	☐	☐
	Hypocalcaemia: calcium (2.15-$2.50\,mmol/L$): osteomalacia, ? vitamin D deficiency/insufficiency	☐	☐	☐	☐
	Hyperglycaemia: glucose (random) (4-$6\,mmol/L$): if symptoms then diabetes mellitus	☐	☐	☐	☐
	High total cholesterol, high LDL, low HDL: high cardiovascular disease (CVD) risk with elevated LDL:HDL	☐	☐	☐	☐
	High U/AC R: microalbuminuria, indicates high risk of CVD and risk of end-stage renal disease	☐	☐	☐	☐
		☐	☐	☐	☐
Haematology: Hb 10.2, MCV 104 , B₁₂ 84, CRP 4	**Haemoglobin** (13-$17\,g/dL$): **Low**: anaemia	☐	☐	☐	☐
	MCV (80-$100\,fL$): **macrocytic** B₁₂ deficiency	☐	☐	☐	☐
	B₁₂ (150-$800\,ng/L$): deficiency causes macrocytosis, ? pernicious anaemia	☐	☐	☐	☐
	CRP normal: test probably not indicated routinely at admission	☐	☐	☐	☐
		☐	☐	☐	☐
Immunology: rheumatoid factor 39 kU/L, TPO 378 IU/L, protein electrophoresis normal	**Rheumatoid screen** ($<15\,kU/L$): **raised** ? rheumatoid arthritis	☐	☐	☐	☐
	Protein electrophoresis: diagnosis of multiple myeloma probably considered but would be needed in hypercalcaemia	☐	☐	☐	☐
	Thyroid peroxisome antibody (TPO): **Raised** Hashimoto's thyroiditis	☐	☐	☐	☐
		☐	☐	☐	☐
Endocrinology and diabetes: HbA₁c %8.77, TSH 24.8, FT₄ 5, Synacthen test 223 rising to 278, LH 78, FSH 66	**HbA₁c** ($<6.5\%$): **Raised** indicates diabetes presents for several months and poorly controlled	☐	☐	☐	☐
	TSH (0.3-$4.0\,mU/L$): elevated indicated hypothyroidism- Hashimoto's hypothyroidism	☐	☐	☐	☐
	FT₄ (11-$26\,pmol/L$): low T₄ indicates hypothyroidism	☐	☐	☐	☐
	Synacthen (tetracosactrin) test: rise by less to 200 and above 550 nmol/L indicates adrenal insufficiency	☐	☐	☐	☐
		☐	☐	☐	☐
LH raised (post menopausal: LH >16 IU/L, FSH >29 IU/L)	Patient expected to be postmenopausal at this age, not indicated	☐	☐	☐	☐
Seeks help as appropriate	Considers seeking expert help, e.g. clinical biochemist, clinical haematologist	☐	☐	☐	☐
Post-procedure management and professionalism	Documents abnormal results, produces management plan, and plans follow up for re-testing and review	☐	☐	☐	☐
Explanation to patient	Explains result to patient as appropriate and explains management plan. Allows patient opportunity to questions	☐	☐	☐	☐
Self-assessed as at least borderline:	Signature: Date:	U B S E	U B S E	U B S E	U B S E
Peer-assessed as ready for tutor assessment:	Signature: Date:	U B S E	U B S E	U B S E	U B S E
Tutor-assessed as satisfactory:	Signature: Date:	U B S E	U B S E	U B S E	U B S E

Notes

15.3 Surgical safety checklist

Background

In industrialized countries, major complications with permanent disability or death are reported to occur in 0.4–0.8% of inpatient surgical procedures. In 2007, 129 419 incidents were reported to the National Patient Safety Agency (NPSA) across England and Wales, of which 271 resulted in death. In June 2008, the World Health Organization (WHO) launched a Global Patient Safety Challenge, *Safe Surgery Saves Lives* to reduce the number of surgical deaths across the world. A core set of safety checks were identified in the form of a WHO Surgical Safety Checklist. A multicentre, international study found a significant reduction in postoperative morbidity and mortality following implementation of the surgical safety checklist. This was carried out in eight countries in 3733 surgical procedures. Mortality was reduced from 1.5% to 0.8% (46% reduction) and complications from 11% to 7% (36% reduction).

Clinical indications

The surgical safety checklist should be used for all patients undergoing a surgical procedure under general/regional/local anaesthesia or sedation. This includes interventions performed in specialist areas such as endoscopy, radiology, and dermatology. Adaptation of the WHO checklist is encouraged to ensure it is effectively integrated into *local* clinical practice. It has also been translated into different languages to improve its accessibility worldwide.

Contraindications

There are no contraindications to the use of the surgical safety checklist. It is important to use it in emergency situations where it provides prompts for clinical staff to ensure mistakes are not made in a highly pressurized, stressful environment.

Sequence

The exact form of the checklist varies between different hospitals but the general process is similar. There are five steps, which include:

1 **Preoperative briefing – including site of surgery**
2 **Sign in** – before induction of anaesthesia
3 **Time out** – before start of surgical intervention
4 **Sign out** – before the patient leaves the operating
5 **Post-operative de-briefing**.

Organizational preparation

Each organization is responsible for identifying an executive and a clinical lead who are then responsible for implementation of the surgical safety checklist. Clinical audits should be conducted on the appropriate use of the surgical checklist. Any problems in relation to non-implementation will need to be sorted out urgently. In some hospitals, the checklist is performed using a paperless version, for example, using a whiteboard or computer. In other hospitals, it forms part of the written documentation within the patient records.

Explanation and consent

Clinical staff working in any environment where the surgical safety checklist is to be used should be trained to use it appropriately. The patient is not required to give consent but needs to participate in the first phase. It is important to explain the process to the patient, especially if it is to be conducted with the patient awake for a procedure under regional/local anaesthesia. It will act to reassure the patient further.

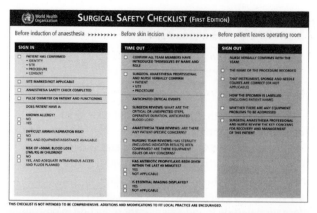

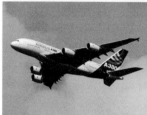

Aviation has used the 'safety checklist' for at least the last 75 years. It is used in every flight and is multi-professional

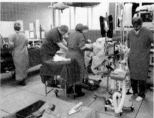

In the seminal paper, the multi-professional use of the checklist in eight countries resulted in significant reduction in mortality (by 46%) and complications (by 36%)

Figure 15.2 Images in use of the surgical safety checklist. Left © apply pictures; middle © WHO 2011.

Procedure: before surgery

- **Preoperative briefing**: The briefing session takes place between the anaesthetist, surgeon, scrub nurse and the operating department professional (ODP) before the theatre session is commenced. It is designed to determine the requirements for the operating list and identify any safety concerns. **All new members must be introduced to each other**.

- **Sign-in**: During 'sign-in', the anaesthetist and anaesthetic assistant run through a series of checks to confirm:

  ○ **Identity of the patient**: check name, hospital number, date of birth, and address

  ○ **Site of the operation**: mark clearly if needed. Especially careful about **right vs left**

  ○ **Allergies**: if any, are known

  ○ **Safe administration of anaesthesia**: both the anaesthetic equipment and availability of anaesthetic agents are checked

  ○ **Airway check**: It is important to determine if the patient has a difficult airway as this may require additional equipment such as a fibreoptic endoscope

  ○ **Blood products and venous access**: the volume of anticipated blood loss also needs to be determined to ensure that adequate venous access is sited and that blood products are available before commencing with surgery. The surgeon does not necessarily have to be present.

- **Time-out**: a team member in theatre is allocated responsibility for going through all the steps described in the 'time-out' phase:

  ○ **Introductions**: the team members introduce themselves

  ○ **Confirm identity of patient and operation planned**: the surgeon and or anaesthetist verbally confirm the identity of the patient and the site of the surgical procedure planned

  ○ **Critical event review**: the surgeon, anaesthetist, and scrub nurse are asked specific questions to determine if there are any critical events

- ○ **Surgical site infection bundle** is then carried out. This includes checking if antibiotic prophylaxis is given, patient warming, hair removal, and glycaemic control
- ○ **VTE prophylaxis**: the leading team member must then check if VTE prophylaxis has been given or planned
- ○ **Essential imaging available**: determine if any essential imaging such as CT or X-ray has been seen and is available.

The surgical procedure is then performed.

- **Sign-out**: Before the patient leaves the operating theatre, the leading team member goes through the steps in the sign out phase:
  - ○ **Procedure documented**: *This* involves checking that the procedure has been documented
  - ○ **Swab/instrument count**: This is confirming that the instruments, swabs, and sharps count is correct
  - ○ **Specimen** correctly labelled and dispatched to histology, microbiology, etc.
  - ○ **Key concerns** for the postoperative recovery of the patient identified.
- **Debriefing session**: ideally this should be conducted between all members involved in the care of the patients at the end of the operating session. It aims to evaluate the entire process to determine if there were any problems with the ability to perform the procedures or in the implementation of the surgical safety checklist. Any deficiencies identified can be addressed in subsequent sessions to improve the process.

Post-procedure management

Once the checklist has been completed, if it is in written form, it should be inserted within the patient records. If it is conducted in paperless form, a record is kept to confirm that it has been completed for that patient. At present there is a legal requirement to implement the checklist in the UK as each hospital trust must show to the Care Quality Commission that it complies with the NPSA requirements.

Professionalism

Communicate effectively and listen to others. Identify a team member who will lead the process and is responsible for the checks. Address any concerns or failures as a team. Conduct regular audit to determine compliance with NPSA requirements and thereby improve clinical practice.

Complications

There are no specific complications in association with the checklist. A finite additional amount of time is likely to be needed and this must be taken into account when planning size of operating lists.

Patient safety tip

- ✔ **Patient identity, site of surgery, and antibiotic therapy are still major correctable areas of avoidable complications**: ensure the patient has a wristband or equivalent to identify them and are accompanied by all relevant documentation of planned procedure prior to transfer to the operating theatre. When confirmation by the patient is not possible, carers or significant others can support the process.
- ✔ **Allergies**: check notes very carefully for allergies in notes – do not rely on a sedated patient.

Student name:	Medical school:	Year:

Surgical safety checklist

Describe how you would perform the surgical safety checklist for a diabetic patient undergoing right above-knee amputation.

		Self	Peer	Peer/tutor	Tutor
Equipment and preparation	• Introduces all team members involved in theatre session	☐	☐	☐	☐
	• Identifies the correct patient by name, hospital number, date of birth, and address	☐	☐	☐	☐
	• Identifies team lead responsible for conducting surgical safety checks	☐	☐	☐	☐
	•	☐	☐	☐	☐
Explanation and consent	• Explains to patient that checklist will be conducted	☐	☐	☐	☐
	• Collates all necessary documentation including written consent form	☐	☐	☐	☐
	•	☐	☐	☐	☐
Sign-in phase	• Confirms identity of patient	☐	☐	☐	☐
	• Determines site of operation is marked	☐	☐	☐	☐
	• Records any drug allergies	☐	☐	☐	☐
	• Ensures appropriate anaesthetic equipment and anaesthetic agents are available	☐	☐	☐	☐
	• Checks airway to determine if additional equipment such as a fibreoptic endoscope is required	☐	☐	☐	☐
	• Checks for availability of blood products if necessary	☐	☐	☐	☐
	•	☐	☐	☐	☐
Time-out phase	• Introduces all team members	☐	☐	☐	☐
	• Confirms identity of patient and operative procedure	☐	☐	☐	☐
	• Performs critical event review with anaesthetist and surgeon	☐	☐	☐	☐
	• Ensures that surgical site infection bundle is implemented	☐	☐	☐	☐
	• Ensures that VTE prophylaxis bundle is implemented	☐	☐	☐	☐
	• Checks that any necessary imaging is displayed	☐	☐	☐	☐
	•	☐	☐	☐	☐
Sign-out phase	• Ensures that details of procedure are documented	☐	☐	☐	☐
	• Checks that swab/instrument count is correct	☐	☐	☐	☐
	• Records appropriate details of specimen and ensures it is dispatched	☐	☐	☐	☐
	• Communicates any key concerns for recovery of patient to staff	☐	☐	☐	☐
	•	☐	☐	☐	☐
Post-procedure management	• Conducts debriefing to identify any issues/concerns raised during the procedure	☐	☐	☐	☐
	• Understands the rationale for the surgical safety checklist	☐	☐	☐	☐
	•	☐	☐	☐	☐
Professionalism	• Communicates effectively and directs team members to ensure that all aspects of surgical safety checklist are implemented appropriately	☐	☐	☐	☐
	• Completes all documentation legibly and unambiguously	☐	☐	☐	☐
	• Communicates appropriately with nursing staff.	☐	☐	☐	☐
	•	☐	☐	☐	☐

			Self	Peer	Peer/tutor	Tutor
Self-assessed as at least borderline:	Signature:	Date:	U B S E	U B S E	U B S E	U B S E
Peer-assessed as ready for tutor assessment:	Signature:	Date:	U B S E	U B S E	U B S E	U B S E
Tutor-assessed as satisfactory:	Signature:	Date:	U B S E	U B S E	U B S E	U B S E

Notes

15.4 Referral letters

Background

There will always be clinical cases where specialist input is needed from more than one clinical discipline. Consultants will refer to other specialties for advice, opinion, or request for a colleague to take over or give assistance in management. In such instances a referral letter is written to the specialist, which conveys the salient points of the case and has a particular question that needs to be answered or an action that the referred team is best able to undertake.

Clinical indications

High standards of clinical care and safety are promoted by timely and relevant referral. No single clinical team will have the prerequisite knowledge and skills to manage all aspects of care for a patient. The rigor advised in relation to clinician to clinician referral should also be applied to referrals for other reasons such as occupational therapy, physiotherapy, social care, pathology, and radiology requests.

Physiological and professional principles

Often key facts and assessments are missing in the referral letter. It cannot be stressed enough that abnormal results and concerns should be clearly expressed. Without the correct level of detail, the referred clinician is unlikely to be able to make the best judgement as to the urgency or need for the request.

Patient details given	**Mr Stephen Boylan** **Hosp No. N123456** **DoB: 15/5/50** **Location: ElizabethWard**
Specialist to whom referral is going to	*Mr G. Bilroth: Consultant Upper GI surgeon*
Case history Presenting complaint - brief history Investigations and results	*We would appreciate a review of the above patient, a 57-year-old gentleman who presented with a 3-week history of increasingly severe epigastric pain and an episode of haematemesis. He has also had around 7 kgs of weight loss over the past 2 months and has been passing maleana. Routine investigations on admission showed haemoglobin of 8g/dl. This was corrected by transfusion of 2 units of blood. An OGD revealed the presence of a possibly malignant ulcer. He has had a staging CT scan, results are still pending.* *This patients case has been submitted to the upper GI Multi-Disciplinary Team and currently his treatments have been optimised to reduce the risk of any further GI bleeds. His current active co-morbidities are hypertension and asthma – both of which are well controlled.*
Request for a review	*Dr Sushraton would appreciate a review of this patient in case surgery is a viable management option.* *Many thanks and kind regards*
Signed off correctly	*Glen Jackson* Dr Glen Jackson: Bleep 1234 House Officer to Dr Sushraton

Figure 15.3 Referral letter example.

Contraindications

Clinical time is always pressured and valuable. Be sure that the referral is actually needed! (See Figure 15.3 for an example.)

Sequence

Documentation and preparation

All referral letters should have information on it relevant to the specialty to which you are referring, and should be polite and courteous. Be sure to include all relevant patient identifiers and your own details. Once completed fax or mail the referral to the appropriate department as quickly as possible. Ideally, deliver it by hand to a team member so that the request can be actioned as soon as possible. Handing a referral letter over to the junior doctor of a consultant should ensure that your patient is seen on the next consultant ward round.

Explanation and consent

The most common referral is to the radiology department requesting a scan. Be clear about what scan you want and why you want it. Different scans ask different questions, e.g. when requesting X-rays – exclude pregnancy in women, computed tomography (CT) scans often use contrast agents which may cause lactic acidosis in patients on metformin. For magnetic resonance imaging (MRI) patients have to have clearance with respect to any metal implants or fragments.

Protocol

Other specialties also ask specific questions, e.g. when referring to cardiology include details of current symptoms and examination findings, past cardiac history, previous investigations, and relevant results. Make sure that up-to-date investigations are ready for the cardiologists to assess, i.e. recent ECG, cardiac enzymes, echocardiograms. In doing so, the cardiologist will receive a succinct referral letter for a case with up-to-date results of any investigations. This will allow the cardiologist to have a reasonable idea of what is going on with the patient and assess the degree of urgency.

Key details to include:

- Patient details – name, date of birth, hospital number, and location in hospital if inpatient or address if outpatient
- Name of the current consultant
- Name of the specialist to whom you are referring
- Details of case: specific history, examination findings, investigation results, significant other history
- Request: why is specialist input needed? Is a routine review needed or is there something specific that needs to be done?
- Urgency (mark the referral urgent if necessary)
- Signing off: polite end to letter, signature, name and bleep number, date.

Post-protocol management

Once the referral letter has been completed, deliver the referral to the appropriate department (usually the secretary of the specialist or the junior doctors if urgent). In many hospitals referrals will be done electronically, fax or direct discussion.

Professionalism

In most hospitals radiology requests are usually made in the form of a request card. Completing these cards is no different to completing a referral letter. Consult local guidelines for radiology and other referrals if they exist.

Patient safety and clinical governance tips

✔ **Avoid late referrals**: specific examples abound in relation to late referrals for abnormal biochemistry, worsening sepsis, uncontrolled bleeding and increasing confusion, and coma in patients. Concerns in relation to necessity for referrals and ensuring patient safety should always be expressed appropriately usually to the more senior doctors and especially the clinical supervisor, who will usually be the consultant.

✔ **Appropriate referrals**: it will be obvious that late or inappropriate referrals will delay discharge, result in substandard care and compromise patient safety.

Student name: Medical school: Year:

Referral letters

Please refer the following patient to the appropriate speciality. Please write out a referral letter to facilitate this.

50-year-old obese gentleman, past medical history of angina, myocardial infarction, asthma, bilateral knee arthritis. Presented with raised blood glucose levels that are difficult to control. Blood results are still pending.

		Self	Peer	Peer /tutor	Tutor
General questions	To whom would you refer?	☐	☐	☐	☐
	What history and examination would you give?	☐	☐	☐	☐
	What other investigations might you do?	☐	☐	☐	☐
	What investigation results would you give?	☐	☐	☐	☐
	What question will you be asking?	☐	☐	☐	☐
		☐	☐	☐	☐
Patient details	Name	☐	☐	☐	☐
	Hospital number	☐	☐	☐	☐
	Date of birth	☐	☐	☐	☐
	Address	☐	☐	☐	☐
	Ward if inpatient	☐	☐	☐	☐
		☐	☐	☐	☐
Name of consultant	Referring consultant	☐	☐	☐	☐
	Consultant to whom patient is referred	☐	☐	☐	☐
		☐	☐	☐	☐
Brief history of the patient's problems	Date of admission	☐	☐	☐	☐
	Reason for admission	☐	☐	☐	☐
	Ongoing problem requiring consultation	☐	☐	☐	☐
	Results of relevant investigations	☐	☐	☐	☐
	Current treatment	☐	☐	☐	☐
		☐	☐	☐	☐
Reason for referral	Should be concise	☐	☐	☐	☐
	Reason for referral should be clear	☐	☐	☐	☐
		☐	☐	☐	☐
How urgent and why?	Urgent	☐	☐	☐	☐
	Routine	☐	☐	☐	☐
		☐	☐	☐	☐
Doctor's details	Full name	☐	☐	☐	☐
	Bleep	☐	☐	☐	☐
	Signature	☐	☐	☐	☐
	Date of referral	☐	☐	☐	☐
		☐	☐	☐	☐

				Self	Peer	Peer/tutor	Tutor
Self-assessed as at least borderline:	Signature:	Date:		U B S E	U B S E	U B S E	U B S E
Peer-assessed as ready for tutor assessment:	Signature:	Date:		U B S E	U B S E	U B S E	U B S E
Tutor-assessed as satisfactory:	Signature:	Date:		U B S E	U B S E	U B S E	U B S E

Notes

15.5 Clinical discharge summary

Background

At the end of a patient's stay in hospital, a discharge summary must be completed. It is an important medium of communication between the hospital and primary care. It should relay clinical information for continued safe management and include details that will be relevant to a number of healthcare professionals who will take over the care of the patient, including the general practitioner (GP), practice nurse, district nurse, social worker, and others. The discharge summary contains details of the patient's current admission, investigations, and treatments received in hospital and may also contain future management plan for the patient. It also serves as a prescription for medications that the hospital pharmacy supplies and sends the patient home with. The discharge summary is usually sent to the patient's GP and to other agencies such as social services.

Professional principles

Like any other hospital document, a discharge summary (Figure 15.4) is also a legal document stating that the patient has received clinical treatment and is being sent home safely with an appropriate care plan. The care plan is not just medications, but includes arrangements for follow-up and multiprofessional care. In more complex cases, an additional detailed discharge letter rather than just the typical brief form will be desirable. The prescription component has to be given the same care and attention as all prescriptions: clearly legible, dose and duration stated, and reviewed for interactions and side effects, with adequate patient information and explanation.

Discharge/Transfer Advice Note % Prescription Sheet
Write whilst pressing hard & using black ballpoint pen only

Directorate of: *MEDILINE*
Consultant Name: *Dr T. Jones*

	DATE	WARD	WEIGHT
Admission	12/10/07	A & E	
Discharge/Transfer	15/10/07	B12	

Time TTO required by (only if urgent):

Pharmacist Prof. Check by:
Your patient Mr Mrs Ms
Name *STEWART GRIFFIN*
Address *32 ALBANY TERRACE, WICKBY*
LANCASHIRE Postcode *WI3 1JL*
DOB 1/2/49 Hospital No: N12345 GP Dr Smith

Main diagnosis: NON SPECIFIC CHEST PAIN
Other diagnosis: ANXIETY, DEPRESSION, ARTHRITIS

Main Procedure/Treatment: *Addressed risk factors for cardiac events*

Comments: *This gentleman presented with chest pain that started 2 days proir to admission*

Investigations: *ECG -ve for ischeamic changes*
Exercise tolerance Test -ve
Troponon T -ve *CTPA -ve for PE*

Follow Up	Yes	No		Yes	No	Weeks
District nurse:		X	Sick note issued:		X	
Social Services:		X	Further Inverstigations		X	
Named Social Worker:		X				

Hospital Appointment: Yes ☐ No ☐ Weeks.......... Further Summary letter to follow Yes ☐ No ☐
Anti-coagulant clinic appointment: Yes ☐ No ☐ Weeks..........

Advice to GP/Review arrangements *Please refer to anxiety management services thank you*

Drugs on Discharge - Name & form (IN BLOCK CAPITALS)	Dose & Frequency (IN BLOCK CAPITALS)	Supply for ....days to a max of 28 then	Pharmacy use only		
			Quantity	Disp by	Check by
CITALOPRAM	*20mg BD*	Continue/Stop			
PARACETAMOL PRN	*1g QDS*	Continue/Stop			
IBUPROFEN PRN	*200mg ODS*	Continue/Stop			
ASPIRIN	*75mg OD*	Continue/Stop			
OMEPRAZOLE	*30mg OD*	Continue/Stop			
		Continue/Stop			
		Continue/Stop			
		Continue/Stop			
		Continue/Stop			
		Continue/Stop			
		Continue/Stop			

Signed [signature] Name HARRY SHILL Blep No: #1234 cons Reg SHO HO
Date 15/10/07

Figure 15.4 A discharge form.

Full patient details: including name, address, date of birth, hospital number and GP name.

Reason for admission: Enter the main reason for the current admission with other significant co-morbidities.

Concise, accurate outline of the clinical case: including presentation, management, investigations and results.

Follow up plans: Any intervention in the community and/or follow up should be indicated here. Advice for the GP will allow appropriate community follow up.

Medications: All medications the patient is taking should be stated. Medications should be on this list even if they are not supplied by the hospital due to existing supplies (such as inhalers, insulins). This section informs the GP of any change in intervention. If any drug is missed off, then the GP may not continue to prescribe it and pharmacy may not dispense any to the patient.

Sign off: The document should have the doctor's name, signature, and bleep number, rank and date

Sequence

Documentation and preparation

As always, any document about a patient should have identifying details on it (patient name, address, date of birth and hospital number). As a minimum the discharge summary should have on it the following details:

- Directorate (e.g. medicine, surgery, psychiatry), consultant's or senior clinician's name
- Admission and discharge/transfer dates
- History of current admission including investigations and treatments
- Follow-up (any outpatients appointments, district nurse/social service involvement)
- Advice for primary care team: GP, practice/district nurse, social worker and others
- Full current prescription.

Explanation and consent

Take time to explain what has happened during admission and the discharge plan. Give explanation with respect to the medications, particularly changes in treatment and new medications.

Key points

- Ensure that any further hospital appointments/referrals are made prior to the patient leaving the hospital
- Give as much information as possible about the current admission, including significant positive and negative results

Patient safety and clinical governance tips

✔ **Legibility**: is still the commonest complaint from general practice in relation to discharge letters. The implication of illegibility for unsafe practice is obvious. In addition, this can result in dispensing errors.

✔ **Patients who self-discharge**: phone GP for self-discharge cases, these patients are at particularly high risk of further morbidity and even mortality.

✔ **Contact GP**: contact the GP if review is needed in a matter of days, in case the letter is delayed.

✔ **Write the discharge letter as soon as the patient is declared ready for discharge**: this allows an optimal amount of time for the medications to be dispensed and for the medications to be discussed with the patient. Anything that can be done to prevent a delayed discharge, with consequent pressure on beds and throughput of patients should be prioritized. The mathematics are clear if there are 100 hospital beds with an average length of stay of 5 days then preventing, for example, the 6-hour delay for the discharge letter and dispensing of medications, would result in freeing up of 5 beds. This is 5 fewer beds that the hospital needs to look after on average! In UK each bed costs at least £100 000 per year.

✔ **Care planning and self-management**: Ideally, through a process of care planning, a written care plan should be given to patients with long-term conditions to prevent future admissions and optimize care and aid self-management. For example, hypoglycaemia admission avoidance would entail the involvement of the diabetes nurses with patients better able to manage home blood glucose monitoring and hypoglycaemia avoidance and treatment. Similarly, a patient with asthma would be educated to look out for the early signs of an exacerbation with peak expiratory flow rate (PEFR) monitoring and be advised to increase inhaler treatment at home and perhaps consult the community pharmacist or GP for steroids or antibiotics or both.

Student name:	Medical school:	Year:

Discharge summary

Please complete this patient's discharge summary

Mrs Nailia Hutt, an 85-year-old woman (hospital number N1234), presented with acute shortness of breath, green sputum and some right sided chest discomfort. She was also confused. (Admission details) She has hypertension that is controlled by amlodipine 5 mg od. She has been in hospital for 3 days, and she is stable. Your consultant, Dr Hari, has asked you to complete the discharge summary for this patient and ensure that she is on appropriate antibiotics for 4 more days (erythromycin and amoxicillin) and also additional medication (omeprazole, paracetamol prn). Dr Hari also emphasizes that the GP needs to follow up in 6 weeks. Mrs Hutt lives in a nursing home (Poplar House Nursing Home, Carlton). Her birthday was on the 5th August.

CXR	Right basal shadowing	ECG	No acute changes	Bloods	WCC ↑, CRP ↑, Urea ↑	Self	Peer	Peer /tutor	Tutor
Identifiers	Attaches correct label to discharge sheets					☐	☐	☐	☐
	or								
	Writes correct patient details on discharge sheet including					☐	☐	☐	☐
	○ Name								
	○ Address								
	○ Date of birth								
	○ Hospital number								
	○ GP name								
	•					☐	☐	☐	☐
Admission Details	Admission date					☐	☐	☐	☐
	Discharge date					☐	☐	☐	☐
	Consultant names					☐	☐	☐	☐
	Department					☐	☐	☐	☐
	•					☐	☐	☐	☐
Diagnosis	Current admission diagnosis					☐	☐	☐	☐
	Significant co-morbidities					☐	☐	☐	☐
	•					☐	☐	☐	☐
Summary	Presenting complaint					☐	☐	☐	☐
	Investigations					☐	☐	☐	☐
	Significant results					☐	☐	☐	☐
	•					☐	☐	☐	☐
Follow-up	Appropriate follow-up					☐	☐	☐	☐
	Outpatient appointment					☐	☐	☐	☐
	Sick note issued					☐	☐	☐	☐
	Social services/district nurses involvement					☐	☐	☐	☐
	Advice to GP					☐	☐	☐	☐
	•					☐	☐	☐	☐
Prescription	Correct drug					☐	☐	☐	☐
	Correct spelling					☐	☐	☐	☐
	Correct dose					☐	☐	☐	☐
	Correct method of delivery					☐	☐	☐	☐
	Correct frequency of dose					☐	☐	☐	☐
	Appropriate length of prescription					☐	☐	☐	☐
	Clear instructions if necessary					☐	☐	☐	☐
	•					☐	☐	☐	☐
Awareness	Consults the BNF to confirm doses					☐	☐	☐	☐
	States that will consult pharmacy or senior if doubt					☐	☐	☐	☐
	•					☐	☐	☐	☐
Language	Handwriting legible					☐	☐	☐	☐
	Spelling correct					☐	☐	☐	☐
	•					☐	☐	☐	☐

			Self	Peer	Peer/tutor	Tutor
Self-assessed as at least borderline:	Signature:	Date:	U B S E	U B S E	U B S E	U B S E
Peer-assessed as ready for tutor assessment:	Signature:	Date:	U B S E	U B S E	U B S E	U B S E
Tutor-assessed as satisfactory:	Signature:	Date:	U B S E	U B S E	U B S E	U B S E

Notes

15.6 Evidence-based healthcare and clinical audit

....

Evidence-based healthcare background

Evidence based medicine is the conscientious, explicit and judicious use of current best evidence in making decisions about the care of individual patients.

This definition by Sackett has served us well and concords with patient-centred care, high standards of clinical care, and best utilization of resources. There are five steps to evidence-based practice:

1 **Defining the question**
2 **Finding the best available evidence**
3 **Critical appraisal of that evidence**
4 **Application of the evidence in practice**
5 **Audit of performance.**

....

Defining the question

Once a need for evidence has been recognized, the question must be defined to focus the search and to recognize relevant evidence when it is found. To help with this the PICO formula has been developed:

- **P** Patient, population, condition, disease, problem
- **I** Intervention or exposure
- **C** Comparison
- **O** Outcome

So for the question 'Is ibuprofen or paracetamol better at relieving pain from headaches?' the PICO would be:

- **P** Headaches
- **I** Ibuprofen
- **C** Paracetamol
- **O** Pain relief

Finding the best available evidence

The first step is defining what you want to find. Not every research design is as robust as others. If a high-quality guideline for a therapy question is not available, then the following hierarchy of evidence should be observed:

1 **Systematic review**: a combination of all the evidence for a particular question found with an exhaustive search strategy. Sometimes the data of the constituent studies may be combined in a **meta-analysis**.

2 **Randomized controlled trial (RCT)**: patients with a particular condition are randomly allocated to an intervention group(s) or a control group(s). Outcomes are then compared. This is the gold standard for whether a treatment intervention works.

3 **Cohort study**: a population is either prospectively followed or retrospectively analysed to see whether any differences affect outcomes. This is the gold standard for causation studies.

4 **Case–control studies**: the outcomes of cases are matched with controls. Useful for rare diseases, where larger studies would be impractical.

5 **Case reports/series**: reports of individual cases, especially useful for adverse drug events.

6 **Expert opinion**: often anecdotal and based on poorly reported outcomes. Should not be dismissed if sources of evidence above are not available or not robust.

The objective is to find the best available evidence that answers our question.

There are a variety of sources of clinical evidence available, depending on what you are looking for:

- **NHS Evidence**: is part of NICE (National Institute for Health and Clinical Excellence) and is an excellent search engine for guidelines and high-quality research. It is possible to filter by type of research.
- **Trip Database**: an independent search engine for clinical evidence
- **Cochrane Library**: database of full-text systematic reviews and abstracts of RCTs and economic evaluations. Freely available to all residents of the UK, Ireland, Australia, New Zealand, India, and some other countries.
- **Medline**: the main medical literature database. It is available in a free version as PubMed and from different providers for universities and NHS trusts.

The Cochrane Library and Medline both use MeSH (Medical Subject Headings) to index abstracts. The advantages of using MeSH is that it avoids finding irrelevant results and allows searching by several synonyms, e.g. searching for neoplasms will also include cancer.

Whatever interface you are using, practice is the best way to learn. Contact your local clinical librarian to see what training is available to you.

Critical appraisal of the evidence

Once a possible piece of evidence has been located, we must decide whether it can be used. Possible problems include:

- The paper is not relevant
- The paper has methodological flaws
- The results are not statistically or clinically significant.

The first step is to see whether the question that the study sought to answer is the same as your question. From analysing the abstract of a paper, we should be able to determine the original PICO question. We can then see whether it was the same as our earlier one.

Once we have established relevance, we need to see whether the research is valid and so can be used. There are various checklists available that can be used, including the Critical Appraisal Skills Programme (CASP) and the one from the Centre for Evidence Based Medicine at Oxford University.

Key questions to ask include:

- In an RCT, was the allocation to groups genuinely random?
- Were all involved in the trial 'masked' to the treatment received?
- In a systematic review, was the literature search comprehensive enough?
- In a meta-analysis are the studies similar enough in their PICO or results to make combination meaningful?

If we have established that the paper is methodologically sound, we can then turn to the results. In therapy trials these can be presented in a variety of different ways.

Analysis of results

A good knowledge of clinical statistics is a requirement to afford even a basic understanding of results of clinical studies. This is outside the scope of this unit and the student is referred to the many excellent books published and courses established. As an absolute minimum, the following should be well known: parametric and non-parametric testing, qualitative versus quantitative studies, risk ratios, basics of meta-analysis, and multifactorial analysis. The material below is included as it is very useful when defining the effectiveness of an intervention in terms of clinical events and healthcare resource needed.

- **Trial A**: drug A reduces CVD from 30% to 20% (similar to CVD prevention with statin for secondary prevention). Assume drug cost £300 per year; 5-year trial.

- **Trial B**: drug B reduces CVD from 3% to 2% (similar to certain anti-platelets agents in primary prevention). Assume drug cost £300 per year; 5-year trial.

Table 15.1 Relative risk reduction (RRR), absolute risk reduction (ARR), and number needed to treat (NNT)

	RRR	ARR	NNT
Trial A, drug A	**33%**	**10%**	**10 people for 5 years of the trial**
	30%–20%=10% *10%/30% = 33%*	*30%–20%=10%*	*ARR 10% means 100 people treated results in 10 fewer events for the duration of the trial*
Trial B, drug B	**33%**	**1%**	**100 people for 5 years of the trial**
	3%–2%=1% *1%/3% = 33%*	*3%–2%=10%*	*ARR 1% means 100 people treated results in 1 less event for the duration of the trial*

- **Number needed to treat**: This is the number of people who needed to be treated with the intervention to see one additional positive outcome compared to the control. It is calculated by dividing 100% by the absolute risk reduction %. So for trial A: 100/10 = 10, Trial B 100/1 = 100. With the latter, 100 people must be treated with drug B, for 5 years, to see the CVD benefit.

- **Relative risk reduction versus absolute risk reduction**: Clearly, if there is a particular vested interest in showing a large treatment effect, the relative risk reduction will be promoted. Note that the RRR is exactly the same in both studies above (Table 15.1). From a health resource (and clinical intervention, patient medicalization stance), the ARR might be more important as the data clearly show that:

  - **Drug A**: 10 patients will need treatment for 5 years to save one CVD event. This will cost £300 × 10 patients × 5 years = £15 000

  - **Drug B**: 100 patients will need treatment for 5 years to save one CVD event. This will cost £300 × 100 patients × 5 years = £150 000 (not so affordable!).

- **Statistical significance**: once we have determined the 'bottom line' result of the study, we must see whether the result is large enough to be statistically significant. There are two main ways to measure this:

  - **P value**: this is the probability that the result is down to chance. The convention is that a p value of less than 5% or 0.05 is significant.

  - **Confidence interval**: this is often more useful than the p value because it shows the margin of error where the real result has a 95% probability to be. If the range includes the possibility that the control might be better than the intervention, then the result is not statistically significant. Even if the result is statistically significant, the bottom of the range might not be a clinically significant result. A cure for the common cold might show a range of reduction of symptoms from 5 days to 1 hour. Clearly the latter is not clinically significant.

Application of the evidence in practice

There are a variety of factors which need to be taken into account when applying evidence:

- Does my patient/population match the inclusion criteria of the study?

- Are there any harms that outweigh the benefits?

- Is the intervention affordable or organizationally possible?
- What are the patient's views, perspective, and values?

Audit of performance

The final step in evidence based practice is to audit clinical performance against the evidence and accepted clinical standards. Clinical audit is the systematic process of evaluating clinical practice. Audit is necessary to assess the quality of care currently provided, to compare current practice with recommended standards, and to drive improvement. Increasingly, clinical audit is seen as one the most important drivers in improvement of clinical quality and to safeguard existing clinical standards achieved.

The audit cycle (Figure 15.5) consists of:

- Identification of the problem or issue
- Setting the criteria and standards
- Collecting data on performance locally
- Comparing performance with the criteria and standards
- Identification and implementation of changes and reaudit.

This is known as standards-based audit. Other types of clinical audit include:

- **Adverse occurrence screening and critical incident monitoring**: individual cases are re-examined when there has been cause for concern or an unexpected outcome. In the UK community-based teams term this 'significant event audit'.
- **Peer review**: experienced peers from other institutions discuss individual cases in order to determine whether, with hindsight, the best possible care was provided.
- **Patient surveys and focus groups**: service users are asked for their views on the quality of care they received.

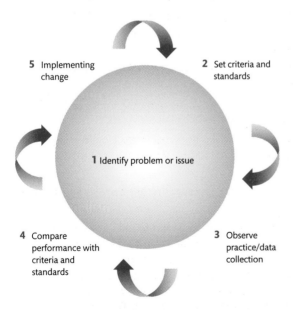

Figure 15.5 Clinical audit cycle.

When an audit is completed it is necessary to produce a **report**. Ideally, the bulk of the initial parts of the report are written when the audit is started. In general, senior clinical advice and consent should be sought prior to undertaking clinical audit. At minimum, the report should include:

- **Title**: a title for the audit which clearly states its focus
- **Introduction or background**: why the audit is being done ? recent events or guidelines

- **Anticipated benefits**: of undertaking the audit
- **Criteria and standards audited against**: ? national, ? additional local standards
- **Method**: sample selection and size, data collection methods
- **Results**: comparison of the data with the criteria and standards
- **Discussion**: if applicable, why the standards were not met, key changes needed
- **Recommendations**: for changes to current practice, these must be specific, realistic, and achievable. Include: how the results of the audit will be disseminated
- **Phase 2 reaudit plan**: any ideas on changes to practice must be reaudited to prove that they have been implemented.

Patient safety tips

✔ **Evidence-based practice**: most changes to practice happen due to implementation of best clinical research into clinical practice. It is incumbent upon us to practise the highest standards of evidence-based healthcare that resources (financial and professional) and personal skills allow. Personalized care for the patient will always be the major overriding factor in all care.

✔ **Clinical audit**: the role of this in improving care and safety is difficult to over-emphasize. Clinical audits in everyday practice often indicate that clinical standards may not be as high as we perceive. Audits are also important for teaching clinical management, leadership skills, service management skills, and health economics.

Assessments

Evidence-based healthcare and clinical audit

on a topic to be specified by the tutor. Questions will be asked as evidence-based medicine and clinical audit. Please perform a literature search.

		Self	Peer	Peer/tutor	Tutor
Defines the question	● Able to define evidence-based practice	☐	☐	☐	☐
	● Uses PICO to produce an answerable question	☐	☐	☐	☐
	●	☐	☐	☐	☐
Searches for evidence	● Can list the different levels of evidence	☐	☐	☐	☐
	● Demonstrates awareness of different sources of evidence.	☐	☐	☐	☐
	● Can find a guideline using NHS Evidence	☐	☐	☐	☐
	● Uses MeSH to find articles in Medline	☐	☐	☐	☐
	● Applies quality filters to searches	☐	☐	☐	☐
	●	☐	☐	☐	☐
Critically appraises the evidence	● Can determine the PICO of an abstract	☐	☐	☐	☐
	● Critically appraises the evidence	☐	☐	☐	☐
	● Can discuss the difference between relative risk, absolute risk and number needed to treat	☐	☐	☐	☐
	● Can discuss the meaning of p values and confidence intervals	☐	☐	☐	☐
	●	☐	☐	☐	☐
Applies best evidence	● Can list the factors to be taken into consideration when applying evidence in practice	☐	☐	☐	☐
	●	☐	☐	☐	☐
Audits practice against best evidence	● Can define clinical audit	☐	☐	☐	☐
	● Can discuss why clinical audit is important	☐	☐	☐	☐
	● Can list the types of clinical audit	☐	☐	☐	☐
	● Can list the stages of the clinical audit cycle	☐	☐	☐	☐
	●	☐	☐	☐	☐

				Self	Peer	Peer/tutor	Tutor
Self-assessed as at least borderline:	Signature:		Date:	U B S E	U B S E	U B S E	U B S E
Peer-assessed as ready for tutor assessment:	Signature:		Date:	U B S E	U B S E	U B S E	U B S E
Tutor-assessed as satisfactory:	Signature:		Date:	U B S E	U B S E	U B S E	U B S E

Notes

Unit 16 Radiology

16.1 Chest radiography

.....

Background

The **chest radiograph** (CXR) is an essential primary investigation for the diagnosis and assessment of intrathoracic pathology. The most commonly performed frontal CXR is the posteroanterior (PA) examination: since the heart is close to the detector or film it is not magnified and its size is more accurately measured. The anteroposterior (AP) radiograph may have to suffice in ill patients who need portable radiography. The lateral radiograph of the chest is rarely performed nowadays. Radiography in inspiration is ideal but in pneumothorax an additional expiratory view is useful since the pneumothorax is better demonstrated.

Spiral computed tomography (CT) or **high-resolution CT** (HRCT) constitute the next line of investigation and assess pathology in the chest in much greater detail. **Cardiac CT scan** is being increasingly performed to assess the coronary arteries. **Radionuclide scan** was previously used for the diagnosis of pulmonary embolism but has now been replaced by **CT pulmonary angiography** (CTPA). **Ultrasonography** of the chest is sometimes performed to assess pleural effusion and guide its aspiration. **Echocardiography** of the heart is commonly performed for a number of cardiac conditions. **Magnetic resonance imaging (MRI)** of the chest is occasionally used as a complementary investigation to CT to answer specific questions and **cardiac MRI** is also now increasingly performed.

.....

Clinical indications for chest radiography

The most commonly encountered indications for chest radiography are: chest pain, breathlessness, haemoptysis, suspected lower respiratory tract infection, and acute abdomen.

Chest radiography may be useful in a wide range of clinical situations including:

- Pneumonia
- Lung metastases
- Pneumothorax or pleural effusion
- Asthma or chronic obstructive pulmonary disease (COPD)
- Cardiomegaly, valvular heart disease, or aortic aneurysm
- Pneumoperitoneum due to perforation of a hollow viscus
- Tumours or masses in the lungs, mediastinum or chest wall
- Chest trauma
- Lung collapse
- Lymphadenopathy
- Left heart failure and pulmonary oedema
- Assessment of the position of tubes, lines, catheters, or pacemaker leads.

General and film quality check

- **Patient details**: check the name, date of birth, and gender of the patient, the date of the radiograph and that the sides are clearly marked.

- **Centring check**: for centring of the radiograph: the distance from the medial end of the clavicle to the spinous process should be equal on both sides.

- **Penetration of the film**: is the film normal, over-penetrated or under-penetrated? In a normally penetrated film the lower thoracic vertebral margins should be just visible through the heart shadow. If over-penetrated the vertebrae can be seen more clearly and the lungs look blacker. If under-penetrated the margins of the vertebrae are not visible and the lungs look whiter.

Anatomical principles

Figures 16.1 and 16.2 show the features of a normal CXR.

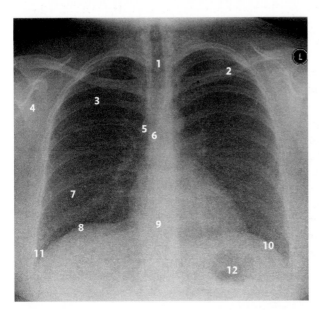

1	Trachea
2	Clavicle
3	Posterior rib
4	Scapula
5	Right main bronchus
6	Carina
7	Anterior rib
8	Right dome of diaphragm
9	Disc space
10	Left dome of diaphragm
11	Costophrenic angle
12	Gastric air

Figure 16.1 Normal CXR: anatomical features (non-cardiovascular).

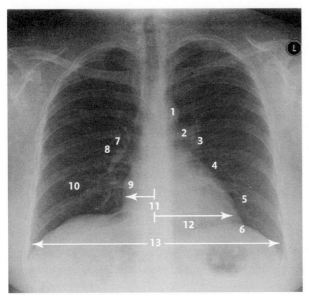

1	Aortic knuckle
2	Left main pulmonary artery
3	Left hilum
4	Left atrial appendage
5	Left ventricle
6	Left cardiophrenic angle
7	Right hilum
8	Right main pulmonary artery
9	Right atrium
10	Segmental pulmonary vessel
11	Cardiac diameter
12	Right ventricle
13	Thoracic diameter

Figure 16.2 Normal CXR: anatomical features (cardiovascular structures).

Analysis by alphabet strategy: *A, B, C, D and review areas*

- **A – Airway**: the trachea and main bronchi.
  - ○ Check whether the trachea is central or not. The right main bronchus is normally straighter than the left. The angle of the carina is usually around 70°.
- **B – Breathing**: the lungs
  - ○ With a good inspiratory effort the mid-part of the diaphragm should be between the anterior ends of the fifth and sixth ribs. With poor inspiration it will be higher and with increased inspiratory effort lower. The lungs are divided into upper, mid, and lower zones demarcated by the anterior ends of the second and fourth ribs.
- **C – Cardiac**: the heart shadow
  - ○ One third of the heart should be to the right of the midline and two-thirds to the left. The heart is enlarged when the cardiothoracic ratio, the ratio of the maximum cardiac diameter to the maximum thoracic diameter, is greater than 50%. The borders of the heart are formed by the right atrium on the right side, right ventricle on the diaphragmatic surface, left ventricle forming the apex and left heart border, left atrial appendage forming the upper left heart border.
- **D – Diaphragm**:
  - ○ The right dome of the diaphragm is normally one rib space higher than the left. Evaluate below the diaphragm, especially for evidence of pneumoperitoneum, and above the diaphragm for pathology.

Check these review areas:

- Behind the heart for mass, hiatus hernia, lower lobe collapse
- The mediastinum: is it widened?
- The hilar regions
- The apices
- The bones
- Any lines or tubes.

Study these CXRs, report on them using the above sequence and answer the questions. Check your answers against the correct ones later in this chapter. Then return to the radiographs to ensure you can recognize and understand the abnormalities shown.

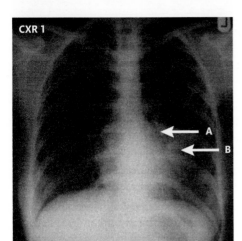

This 48-year old man presented with fever, cough and rusty sputum.
What is the diagnosis?
Which lobe is involved?
What do the arrows A and B indicate?

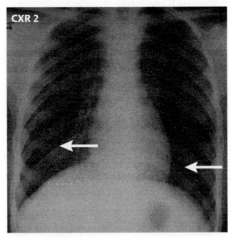

This 20-year old South Asian man had been in contact with a relative diagnosed with an infectious disease. What radiological feature is indicated by the arrows?
What is the diagnosis?

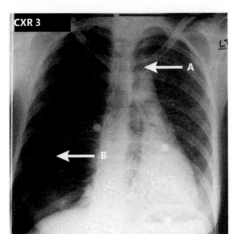

This 43-year old woman presented acutely with chest pain and severe breathlessness.
What radiological features are indicated by the arrows A and B?
What is the diagnosis?

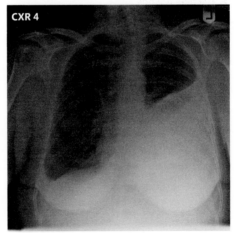

This 72-year old woman presented with progressively worsening shortness of breath.
What are the main radiological findings?
What is the diagnosis?

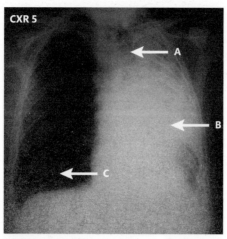

This 76-year old male presented with acute breathlessness.
What radiological features are indicated by arrows A, B and C?
What is the diagnosis?

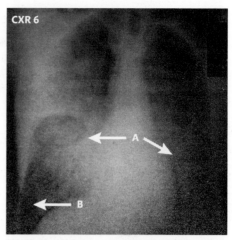

This 60-year old man presented with the sudden onset of severe central chest pain.
What radiological features are indicated by arrows A and B?
What is the diagnosis?

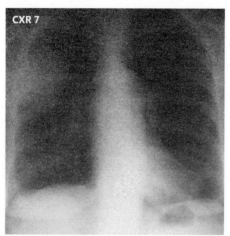

This 70-year smoker presented with haemoptysis
What does the X-ray show?
What is the next appropriate investigation?

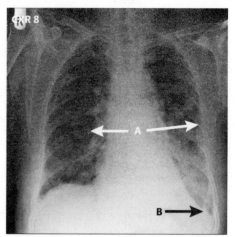

This 81-year old man gentleman presented with general malaise and recent significant weight loss. He had no specific respiratory symptoms.
What are the abnormalities indicated by arrow A?
And by arrow B?

Patient safety tips

✔ **Ionizing radiation**: Since chest radiography involves ionizing radiation it is important to check whether the investigation is needed and the result will affect management, and whether it has already been performed recently and if so whether repeating it is really necessary.

✔ **Pregnant state**: carefully assess whether the patient might be pregnant and the risk-benefit ratio in pregnancy.

Diagnoses and commentary on the CXRs

- **CXR 1**: Area of shadowing in the left mid and lower zones obscuring the left heart border but sparing the left dome of the diaphragm. An air bronchogram is seen. The appearances are consistent with consolidation of the lingular segment of the left lung. The left heart border, to which the lingular segment is adjacent, is obscured. A: air bronchogram due to air in bronchus accentuated by surrounding consolidation. B: air space shadowing due to fluid in the alveoli.

  Diagnosis: left lung consolidation (lingular lobe). Consistent with lobar pneumonia.

- **CXR 2**: Discrete miliary ('millet-seed like') nodules 1–5 mm in size are scattered throughout both lungs, in keeping with miliary tuberculosis. Other differential diagnoses include miliary metastases from, for example, thyroid or breast cancer. Feature arrowed is miliary nodules.

  Diagnosis: miliary tuberculosis.

- **CXR 3**: There is complete collapse of the right lung and no lung markings are seen, with replacement by air in the right pleural space. There is shift of the mediastinum to the left and the right dome of the diaphragm is depressed. These appearances are in keeping with a right-sided tension pneumothorax. A: shift of the trachea to the left. B: absence of lung markings. This is a medical emergency and diagnosis should not wait on a CXR. Consequent upon the mediastinal shift the superior and inferior vena cava are kinked and obstructed. Lack of input to the heart results in catastrophic loss of output.

  Diagnosis: right tension pneumothorax. Treatment comprises urgent insertion of a chest drain.

- **CXR 4**: there is homogeneous opacification in the left mid and lower zones with an S-shaped upper border which reaches its highest level in the axilla. There are no visible bronchopulmonary markings. There is no clear evidence of mediastinal shift but the patient is slightly rotated. The appearances are in keeping with a large left pleural effusion. Blunting of the right costophrenic angle is also present.

  Diagnosis: Large left pleural effusion with a smaller one on the right ? malignancy ? infection.

- **CXR 5**: There is complete opacification of the left hemithorax with mediastinal shift to the left and raised left dome of the diaphragm. The right lung appears normal. The appearances are in keeping with collapse with loss of volume of the left lung. A: mediastinal shift to the left. B: complete opacification of the left hemithorax with loss of lung volume. C: normal right lung.

  Diagnosis: left lung collapse, most likely malignancy.

- **CXR 6**: There is extensive bilateral air space shadowing concentrated in the hilar regions. There are also interstitial lines in the right lower zones peripherally (Kerley B lines). These features are in keeping with pulmonary oedema. A: 'bat's wing' opacities. B: Kerley B line. Other radiological features of pulmonary oedema due to left heart failure include upper lobe vascular prominence, interstitial lines signifying fluid in the interstitium, air space shadowing due to fluid in the alveoli, small pleural effusions and cardiomegaly. In this case the heart was not enlarged because of the acute onset of the heart failure.

  Diagnosis: acute pulmonary oedema.

- **CXR 7**: There is large rounded opacity peripherally situated in the right upper/mid zone measuring approximately 4–5 cm in diameter. There is some associated pleural thickening. There is no evidence of metastases elsewhere in the lungs or the bones. A peripheral mass in the upper and mid-zone of the right lung adjoining the pleura, is most likely to be lung cancer.

  Diagnosis: lung cancer. The next appropriate investigations are CT scan of thorax and abdomen for staging the disease followed by CT-guided biopsy.

- **CXR 8**: there are multiple nodules 1–1.5 cm in diameter throughout both lungs in keeping with multiple metastatic deposits. There is also triangular opacification in the left lower lobe obscuring the medial part of the left dome of the diaphragm in keeping with left lower lobe collapse. A central obstructing mass lesion should be considered. A: multiple pulmonary nodules likely to be metastases. B: left lower lobe collapse possibly due to an underlying centrally obstructing mass lesion.

  Diagnosis: multiple metastatic deposits ? location of primary tumour could be lung, breast, colon, pancreas or kidney.

Student name:	Medical school:	Year:

Chest radiography

Please interpret this CXR provided by the assessor.

		Self	Peer	Peer /tutor	Tutor
General check	● Checks the name, date of birth, and gender of the patient, the date of the X-ray and that the sides are clearly marked	☐	☐	☐	☐
	●	☐	☐	☐	☐
Film quality check	● Comments on whether the film is properly centred	☐	☐	☐	☐
	● Comments on the penetration of film	☐	☐	☐	☐
	●	☐	☐	☐	☐
Alphabet strategy analysis	Comments on the following structures, noting any abnormality:	☐	☐	☐	☐
	● The trachea and right and left main bronchi	☐	☐	☐	☐
	● Right and left lungs	☐	☐	☐	☐
	● The cardiac shadow	☐	☐	☐	☐
	● The diaphragm, and above and below it	☐	☐	☐	☐
	●	☐	☐	☐	☐
Review areas	Comments on the following areas, noting any abnormality:	☐	☐	☐	☐
	● Behind the heart	☐	☐	☐	☐
	● The mediastinum	☐	☐	☐	☐
	● The hilar regions	☐	☐	☐	☐
	● The bones	☐	☐	☐	☐
	● Any lines or tubes	☐	☐	☐	☐
	●	☐	☐	☐	☐
Summary	● Summarizes findings accurately and concisely	☐	☐	☐	☐
	●	☐	☐	☐	☐

	Signature:	Date:	Self	Peer	Peer/tutor	Tutor
Self-assessed as at least borderline:	Signature:	Date:	U B S E	U B S E	U B S E	U B S E
Peer-assessed as ready for tutor assessment:	Signature:	Date:	U B S E	U B S E	U B S E	U B S E
Tutor-assessed as satisfactory:	Signature:	Date:	U B S E	U B S E	U B S E	U B S E

Notes

16.2 Abdominal radiography

Background

Abdominal radiographs are now performed mainly to image the bowel in acute abdominal conditions. In investigation of the newly presenting acute abdomen the two radiographs needed are a supine abdominal X-ray and an erect X-ray of the chest. Erect abdominal X-rays are no longer performed.

The information provided by the plain abdominal radiograph is limited. A relatively normal radiograph does not exclude an acute abdominal emergency. The plain X-ray may suggest small or large bowel obstruction but CT scan can more accurately identify the site and the cause. However, the availability of urgent and out-of-hours CT scanning may vary between hospitals, although it is widely available in the UK.

Careful study of an abdominal X-ray may occasionally reveal other abnormalities: for example, previously unsuspected calcified aortic aneurysms are not uncommon. However, almost all intra-abdominal pathology is best imaged by other means, usually by ultrasonography or CT.

Clinical indications

- Mainly suspected small or large bowel obstruction
- Perforation with gas under the diaphragm (CXR better)
- Psoas abscess may be suspected
- Constipation (rarely used, unnecessary in most cases)
- Stones: not all opacify and ultrasound is best

Anatomical principles

Figure 16.3 shows the features of a normal abdominal radiograph with incidental spinal osteoarthritis.

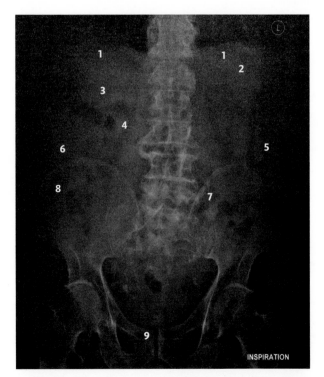

1	Diaphragm
2	Spleen
3	Liver
4	Psoas shadow
5	Descending colon
6	Right kidney
7	Small bowel
8	Caecum
9	Pubic Symphysis

INSPIRATION

Figure 16.3 Normal abdominal radiograph: anatomical features.

Interpretation sequence

General and film quality check

- **Patient details**: check the name, date of birth, and gender of the patient, the date of the radiograph, and that the sides are clearly marked
- **Film quality check**: an adequate abdominal X-ray should include the diaphragm superiorly, the abdominal walls laterally, and the pubic symphysis inferiorly.

Small and large bowel

Distinguishing between small and large bowel is usually straightforward (see Table 16.1). After analysis of intraluminal air look for air outside the bowel lumen in the peritoneum, biliary and urinary tracts, and the bowel wall.

Table 16.1 Distinguishing between the small and large bowel

Small bowel	Large bowel
Centrally situated	Peripherally situated
Valvulae conniventes visible around full circumference of bowel	Haustrae visible around part circumference of bowel
In obstruction, more secretions	In obstruction, more air
Smaller diameter : >2.5 cm suggests dilatation	Larger diameter: >5 cm suggests dilatation

Other intra-abdominal structures

- **Solid organs**: liver, spleen, kidneys, uterus
- **Fluid-filled organs**: gallbladder, urinary bladder
- **Muscle and fat**: **diaphragm**: psoas shadow, flank stripe
- **Calcification and radio-opaque calculi**: arterial, venous (phleboliths), lymph nodes, pancreas, urinary tract stones, gallstones
- **Bones**: spine, pelvis, sacroiliac joints, hips

Study these abdominal radiographs, report on them using the above sequence and answer the questions. Check your answers against the correct ones later in this chapter. Then return to the radiographs to ensure you can recognize and understand the abnormalities shown. One CXR and pelvic X-ray have also been included in this section, as they have important patient safety implications if missed.

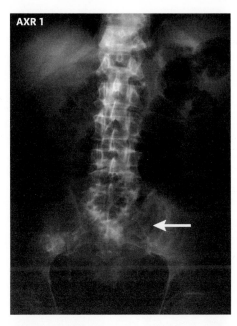

AXR 1

This 47-year old patient presented with a 24-hour history of abdominal pain and vomiting.
What is the diagnosis?
What structure does the arrow indicate?

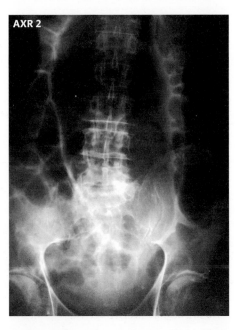

AXR 2

This 70-year old patient presented with abdominal distension and constipation.
What is the diagnosis?

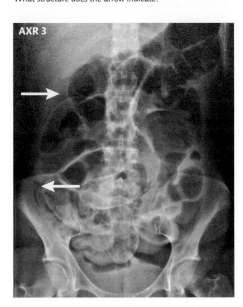

AXR 3

This 65-year old woman presented with abdominal pain and vomiting: examination of the abdomen revealed tenderness, guarding and rigidity.
What radiological sign is demonstrated?
What do the arrows indicate?

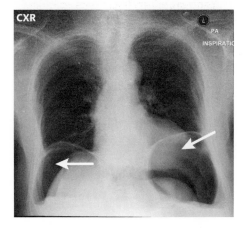

CXR

This is the erect chest radiograph of a 42-year old patient who presented with the sudden onset of severe abdominal pain.
What do the arrows indicate?
What is the diagnosis?

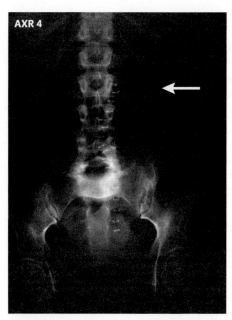

AXR 4

This 73-year old patient developed diarrhoea several days after abdominal surgery and had received antibiotics.
What radiological sign is indicated by the arrow?
What is the likely diagnosis?

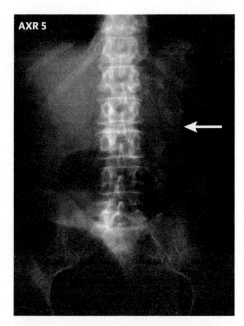

AXR 5

This 84-year old man presented to the Accident and Emergency Department with severe back pain.
What abnormality is indicated by the arrow?
What serious complication may have occurred?

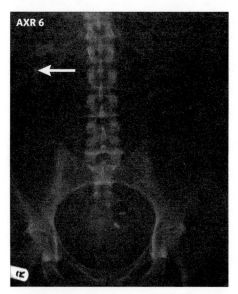

AXR 6

This 58-year old patient presented with right loin pain and haematuria.
What abnormality does the arrow indicate?

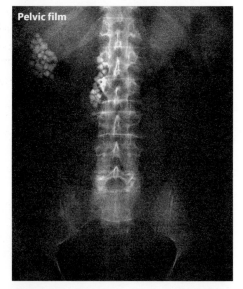

Pelvic film

This patient presented with a 4-year history of episodes of right upper quadrant pain. Her stools were also noted to be pale on several occasions.
What diagnosis can be made from the X-ray shown?

Patient safety tips

✔ **Ionizing radiation**: since abdominal radiography involves ionizing radiation it is important to check whether the investigation is needed and the result will affect management, and whether it has already been performed recently and if so whether repeating it is really necessary. Often other forms of imaging such as ultrasound will be more valuable.

✔ **Pregnant state**: carefully assess whether the patient might be pregnant and the risk-benefit ratio in pregnancy.

- **AXR 1**: This supine abdominal radiograph shows centrally situated dilated loops of bowel: the appearances are suggestive of small bowel obstruction. The flanks and lower pelvis are not included on this radiograph so no comment can be made on the large bowel.

  1 Small bowel obstruction

  2 Valvulae conniventes.

  Diagnosis: small bowel obstruction.

- **AXR 2**: This supine abdominal radiograph shows peripherally situated widely dilated air-filled loops of bowel. There is no air seen in the rectal region which would suggest large bowel obstruction at the site of the sigmoid colon. The centrally situated bowel loop is the dilated sigmoid colon.

  Diagnosis: sigmoid volvulus, which was confirmed on Gastrografin enema.

- **AXR 3**: This radiograph shows extraluminal air in the abdomen suggesting pneumoperitoneum. Rigler's sign, in which the bowel wall is clearly visualized due to the presence of air both inside and outside the bowel lumen. There is free air in the peritoneal cavity.

  Diagnosis: bowel perforation.

- **CXR**: This erect PA CXR shows air beneath both hemidiaphragms.

  Air under the diaphragm.

  Pneumoperitoneum due to perforation of an air-filled hollow viscus, probably bowel.

  Diagnosis: bowel perforation.

- **AXR 4**: This supine abdominal radiograph shows thickening of the wall of the transverse and descending colon suggesting bowel wall oedema. Metallic surgical clips are also noted in the mid abdomen. There is 'thumb printing' in the transverse colon indicating bowel wall oedema: this may be seen in infection, inflammation, and ischaemia.

  Diagnosis: Pseudomembranous colitis due to *Clostridium difficile* infection caused by prolonged antibiotic use.

- **AXR 5**: There is a thin rim of calcification in the mid-abdomen to the left side of the spine which is a large calcified abdominal aortic aneurysm. The radiograph is otherwise unremarkable.

  Diagnosis: calcified abdominal aortic aneurysm. The back pain suggests the aneurysm may be leaking.

- **AXR 6**: This abdominal radiograph for kidneys, ureters, and bladder ('KUB') shows a large calcified area corresponding to the pelvicalyceal system of the right kidney in keeping with a staghorn calculus. Sterilization clips noted in the pelvis. The plain abdominal radiograph is no longer the investigation of choice for renal calculi: non-contrast CT KUB is preferred.

  Diagnosis: staghorn calculus.

- **Pelvic film**: The X-ray shows multiple gallstones in the gallbladder and common bile duct. Radio-opacification of gallstones is only seen in 10% of such cases.

Student name:	Medical school:	Year:

Abdominal radiography

Please interpret this abdominal X-ray provided by the assessor.

		Self	Peer	Peer /tutor	Tutor
General check	● Checks the name, date of birth, and gender of the patient, the date of the X-ray, and that the sides are clearly marked	☐	☐	☐	☐
	●	☐	☐	☐	☐
Quality check	● Checks that the X-ray includes the diaphragm, the abdominal walls, and the pubic symphysis	☐	☐	☐	☐
	●	☐	☐	☐	☐
Bowel	● Accurately identifies the small bowel and comments on any abnormality	☐	☐	☐	☐
	● Accurately identifies the large bowel and comments on any abnormality	☐	☐	☐	☐
	● Accurately identifies any extraluminal air	☐	☐	☐	☐
	●	☐	☐	☐	☐
Other structures	● Comments on any abnormality in the liver, spleen, kidneys, or uterus	☐	☐	☐	☐
	● Comments on any abnormality in the gallbladder or urinary bladder	☐	☐	☐	☐
	● Comments on any abnormality in the diaphragm, psoas shadow, or fat deposition	☐	☐	☐	☐
	● Comments on any calcification in the arteries, veins, lymph nodes, or pancreas, and any radio-opaque calculi in the urinary tract or gallbladder	☐	☐	☐	☐
	● Comments on any bony abnormality in the spine, pelvis, sacroiliac joints, or hips	☐	☐	☐	☐
	●	☐	☐	☐	☐
Summary	● Summarizes findings accurately and concisely	☐	☐	☐	☐

				U B	U B	U B	U B
Self-assessed as at least borderline:	Signature:	Date:		S E	S E	S E	S E
Peer-assessed as ready for tutor assessment:	Signature:	Date:		U B	U B	U B	U B
				S E	S E	S E	S E
Tutor-assessed as satisfactory:	Signature:	Date:		U B	U B	U B	U B
				S E	S E	S E	S E

Notes

16.3 CT brain scanning

Background

The CT brain scan facilitates the rapid, effective and safe diagnosis of many intracranial pathologies. The CT scan shows axial slices through the brain represented on a grey scale. While originally the investigation took many minutes to perform, modern multislice scanners can obtain the entire scan in a few seconds. This is ideal for unstable acute patients and in those who find it difficult to keep still.

Clinical indications

There are many indications for a brain CT, but the main categories are:

- Acute or subacute neurological deficit when the clinical differential diagnosis includes ischaemic stroke, haemorrhage, or space-occupying lesion
- Major trauma or assessment of intracranial injury: in the UK the National Institute for Health and Clinical Excellence (NICE) guidelines apply
- Sinister headache, when the clinical question is often to exclude a space-occupying lesion
- Memory loss, to assess the cerebral volume and the presence of ischaemia or atrophy
- Sepsis or meningitis, to assess for hydrocephalus or cerebral abscess.

For some clinical conditions an MRI brain is the preferred initial investigation. These include:

- Encephalitis
- Demyelination
- Investigation of epilepsy: NICE guidelines apply in the UK.

Anatomy

Figures 16.4 and 16.5 show the features of a normal CT brain scan.

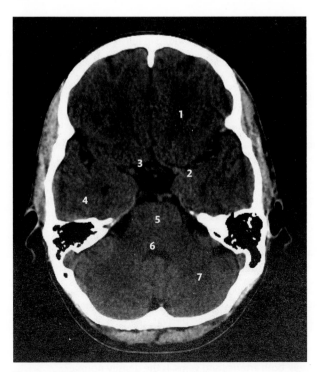

1	Left frontal lobe
2	Left internal carotid artery
3	Optic chiasm
4	Right temporal lobe
5	Pons
6	Fourth ventricle
7	Left cerebellar hemisphere

Figures 16.4 CT head: slice at the level of the pons.

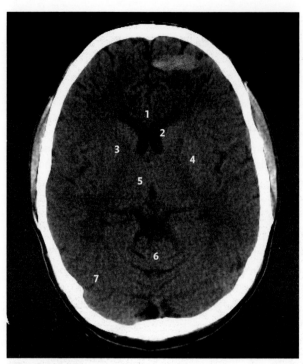

1	Corpus callosum
2	Lateral ventricle
3	Internal capsule
4	Lentiform nuclei
5	Thalamus
6	Superior cerebellar vermis
7	Right occipital lobe

Figure 16.5 CT head: higher slice at the level of the internal capsule.

Interpretation sequence

General check

- Check the name, date of birth, and gender of the patient, the date of the scan and that the sides are clearly marked.

- Check whether or not contrast has been given. This may variously be denoted by 'contrast', the name of the contrast used or the letter 'c' on the scan.

Quality of examination

- Is the examination complete? Is the foramen magnum included in full and do the images go all the way to the vertex?

- Are there any movement artefacts?

- Is there any rotation of the patient's head in the scanner?

Main interpretation

- Take into account the age of the patient and assess the overall brain volume for cerebral atrophy. Look at the ventricles and the sulci. Is there hydrocephalus?

- Is the brain symmetrical across the midline?

- Assess the differentiation between the white and grey matter and look for focal areas of low density and loss of grey/white matter differentiation. Look for areas of acute infarction which show as regions of low density.

- Look for any surface haemorrhage: extradural, subdural, or subarachnoid. Do the sulci extend all the way to the inner table of the skull? Look for intracerebral haematoma. Acute haemorrhage shows as white areas of high density.

- Is there any calcification or other high density? Could this be a variant of normal, for example calcification in the basal ganglia, pineal gland or choroid plexus?

Review areas

- Assess the major intracranial vessels, both arteries and veins. Is the density normal?

- Review the pituitary and supra-sellar regions. Is there a mass lesion?
- Assess basal cisterns and cerebellar tonsils. Is there brain swelling or subtle haemorrhage?
- Assess the bones and soft tissues included on the scan. Is there any fracture or bone lesion?

Assessment exercises

Study these CT scans and answer the questions. Check your answers against the correct ones later in this chapter. Then return to the images to ensure you can recognize and understand the abnormalities shown.

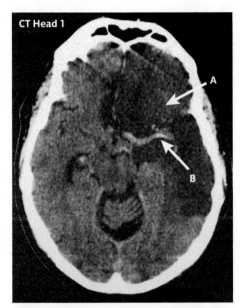

CT Head 1

This 76-year old woman presented to the Accident and Emergency Department with the sudden onset of weakness in the right arm and leg. She did not complain of headache.
What does arrow A indicate?
And arrow B?
What is the diagnosis?

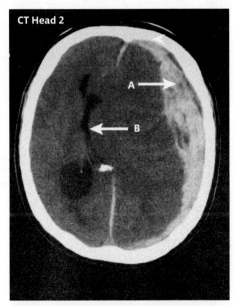

CT Head 2

This elderly man developed headache, confusion and vomiting following a fall.

What does arrow A indicate?
And arrow B?
What is the diagnosis?

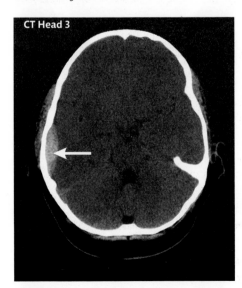

CT Head 3

This 45 year old man fell off his motorcycle, struck his head and subsequently developed headache and vomiting.
What does the arrow indicate?

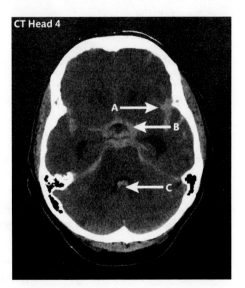

CT Head 4

This 30 year old woman presented with the sudden onset of headache, vomiting, photophobia and neck stiffness.
What is the diagnosis?
To what are the arrows pointing?

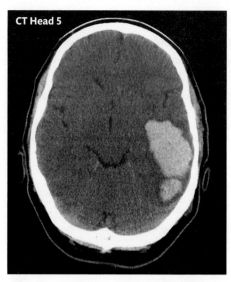

CT Head 5

This 65 year old man with a past history of hypertension and taking warfarin for a recent deep vein thrombosis presented with headache, drowsiness and right-sided weakness.
What is the diagnosis?

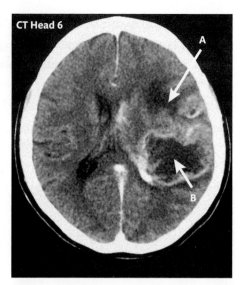

CT Head 6

This 55 year old man presented with fits and progressively worsening headaches.

What is the diagnosis?
What do arrows A and B indicate?

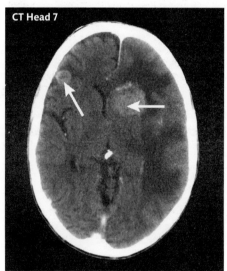

CT Head 7

This 63 year old woman with known breast cancer presented with headaches and confusion.
What are the lesions arrowed ?

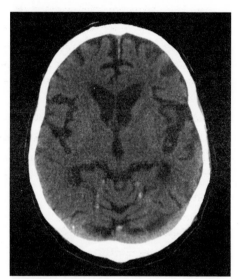

This 74 year old man presented with confusion and declining abilities to perform normal activities of daily living.
What abnormalities can be seen and what is the likely diagnosis?

Patient safety tips

✔ **Ionizing radiation**: Since CT head involves ionizing radiation it is important to check whether the investigation is needed and the result will affect management.

✔ **X-ray dose to the orbit and lens can be reduced**: by angulating the imaging plane to avoid these structures.

✔ **Contrast agent**: If the patient requires a contrast examination then careful questioning to assess for prior contrast allergy is needed. Intravenous contrast should also be avoided in acute or chronic renal failure unless the patient is already on replacement therapy.

- **CT head 1**: This non-contrast CT scan of brain shows a large low-attenuation (low-density) area in the left middle and anterior cerebral artery territories in keeping with acute infarction. There is no evidence of acute haemorrhage.

  1 Area of infarction in the left middle cerebral artery (MCA) and anterior cerebral artery (ACA) territories

  2 Thrombus in MCA

  3 Thrombotic stroke.

  Diagnosis: Left MCA stroke.

- **CT head 2**: There is a large acute subdural haemorrhage on the left side with significant midline shift to the right.

  1 A high-density crescent-shaped haemorrhage in the subdural space

  2 Midline shift of the ventricles

  3 Acute subdural haemorrhage.

  In elderly patients with cerebral atrophy subdural haemorrhage may occur after apparently minor head injury. Urgent neurosurgical referral for drainage is recommended.

  Diagnosis: subdural haematoma.

- **CT head 3**: There is a right sided lens-shaped high density area consistent with an acute extradural haematoma causing a localized mass effect. This is frequently associated with skull fractures and it is important to assess the bones in bone windows.

  Diagnosis: right sided acute extradural haematoma.

- **CT head 4**: this CT scan demonstrates extensive acute subarachnoid haemorrhage. There is also some blood seen in the fourth ventricle and there is dilatation of the temporal horns of the lateral ventricles.

  1 Acute subarachnoid haemorrhage

  2 Blood in the left Sylvian fissure (A), the suprasellar cistern (B), and the fourth ventricle (C).

  Diagnosis: Extensive subarachnoid haemorrhage.

- **CT head 5**: this CT scan of the brain shows a left-sided acute intracerebral haematoma.

  Haemorrhagic stroke

  Common causes of intracerebral haematoma are hypertension, ruptured aneurysm, anti-coagulation therapy, and amyloidosis.

  Diagnosis: Haemorrhagic stroke.

- **CT head 6**: this post-contrast CT scan demonstrates a heterogeneously enhancing left hemispheric intrinsic mass lesion. Appearances are typical of a glioblastoma multiforme.

  1 Intracerebral tumour

  2 A: localized white matter oedema. B: tumour.

  Diagnosis: glioblastoma multiforme.

- **CT head 7**: this post-contrast CT scan of the brain shows multiple (two) enhancing nodules in the frontal regions causing local mass effect. There is also white matter oedema noted on the left side. The appearances are in keeping with metastatic deposits. Common brain parenchymal metastases are from cancers of the breast, lung, kidney, and gastrointestinal tract, and melanoma.

  Diagnosis: cerebral metastases from breast cancer.

- **CT head 8**: lateral ventricles are larger than normal with blunting of the anterior horns. The sulci are prominent. The appearances are consistent with reduction in overall brain volume.

  Diagnosis: dementia with cerebral atrophy.

Student name:	Medical school:	Year:

CT head

Please interpret this CT brain scan.

	Self	Peer	Peer/tutor	Tutor
General check				
Checks the name, date of birth, and gender of the patient, the date of the scan, and that the sides are clearly marked	☐	☐	☐	☐
Checks whether contrast has been given	☐	☐	☐	☐
	☐	☐	☐	☐
Quality check				
Checks that the scan includes the foramen magnum and that the images go all the way to the vertex	☐	☐	☐	☐
Checks for movement artefact and any rotation of the patient's head	☐	☐	☐	☐
	☐	☐	☐	☐
Main interpretation				
Assesses overall brain volume, symmetry, and checks for hydrocephalus	☐	☐	☐	☐
Assesses white/grey matter differentiation and notes the presence of any tumour(s) or areas of acute infarction	☐	☐	☐	☐
Checks for any surface haemorrhage or intracerebral haematoma	☐	☐	☐	☐
Notes any areas of calcification	☐	☐	☐	☐
	☐	☐	☐	☐
Review areas — Checks for any abnormality in:				
The intracranial vessels	☐	☐	☐	☐
The pituitary and suprasellar regions	☐	☐	☐	☐
The basal cisterns and cerebellar tonsils	☐	☐	☐	☐
The bones and soft tissues	☐	☐	☐	☐
	☐	☐	☐	☐
Summary				
Summarizes findings accurately and concisely	☐	☐	☐	☐
	☐	☐	☐	☐

			Self	Peer	Peer/tutor	Tutor
Self-assessed as at least borderline:	Signature:	Date:	U B S E	U B S E	U B S E	U B S E
Peer-assessed as ready for tutor assessment:	Signature:	Date:	U B S E	U B S E	U B S E	U B S E
Tutor-assessed as satisfactory:	Signature:	Date:	U B S E	U B S E	U B S E	U B S E

Notes

Unit 17 **Advanced clinical skills**

17.1 **Advanced communication skills**

Background

Patients expect to be treated with respect and compassion by their doctors. Good communication improves health outcomes, enhances patient satisfaction, and reduces litigation. This chapter will summarize some important principles in relation to consultation with patients. The focus is on dealing with patients in special circumstances and a tool that serves as a simple but effective reminder of how to conduct an effective clinical consultation, even if seeing many patients in a session such as an outpatient clinic or in general practice.

Clinical indications and key skills

Good communication skills are a key part of every interaction with a patient.

Excellent communicators demonstrate the following skills:

- **Timing and location**: allow adequate time to talk with patient. Choose a location that is quiet and where patient confidentiality can be respected.

- **Patient at ease**: invite patient to bring someone along for support where appropriate. Consider whether a chaperone might be helpful. Attend to the patient's needs (Are they comfortable? In pain?).

- **Introduction**: introduce self fully, and provide contact details in case of follow-up questions later.

- **Demonstrate attentiveness, benevolence and compassion/empathy**: be mindful of potential blocks to good communication, e.g. cultural/language issues (if in doubt, find out more about the patient's cultural background).

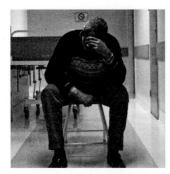
Perception in relation to difficult consultations is vital: imagine what it must be like to have to receive bad news or to have had to express anger due to a concern in delivery of health services.

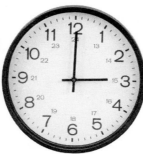
In difficult or special consultations, time is vital. These consultations cannot be rushed. At least 30 minutes are usually required.

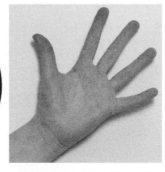
Neighbour's Consultation Checkpoints: **Connecting with the patient** (little finger), **Summarising** (ring finger), **Handing over** (middle finger), **Safety-netting** (index finger), **Housekeeping** (thumb)

Figure 17.1 Images in advanced communication skills. Left © poco_bw/iStockphoto; right © Ingram

- **Allow patients to freely communicate their problems**: studies indicate that on average doctors interrupt their patients after only 24 seconds yet patients rarely need more than 2.5 minutes to express their problems.
- **Explain in jargon-free language**: check that patient has understood and encourage questions at all stages.
- **Explore ideas, concerns, and expectations**: it will be obvious to all clinicians that these are the main reasons why a patient presents with a clinical problem, however, these are often not aired sufficiently.
- **Provide both verbal and written information** where appropriate. Be prepared to repeat information several times if needed, or to offer a further meeting for further clarification.
- **Finish the consultation** by providing information on 'what next' (i.e. do not just deliver information and leave).

Factors that negatively affect ability to communicate effectively:

- Feeling angry or stressed
- Not prepared
- No time
- Talking in corridors or in public places.

Interestingly doctors who have never been sued are skilled in all of the above and use humour and laughter appropriately in their consultations!

Sequence

This section will explore four scenarios requiring excellent communication skills:

- Breaking bad news
- Talking with an angry patient
- Explaining a complex procedure
- Communicating with people with learning difficulties.

Breaking bad news

Breaking bad news is one of the most challenging communication tasks for doctors. The mnemonic SPIKES may be helpful when breaking bad news: **S**etting, **P**erception, **I**nvitation, **K**nowledge, **E**mpathy, and **S**trategy and **S**ummary.

Setting

- Prepare a quiet room and adequate time with no interruptions.
- Attend to your own feelings, and think of what the family/patient might be feeling.
- Give your name, your job title, and the role you played in the patient's care: 'I am Doctor X, I am the registrar on the team that has been caring for your father. I have just come from the operating room, where I was helping the consultant perform your father's operation'

Perception

- Find out what the patient/family knows so far, so that you can tailor your explanation to their knowledge.

Invitation

- Invite the family/patient to let you know how much detail they want at this stage, offering to give more information later as needed.

Knowledge

- Explain in simple language what has occurred: 'I'm very sorry to say that ...died during the operation. We tried to resuscitate him but we did not succeed. I'm very sorry', or, 'I'm afraid the test results have come back, and it looks more serious than we had hoped'.
- Then leave a silence, so that the patient/family can absorb the information.

- Answer any questions asked in simple language, and in a non-defensive manner. Be guided by what the family wants when deciding how much information to give.
- Avoid technical jargon.

Empathy

- Show your concern, allow patient/family to absorb what is happening, proceed at their pace.
- Attend to their needs: 'Do you need to call anyone to be with you?' 'Is there anything you need?'.

Strategy and summary

- Check understanding, and offer written information.
- Orientate the patient/family: tell them what will happen next: 'The consultant will come as soon as she can to speak with you: you can stay here in the meantime. Can we offer you a cup of tea?'.
- Offer your contact details so that the team can be contacted in the event of further questions.
- Offer a follow-up appointment, and document what has been discussed.

Talking with an angry patient

This can be particularly challenging for most clinicians.

Setting

- Prepare in advance. Get patient's file and read it.
- Pay attention to your own state of mind. It is difficult to deal sympathetically with an angry patient if you are also feeling stressed and annoyed.
- Set aside adequate time, and find a quiet location.
- Ask if patient would like to bring someone with them for support.

Perception

- When planning a 'difficult' consultation, put yourself in the patient's shoes: what might they be feeling? What might they want from the consultation?

Invitation

- When opening the consultation, orientate the patient: 'We have 30 minutes to talk together today, and if you feel that we haven't covered everything in that time, we can arrange a further meeting'.
- Then, let the patient talk without interruption: allow them to express their anger. If they are very angry, it is likely that they have felt ignored or disrespected by previous doctors, so your ability to listen and take them seriously will be much appreciated. Make notes in brief if you need.
- Acknowledge and apologize for the difficulties they have faced. Even if nothing could have been done differently for the patient, it is still appropriate to apologize for the fact that they have felt let down.

Knowledge

- Explain in simple language what has occurred: 'I'm very sorry to hear from you that X did not happen'. Then honestly explain and offer reasons if relevant.
- Then leave a silence, so that the patient/family can absorb the information.
- Answer any questions asked in simple language, and in a non-defensive manner. Avoid technical jargon.
- If you do not have a piece of information that the patient requires, undertake to find it out for them: 'I don't know the answer to that right now but I will find out for you, and tell you at our next meeting. Is there anything else you would like me to find out for you?'

Empathy

- Show your concern, allow patient/family to absorb what is happening, proceed at their pace.

Strategy and summary

● Ensure that main points of concern have been covered: 'Have you found out what you needed to know?' And/or 'Have we explained and apologized for all your concerns?' And 'is there anything that you want to ask about?'

● If they wish to make a complaint, offer them advice on the best way to do this according to local protocols such as support provided by the NHS Patient and Liaison Service (PALS).

● At the close of the meeting, summarize the main issues, and what you are proposing to do to address them. Check that the patient agrees with your summary and plan. State (if relevant) that learning will take place and that other patients/relatives will be unlikely to suffer from the same situation.

● Thanks the patient/family and offer your contact details and ensure that the patient knows what is going to happen next to address their concerns.

Explaining a complex procedure

An inadequate explanation, especially in relation to consent, has immense potential to lead to fear and anxiety in a patient, and needless complaints and even litigation thereafter.

Setting

● Introduce self, offer the patient the opportunity to bring someone with them for support.

Perception

● Check what the patient already knows about the procedure (which may reveal misconceptions or fears that you can address): 'What do you know about this procedure?' or 'Do you know anyone who has had this procedure before?' or 'How did they get on?' or 'Do you have any particular questions or concerns about it that you would like answered before we start?'

Knowledge

● 'I am now going to talk you through the whole procedure from start to finish. If anything I say is unclear, please stop me and ask'.

● Talk the patient through the procedure, using jargon-free language, and focusing on what the patient will experience. Some patients may find a diagram helpful, if appropriate.

● Explain the positive benefits of having the procedure, and the side effects that may occur (both common side effects, and rare but serious side effects must be explained).

● Explain what other options the patient may have, and what the implications of choosing one option over another would be.

● Check understanding at regular intervals and ensure that the patient has the chance to ask questions and clarify any issues which may cause concern.

Empathy

● Show concerns about any anxieties expressed. Allay anxieties by exploring the concern and giving time for questioning and explanation.

Strategy and summary

● Signpost important points and empower patient to take an active role in their care: 'There is a risk of blood clots in the legs after a big operation, but you can minimize this risk by regular walking once you are steady on your feet after the operation'.

● At the end, provide written information, if available, on the procedure, and ask for questions.

People with learning difficulties

Many people who are labelled as having learning disability prefer the term people with learning difficulties. This is also the preferred term used by People First, an international advocacy organization for people who fall into several definitions of learning impairment.

The World Health Organization (WHO) defines learning disabilities as 'a state of arrested or incomplete development of mind' with 'significant impairment of intellectual functioning' and 'significant impairment of adaptive/social functioning'. This means that the person will have difficulties understanding, learning, remembering new things, and in using any learning to new situations. The person may well have difficulties with communication, health needs and self-care. The definition assumes that the condition started and developed in childhood, not from any clinical condition or injury in adulthood.

Key principles

- **Person-centred care**: this should apply to all clinical communication and care. Specifically with this group of patients:
  - ○ Does things *with* the person, not *to* them or *for* them
  - ○ Understands the person's perspective, abilities, needs, and interests
  - ○ Seeks to help the person make choices and decisions to get the best out of life.
- **Consider health needs that affect communication**: mental agility, sight, hearing, distress, effect of medications (for example, antiepileptic medication)
- **Difficulty checking understanding**: common responses from the clinician or patients may be misinterpreted. For example; is a nod a yes?
- **Different modes of communication**: eye gaze, facial expressions, body language and posture, signs, verbalizing without distinct words being used, charts with pictures or symbols, electronic devices.
- **Time and patience**: extra time will be needed, often two to five times longer than standard clinical time allocations.

Patient and professional safety tips

Roger Neighbour describes the consultation as a journey with 'checkpoints' along the way. His 'inner consultation' model provides a useful patient safety-focused checklist. It is best remembered, as espoused by the author, by recalling the fingers of the hand.

- ✔ **Connecting with the patient** (little finger): developing rapport and empathy, gambits and curtain raiser, non-verbal cues
- ✔ **Summarizing** (ring finger): information gathering, summarizing their reasons for attending; their ideas, concerns, and expectations.
- ✔ **Handing over** (middle finger): negotiating-patient options, explain diagnosis and management, gift wrap, chunk, and check.
- ✔ **Safety-netting** (index finger): making contingency plans in case the clinician is wrong or something unexpected happens, go through red-flag symptoms.
- ✔ **Housekeeping** (thumb): taking measures to ensure the clinician stays in good shape for the next patient. Keeping time for yourself between patients, and during consultation.

Student name:	Medical school:	Year:

Communication skills in special circumstances

Please consider the following scenarios. Use role play and discussion to assessment whether aspects of good communication skills are demonstrated and known by the candidate.

				Self	Peer	Peer /tutor	Tutor
Breaking bad news Vignette 1 You are a newly qualified doctor, working in the accident and emergency department of a large hospital. A 56-year-old patient is brought in following a myocardial infarction. You and your team attempt resuscitation, but are unsuccessful and the patient dies. You are now asked to speak with his wife and 18-year-old daughter, to explain to them what has happened	1	Explains and elaborates upon the SPIKES model as template for communicating bad news (Setting, Perception, Invitation, Knowledge, Empathy, Strategy and Summary)		☐	☐	☐	☐
	2	Demonstrates above skills in role play with the assessor in the role of patient		☐	☐	☐	☐
	3	Notices emotional state of relatives, e.g. 'I can see this is a real shock for you'.		☐	☐	☐	☐
Breaking bad news Vignette 2 You are asked to speak with a 45-year-old woman who is awaiting the results of a breast biopsy. The biopsy shows cancerous cells. You have been asked to deliver this news to her. Alternatively for a male assessor, the gastric ulcer biopsy shows malignant cells.	1	Explains and elaborates upon the SPIKES model as template for communicating bad news (Setting, Perception, Invitation, Knowledge, Empathy, Strategy and Summary)		☐	☐	☐	☐
	2	Demonstrates above skills in role play with the assessor in the role of patient		☐	☐	☐	☐
	3	Notices emotional state of patient, e.g. 'I can see this is a real shock for you'.		☐	☐	☐	☐
Talking with an angry patient Vignette 3 You are working as a surgical trainee at a busy outpatient clinic. Your next patient is a 27-year-old man who has suffered complications from a recent appendicectomy operation and an MRSA infection and who feels he has had no explanation or apology for what has happened. He has come today to the clinic to complain	1	Explains and elaborates upon the SPIKES model as template for communicating bad news (Setting, Perception, Invitation, Knowledge, Empathy, Strategy and Summary)		☐	☐	☐	☐
	2	Reacts non-defensively to anger, e.g. 'I can see you are very upset about this, can you explain exactly what happened from your point of view'.		☐	☐	☐	☐
Explaining a complex procedure Vignette 4 Your patient, Mr Smith, has significant atherosclerosis in his carotid arteries, and has suffered several transient ischaemic attacks in the last 6 months. His consultant is considering performing a carotid endarterectomy, and you have been asked to explain this procedure to him in full	1	Explains and elaborates upon the SPIKES model as template for communicating bad news (Setting, Perception, Invitation, Knowledge, Empathy, Strategy and Summary)		☐	☐	☐	☐
	2	Provide written information appropriate to understanding by the patient.		☐	☐	☐	☐
Communication with people with learning difficulties Vignette 5 Your patient, Ronni Green has been admitted with a community-acquired pneumonia. You have been called to put in a venous cannula for intravenous antibiotics	•	Explains specific concerns in relation to managing people with learning difficulties in hospitals (more health problems, die at earlier age, limitation in communication is one of the causes of deficiency in care)		☐	☐	☐	☐
	•	Lists tips from people with learning difficulties on how they like to be treated (respect, talk to people with learning difficulties directly, talk in a way that the individual understands, listen, do not rush)		☐	☐	☐	☐
	•	Checks understanding		☐	☐	☐	☐

			Self	Peer	Peer /tutor	Tutor
Self-assessed as at least borderline:	Signature:	Date:	U B S E	U B S E	U B S E	U B S E
Peer-assessed as ready for tutor assessment:	Signature:	Date:	U B S E	U B S E	U B S E	U B S E
Tutor-assessed as satisfactory:	Signature:	Date:	U B S E	U B S E	U B S E	U B S E

Notes

17.2 On the job teaching

Background

To study the phenomenon of disease without books is to sail an uncharted sea, whilst to study books without patients is not to go to sea at all

Sir William Osler (1849-1919)

Learning in the real-life clinical environment is fundamental to medical education. The great physician and medical educator Sir William Osler once said he hoped his tombstone would say only, 'He brought medical students into the wards for bedside teaching'. Essential learning outcomes for students from contact with real patients include:

- Acquisition of history taking and physical examination skills
- Acquisition of communication skills and professional attitudes
- Acquisition of core knowledge
- Understanding the patient's experience and perspective
- Understanding the social context of disease
- Understanding health service organization and health care delivery
- Pre-qualification experience in preparation for work.

Elements of effective teaching

The following principles apply to any teaching, but are particularly relevant in the busy and time-restricted clinical environment:

- Discover what students want and need to learn, and can be taught
- Consider the constraints of the situation and the time available
- Provide an environment that is conducive to learning
- Establish a relationship with the trainee
- Use teaching methods appropriate to the learners and the situation
- Review what has been learnt and plan for further learning
- Evaluate the teaching.

Experiential learning

Medicine is learned from experience. The process of experiential learning is summarized in the four-stage Kolb's learning cycle:

- Concrete experience
- Reflective practice
- Abstract conceptualization
- Active experimentation.

The concrete experience might be, for example, a busy night on call in the Accident and Emergency Department. The student should be encouraged to reflect on the experience and what was learnt. A tutor or peer will then be able to provide an educational prescription how to continue that learning: this might include recommended reading to remedy gaps in knowledge or further supervised practice in a procedural skill. The final stage of active experimentation is the student revisiting the clinical environment with the newly acquired skills and knowledge. The cycle is then repeated numerous times, ideally over an entire professional lifetime.

Helping learners to think for themselves

The use of open-ended questions encourages learners to think about the subject and develop ideas for themselves. Socrates is believed to have developed the method whereby such questioning by the tutor enables the learner to reach a true conclusion without being informed of it directly, for example:

- Seeking clarification: 'Can you explain that?'
- Probing reasoning: 'Why do you think that?'
- Exploring alternatives: 'What would be an alternative explanation?'
- Testing implications: 'So what would your management plan be?'
- Inviting questions and discussion: 'Who can summarize so far?'

The one-minute preceptor model enables the tutor to combine several teaching microskills to deliver a brief but highly effective educational package:

- Get a commitment: 'What do you think is going on here?'
- Probe for supporting evidence: 'What led you to that conclusion?'
- Teach general rules and principles: 'When this happens always consider...'
- Reinforce what was right: 'Specifically you did an excellent job of ...'
- Correct mistakes: 'Next time quickly consider life-saving treatment first...'

Giving effective feedback

One of the most useful contributions a peer or tutor can make to a trainee's learning is to give meaningful, effective feedback. Many structured methods have been devised for this but Pendleton's is the one most commonly employed. It can be used, for example, after a trainee has been observed taking a history, performing a physical examination, or executing a practical procedure:

- Clarification of matters of fact
- The student identifies what went well
- The tutor identifies what went well
- The student discusses what did not go well and how to improve
- The tutor identifies areas for improvement
- Agreement between student and tutor on areas for improvement and formulation of an action plan.

Practical tips for teaching on the ward

- Maintain a list of patients whom students must see
- Give students responsibility for daily review of a few patients
- If time is pressing ask the student to take just one part of the history, for example the treatment history, or one element of the physical examination, percussion of the chest, say, rather than a full respiratory examination.
- Use students as a resource, e.g. filling in forms and recording observations
- On ward rounds teach on some but not all patients
- Debrief at the end of a teaching session with an open question: 'What did you learn today?'

Two practical aids to teaching

A handheld tips reminder

This folds to credit card size and includes six key reminders for teaching on the job, selected by a group of students on a teaching course:

- Teaching tips and tools: an ideas box with tips for teaching
- Suggestions for Socratic questioning
- A summary of the one-minute preceptor model
- Pendleton's rules of feedback
- History outline: a box diagram which deconstructs the clinical history into several 2-4 minute chunks
- The Warwick Four-Point Presentation (See Suite 1, *Summary: the Complete Consultation*, page 108).

A clinical logbook

Often students have sat in on a clinic of 15-20 patients and made notes that would be indecipherable for purposes of revision and reflection. The clinical logbook encourages students to make a structured record of 2-3 patient encounters per clinic. The student is required to note not only what is *present* in the history, physical examination, and investigations but also what are the important *negative* findings. For example, in a patient with psoriasis presenting with a rash alone the more advanced student will look for arthritis and nail changes. These features of the disease are entered in (brackets) if thought about but not found. An increasing number of (bracketed) entries is evidence of improving knowledge and clinical reasoning. The logbook also asks for alternative diagnoses at each of the stages of history, physical examination, and investigation to stretch individual students to the limit of their current competence.

These two practical aides to teaching are reproduced on the Online Resource Centre accompanying the book at www.oxfordtextbooks.co.uk/orc/patel_skills/.

Conclusion

Teaching should be both a professional duty and a personal pleasure. Every day in clinical practice offers numerous opportunities to teach and to learn. There are many ways to overcome the time constraints imposed by the clinical environment. Welcome students as members of the team, ask them to take responsibility for some of the day-to-day work, and let the junior doctors, students, and patients learn from each other. Create a community of learning in the workplace.

Student name:	Medical school:	Year:

On the job teaching

Teaching observation form

	Self	Peer	Peer /tutor	Tutor
• States a clear aim for the teaching session	☐	☐	☐	☐
• Discovers what the students want and need to learn	☐	☐	☐	☐
• Sets objectives appropriate to the level of learners	☐	☐	☐	☐
• Provides an environment conducive to learning	☐	☐	☐	☐
• Structures the session appropriately	☐	☐	☐	☐
• Content is accurate and relevant	☐	☐	☐	☐
• Involves students with different learning styles	☐	☐	☐	☐
• Facilitates a high level of student participation	☐	☐	☐	☐
• Uses high-quality visual aids	☐	☐	☐	☐
• Speaks audibly, clearly and at an appropriate pace	☐	☐	☐	☐
• Keeps the session to time	☐	☐	☐	☐
• Reviews what has been learnt	☐	☐	☐	☐
• Responds to students' questions	☐	☐	☐	☐
• Makes suggestions about further learning	☐	☐	☐	☐
• Makes arrangements for evaluation of teaching	☐	☐	☐	☐
•	☐	☐	☐	☐

			Self	Peer	Peer /tutor	Tutor
Self-assessed as at least borderline:	Signature:	Date:	U B S E	U B S E	U B S E	U B S E
Peer-assessed as ready for tutor assessment:	Signature:	Date:	U B S E	U B S E	U B S E	U B S E
Tutor-assessed as satisfactory:	Signature:	Date:	U B S E	U B S E	U B S E	U B S E

Notes

17.3 Care of the dying patient

Background

Care of the dying is a vital part of the work of doctors. When patients are diagnosed with a terminal illness, they and their families experience a wide range of emotions. There is a lot of fear and uncertainty that surrounds dying, especially as it is associated with a great deal of pain and suffering. Palliative care is a multiprofessional approach that focuses on the patient with life-limiting illness. It was recognized only relatively recently as a medical subspecialty in 1987 by the Royal College of Physicians.

The WHO defines palliative care as:

An approach that improves the quality of life of patients and their families facing the problems associated with life-threatening illness, through the prevention and relief of suffering by means of early identification and impeccable assessment and treatment of pain and other problems, physical, psychosocial and spiritual. Palliative care:

- provides relief from pain and other distressing symptoms;
- affirms life and regards dying as a normal process;
- intends neither to hasten or postpone death;
- integrates the psychological and spiritual aspects of patient care;
- offers a support system to help patients live as actively as possible until death;
- offers a support system to help the family cope during the patient's illness and in their own bereavement;
- uses a team approach to address the needs of patients and their families, including bereavement counselling, if indicated;
- will enhance quality of life, and may also positively influence the course of illness;
- is applicable early in the course of illness, in conjunction with other therapies that are intended to prolong life, such as chemotherapy or radiation therapy, and includes those investigations needed to better understand and manage distressing clinical complications.

NICE has published guidelines in an attempt to streamline palliative care services, as traditionally hospitals have been regarded as poor providers compared with hospices. As the population is living longer, the burden of chronic illness and demand for palliative care services is increasing. While hospices and specialist palliative care services focus their limited resources on patients and families with complex palliative care needs, all healthcare professionals need to know how to provide these services in hospitals or in the community.

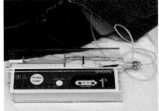

Many components of the Liverpool Care Pathway rely on a syringe driver for the safe and timely delivery of drugs.

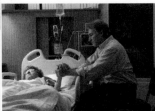

An individualised approach is needed to each patient for the prevention and relief of suffering.

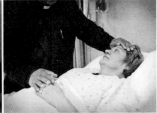

Spiritual needs have to be addressed in the patients who require this. The Hospital chaplaincy team will be able to access help for all the main religions in the local community.

Figure 17.2 Images in care of the dying patient. Middle © Claudio Rossol; right © Nancy Louie.

Clinical indications

The palliative care approach may often be appropriate for patients with life-limiting disease at a relatively early stage in order to maximize quality of life. However, in recent years, particular attention has been focused on improving the management of patients during the last days and hours of life.

The Liverpool Care Pathway (LCP) is a care template that was developed to enable hospice quality care for the dying to be used in other environments such as acute general hospitals, nursing homes and patients' own homes. To be placed on the LCP, the patient should be diagnosed as actively dying, i.e. in the last days or hours of life. This usually follows a gradual deterioration in function over time. It is often hard to recognize when a patient is in the terminal phase of their illness, but the Ellershaw–Ward signs have been identified as prognostically significant:

- The patient is mostly bedbound
- The patient is asleep for most of the time
- The patient loses interest in food and will only take sips of fluid
- The patient cannot swallow their oral medication.

In a hospital setting, heart failure is the single most common cause of death on the wards and these patients often die in distress. Causes of heart failure are often reversible, such as anaemia or arrhythmias, and it is important that these causes are ruled out before committing them to terminal care. It is very hard to identify the terminal phase in heart failure patients, as they go through periods of acute deterioration and recovery and they may die suddenly. However, there are features that predict early mortality:

- Frequent admissions with worsening heart failure
- Renal function deteriorating
- Systolic blood pressure less than 100 mmHg and/or pulse greater than 100
- Decreased left ventricular ejection fraction (linear relationship with survival at 45% or less)
- Anaemia or cachexia.

Owing to the difficulties in identifying the terminal phase in heart failure, end of life care is often not initiated and patients continue to receive active treatment. Patients are not given the opportunity to discuss dying and have less access to specialist palliative care services when compared with patients with malignant disease. Heart failure patients can suffer from severe breathlessness, pain, and fatigue, which require palliation. Depression and other psychological problems are also common and should not be neglected.

Non-malignant chronic lung disease is another area which can be neglected in terms of palliative care. Many resources are available for patients with advanced lung cancer, but there is not so much available for other conditions such as idiopathic lung fibrosis and COPD. Mortality is just as high in these conditions but they have less well-defined end of life pathways and less access to specialist palliative care services. The BODE index (Table 17.1) is promoted to predict mortality (body mass index (BMI), obstruction (forced expiratory volume in one second [FEV_1]), dyspnoea, exercise tolerance) but is still not precise. The higher the score (maximum 10), the higher the risk of death.

Table 17.1 Calculation of the BODE index

Variable	Points on BODE index			
	0	1	2	3
FEV_1 % of predicted	≥65	50–64	36–49	≤35
Distance walked in 6 min (m)	≥350	250–349	150–249	≤149
MMRC dyspnoea scale (See Table 17.2)	0–1	2	3	4
Body mass index	>21	≤21	–	–

Table 17.2 Modified Medical Research Council (MMRC) dyspnoea scale

Grade	Description
0	Breathlessness only on severe exercise
1	Breathlessness when hurrying on the flat or walking up a slight incline
2	Walks slower than others or has to stop for breath when walking at their own pace on the flat
3	Needs to stop for breath after walking for 100 yards/a few minutes on the flat
4	Breathless when dressing/undressing, unable to leave the house

Management

Social and spiritual

It is vital to discuss the overall plan with the patient and their carer or relatives and ensure, while remaining sensitive to individual needs, that they understand they are dying. It should be stated that the pathway is designed to make them more comfortable. You should also discuss with the patient where they want to die. Ideally, discussion of patients' wishes for symptom control and preferred place of care for their dying phase will have been broached prior to the terminal illness or admission, but this is often not the case, particularly among patients dying from a non-cancer diagnosis. The situation may be further complicated by denial.

Having ascertained patients' wishes and taken into account the needs of family members, you need to work with the multiprofessional team to make arrangements for the patient to be transferred to a hospice (if they have complex needs) or discharged home if this is appropriate and feasible. However, it must be recognized that for some patients with a longer or unpredictable terminal phase (particularly those living alone or with elderly or frail partners) a nursing home may be the only viable alternative, which needs to be broached sensitively but realistically. The patient and their relatives may not take in all of the information when you first discuss it with them, so it is important to offer them the opportunity to come back to you with any further questions they may have.

Psychological care of patients and their families/carers is an essential feature of the palliative care approach. In exploring psychological issues, you need to be aware that patients' needs and coping strategies as they approach the terminal phase may change, and may be very different from those of their carers. It may be helpful to involve clinical psychology or counselling services, if this has not already been initiated. If the patient him/herself is too unwell at this point, it may still be valuable to signpost carers, particularly for onward bereavement support of both adults and children.

The patient and relatives' values and spiritual needs should not be neglected. They should be discussed and if you feel uncomfortable in this area, you should refer them to the hospital chaplaincy team. The family should also be given information about dying and contacts for bereavement support following the death.

Therapeutic

The multidisciplinary team must all be in agreement that the patient is dying. The patient's condition should be reviewed regularly, and if there is an improvement in their condition then it may be appropriate to remove them from the LCP. At any time, advice can be sought from the specialist palliative care team if you are unsure. When a patient is identified as actively dying, their medication must be reviewed and all non-essential medications stopped, e.g. antihypertensives and antibiotics. All inappropriate interventions should also be stopped, e.g. blood tests and IV fluids. The patient must be documented as not for cardiopulmonary resuscitation. If they have an implantable cardioverter defibrillator (ICD) in place, this should be deactivated.

The only medications prescribed should be for comfort and symptom control (see Table 17.3). You should consider subcutaneous administration of analgesics, antiemetics, and anxiolytics using a syringe driver or injection as patients are often unable to swallow tablets. You should also prescribe 'as required' medication for pain, nausea, agitation, and respiratory secretions. This will prevent any delay in the patient receiving symptom relief, even if they do not present with these symptoms at first. The key to symptom management in the dying phase is regular review and latest guidelines should be used.

Pain

- Pain affects the majority of dying patients. While this is clearly recognized among health professionals caring for cancer patients, it may receive less emphasis among patients with non-cancer diagnoses, but is equally prevalent (Johnson, 2007). However, as long as it is considered and adequately treated, pain can be controlled in the vast majority of patients. Pain from progressive disease is continuous, and should be managed continuously by continuous subcutaneous infusion (CSCI) if severe. Syringe driver medication will usually involve conversion of a previous oral opioid, although patients requiring adjunct analgesics may need these continued if pain has been previously difficult to control. If in doubt about subcutaneous alternatives, refer to the palliative care team for advice. Breakthrough episodes of pain can be managed by giving one-sixth of the total 24-hour opioid dose. If the patient is having several breakthrough episodes in 24 hours, you should increase the background dose in the syringe driver. There is no 'ceiling dose', and you should continue to raise it until the patient is comfortable (as long as the pain appears to be opioid responsive). Remember that patients who are debilitated are equally likely to suffer pain and discomfort from sore muscles, pressure areas, and dry or sore mouths, and that these aspects of symptom control and nursing care are equally important.

- Remember also that pain has a large psychological component; for patients who are still able to concentrate on verbal conversation, counselling or specialist psychological or spiritual input may be helpful; for patients who are dying, touch therapies such as simple massage or aromatherapy can be effective for reducing anxiety and distress that the patient may no longer be able to verbalize.

Nausea and vomiting

- The cause of nausea and vomiting needs to be considered in prescribing during the dying phase, although decisions on potential reversibility of any underlying causes such as hyper-calcaemia should have been made before placing the patient on the LCP. Table 17.3 shows the antiemetics that can be used to treat different causes of nausea and vomiting and will usually involve administration via subcutaneous syringe driver. Vomiting tends to decrease in patients in their dying phase as they take less in orally, except in cases of high gastrointestinal obstruction, which should be managed in consultation with the palliative care team.

Agitation

- Restlessness and agitation are common when patients are dying. This may have a treatable underlying cause, such as constipation or urinary retention. It may also be caused by hyper-calcaemia, uraemia, infection, or brain metastases, which will not be treated actively if the patient is in the terminal stage. It is important to treat symptomatically to make the patient more comfortable, and also reduce anxiety of the patient's relatives who find it distressing to witness.

Respiratory secretions

- Retained respiratory secretions are also common in the terminal phase, and this causes noisy, bubbly breathing. This may be more distressing for carers than for an unconscious patient. It may be managed by positioning of the patient, but if it appears to be causing distress, the use of anticholinergic drugs such as hyoscine hydrobromide may be helpful.

Breathlessness

- Breathlessness is very distressing for patients. It can be helped with 1–2 L/min of oxygen. Opioids can also relieve breathlessness. If the patient is already prescribed opiates for pain, the dose can be increased by 25–50%. Midazolam can also be used, at 10–20 mg/24 h, if the patient has not already been prescribed it for agitation. Clinical evidence shows that a simple fan can be helpful in relieving breathlessness.

Table 17.3 Prescribing for the dying patient: refer to local protocols if available

Pain

Diamorphine: first choice for subcutaneous administration as it is more water soluble than morphine	*Mode of action*: broken down into morphine and 6-MAM in the brain, which bind to μ-opioid receptors to result in analgesia *Dose*: one-third total daily dose of oral morphine *Side effects*: constipation (always prescribe with stimulant laxative), sedation (lessens after first few doses), nausea (always prescribe with anti-emetic), dry mouth, itching, sweating Hallucinations – may need to change to an alternative opioid, such as oxycodone or alfentanil
Morphine: subcutaneous use	*Mode of action*: mainly binds to the μ-opioid receptor in the central nervous system (CNS) to result in analgesia *Dose*: half total daily dose of oral morphine *Side effects*: as for diamorphine

For patients in renal failure consult Palliative Care Team regarding alternative opioids.

Nausea and vomiting

Metoclopramide	*Indication and mode of action*: impaired gastric emptying – aids gut motility, D_2 receptor antagonist at the chemoreceptor trigger zone *Subcutaneous starting dose and range in 24 hours*: 30–40 mg (range 30–80 mg) *Side effects*: restlessness, drowsiness, extrapyramidal effects, hyperprolactinaemia
Haloperidol	*Indication and mode of action*: nausea with a metabolic or drug-induced cause, D_2 receptor antagonist at the chemoreceptor trigger zone *Subcutaneous starting dose and range in 24 hours*: 2.5–5 mg (range 2.5–10 mg) *Side effects*: drowsiness, dizziness, extrapyramidal effects
Cyclizine	*Indication and mode of action*: intestinal obstruction, antagonist of central H_1 and muscarinic receptors *Subcutaneous starting dose and range in 24 hours*: 100–150 mg (range 50–150 mg) *Side effects*: drowsiness, dry mouth, anticholinergic effects NB: May precipitate in syringe driver if used alongside high doses of bromide
Levomepromazine	*Indication and mode of action*: general nausea or agitation – also acts as sedative. Acts at multiple receptor sites *Subcutaneous starting dose and range in 24 hours*: 2.5–12.5 mg *Side effects*: drowsiness, dizziness, blurred vision

Agitation

Midazolam: subcutaneous use	*Mode of action*: enhances effect of γ-aminobutyric acid (GABA) on $GABA_A$ receptors causing sedation *Subcutaneous dose*: 10–30 mg (range 10–90 mg) *Side effects*: confusion, drowsiness
Levomepromazine: *see above*	*Mode of action*: acts as sedative. Acts at multiple receptor sites *Subcutaneous dose*: 2.5–12.5 mg. Range in 24 hours: 12.5–100 mg *Side effects*: confusion, drowsiness

Respiratory secretions

Hyoscine hydrobromide (also antiemetic)	*Mode of action*: anticholinergic *Subcutaneous dose*: 0.6–1.2 mg in 24 hours *Side effects*: constipation, dry mouth, urinary retention
Glycopyrronium	*Mode of action*: anticholinergic *Subcutaneous dose*: 0.6–1.2 mg in 24 hours *Side effects*: constipation, dry mouth, urinary retention
Hyoscine butylbromide (also antiemetic)	*Mode of action*: anticholinergic *Subcutaneous dose*: 60–180 mg in 24 hours *Side effects*: constipation, dry mouth, urinary retention

Constipation

- Constipation should be prevented by regular laxatives. It is important to treat because it causes a great deal of discomfort and can also cause agitation, nausea, and vomiting. In patients who are earlier in their palliative phase and who are still able to swallow you may prescribe a faecal softener with a peristaltic stimulant such as co-danthramer or lactulose with senna (although the latter combination can be unpalatable for some patients and also causes increased flatulence which may cause discomfort). You can also prescribe methylnaltrexone for constipation induced by opiates. In more severe cases, a phosphate enema may be required.

- For debilitated patients who have minimal oral intake a mild faecal softener such as sodium docusate may be sufficient.

Ethical aspects

Patient autonomy should always be considered, especially when a patient is dying. It is important to discuss their views on death and how they want to be treated. When a patient is identified as actively dying, they will need documentation of the decision not to attempt resuscitation (DNAR form) as it is futile, but this should be agreed with them if at all possible. For patients with a less predictable illness trajectory, it may be important to differentiate between full CPR and active management of a potentially reversible problem (e.g. intravenous antibiotics for an episode of infection) as patients and families may be concerned that all active management will cease once a DNAR form is signed. However, the patient may have set up an advance directive which will dictate what treatments they do not want to receive and this can guide your management if the patient lacks capacity. Remember that the aim of palliative care is neither to hasten nor postpone death and patients and their relatives need to be aware of this.

It is also important to consider the needs of patients with dementia, as they now form a growing proportion of elderly patients. Patients with dementia are vulnerable as they may be unable to express their symptoms or their wishes regarding terminal care. It has been found that patients with dementia are less likely to be referred to specialist palliative care services, be prescribed appropriate palliative drugs or have their carers involved in the decision-making process. Because of this, it is important to seek specialist help when dealing with these patients.

Patient safety and professional tips

✔ **Prescribing**: when it comes to prescribing, always refer to the LCP and your local guidelines.

✔ **Palliative care team**: always consult the specialist palliative care team if you are unsure.

✔ **Multidisciplinary team**: always work closely with the multidisciplinary team and make decisions together. Provide information to family/friends/carers regularly.

✔ **Nursing care**: all aspects of care should be of the highest standard ensuring dignity, comfort and relief of distress.

✔ **Aspects of care**: remember that palliative care is for specialist symptom control and psychological support as well as terminal care.

✔ **Syringe driver**: the use of a syringe driver is determined by the need for reliable administration of drugs that cannot be taken or absorbed orally at any point in time. It is not synonymous with terminal care; equally, not all dying patients require syringe drivers. Ensure that you are familiar with the use of a syringe driver.

✔ **Bereavement services**: often invaluable in providing support for relatives and friends of the dying or deceased. They are also expert in providing support to carers and healthcare professionals if needed.

Student name: **Medical school:**   **Year:**

Care of the dying patient

Please could you consider the following case history and advise on various aspects of treatment.

Douglas Smith (24b Fox Lane, Adamtown, CB1 7TP; date of birth 23 September 1944, hospital number GE7360, Spenser Ward) was admitted because of severe abdominal pain, nausea, vomiting, and intense low back pain. He is known to have carcinoma of the pancreas with metastatic deposits, severe COPD, and is dying. He has expressed a wish not to have resuscitation but would like to be 'kept alive' until his son arrives from the USA in 3 days. His investigations were all normal apart from those below:

			Self	Peer	Peer /tutor	Tutor
Hb 11.8 g/dL	Potassium 5.1 mmol/L	Calcium 3.4 mmol/L				
Urea 17.4 mmol/L	Creatinine 167 μmol/L					

What clinical aspects of care are encompassed by the WHO definition of palliative care?

'... improve quality of life of patients and their families ... through the prevention and relief of suffering by means of early identification and impeccable assessment and treatment of pain and other problems, physical, psychosocial and spiritual' The Palliative Care Team:
- affirms life and regards dying as a normal process;
- intends neither to hasten or postpone death;
- integrates the psychological and spiritual aspects of patient care;
- offers a support system to help patients live as actively as possible until death;
- offers a support system to help the family cope during the patient's illness ... [and] ... bereavement;
- will enhance quality of life, and may also positively influence the course of illness...'

(checkboxes: Self / Peer / Peer /tutor / Tutor)

Identifies main aspects of care in this patient
- Social and spiritual needs
- Pain: morphine based treatment with caution re dose to avoid excessive accumulation in renal failure. Via syringe driver if vomiting
- Nausea: cyclizine if most likely cause is metabolic or metoclopramide if symptoms and signs suggest squashed stomach syndrome. Do not give both together.
- Consider correcting underlying cause of nausea: hypercalcaemia: intravenous fluids followed by bisphosphonate, e.g. pamidronate

Interprets clinical data and diagnosis correctly
- Patient has hypercalcaemia with dehydration plus or minus acute renal failure

Is able to discuss and list the four clinical parameters in the Bode Index
- FEV$_1$% of predicted, distance walked in 6 minutes, MMRC Dyspnoea Scale, BMI

Suggests suitable common drugs for the treatment of symptoms in the LCP
- **Pain**: morphine, diamorphine,
- **Nausea and vomiting**: cyclizine, metoclopramide, haloperidol; levomepromazine
- **Agitation**: midazolam, levomepromazine
- **Respiratory secretions**: hyoscine, glycopyrronium (if trying to avoid sedation)
- **Breathlessness**: oxygen, opioids, midazolam
- **Constipation**: co-danthramer or sodium docusate
- **Poor appetite**: steroids

Discussions ethical aspects of care in relation to an actual patient
- Role of advance directive and patient autonomy
- Do not resuscitate orders (DNAR forms)
- Categories of DNAR reasons

Understands role of multidisciplinary team in palliative care and how referral is made
- Core palliative care team: pharmacist, dietician, ward nurses, family and carers, chaplaincy team, bereavement counsellor; discharge co-ordinator; community Macmillan team; hospice at home

	Signature:	Date:	Self	Peer	Peer /tutor	Tutor
Self-assessed as at least borderline:			U B S E	U B S E	U B S E	U B S E
Peer-assessed as ready for tutor assessment:			U B S E	U B S E	U B S E	U B S E
Tutor-assessed as satisfactory:			U B S E	U B S E	U B S E	U B S E

Notes

17.4 Clinical leadership skills

Background

Clinical leadership is likely to be perceived as a low priority skill for a clinical student or newly qualified healthcare professional. However, all innovation and major changes in a health service relies on leaders of the future. Leadership is not just the skill in leading others, which is often needed, but also, the ability to follow and help others when necessary. Leadership operates on many levels, it is often seen just as an ability to lead others but the essential core of leadership is to lead yourself to become the healthcare professional you wish to be in terms of education, clinical service, personal aspirations, and the overarching aim of improving the lives of patients and the community. Leadership and management have overlapping competencies but must not be confused.

Leadership versus management

Management is doing things right, leadership is doing the right thing.

Peter F Drucker

- **Leadership** takes people in a specific direction, and has vision and awareness of context, innovates, develops, asks why and what, challenges, focuses on people, establishes direction, motivates. Leadership involves power by influence.

- **Management** is enabling people to achieve specific goals via establishment, administrating structures, maintaining governance in committees, implementing accepted new ways of doing things. The goals are achieved through planning and solving problems in real time. Management involves power by position.

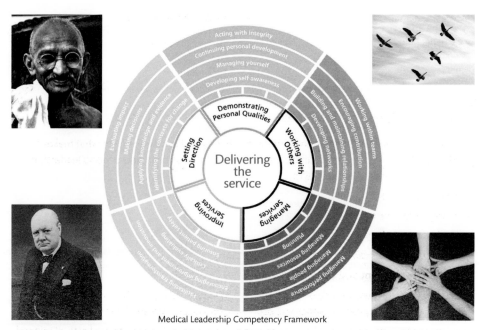

Medical Leadership Competency Framework

Personal ideas of leadership will depend on the very many values in leadership that you consider important

The wisdom of geese: a powerful metaphor of human leadership, followership and teamwork.

Figure 17.3 Images in clinical leadership. Top left licensed under Creative Commons; top right © scol22/ iStockphoto; middle © NHS Institute for Innovation and Improvement and Academy of Medical Royal Colleges 2010.

From Table 17.4 it is immediately obvious that all clinicians would need to have a degree of competency in most domains.

Table 17.4 Managers and leaders: adapted from Bennis (1997)

Managers		Leaders
Build and maintain organizational structures	↔	Build and maintain organizational cultures
Path follow, do things right	↔	Path find, do the right things
Undermined by setbacks	↔	See setbacks as opportunities
Maintain and rely on control	↔	Develop and inspires trust
Focus on 'here and now' of goal attainment	↔	Focus on the creation of vision about a desired future state
Maintain a low level of emotional involvement	↔	Have empathy with others, attend to meaning and interpretation
Design and carry out plans	↔	Establish a mission and a sense of direction
Administer	↔	Innovate
Ask how and when	↔	Ask what and why
Focus on systems	↔	Focus on people
Do things right	↔	Do the right things
Maintain	↔	Develop
Rely on control	↔	Inspire trust
Short-term perspective	↔	Longer-term perspective
Accept status quo	↔	Challenge the status quo
Eye on the bottom line	↔	Eye on the horizon
Imitate	↔	Originate

Qualities of effective leadership

Table 17.4 helps us towards an understanding of what a good leader does. But what makes a good leader? There are several qualities that we all recognize as hallmarks of good leadership. These qualities include (Bennis, 1989):

- **Self-awareness**
- **Being reflective and reflexive**
- **Understanding change and transition**
- **Ability to teach, train, and provide consultancy**
- **Readiness to adapt and innovate**
- **Political astuteness**: identify power holders, understand their position, work out how their views fit with their position, anticipate problems, find allies, plan and have contingency plans.

Good leadership and especially charisma must never become an excuse for low levels of general clinical competency and inefficiency.

Competencies in clinical leadership

Statements and documents from learned bodies in relation to clinical training now emphasize the need for development of leadership skills. *Tomorrow's Doctors* (2009), by the General Medical Council, specifically articulates the role of leadership:

> It is not enough for a clinician to act as a practitioner in their own discipline. They must act as partners to their colleagues, accepting shared accountability for the service provided to their patients. They are also expected to offer leadership and to work with others to change systems when it is necessary for the benefit of patients.

Competencies for clinical leadership are difficult to define. The Medical Leadership Competency Framework (MLCF) was first published in 2008, with the undergraduate guidance published in 2010. The MLCF is part of a wider UK project to promote medical leadership, which was commissioned by the Academy of Medical Royal Colleges and delivered by the NHS Institute for Innovation and Improvement. The MLCF is applicable for all doctors and incorporates undergraduate, postgraduate and continuing practice training and development. The MLCF describes the leadership competences doctors need to become more actively involved in the planning, delivery and transformation of health services. The MLCF incorporates the following five domains:

- **Demonstrating personal qualities**: developing self-awareness, managing yourself, continuing personal development, acting with integrity.
- **Working with others**: developing networks, building and maintaining relationships, encouraging contribution, working within teams.
- **Managing services**: planning, managing resources, managing people, managing performance.
- **Improving services**: ensuring patient safety, critically evaluating, encouraging improvement and innovation, facilitating transformation.
- **Setting direction**: identifying the contexts for change, applying knowledge and evidence, making decisions, evaluating impact.

The skills accrued, it is hoped, would result in greater competence in any sphere, whether in a large team at a national level or small team in a local specific service. All these competencies also have a vital function at the level of the individual student or clinician. The competencies are generic and can apply to most clinical posts and also have substantial potential for use in undergraduate education. In July 2010 a further document, *Guidance for Undergraduate Medical Education: Integrating the Medical Leadership Competency Framework* was produced, to support medical schools in the integration of leadership competencies into undergraduate curriculum. The MLCF is built on the concept of shared leadership. This is:

> Where leadership is not restricted to those who hold designated leadership roles ... (but also) ... where there is a shared sense of responsibility for the success of the organization and its services. Acts of leadership can come from any individual in the organization, as appropriate, at different times.

MLCF, 2010

What do we do in human healthcare?

Having discussed what the generic skills and qualities a competent leader in healthcare is expected to have was relatively easy. The answer to the question posed in this sub-heading is surprisingly difficult to locate in the available literature or within the outputs of learned societies and institutions. Box 17.1 offers a summary of points made in several tutorials and interactive lectures with trained or training healthcare professionals. This is by no means an exhaustive or a definitive definition. It is necessary to define what we do or should do in human healthcare so that our clinical skills and competencies can specifically focus on delivering these outcomes.

> **Box 17.1** Human healthcare
>
> In human healthcare we work to relieve suffering, morbidity, and mortality by preventing illness, treating disease, rehabilitation, and appropriate end of life care.
>
> For this work, high standards of clinical care and competence are considered to be:
>
> - Being kind, acting in an ethical manner and ensuring human rights
> - Regarding patients as individuals and respecting their dignity
> - Personal continuous professional development and continuous innovative development of services taking into account local conditions
> - Working effectively in partnership with patients/carers on decision making
> - Addressing health inequalities
> - Promoting health in individual patients, local communities and the wider public
> - Working well and effectively with other healthcare professionals particularly in sharing best practice to reduce duplication of effort
> - Managing services optimally with leadership & follower-ship skills
> - Teaching, innovation and research
> - Being cost efficient and cost effective but always clinically governed

An algebra of effective healthcare: the POETIC vision

The shift towards more integrated public services, espoused in the 2010 White Paper *Equity and Excellence: Liberating the NHS*' requires that health professionals of the future must increasingly work effectively with and alongside other health and social care professionals, stakeholders, community organizations, and professional, regulatory, and statutory bodies. Most healthcare professionals tend to work within specific professional domains and also have a duty to implement reports and guidance from their learned societies.

This has the potential to lead to a vast array of reports and guidance that needs to be implemented with very little attention given to the overall intended vision. In the West Midlands (UK), a multidisciplinary clinical pathway group considering long-term conditions derived a model for effective healthcare: the *POETIC vision*. The vision encompassed what the team saw as an enabler for all those involved in healthcare, managers, and clinicians alike, to help create an outstanding service that improved the care and the lives of people. Such vision statements are not unusual; however, the acronym provides a structure and vision for what we might aspire towards to enable a shared approach to health service delivery and education.

This approach promotes an holistic platform derived from health and educational philosophies and is intrinsically linked to the way in which health and public services are designed, shaped, and delivered. It provides all stakeholders (patients, carers, healthcare professionals, voluntary groups and charities, industry and social enterprise (including pharmaceuticals, delivery and devices), educational institutes, managers, politicians, students, local communities) with a simple acronym which incorporates an approach to healthcare delivery, teaching and learning, and innovation.

Overall, the *POETIC Vision* is an 'algebra' of effective healthcare. The idea of an algebra was inspired by a book title by Arundhati Roy. The POETIC Vision is summarized in Table 17.5. Diabetes care is used as an example to elaborate the idea clinically but can be applied to most clinical services and conditions.

Excellent leadership in healthcare has the potential to create a world-class service for our patients, current and future, and which improves the lives of patients, carers, and the community as a whole. This is a difficult challenge but a mantle that we must all take up in great or small measure.

Table 17.5 shows how the POETIC Vision could be applied to diabetes care.

Table 17.5 POETIC vision and diabetes care

		Notes in relation to diabetes care
P	**Patient-centred and safe Public health driven Prevention-focused Professionally inspired**	• Patient education and care planning essential to effective care. Care must be individualized and patient-led. The central of the carer is emphasized. Care should be culturally sensitive. • Remember healthcare professionals on average only provide 3 hours of direct care a year, the other 8757 hours are self-care or care by family and others! • Diabetes remains a major public health challenge consuming 10% of NHS resources • Health inequalities must be addressed alongside prevention strategies, especially as 90% of type 2 diabetes can be prevented by addressing lifestyle factors • Inspired professionals will always deliver higher standards. Supporting and promoting innovation is essential
O	**Objectives clear Outcome driven**	• Patient-related outcome measures would include reduction in diabetes interfering with everyday life and employment, reducing admissions for hypoglycaemia, and diabetic ketoacidosis (DKA), improving emotional wellbeing • Specific complications such as cardiovascular disease (CVD), renal failure, amputation, and blindness need and can be prevented
E	**Evidence based**: informed by clinical audit, quality assurance, research and evaluation of innovation	• Clear guidelines have been produced by well-recognized bodies especially NICE, based on the many well-conducted randomized controlled trials that have taken place in diabetes care such as UKPDS, CARDS, STENO-2, Diabetes Prevention Programme. Further research is desirable • Clinical audit is a major driver to improved care with the emphasis on implementation of audit finding and repeating the audit after a period of change to improve standards to create a constant dynamic of improvement
T	**Team delivered**: multi- disciplinary, well trained and accredited	• Diabetes care requires coordinated partnership of many health-care professionals, for example: nurses, healthcare support workers including administration staff, doctors, pharmacists, dietitians, podiatrists • The team should train together and be accredited by external review
I	**Integrated**: Across all health and social care sectors	• Partnership oriented: especially through sharing of good practice. • Effectively integrating primary and secondary care, community organizations and health, education, and social care agencies • The patient and carer should be facilitated in 'navigating' through these agencies for their specific health needs
C	**Cost efficient and effective but clinically governed***	• Although there are many expensive treatments in diabetes care that are effective and need to be used, it will be most cost-effective to use these where there is greatest clinical benefit • Organization of care should be considered in detail and will often lead to greater effectiveness and cost-efficiency. • A multifactorial approach is best at reducing complications. Thankfully, the most effective treatments (for type 2 diabetes) are generic: blood pressure (angiotensin-converting enzyme inhibitors, angiotensin receptor blockers), cholesterol (statins), glycaemic control (metformin), CVD prophylaxis (aspirin)

****Clinical governance** formal definition in the NHS: 'A framework through which NHS organisations are accountable for continually improving the quality of their services and safeguarding high standards of care by creating an environment in which excellence in clinical care will flourish', Scally and Donaldson, 1998.

Student name: Medical school: Year:

Leadership

You are the healthcare professional tasked to look after Mr Feroz Khan, a 72-year-old man admitted with collapse. His blood pressure on arrival is 74/52, urea 15.6 mmol/L, creatinine 268 µmol/L. His drugs on admission were lisinopril 40 mg od in the morning and metformin 1 g bd.

Previously, 3 months ago all his results were normal. There is a past medical history of type 2 diabetes and a previous myocardial infarction.

Mr Khan has been fasting during Ramadan and has already undertaken 14 of an estimated 28 fasts. Your senior clinical colleagues have told you that this often happens during Ramadan. You have been asked by a tutor to see this patient and come for a detailed discussion focusing on the clinical aspects and MLCF domains. You have been advised to consult the full guidance in preparation.

		Self	Peer	Peer/tutor	Tutor
Discuss the five domains of the MLCF leadership wheel generally and in relation to the above vignette where possible	**Developing self-awareness**: multisource feedback, own values, emotions, and behaviours, role in teaching or clinical placement, respect for rights of patients, respect for diversity	☐	☐	☐	☐
	Managing yourself: personal health and impact of effectiveness, access healthcare, maintain own health and safety, good time management, balances work and home life, professional	☐	☐	☐	☐
	Continuing personal development (CPD): approaches to CPD, critical incident and complaints reporting, development goals, self-directed of learning and reflection, learns from mistakes	☐	☐	☐	☐
	Acting with integrity: GMC good medical practice, effective and respective relationships with others, identify and manage ethical issues, respect for professional regulation and standards	☐	☐	☐	☐
		☐	☐	☐	☐
Working with others	**Developing networks**: roles of multidisciplinary team, roles of other agencies, involve others in problem solving, understand importance of teamwork and collaboration	☐	☐	☐	☐
	Building and maintaining relationships: factors that demonstrate effective team working, different leadership styles, gain respect from colleagues, healthcare professionals, and patients, respect others	☐	☐	☐	☐
	Encouraging contribution: encourage patient participation, values views of all team, seek others views including patients and carers, encourage diverse views, acknowledge others	☐	☐	☐	☐
	Working within teams: understand shared leadership, team dynamics and addressing problems, lead and be led, flexibility in role in teams, respect team decisions, partnerships	☐	☐	☐	☐
		☐	☐	☐	☐
Managing services	**Planning**: current NHS strategy, steps in planning change, consider quality improvement project and work to time, views of patients and service users, consider alternative approaches	☐	☐	☐	☐
	Managing resources: understand resource allocation in healthcare, how extra resources can be acquired, ideas for improving cost-effectiveness, awareness of limited resources	☐	☐	☐	☐
	Managing people: analysis of personal and team performance, principles of effective feedback, support others to take on new roles, learn from feedback, readiness to seek advice	☐	☐	☐	☐
	Managing performance: role of appraisal, addressing cause for concern in healthcare professionals, support and motivate team, learn from good and poor performance, how to take action if concerns re healthcare professional	☐	☐	☐	☐
		☐	☐	☐	☐
Improving services	**Ensuring patient safety**: role of risk management, sources of risk and medical error, identify and analyse significant incidents, systematic approach to reduction of risk and error, commitment to patient safety agenda, assessing and communicating risk to patients	☐	☐	☐	☐
	Critically evaluating: principles of clinical governance, evaluation of quality by clinical audit, significant event analysis and patient feedback, evidence-based practice, clinical audit	☐	☐	☐	☐
	Encouraging improvement and innovation: change management theory, innovations to improve healthcare or education, improving patient experience, open to new ideas, changes status quo	☐	☐	☐	☐
	Facilitating transformation: strategies for motivating change, present results and recommendations (? audit) to influence change, positive attitude to implementing change	☐	☐	☐	☐
		☐	☐	☐	☐

Setting direction					
	● **Identifying the contexts for change**: awareness of national and local healthcare policies for change, understand how this influences patient care, willing and ability to keep up to date	☐	☐	☐	☐
	● **Applying knowledge and evidence**: sources of and accessing evidence-based care, use of patient reporting systems, use of proven good practice, understand healthcare strategy	☐	☐	☐	☐
	● **Making decisions**: decision-making processes at various levels, influencing and negotiating skills, preparing for meetings, involving patients and communities in developing healthcare	☐	☐	☐	☐
	● **Evaluating impact**: barriers to implementation, effective dissemination, participate in clinical audit, service change impact on patient care, openness to new ways of working	☐	☐	☐	☐
	●	☐	☐	☐	☐

What is does leadership mean to you?	☐	☐	☐	☐
Who do you consider to be good leaders in the health service?	☐	☐	☐	☐

Compare and contrast the attribute of management and leadership in relation to a clinical service	☐	☐	☐	☐

What is that we do in healthcare? Discuss in relation to Table 17.4. Is there anything that you would add or take out or simplify?	☐	☐	☐	☐

Discuss the POETIC Vision template in relation to the management of a patient you have seen recently. Consider any suitable patient or one with a long-term condition.	☐	☐	☐	☐

Self-assessed as at least borderline:	Signature:	Date:	U B S E	U B S E	U B S E	U B S E
Peer-assessed as ready for tutor assessment:	Signature:	Date:	U B S E	U B S E	U B S E	U B S E
Tutor-assessed as satisfactory:	Signature:	Date:	U B S E	U B S E	U B S E	U B S E

Notes

Appendix A Adult life support algorithms

Adult Basic Life Support

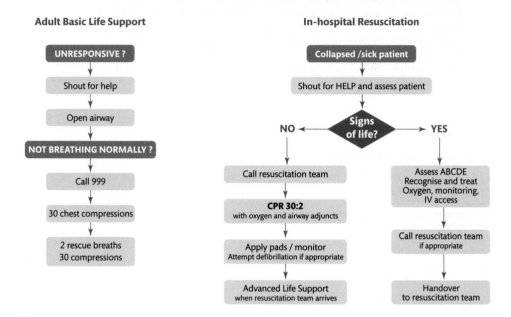

UNRESPONSIVE ?

↓

Shout for help

↓

Open airway

↓

NOT BREATHING NORMALLY ?

↓

Call 999

↓

30 chest compressions

↓

2 rescue breaths
30 compressions

In-hospital Resuscitation

Collapsed /sick patient

↓

Shout for HELP and assess patient

↓

Signs of life?

NO ←   → YES

NO branch:

Call resuscitation team

↓

CPR 30:2
with oxygen and airway adjuncts

↓

Apply pads / monitor
Attempt defibrillation if appropriate

↓

Advanced Life Support
when resuscitation team arrives

YES branch:

Assess ABCDE
Recognise and treat
Oxygen, monitoring,
IV access

↓

Call resuscitation team
if appropriate

↓

Handover
to resuscitation team

Adult Advanced Life Support

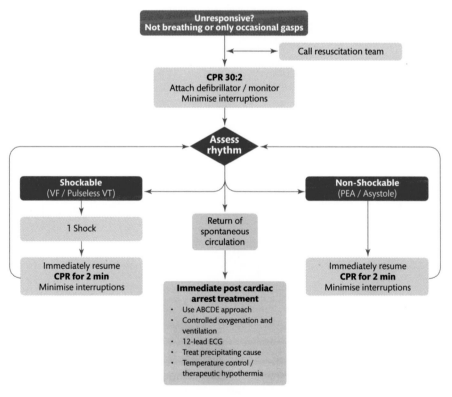

**Unresponsive?
Not breathing or only occasional gasps**

↓ ← → Call resuscitation team

CPR 30:2
Attach defibrillator / monitor
Minimise interruptions

↓

Assess rhythm

Shockable
(VF / Pulseless VT)

↓

1 Shock

↓

Immediately resume
CPR for 2 min
Minimise interruptions

**Return of
spontaneous
circulation**

↓

**Immediate post cardiac
arrest treatment**
· Use ABCDE approach
· Controlled oxygenation and
  ventilation
· 12-lead ECG
· Treat precipitating cause
· Temperature control /
  therapeutic hypothermia

Non-Shockable
(PEA / Asystole)

↓

Immediately resume
CPR for 2 min
Minimise interruptions

During CPR
· Ensure high-quality CPR: rate, depth, recoil
· Plan actions before interrupting CPR
· Give oxygen
· Consider advanced airway and capnography
· Continuous chest compressions when advanced
  airway in place
· Vascular access (intravenous, intraosseous)
· Give adrenaline every 3-5 min
· Correct reversible causes

Reversible Causes
· Hypoxia
· Hypovolaemia
· Hypo- / hyperkalaemia / metabolic
· Hypothermia

· Thrombosis - coronary or pulmonary
· Tamponade - cardiac
· Toxins
· Tension pneumothorax

Appendix B   Paediatric life support algorithms

Paediatric Basic Life Support
(Healthcare professionals with a duty to respond)

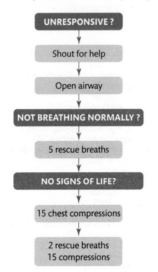

```
UNRESPONSIVE ?
        ↓
Shout for help
        ↓
Open airway
        ↓
NOT BREATHING NORMALLY ?
        ↓
5 rescue breaths
        ↓
NO SIGNS OF LIFE?
        ↓
15 chest compressions
        ↓
2 rescue breaths
15 compressions
```

Paediatric Advanced Life Support

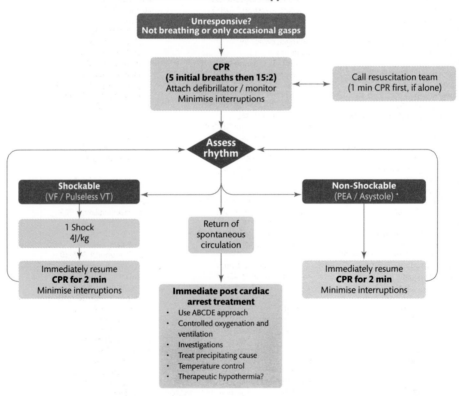

```
Unresponsive?
Not breathing or only occasional gasps
        ↓
CPR
(5 initial breaths then 15:2)    ←→   Call resuscitation team
Attach defibrillator / monitor          (1 min CPR first, if alone)
Minimise interruptions
        ↓
Assess rhythm
```

Shockable
(VF / Pulseless VT)

1 Shock
4J/kg

Immediately resume
CPR for 2 min
Minimise interruptions

Return of spontaneous circulation

Immediate post cardiac arrest treatment
- Use ABCDE approach
- Controlled oxygenation and ventilation
- Investigations
- Treat precipitating cause
- Temperature control
- Therapeutic hypothermia?

Non-Shockable
(PEA / Asystole) *

Immediately resume
CPR for 2 min
Minimise interruptions

During CPR
- Ensure high-quality CPR: rate, depth, recoil
- Plan actions before interrupting CPR
- Give oxygen
- Vascular access (intravenous, intraosseous)
- Give adrenaline every 3-5 min
- Consider advanced airway and capnography
- Continuous chest compressions when advanced airway in place
- Correct reversible causes

Reversible Causes
- Hypoxia
- Hypovolaemia
- Hypo- / hyperkalaemia / metabolic
- Hypothermia
- Tension pneumothorax
- Toxins
- Tamponade - cardiac
- Thromboembolism

Index